EMOTION REGULATION
AND PSYCHOPATHOLOGY

Emotion Regulation and Psychopathology

A TRANSDIAGNOSTIC APPROACH TO ETIOLOGY AND TREATMENT

Edited by

Ann M. Kring
Denise M. Sloan

THE GUILFORD PRESS
New York   London

© 2010 The Guilford Press
A Division of Guilford Publications, Inc.
72 Spring Street, New York, NY 10012
www.guilford.com

Printed in the United States of America

This book is printed on acid-free paper.

Last digit is print number: 9   8   7   6   5   4   3   2   1

Library of Congress Cataloging-in-Publication Data

Emotion regulation and psychopathology : a transdiagnostic approach to
etiology and treatment / edited by Ann M. Kring, Denise M. Sloan.
   p. cm.
  Includes bibliographical references and index.
  ISBN 978-1-60623-450-1 (hbk.)
  1. Emotions.   2. Mental illness—Etiology.   3. Psychology,
Pathological.   I. Kring, Ann M.   II. Sloan, Denise M.
  BF531.E4954 2010
  616.89—dc22

               2009016164

To Angie for her patience, love, and support
and to Lisa Feldman Barrett
for her friendship and intellectual inspiration.
—A. M. K.

To Brian and Colin for their love and support,
and to my father, William, for instilling in me
the importance of work ethic and perseverance.
—D. M. S.

About the Editors

Ann M. Kring, PhD, is Professor of Psychology at the University of California, Berkeley, and former Director of the Clinical Science Program and Psychology Clinic. Her current research focus is on emotion and psychopathology, with a specific interest in the emotional features of schizophrenia, assessing negative symptoms in schizophrenia, and the linkage between cognition and emotion in schizophrenia. Dr. Kring has received numerous awards, including a Young Investigator award from the National Alliance for Research on Schizophrenia and Depression, the Joseph Zubin Memorial Fund Award, and a Distinguished Teaching Award from UC Berkeley. She is currently a member of the Executive Board for the Society for Research in Psychopathology, Associate Editor for the *Journal of Abnormal Psychology*, and a member of the editorial board for the journals *Emotion, Applied and Preventive Psychology*, and *Psychological Science in the Public Interest*.

Denise M. Sloan, PhD, is Associate Director in the Behavioral Science Division at the National Center for PTSD and Associate Professor of Psychiatry at the Boston University School of Medicine. Her current research focus is on emotion and psychopathology, with a specific interest in emotional processes in traumatic stress disorders and integration of methods to assess and treat emotional disturbances related to traumatic stress. Dr. Sloan has received funding for her work from the National Institute of Mental Health and the U.S. Department of Defense, among other organizations. She is a member of the editorial board for the journals *Behavior Therapy, Psychosomatic Medicine*, and *Journal of Contemporary Psychotherapy*.

Contributors

Michael E. Addis, PhD, Department of Psychology, Clark University, Worcester, Massachusetts

Nader Amir, PhD, Center for Understanding and Treating Anxiety and Department of Psychology, San Diego State University, San Diego, California

Adam Anderson, PhD, Department of Psychology, University of Toronto, Toronto, Ontario, Canada

David H. Barlow, PhD, Center for Anxiety and Related Disorders, Boston University, Boston, Massachusetts

Lian Bloch, MA, Department of Psychology, University of California, Berkeley, Berkeley, California

Christina L. Boisseau, MA, Center for Anxiety and Related Disorders, Boston University, Boston, Massachusetts

George A. Bonanno, PhD, Teachers College, Columbia University, New York, New York

Jennifer L. Boulanger, MA, Department of Psychology, University of Nevada, Reno, Reno, Nevada

Charles S. Carver, PhD, Department of Psychology, University of Miami, Coral Gables, Florida

Karin G. Coifman, PhD, Department of Psychology, Columbia University, New York, New York

Kathleen M. Corcoran, PhD, Centre for Addiction and Mental Health and Department of Psychiatry, University of Toronto, Toronto, Ontario, Canada

Bryan T. Denny, BA, Department of Psychology, Columbia University, New York, New York

Daniel G. Dillon, PhD, Department of Psychology, Harvard University, Cambridge, Massachusetts

Jill T. Ehrenreich, PhD, Department of Psychology, University of Miami, Coral Gables, Florida

Kristen K. Ellard, MA, Center for Anxiety and Related Disorders, Boston University, Boston, Massachusetts

Christopher P. Fairholme, MA, Center for Anxiety and Related Disorders, Boston University, Boston, Massachusetts

Norman Farb, MA, Department of Psychology, University of Toronto, Toronto, Ontario, Canada

John P. Forsyth, PhD, Department of Psychology, University at Albany, State University of New York, Albany, New York

David M. Fresco, PhD, Department of Psychology, Kent State University, Kent, Ohio

Daniel Fulford, MS, Department of Psychology, University of Miami, Coral Gables, Florida

Miranda Goodman, MA, Department of Psychology, University of California, Davis, Davis, California

James J. Gross, PhD, Department of Psychology, Stanford University, Stanford, California

June Gruber, MA, Department of Psychology, Yale University, New Haven, Connecticut

Allison G. Harvey, PhD, Department of Psychology, University of California, Berkeley, Berkeley, California

Steven C. Hayes, PhD, Department of Psychology, University of Nevada, Reno, Reno, Nevada

Sheri L. Johnson, PhD, Department of Psychology, University of California, Berkeley, Berkeley, California

Jutta Joormann, PhD, Department of Psychology, University of Miami, Coral Gables, Florida

Ann M. Kring, PhD, Department of Psychology, University of California, Berkeley, Berkeley, California

Brett T. Litz, PhD, National Center for PTSD, VA Boston Healthcare System, and Department of Psychiatry, Boston University School of Medicine, Boston, Massachusetts

Christopher R. Martell, PhD, private practice and Department of Psychology, University of Washington, Seattle, Washington

Eleanor McGlinchey, BA, Department of Psychology, University of California, Berkeley, Berkeley, California

Douglas S. Mennin, PhD, Department of Psychology, Yale University, New Haven, Connecticut

Erin K. Moran, BA, Department of Psychology, University of California, Berkeley, Berkeley, California

Kevin N. Ochsner, PhD, Department of Psychology, Columbia University, New York, New York

Jacqueline Pistorello, PhD, Department of Psychology, University of Nevada, Reno, Reno, Nevada

Diego A. Pizzagalli, PhD, Department of Psychology, Harvard University, Cambridge, Massachusetts

Kristalyn Salters-Pedneault, PhD, National Center for PTSD, VA Boston Healthcare System, and Department of Psychiatry, Boston University School of Medicine, Boston, Massachusetts

Zindel V. Segal, PhD, Centre for Addiction and Mental Health and Department of Psychiatry, University of Toronto, Toronto, Ontario, Canada

Sean C. Sheppard, BA, Department of Psychology, University at Albany, State University of New York, Albany, New York

Matthias Siemer, PhD, Department of Psychology, University of Miami, Coral Gables, Florida

Jennifer A. Silvers, BA, Department of Psychology, Columbia University, New York, New York

Denise M. Sloan, PhD, Behavioral Science Division, National Center for PTSD, VA Boston Healthcare System, and Department of Psychiatry, Boston University School of Medicine, Boston, Massachusetts

Maria Steenkamp, MA, Department of Psychology, Boston University, Boston, Massachusetts

Matthew R. Syzdek, MA, Department of Psychology, Clark University, Worcester, Massachusetts

Charles T. Taylor, PhD, Center for Understanding and Treating Anxiety and Department of Psychology, San Diego State University, San Diego, California

Ross A. Thompson, PhD, Department of Psychology, University of California, Davis, Davis, California

Sonsoles Valdivia-Salas, PhD, Department of Psychology, University at Albany, State University of New York, Albany, New York

Els van der Helm, MSc, Department of Psychology, University of California, Berkeley, Berkeley, California

Matthew P. Walker, PhD, Department of Psychology, University of California, Berkeley, Berkeley, California

Kelly Werner, PhD, Department of Psychology, Stanford University, Stanford, California

K. Lira Yoon, PhD, Department of Psychology, University of Miami, Coral Gables, Florida

Contents

Introduction and Overview

Denise M. Sloan and Ann M. Kring

The past two decades have witnessed tremendous advances in theory and research on emotion regulation. Specifically, we have gained a more thorough understanding of its developmental trajectory, neuroanatomy, genetic and environmental influences, and interface with cognition. A recent edited book by James J. Gross (2007), *Handbook of Emotion Regulation*, encapsulates the current state of the field. With this advanced knowledge of emotion regulation, the field has begun to turn its attention toward understanding the circumstances under which emotion regulation goes awry.

Psychopathologists have long speculated that problems in emotion regulation play a central role in the development and maintenance of psychiatric disorders and maladaptive behaviors. Indeed, the majority of the disorders found in the current *Diagnostic and Statistical Manual of Mental Disorders* (DSM-IV-TR; American Psychiatric Association, 2000) include at least one symptom reflecting a disturbance in emotion. Theories of how emotion regulation manifests in, maintains, and contributes to psychiatric problems are now gaining empirical support, which, in turn, has stimulated treatment development.

The goals of our edited book are to (1) provide a compilation of the state-of-the-art frameworks for understanding how problems in emotion regulation characterize, maintain, or cause psychiatric problems that transcend current diagnostic boundaries; (2) describe empirical support for these frameworks, and (3) provide an overview of psychosocial treatments that target these causal and sustaining mechanisms.

Although psychopathology can be classified using a categorical approach, such as that used in the DSM-IV-TR (American Psychiatric Association, 2000), there is a growing consensus that this approach may not

1

be ideal for all psychiatric disturbances (e.g., Helzer, Wittchen, Krueger, & Kraemer, 2008; Widiger & Clark, 2000; Widiger & Samuel, 2005). For instance, the DSM-IV-TR classification system does not readily accommodate the large percentage of individuals that have comorbid psychiatric diagnoses (Krueger, 2002). There is also evidence that individuals who exhibit subthreshold levels of symptoms for a given disorder appear to be equally impaired and require the same treatment as those who meet diagnostic criteria for the same disorder (e.g., Blanchard et al., 2003; Krug et al., 2008). Another common occurrence that underscores problems with the categorical approach to psychopathology is that some individuals meet diagnostic criteria for one disorder but later in the course of their illness they meet diagnostic criteria for another disorder. An example of this scenario is with the eating disorders, in which a substantial percentage of women who initially meet diagnostic criteria for anorexia nervosa later meet diagnostic criteria for bulimia nervosa (e.g., Fichter, & Quadflieg, 2007; Eddy et al., 2007). There is some evidence that anorexia nervosa and bulimia nervosa are manifestations of the same disorder at differing points in the trajectory (e.g., Eddy et al., 2007). As a result of these and other issues that highlight the problems of using a categorical conceptualization of psychopathology, there has been a call for adopting a different approach to classifying psychopathology. One possible alternative is a transdiagnostic approach. This scheme categorizes disorders based on underlying mechanisms or core disturbances (e.g., attention, emotion; see Harvey, Watkins, Mansell, & Shafran, 2004), and cuts across current DSM-IV-TR disorders.

In this edited volume, we have adopted a transdiagnostic approach to psychiatric disorders by focusing on common manifestations and difficulties in emotion regulation that cut across current diagnostic boundaries. One advantage to this approach is that treatments can be developed to target mechanisms, not disorders, thus potentially reducing the number of evidence-based treatment protocols to sort through. In addition, focusing on mechanisms of action eliminates problems that arise in selecting treatments when patients present with comorbid diagnoses, which is the typical patient presentation in treatment settings (e.g., Harvey et al., 2004).[1]

Although we have asked contributors to focus on emotion regulation manifestations and mechanisms rather than specific psychiatric disorders, the contributors have primarily highlighted mechanisms as they relate to mood and anxiety disorders, because the majority of empirical work on problems in emotion regulation has been done in the mood and anxiety disorders. However, contributors have pointed to the relevance of these emotion regulation mechanisms and treatments across a wide swath of

---

[1]The importance of considering mechanisms rather than disorders has also been emphasized by Jacqueline Persons in her book *The Case Formulation Approach to Cognitive-Behavior Therapy* (2008).

disorders, such as eating disorders and psychotic disorders, with an eye toward the need for future research.

Structure of the Book

The book is divided into three sections. Each section reflects our intent to link theories of emotion regulation, mechanisms of emotion regulation that contribute to psychopathology, and treatment approaches that target these mechanisms. One lingering issue in the emotion regulation field relates to defining *emotion* and *emotion regulation*. Because these terms reflect broad areas, varying definitions exist. In order to provide clarity and continuity to the book, we asked each of the contributors to describe how they define emotion and emotion regulation as well as to describe how their conceptualization of emotion and emotion regulation situate emotion regulation problems across disorders. In addition, Bloch, Moran, and Kring (Chapter 4) delineate several definitions of emotion and emotion regulation that are currently used in the field, and they go on to offer a synthesis of these definitions, with an eye toward unifying the next generation of research in this area.

The first section of the book is devoted to models of emotion regulation. Werner and Gross (Chapter 1) start off the section by presenting the "modal model" of emotion, which they use as a framework for understanding emotion regulation. The modal model describes a situation–attention–appraisal–response sequence. More specifically, a psychologically relevant stimulus draws a person's attention, which then requires the person to appraise the stimulus. One's appraisal of the situation will help determine his or her emotional response. Because emotional responses can, in turn, modify the situation the person was initially responding to, a feedback loop is created in which emotional response tendencies can alter the environment. Werner and Gross define emotion regulation as processes that serve to decrease, increase, or maintain one or more aspects of emotion. Many of the contributors in this volume use the same definition of emotion regulation that is used by Werner and Gross.

The next chapter, by Thompson and Goodman, concerns the development of emotion regulation through the lifespan. Thompson and Goodman's chapter provides a developmental framework to understanding emotion regulation, which is helpful in determining whether emotion regulation observed in a specific context is problematic or not. Next, Denny, Silvers, and Ochsner (Chapter 3) present current evidence on the functional neural architecture of emotion regulation. Denny and colleagues' chapter provides a useful overview of brain mechanisms that are involved in emotion and the regulation of emotion. The first section of the book concludes with Chapter 4, by Bloch, Moran, and Kring, who emphasize the importance of achieving conceptual and definitional clarity in the construct of emotion regulation in order to advance our understanding of the role of emotion regulation in psychopathology. The authors highlight the similarities and differences of the most prominent definitions of emotion regulation used by psychopathology researchers. Bloch and colleagues also provide suggestions regarding what features of an emotion regulation definition are most useful and can be broadly applied to the study of psychopathology mechanisms and treatments.

The second section of the book covers specific emotion regulation mechanisms that are relevant to the development and maintenance of psychopathology, with an explicit focus on emotion regulation problems that cut across different disorders. This section starts with Chapter 5, by Boulanger, Hayes, and Pistorello, describing the construct of experiential avoidance. In this chapter, Boulanger and colleagues describe the construct of experiential avoidance and how experiential avoidance impacts emotion regulation. The authors also discuss the implications of experiential avoidance for the development, maintenance, and treatment of psychopathology. The next chapter discusses a specific form of emotional regulation, namely suppression. As Salters-Pedneault, Steenkamp, and Litz (Chapter 6) describe, suppression is an emotion regulation strategy that is used to reduce or down-regulate unwanted emotional experiences. However, the available evidence indicates that suppression is mainly used to reduce negative emotions. Although it is common and can be useful in regulating one's emotions, the habitual use of suppression can lead to emotion regulation difficulties.

Context insensitivity is another mechanism that is implicated in maladaptive emotion regulation. Coifman and Bonanno (Chapter 7) provide an overview of the importance of using the situation to modify one's emotional response, individual differences in context sensitivity and emotional responding, and how context insensitivity can be used to inform clinical treatment. Next, Joormann, Yoon, and Siemer (Chapter 8) highlight how and why cognition plays a critical role in emotion regulation. These authors also provide an overview of individual differences in cognitive processes and describe how these individual differences are linked to psychopathology. The reciprocal relationship between goal regulation and emotion regulation is discussed in Chapter 9 by Johnson, Carver, and Fulford. Evidence that goal dysregulation occurs in psychopathology is provided, and the authors emphasize the way in which some clinical approaches are informed by the importance of addressing goal dysregulation treatment.

Although psychopathology research has mainly focused on the importance of negative emotion, there is accumulating evidence surrounding the critical role of positive emotion in psychopathology. Some of the work in this area discussed in Chapter 9, by Johnson and colleagues, and Chapter 10, by Dillon and Pizzagalli, provides a more comprehensive discussion of how positive emotion can impact psychopathology. These contributors review the importance of positive emotions to the regulation of emotion generally as well as the regulating of negative emotions specifically. Dillon and Pizzagalli also discuss the empirical evidence implicating impairments in positive emotion in psychopathology. Given that the empirical literature concerning the role of positive emotions in psychopathology is in its early stages, Dillon and Pizzagalli provide valuable suggestions for future research in the area. The last chapter of Part II concerns the role of sleep in emotion regulation. In Chapter 11, van der Helm and Walker review findings from both basic science and clinical science, which highlight emotional processing that occurs during sleep and how this processing affects the subsequent day's reactivity of specific brain regions and associated autonomic networks. This chapter provides a valuable overview of how and why sleep can impact psychological processes such as emotion regulation.

After gaining a more thorough understanding of emotion regulation mechanisms that affect psychopathology, readers will be poised to appreciate the chapters included in the third, and last, section of the book, which describe various treatment approaches in which emotion regulation is a target. Fairholme, Boisseau, Ellard, Ehrenreich, and Barlow (Chapter 12) start off Part III by describing their recently developed unified treatment for mood and anxiety disorders. These investigators describe the theories on which the unified treatment was developed, including Gross's modal model of emotion regulation; provide a description of the various components of the treatment; and conclude with a case example that illustrates how the treatment is implemented. As Boulanger and colleagues describe in Chapter 5, experiential avoidance is a maladaptive emotion regulation strategy that has broad psychopathology implications. Chapter 13 describes acceptance and commitment therapy (ACT) approach, which is based on the experiential avoidance model. Valdivia-Salas, Sheppard, and Forsyth describe the basic tenets of ACT and provide an overview of the empirical evidence demonstrating the efficacy of ACT for a variety of psychiatric disorders, emphasizing its impact on emotion regulation difficulties. Another treatment approach that can target experiential avoidance is mindfulness-based therapy. In Chapter 14, Corcoran, Farb, Anderson, and Segal describe this therapy alongside its connections to emotion regulation as well as the efficacy data for various psychiatric disorders. Next, Mennin and Fresco (Chapter 15) describe a treatment approach that they have developed that explicitly targets emotion regulation difficulties in anxiety. Efficacy evidence for the treatment is presented and the promise the treatment holds for multiple forms of psychopathology is considered. As with the ACT and mindfulness-based interventions, the therapy approach developed by Mennin and colleagues targets multiple mechanisms of emotion regulation.

Recent treatment development efforts have been directed toward modulating attention to impact emotional processes. These treatments are reviewed by Taylor and Amir in Chapter 16. Although treatments in this area are in their early developmental stages, the efficacy data are impressive. Given that emotion regulation difficulties can and do involve positive emotions, treatment approaches that target positive emotions are essential. Behavioral activation is one such treatment approach. In Chapter 17, Syzdek, Addis, and Martell describe the behavioral theory underlying behavioral activation treatment, review the essential components of the treatment, and describe the efficacy data for the treatment. Although behavioral activation was developed for the treatment of depression, Syzdek and colleagues describe the available efficacy data for other disorders as well as its potential to impact emotion regulation difficulties.

This volume concludes with Chapter 18 by Harvey, McGlinchey, and Gruber, which describes a psychosocial treatment approach for sleep dysregulation problems. As with the other chapters in Part III, treatment targeting sleep problems has transdiagnostic implications given that substantial sleep problems have been noted to exist in nearly all forms of psychopathology (American Psychiatric Association, 2000). As van der Helm and Walker describe in Chapter 11, sleep problems have a direct effect on emotion regulation processes.

Looking Forward

The chapters in this volume make it clear that substantial progress has been made within the field of emotion regulation and psychopathology in a relatively short period of time. Various emotion regulation mechanisms that have an impact on psychopathology have been identified, and treatments have been developed that specifically target these problems. Although much progress has been made, there are several areas in which continued work will be important. One such area is in the continued translation or application of the basic science of emotion regulation to psychopathology. As described by Bloch, Moran, and Kring in this volume, a number of emotion regulation constructs have been identified as having an impact on psychopathology, although these constructs differ in terms of which aspects of emotion regulation are important to psychopathology and the manner in which emotion regulation problems lead to specific symptoms of psychopathology. To advance our understanding of the mechanisms of emotion regulations that are pertinent to psychopathology, we should draw upon basic science of emotion regulation; doing so would allow the psychopathology field to have a clear theory and definition to guide our research.

Another area that will be important to investigate is the assessment of emotion regulation as an outcome measure in treatments that specifically target emotion regulation. As several chapters in this volume have described, a number of treatments specially state as a goal the improvement of emotion regulation skills. These treatments have demonstrated treatment efficacy with a variety of clinical samples. However, treatment outcome is typically assessed by examining decreases in psychopathology symptom severity. Although there is merit in examining psychopathology as a treatment outcome measure, it is important to investigate whether or not these treatments actually improve the emotion regulation skills that are targeted in the treatment. For instance, it will be important to know whether ACT decreases experiential avoidance and whether mindfulness-based treatments increase mindfulness. It will also be important to examine whether changes in emotion regulation ability mediate psychopathology symptom severity outcome.

As previously described, the current classification system used in DSM-IV-TR has a number of limitations. Within this volume, we have emphasized a transdiagnostic approach to psychopathology, and we have described how this approach can be helpful in understanding emotion regulation problems that occur in a variety of psychiatric diagnoses, and that using such an approach would result in needing only a handful of treatment protocols. Another way to classify psychopathology would be to focus on emotional disturbances, and Berenbaum, Raghavan, Le, Vernon, and Gomez (2003) have argued for such a taxonomy of emotional disturbances. These authors suggest that using a taxonomy for emotional disturbances would result in additional attention to the importance of emotional disturbances in psychopathology as well as provide a framework for understanding emotional disturbances in psychopathology. Berenbaum et al. propose that a taxonomy of emotional disturbances would provide information that is above and beyond (i.e., incremental validity) what is provided with the current DSM classification system. These authors suggest a taxonomy of emotional disturbances that consists of (1) emotional valence disturbances (e.g., excess of unpleasant emotions), (2) emotional intensity/regulation disturbance (e.g., emotional numbing), and (3) emotional disconnections (e.g., emotional awareness). We agree that such taxonomy would foster greater attention to the importance and ubiquity of emotional disturbance in psychopathology, which would, in turn, result in greater research attention to emotion regulation mechanisms in psychopathology and treatment approaches directed at these problems.

Another area where the field could advance is in the assessment methods used to investigate emotion regulation and their applicability to assessing psychosocial treatment outcome (Sloan & Kring, 2007). Research on emotion regulation in psychopathology has most often been conducted in a laboratory setting. Although there are a number of advantages to studying emotion regulation in the laboratory, there are some limitations in terms of ecological validity. To gain a greater understanding of how people regulate their emotions and the context in which emotion regulation may go awry, it is important to study individuals outside of the laboratory. Fortunately, recent technology advances have made it more possible to study emotion regulation outside of the laboratory. For example, ambulatory psychophysiology has substantially progressed over the past several years, and some systems have the ability to integrate psychophysiology recording with experience sampling methodology, and prompts for experience sampling are typically linked with substantial changes in psychophysiology activity (e.g., LifeShirt System; ViVoMetrics, Los Angeles, CA). In addition, developments are being made that allow for unobtrusive video and audio recording (e.g., small camera attached to the side of eye glass frames) to be linked with substantial changes in psychophysiology activity. Such recordings allow researchers to be able to objectively examine situations in everyday life in which emotions are elicited and when emotion regulation strategies are used. Moreover, the integration of experience sampling along with psychophysiological recording would allow for the examination of multiple channels of emotional responding to be investigated.

These are just a few suggestions of the ways in which the field of emotion regulation and psychopathology can further progress. Some of these suggested changes are already underway. Given the current interest level in emotion regulation and the number of empirical studies that are currently published within this area, it seems likely that we will continue to advance in our understanding of emotion regulation mechanisms in psychopathology and how best to treat these mechanisms.

References

American Psychiatric Association. (2000). *Diagnostic and statistical manual of mental disorders* (4th ed. text rev.). Washington, DC: Author.

Berenbaum, H., Raghavan, C., Le, H. N., Vernon, L., & Gomez, J. (2003). A taxonomy of emotional disturbances. *Clinical Psychology: Science and Practice, 10,* 206–226.

Blanchard, E. B., & Hickling, E. J. (2004). *After the crash. Psychological assessment and treatment of survivors of motor vehicle accidents* (2nd ed.). Washington, DC: American Psychological Association.

Eddy, K. T., Dorer, D. J., Franko, D. L., Tahilani, K., Thompson-Brenner, H., & Herzog, D. B. (2007). Should bulimia nervosa be subtyped by history of anorexia nervosa?: A longitudinal validation. *International Journal of Eating Disorders, 40,* S67–S71.

Fichter, M. M., & Quadflieg, N. (2007). Long-term stability of eating disorder diagnoses. *International Journal of Eating Disorders, 40,* S61–S66.

Gross, J. J. (Ed.). (2007). *Handbook of emotion regulation.* New York: Guilford Press.

Harvey, A. G., Watkins, E., Mansell, W., & Shafran, R. (2004). *Cognitive behavioural processes across psychological disorders: A transdiagnostic approach to research and treatment.* New York: Oxford University Press.

Helzer, J. E., Wittchen, H.-U., Krueger, R. F., & Kraemer, H. C. (2008). Dimensional options for DSM-V: The way forward. In J. E. Helzer, H. C. Kraemer, R. F. Krueger, H.-U. Wittchen, & P. J. Sirovatka (Eds.), *Dimensional approaches in diagnostic classification: Refining the research agenda for DSM-V* (pp. 115–127). Washington, DC: American Psychiatric Association.

Krueger, R. F. (2002). Psychometric perspectives on co-morbidity. In J. E. Helzer

& J. J. Hudziak (Eds.), *Defining psychopathology in the 21st century: DSM-V and beyond* (pp. 41–54). Arlington, VA: American Psychiatric Publishing.

Krug, I. Casasnova, C., Granero, R., Martinez, C., Jiménez-Murcia, S., Bulik, et al. (2008). Comparison study of full and subthreshold bulimia nervosa: Personality, clinical characteristics and short-term response to therapy. *Psychotherapy Research, 18,* 37–47.

Persons, J. B. (2008). *The case formulation approach to cognitive-behavior therapy.* New York: Guilford Press.

Sloan, D., & Kring, A. M. (2007). Measuring changes in emotion during psychotherapy: Conceptual and methodological issues. *Clinical Psychology: Science and Practice, 14,* 307–322.

Widiger, T. A., & Clark, L. A. (2000). Toward DSM-V and the classification of psychopathology. *Psychological Bulletin, 126,* 946–963.

Widiger, T. A., & Samuel, D. B. (2005). Diagnostic categories or dimensions: A question for DSM-V. *Journal of Abnormal Psychology, 114,* 494–504.

PART I

Models of Emotion Regulation

INSIGHTS FROM BASIC SCIENCE

CHAPTER 1

• ——— • ——— • ———— •

Emotion Regulation and Psychopathology

A CONCEPTUAL FRAMEWORK

Kelly Werner and James J. Gross

A person with social anxiety clenches her hands to avoid shaking as she tries to answer a professor's question. A person with alcohol dependence drinks himself into oblivion following a bitter divorce. A person with bulimia has a spat with a friend and then gorges herself, all the while feeling out of control. A person with obsessive–compulsive disorder feels intense anxiety and washes his hands until they bleed. A person with depression fights back tears during an unpleasant work meeting.

What do these people have in common? Although each person is suffering from a different psychiatric disorder, all are experiencing high levels of negative emotion and, in varying ways and to varying degrees, all are trying to suppress the experience or expression of these emotions. Emotion regulation strategies such as suppression are appealing because they help in the short term (e.g., they allow one to feel or look less negative in the moment), but they can be costly in the longer term because they often maintain or even increase one's overall experience of negative emotion (Campbell-Sills & Barlow, 2007; Gross & John, 2003).

Problems with emotion or emotion regulation characterize more than 75% of the diagnostic categories of psychopathology in the *Diagnostic and Statistical Manual of Mental Disorders* (Youth edition [DSM-IV]; American Psychiatric Association, 1994; see Barlow, 2000; Kring & Werner, 2004). In some cases, such as the mood and anxiety disorders, emotion dysregulation is so prominent that the disorders are defined primarily on the basis of disturbed emotions (Mineka & Sutton, 1992). In other cases, such as borderline personality disorder, posttraumatic stress disorder, or alcohol intoxication, the pervasiveness of emotion dysregulation across these and other DSM disorders suggests that emotion regulatory difficulties lie at the heart of many types of psychopathology and may be a key to their treatment.

How can we understand the diverse roles played by different forms of emotion regulation in different types of psychopathology? What is needed is a basic framework for organizing the mounting research on emotion and emotion regulation. Our goal in this chapter is to provide such a framework for researchers and clinicians who are interested in understanding the role of emotion regulation processes in psychopathology. In the first section, we describe core features of emotion and emotion regulation and review a process model of emotion regulation that distinguishes among five families of emotion regulatory strategies. In the second section, we use this emotion regulation framework to examine diverse forms of psychopathology and treatment.

Emotion and Emotion Regulation

According to a functionalist perspective, emotions have evolved because they can be—and often are—adaptive responses to the problems and opportunities that we face (Levenson, 1994). Contemporary emotion theories emphasize the importance of emotions in readying behavioral, motor, and physiological responses, in facilitating decision making, in enhancing memory for important events, and in negotiating interpersonal interactions (Gross & Thompson, 2007). Yet emotions can hurt us as well as help. Emotions are problematic when they are of the wrong type, occur in an inappropriate context, are too intense, or last too long. At such moments, an individual may try to influence, or alter, his unfolding emotional responses.

Emotion

Although everyone has intimate firsthand knowledge of emotion, trying to define emotion is surprisingly difficult. The problem is that emotion refers to an extraordinarily wide variety of responses. For example, "emotion" can refer to sadness during a movie, embarrassment at a colleague's behavior, enjoyment of a funny e-mail, annoyance at traffic, fear of the stock market declining, guilt at becoming angry with a parent, or relief at a benign diagnosis. These emotions vary, among other things, in whether they are mild or intense, negative or positive, public or private, short or long, and primary (initial emotional reaction) or secondary (an emotional reaction to an emotional reaction).

To pin down the elusive construct of emotion, researchers have found it useful to characterize several different features of a prototypical emotional response. A prototypical definition emphasizes typical features, which may not be present in every emotional response.

One feature of emotion is its trigger, or situational antecedents. No matter what the emotion, it begins with a psychologically relevant situation, which can be either external (e.g., watching a car crash) or internal (e.g., anticipating a necessary confrontation). A second feature of emotion is attention. Whether external or internal, situations must be attended to in order for an emotional response to occur. A third feature of emotion is appraisal. Once they are attended to, situations are appraised for their bearing on one's currently active goals, a process referred to as appraisal (Lazarus, 1966). Goals are based on one's values, cultural milieu, current situational features, societal norms, developmental stage of life, and personality.

It bears emphasizing that two people could face exactly the same situation, yet have different goals and, therefore, attend to and appraise the situation differently. For example, a boss could say to two different employees: "I know you can do better in this second presentation than you did in the first." The first employee could feel supported, whereas the second could take this as critical and feel depressed that the first attempt was not good enough. The difference between the two is their goals and subsequent appraisals. The first employee's goal is to grow in his presentation skills, and he interprets the feedback in line with his goals and feels positively. The second employee has the goal of performing perfectly in his first attempt, and the feedback indicates a failure to reach this goal, thereby catalyzing negative emotion. Here we see that positive emotions may result when a situation is appraised as proceeding in line with one's goals and negative emotions may result when a situation is appraised to be counter to one's goals. As things change over time—either the person, the situation, or the meaning the situation holds for an individual—the emotion will also change.

Once a situation has been attended to and appraised as relevant to an individual's goals, the appraisal sets in motion an elaborated emotional response, which is the fourth aspect of emotion. This involves a coordinated set of loosely coupled response tendencies, including experiential, behavioral, and central and peripheral physiological systems (Mauss, Levenson, McCarter, Wilhelm, & Gross, 2005). The experiential component is referred to as "feeling" in everyday language and is so compelling that it is often used interchangeably with emotion. Yet we actually do not know how neurobiological processes give rise to emotional contents (Barrett, Ochsner, & Gross, 2006) and how experience can be dissociated from other aspects of the emotion (e.g., Bonanno, Keltner, Holen, & Horowitz, 1995). Emotions also can be associated with behavioral displays, such as smiling in happiness or eyes widening in fear. Furthermore, emotions also often make us more likely to do something (e.g., flee a stressful scene, laugh, or punch someone) than we otherwise would have been (Frijda, 1986). The facial displays of emotions and impulses to act in certain ways are associated with autonomic and neuroendocrine changes that both anticipate the associated behavioral responses (thereby providing metabolic and motor support for the action) and follow it.

A fifth feature of emotion is its malleability. Once initiated, emotional responses do not necessarily follow a fixed and inevitable course. Emotions can interrupt what we are doing and force themselves upon our awareness (Frijda, 1986). Yet they must compete with other responses to our current situation and can be overtaken by those. It is this last aspect of emotion that is most crucial for an analysis of emotion regulation because it is this feature that gives rise to the possibility for regulation.

These core features of emotion (i.e., situational antecedents, attention, appraisals, multifaceted response tendencies, and malleability) are emphasized in many different theories of emotion (Ekman, Friesen, & Ellsworth, 1972; Frijda, 1986; Levenson, 1994). A simple way to describe these core features of emotion is using the "modal model" of emotion (Barrett et al., 2006; Barrett, Ochsner, & Gross, 2007; Gross, 1998; Gross & Thompson, 2007).

In Figure 1.1, we present in schematic form the situation–attention–appraisal–response sequence specified by the modal model of emotion. This sequence begins with a psychologically relevant situation (external happening or internal thought) that is attended to in various ways. This gives rise to appraisals, which involve judgments of the situation's familiarity, valence, and goal relevance among other things (Ellsworth & Scherer, 2003). These appraisals, in turn, give rise to emotion response tendencies, ranging from slight anxious uneasiness to full-scale outbursts of emotion (such as anger) with vivid emotion experience, behavioral displays of flared nostrils, and a whole host of powerful physiological changes (e.g., red face, increased heart rate).

Because emotional responses often change the situation that gave rise to these responses in the first place, the model has an arrow that shows the response feeding back to (and modifying) the situation. For example,

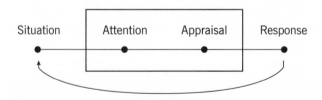

FIGURE 1.1. The modal model of emotion. Recursion is shown with the arrow. From Gross and Thompson (2007). Copyright 2007 by The Guilford Press. Reprinted by permission.

when someone becomes angry after an innocuous incident and others see this anger, it may arouse fear and make them more likely to avoid further interaction. We depict this recursive aspect of emotion with the reentrant arrow. Thus, emotions can change the environment, altering the subsequent instances of emotion.

Emotion Regulation

We have emphasized that emotions are often, but not always, helpful. The idea that emotions can sometimes be harmful brings us to the notion of emotion regulation, which refers to processes that serve to decrease, maintain, or increase one or more aspects of emotion. Such processes range from emigrating from a war-torn country to snuggling with a loved one to watching TV after a stressful day. These processes vary as to whether they are automatic or effortful and whether they are intrinsic (one regulates one's own emotions) or extrinsic (one person regulates another person's emotions, such as when a parent soothes a child). For the purposes of this chapter, which is concerned with adult psychopathology, we focus on intrinsic processes. Emotions can be enhanced (up-regulated) or reduced (down-regulated) (Parrott, 1993). Because psychopathology is largely characterized by excessive negative emotion, much of the discussion in this chapter focuses on the down-regulation of negative emotion. Yet, in some instances, up-regulation may be in need of attention; in bipolar disorder, the down-regulation of positive emotion may be adaptive (Rottenberg & Johnson, 2007), and in depression people may be deficient in their ability to up-regulate positive emotions (Rottenberg, Gross, & Gotlib, 2005).

One additional complexity is that emotion regulation strategies may differentially affect the three components of the emotion response (experiential, behavioral, and physiological) (Mauss et al., 2005). For example, regulation targeted toward experience could involve attempts not to feel an unpleasant feeling, whereas regulation targeted toward behavior could involve smiling although feeling sad. Another important complexity is that emotion regulation typically occurs in social contexts (Gross, Richards, & John, 2006), and these contexts are powerfully shaped by larger societal forces. For example, different cultures encourage different amounts of emotional expression; researchers found that when Japanese and American participants were given the same instructions to pose emotional faces, Japanese participants naturally posed expressions with less intensity than their American counterparts (Matsumoto & Ekman, 1989).

How should we conceptualize the potentially overwhelming number of processes involved in regulating emotions? Gross (1998) has proposed a temporal model of emotion regulation—referred to as the process model of emotion regulation—in which strategies are distinguished in terms of when they have their primary impact on the emotion-generative process: either before the response (antecedent focused) or after the response

(response focused). Antecedent-focused strategies refer to strategies used before the behavioral and physiological emotion response tendencies have become fully activated. For example, a person with borderline personality disorder may avoid an intimate relationship, so that she doesn't have to endure possible rejection and feel abandoned (antecedent focused). By contrast, response-focused strategies refer to things one does once an emotion is underway, after the response tendencies have already been generated. For example, if a person with borderline personality disorder is feeling abandoned because her partner is away on a business trip, she may cut herself in attempt to relieve or distract herself from the painful feelings.

In the process model of emotion regulation, five groups of specific emotion regulation strategies are located along the time line of the emotion process (Figure 1.2). The distinctions made in this model are conceptual, and it is assumed that many emotion regulation attempts will involve multiple regulatory processes. For example, having a few drinks with friends after a stressful day at work may involve regulatory processes at all points in the model. This process model, therefore, provides a conceptual framework useful for understanding the causes, consequences, and mechanisms underlying basic emotion regulatory strategies.

The process model distinguishes five families of emotion regulatory strategies. *Situation selection* refers to choosing whether or not to enter a potentially emotion-eliciting situation. Specifically, it involves choosing to approach or avoid certain people, places, or activities so as to regulate emotion. Once a situation is selected, *situation modification* acts on the situation itself so as to modify its emotional impact. Situations have many different aspects, and *attentional deployment* can be used to choose aspects of situations to focus on. Once focused on a particular aspect of the situation, *cognitive change* refers to changing the way one constructs the meaning of

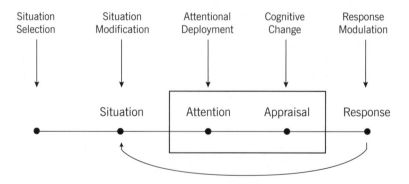

FIGURE 1.2. Process model of emotion regulation. From Gross and Thompson (2007). Copyright 2007 by The Guilford Press. Reprinted by permission.

the situation. These first four families of emotion regulation strategies are initiated before the emotional response ensues and are thus anteced-ent focused. In contrast, *response modulation* refers to attempts to influ-ence emotion response tendencies (e.g., facial behaviors) once they have been elicited; it is thus a response-focused emotion regulation strategy. In attempt to manage unwanted emotions, each of these emotion regulation strategies may be used in adaptive or maladaptive ways.

Emotion regulation is maladaptive when it does not change the emo-tional response in the desired way (e.g., decrease negative affect) or when the long-term costs (decreases work, social functioning, vitality) outweigh the benefits of short-term changes in emotion (relief, temporary decrease in anxiety). In psychopathology, ineffective emotion regulation may occur in many ways. Difficulties may arise when emotions are too intense (e.g., panic usurps access to a typically accessible strategy such as situation modi-fication), when emotion regulation strategies have not yet developed (e.g., a person with social anxiety who has rarely left her house may not have developed socially appropriate expressive suppression), or when emo-tion regulation capabilities have been compromised (e.g., a person with advanced Alzheimer's dementia lacks the neural systems needed to per-form cognitive reappraisal) (Cicchetti, Ackerman, & Izard, 1995; Farach & Mennin, 2007; Kring & Werner, 2004).

Emotion regulation difficulties also may arise when the strategies are intact but they are implemented poorly, in inflexible, context-insensitive ways that are out of line with one's long-term personal goals (e.g., a nature lover with spider phobia avoids all natural settings such as his backyard and parks). In psychopathological populations, inappropriate implementation of intact strategies are often seen in cases where emotion regulation strate-gies that were helpful in childhood are now unhelpful in adulthood. For example, a person with avoidant attachment whose expressions of need, vulnerability, and negative emotion were met with disapproval in her fam-ily of origin may have learned to use an avoidant coping style (e.g., down-play threats and suppression of feelings) (Shaver & Mikulincer, 2007). This coping style may have served her well while growing up but not in her adult intimate relationships.

Another source of difficulty is when people do not allow their primary emotional response to proceed but instead suppress and resist it (e.g., "It is not okay for me to feel angry at my dying mother"), thereby creating a maladaptive secondary emotional response (e.g., guilt). For example, a person with intermittent explosive disorder may immediately resist any feelings of fear (primary response) and express it as anger (secondary response). Mennin, Heimberg, Fresco, and Turk (2005) describe the cre-ation of secondary responses for resisted emotions coming from emotions that are experienced as anxiety producing, as reflected in rigid attentional processes, lack of acceptance, and the activation of negative beliefs about emotions.

If adaptive emotion regulation requires flexible, context-sensitive modulation of emotion in order to meet longer term personal goals (Barrett, Gross, Christensen, & Benvenuto, 2001; Linehan, 1993; McEwen, 2003), how might this be achieved? We believe that adaptive emotion regulation involves choosing and implementing regulation strategies that are appropriate for the context, appropriate for how controllable the internal and external events are, and are in accordance with one's long-term goals (Berenbaum, Raghavan, Le, Vernon, & Gomez, 2003; John & Gross, 2004; Kring & Werner, 2004; Mennin & Farach, 2007). Such regulation often involves the following four steps: (1) pausing, (2) noticing, (3) deciding how controllable the emotion and situation are, and (4) acting in line with long-term goals.

First, adaptive emotion regulation involves not immediately reacting to the external situation or to one's internal primary emotional response, but rather pausing for a moment and giving oneself some breathing room. This involves allowing space for the emotion to begin to arise free of immediate avoidance (e.g., cognitive, behavioral, or emotional avoidance), immediate resistance (e.g., "I shouldn't want to feel this way"), or impulsive behavioral reaction (e.g., yelling in anger, running in fear). This initial moment of mindful awareness reduces the urgency of emotion so that one can selectively control one's behavior (as opposed to trying to globally inhibit all components of the emotional response).

Second, one needs to be aware of one's primary emotional response and be able to identify what emotion one is having (Mennin et al., 2005; Thompson, 1994). This step is important because emotions differ in their experiential, behavioral, and physiological response tendencies as well as their social implications. To effectively control anything, one must first know what it is one is seeking to control.

Third, one needs to determine how controllable the situation that caused the emotion is and how controllable one's internal reaction to the situation is. For controllable external or internal events, one can proactively act on the situation (e.g., if one angered someone else, then apologize) or their internal state in a way to change their emotional experience in the desired direction (e.g., if one is clearly thinking catastrophizing thoughts about the situation, one can reframe them and view the situation more realistically). Thompson and Calkins (1996) discuss how this alteration of the intensity or duration of an emotion rather than changing the discrete emotion that is experienced is adaptive. For situations or internal thoughts or emotions that are out of one's control, adaptive regulation is to accept the situation and experience (Hayes & Wilson, 1994). This prevents the creation of maladaptive secondary emotional responses. For example, if one feels jealous at another's success, one cannot change the other's success nor the fact that he or she is envious of it. Therefore, if one truly accepts his or her feeling of jealousy and does not resist it, it will arise and dissipate and will not be compounded with extra depressive or angry reactions.

Fourth, adaptive emotion regulation involves awareness of one's long-term goals and values regarding the given situation as well as the ability to determine what response is ultimately in line with those goals. This involves the ability to inhibit/control inappropriate or impulsive behaviors and frees up the person to behave in accordance with desired goals, when experiencing negative emotions (Linehan, 1993).

Emotion Regulation and Psychopathology

Many current diagnostic criteria explicitly refer to emotion regulation difficulties. For example, the criteria "persistent avoidance of stimuli associated with the trauma" in posttraumatic stress disorder, "quick angry reactions" in paranoid personality disorder, "difficulty with impulse control" in substance abuse, "fear of gaining weight" in anorexia nervosa, and "elevated, expansive, irritable mood" in bipolar disorder all point to difficulties in regulating emotion.

From the perspective of the process model of emotion regulation, many features of psychopathology may be construed as involving problematic situation selection, situation modification, attentional deployment, cognitive change, or response modulation. Although each of these strategies can be adaptive in certain situations, individuals with mental disorders often display an overreliance or rigidity that maintains symptoms and disrupts functioning. In the following sections, we use the five-way distinction made by the process model of emotion regulation as a conceptual framework for our review of emotion regulation and psychopathology.

Situation Selection

The first family of emotion regulatory strategies is situation selection. By electing to enter (or avoid) a potentially emotion-eliciting situation, one increases (or decreases) the likelihood of an emotion. People often predict the trajectory of their emotional experience in a given situation and can take steps to influence their emotions. This awareness may motivate them to take steps to alter the default emotional trajectory via situation selection. The avoidance of certain situations and the selection of others can be helpful in navigating one's life. If a person with insomnia is barely coherent after a few sleepless nights, he can reschedule an important job interview. Or a war veteran with posttraumatic stress disorder can choose to move away from a gang-ridden neighborhood to avoid hearing sporadic gunshots and retraumatizing himself. Strategically choosing situations in order to care for oneself or choosing enriching, meaningful situations over negative ones can aid in successfully navigating one's emotional life.

Yet the use of situation selection as an emotion regulatory strategy often becomes problematic. When used chronically or inflexibly, it can maintain psychopathology. We see this with avoidant personality disorder, where the disorder is defined by the maladaptive chronic use of avoidance. Persistent avoidance of safe situations maintains pathological fear, negatively affects psychosocial functioning, and diminishes quality of life (Campbell-Sills & Barlow, 2007; see also Fairholme, Boisseau, Ellard, Ehrenreich, & Barlow, Chapter 12, this volume). Situational avoidance causes people to miss out on enriching social, academic, occupational, and leisure activities. People may feel anger, guilt, shame, or sadness at missing out on these aspects of their lives, leading them to feel an overall increase in negative emotion even if they avoided the distress associated with certain situations. The short-term benefits of avoidance of negative emotion-inducing situations do not outweigh the long-term costs of situational avoidance, withdrawal, and concomitant self-defeating thoughts and emotions (Barlow, 2000; Leary, Kowalski, & Campbell, 1988; see also Syzdek, Addis, & Martell, Chapter 17, this volume). For example, if a woman with obsessive–compulsive disorder refuses to kiss and hold hands with her boyfriend because of her disgust of saliva and sweat, this avoidance restricts full engagement with her life, thereby reducing her quality of life.

An important skill needed for adaptive situation selection is the ability to understand which future situations will induce which emotional experiences. People are inaccurate at predicting their emotional responses to future scenarios (Gilbert & Andrews, 1998). In particular, in response to various outcomes, people overestimate how long their negative responses (e.g., becoming confined to a wheelchair) and positive responses (e.g., winning the lottery) will be. This is particularly the case for people with schizophrenia. Researchers have shown that they are poor at predicting how much pleasure they will derive from a future event (anticipatory pleasure). Yet once they experience a rewarding event like having a cigarette or spending time with a family member, persons with schizophrenia report similar amounts of consummatory pleasure as healthy controls (Gard, Kring, Gard, Horan, & Green, 2007). Similarly, persons with depression often underestimate how much they will enjoy a particular event and they avoid it (Jacobson, Martell, & Dimidjian, 2001). Social withdrawal is a common factor in depression used to avoid immediate feelings of sadness or a more prolonged mood that a social event may cause. But the long-term effects of removing oneself from activities and relationships leads to poorer health and well-being.

Techniques in certain therapies directly help clients with the overuse of situation selection strategy of avoidance. In behavior therapy, exposure is a technique used to decrease avoidance (Feske & Chambless, 1995). For example, clients with agoraphobia would build a hierarchy of feared places to frequent outside of their zone of safety. They would successively expose themselves to increasingly anxiety-producing situations and learn to tolerate the associated anxiety in a graded fashion. Exposure allows individuals to (1) experience physiological habituation when they stay in the situation long enough, (2) practice situations that they are currently avoiding, and (3) test dysfunctional beliefs and see how their catastrophic expectations do not come true (Rapee & Heimberg, 1997).

Situation Modification

Once a situation is selected, it can be modified in an attempt to change its emotional impact. If a person with obsessive–compulsive disorder elects to use a germ-filled public restroom, he can use paper towels and refrain from touching anything with bare skin. A person with narcissistic personality disorder may only leave his house wearing the most expensive designer clothes in attempt to receive favorable responses from others. Such efforts to directly modify the situations so as to alter their emotional impact constitute a second family of emotion regulatory strategies. Examples include turning one's head or body to create physical distance with another (Hofmann, Gerlach, Wender, & Roth, 1997), displaying sadness to engender sympathy, displaying anger to express dominance (Davidson et al., 1993), using speech to influence a situation (e.g., telling jokes to make the listener laugh) (Edelmann & Iwawaki, 1987), preparing beforehand (e.g., memorizing a speech, dressing a certain way) (Clark & Wells, 1995), and using a person or thing as a social buffer (e.g., only talking to new people when spouse is included in the conversation) (Clark & Wells, 1995).

Many types of situation modification strategies are adaptive. The use of situation modification is likely adaptive when one is not acting reactively out of fear but rather genuinely and confidently exercising influence over a social situation. The strategies akin to "active coping" from the stress and coping tradition (e.g., assertion) are adaptive (Lazarus & Folkman, 1984). Instead of looking the other way while a partner cheats and enduring an unhappy marriage as a person with dependent personality disorder might, an assertive person could confront the partner. Other examples of genuine or assertive situation modification behaviors are speaking with a confidant voice, taking an authoritative stance, telling jokes or infusing humor, showing caretaking behavior toward another, and directing the situation. Such efforts to directly modify the situation so as to alter its emotional impact constitute a potent form of emotion regulation.

However, situation modification strategies can also be maladaptive, such as when they prevent full exposure to the feared social situations. In the case of social anxiety disorder, Clark (2001) noted how striking it is that individuals expose themselves to anxiety-producing situations on a daily basis, yet their anxiety remains. Individuals likely are not benefiting from these daily exposures because they are using a variety of situation modification strategies, and when the feared results fail to occur, they attribute the nonoccurrence to the safety behavior rather than inferring that the situation is less dangerous. Furthermore, situation modification can be maladaptive when it monopolizes cognitive resources (e.g., when memorizing lines), draws more attention to the person, or increases negative self-focused attention and self-monitoring (Clark, 2001).

Like situation selection, the treatment of choice for maladaptive situation modification is exposure. For example, in the context of social anxiety disorder, the therapist's challenge is to first identify the client's specific situation modification technique and then expose the client to social situations while instructing him or her to keep from engaging in the specific technique. Because situation modification behaviors are not so readily available to the client and the therapist, a detailed interview about the use of safety behaviors may be helpful. For example, if a client's situation modification strategy is identified as overpreparing for a presentation (for instance, by writing out every word), exposing the client to giving the presentation with only bulleted notes could be helpful. With practice, and as the client builds successful experiences at delivering the presentation, such successes will be attributed to his or her skill in giving a presentation and not to the overpreparation. Indeed, in examining exposures, Clark and Wells (1995) found that exposure sessions in which the client was not allowed to use safety behaviors were ultimately more helpful than exposure sessions in which safety behaviors were allowed.

Attentional Deployment

Unlike the first two forms of emotion regulation, attentional deployment does not change the actual person–environment configuration. With attentional deployment, one redirects attention within a given situation to influence emotions. Attentional deployment is thus used to select which of the many possible "internal situations" are active for an individual at any point in time. In the process model, attentional deployment comes after situation modification in the emotion trajectory and is used particularly when it is not possible to change or modify the situation. Specific forms of maladaptive attentional deployment include rumination, worry, and distraction.

Rumination involves attending to and evaluating thoughts and feelings associated with past events. More specifically, rumination typically involves repetitive attentional focus on feelings associated with negative events, along with a negative evaluation of their consequences (Bushman, 2002; Morrow & Nolen-Hoeksema, 1990). Because rumination regarding negative events has been associated with increased levels of negative emotion, Vassilopoulos (2008) sought to tease apart the relative contributions of attentional focus and evaluation (the latter of which is considered in more detail in the following section) in a study in which persons with anxiety engaged with a 7-minute rumination task. Participants were instructed to either "attend to your experience" or "evaluate your experience." Compared with the evaluative condition, the nonevaluative condition was associated with more positive thoughts on a thought-listing exercise and decreased anxious mood pre- to postexercise. This suggests that it may be the evaluative aspect of rumination (which we consider in the following section), in which one judges the experience as good or bad for the self, that is problematic; nonjudgmental attention to situations (attentional deployment) may not have this deleterious effect of compounding negative responding.

Worry, which is akin to rumination but future oriented in anticipation of negative events, is also a problematic type of attentional deployment used by many with anxiety disorders (Borkovec, 1994). When attention is focused on possible future threats, it may have the effect of increasing anxiety and decreased processing of negative emotions. Borkovec and colleagues have found evidence that worry serves as a method for avoiding intense emotion or physiological arousal (Borkovec, 1994). They have shown that worrying reduces physiological arousal to an imagined public speaking task (Borkovec & Hu, 1990). This dampening of physiological arousal is alluring in the short term, as it leads to less distress. Yet it is not advantageous in the long run as it lengthens decision-making times (Metzger, Miller, Cohen, Sofka, & Borkovec, 1990) and prevents habituation to emotional stimuli (Butler & Gross, 2004).

Probably the most common form of attentional deployment is "distraction." Here an individual refocuses attention on nonemotional aspects of the situation or mentally "checks out" of the immediate situation altogether (Rothbart & Sheese, 2007). Distraction also may involve changing internal focus, such as when individuals invoke thoughts or memories that are inconsistent with the undesirable emotional state (Watts, 2007).

When distraction is automatic and chronic, it is likely maladaptive in that it prohibits the ability to habituate to a feared stimuli and learn that some are neutral or not threatening. When used in social situations, distraction also may cause a conversation partner to feel less socially connected. Campbell-Sills and Barlow (2007) note that distraction used in small doses is effective (e.g., deliberately attending to a friend's funny joke rather than remaining caught in negative rumination) (Nolen-Hoeksema, 1993), but the chronic reliance on it is likely a maladaptive strategy because the distraction prevents one from challenging anxious thinking or taking action to solve problems (Hunt, 1998).

An emerging therapeutic technique in the field of psychotherapy that is proving to be useful for attentional deployment problems is "mindfulness." Mindfulness involves the self-regulation of attention where attention is maintained on immediate experience, thereby allowing for increased recognition of mental events in the present moment. This involves adopting an orientation characterized by curiosity, openness, and acceptance (Bishop et al., 2004). Mindfulness exercises of mindfulness-based stress reduction (Kabat-Zinn, 2003), mindfulness-based cognitive therapy (Williams, Russell, & Russell, 2008), acceptance and commitment therapy (Hayes, 2004), and dialectical behavior therapy (Linehan, 1993) hone attentional processes and counter the action tendencies associated with the narrowed focus inherent in threat-based emotions such as fear and anxiety. Mindfulness involves bringing one's awareness back from thinking about the past, the future, or unimportant details of the present situation to permit a fuller appreciation of the present moment. By residing more frequently in the present moment, clients begin to see more readily both inner and outer aspects of reality. This nonevaluative, nonpersonalized allocation of attention helps people to see reality clearly rather than becoming lost in self-referential judgmental thought regarding a given situation (see also Corcoran, Farb, Anderson, & Segal, Chapter 14, this volume; Taylor & Amir, Chapter 16, this volume).

Cognitive Change

Before a situation that is attended to gives rise to emotion, the situation needs to be judged as important to one's goals (i.e., appraisal). This stage of imbuing a situation with meaning can be influenced if one wishes to change the trajectory of the emotional response. Cognitive change refers to changing how we appraise a situation to alter its emotional significance, by changing how we think about either the external or internal situation or our capacity to manage the demands it poses.

In general, reappraisal has been shown to be an adaptive emotion regulatory strategy. For example, in a college student sample, Gross and John (2003) have shown that the habitual use of reappraisal to manage emotions is associated with higher levels of positive affect and lower levels of negative affect. Reappraisal also correlated positively with interpersonal functioning and well-being (Gross & John, 2003). Reappraisers have fewer depressive symptoms and greater self-esteem, life satisfaction, and well-being (Gross & John, 2003).

In other contexts, however, reappraisal can actually maintain negative emotional states (Beck & Dempster, 1976; Nolen-Hoeksema, 2000). Reappraisal may involve changing either (1) appraisals related to the situation or (2) appraisals related to one's emotional responses to that situation. Two categories of reappraisals associated with psychopathology are (1) self-elaboration (Northoff et al., 2006) (e.g., "This means I might lose my job," "Others must think poorly of me") and (2) emotional resistance/non-acceptance of one's current emotional experience (Hayes, Luoma, Bond, Masuda, & Lillis, 2006; see also Boulanger, Hayes, & Pistorello, Chapter 5, this volume) (e.g., "I shouldn't feel bad" or "I'll do anything to not feel like this").

With regard to self-elaboration, activating the self in reference to a situation can substantially increase the duration and complexity of emotional responses. For example, when a young toddler is playing with a toy and his older brother comes and takes it, the 2-year-old feels upset at the loss of the toy and cries. Once the older sister redirects the child to a piece of candy, the tears stop flowing and the incident is forgotten.

Recovery from tears is often not this quick with adults, particularly those with psychopathology. For example, imagine a woman with depression who has an enjoyable assignment taken away from her at work, only to be given to a more seasoned colleague. Like the toddler's response to something enjoyable being taken away, the woman may initially feel upset. Unlike the child, her negative thoughts and feelings are likely to be reignited throughout the day and she will feel negative for hours afterward rather than for just a minute. She may think to herself or complain to coworkers: "It is not fair," "I wonder if my boss thinks I am incompetent." "Is my job in jeopardy?" These thoughts will reignite upset feelings throughout the day. Furthermore, she may have other thoughts that ignite new emotional experiences: "I should have stood up for myself"—guilt; "I might lose my job"—fear; "Others must think I am not a good employee"—embarrassed; "I will never make it in this career"—despair; "I shouldn't feel so bad about this; the other woman has much more experience than me"—depressed. Why is the reaction to something enjoyable being taken away so different in the two cases? The toddler did not think about the stolen toy in terms of her self-concept, yet the woman with depression considered many alternatives in reference to herself. This elaborates the meaning, thereby increasing her emotional responses (e.g., increased intensity, increased number of emotions). Smith and Greenberg (1981) examined the link between depression and private self-consciousness and found that persons who scored higher on a depressed mood questionnaire also scored higher on measures of private self-consciousness. Other studies testing the self-regulatory self-focused theories (Carver & Scheier, 1981; Hull & Levy, 1979) have induced self-focus by placing participants in a room with a mirror and asking them to read or write passages that includes the words "I" and "me" in them (Barden, Garber, Leiman, Ford, & Masters, 1985). These studies found that dysphoric individuals who are made to self-focus by such manipulations tend to experience increased negative affect, whereas when they focus away from the self, they show reductions in negative mood.

The second category of reappraisal that may be particularly important for psychopathology are beliefs about which emotions are okay to have and which are not. These beliefs greatly influence what becomes regulated. Research into the acceptability of emotions has found that an unwillingness to experience negative emotions and the subsequent attempts to avoid feelings such as anxiety or depression maintain psychopathology (Hayes et al., 2006). That is, one's beliefs about the acceptability of emotions lead to emotions about emotions, which, when these emotions about emotions are negative ("I hate myself when I'm anxious!"), may lead to frantic efforts to diminish this second layer of negative emotions.

Western culture impresses upon people that they should feel good, happy, and excited, and it is a personal failing if people have not organized their life so that they are feeling good most of the time. Therefore, many Westerners have an immediate resistance to feeling negatively and start to resist feelings of uneasiness, anxiety, sadness, loneliness, boredom, or irritation just as they appear. Studies are beginning to demonstrate the association between negative reactions to emotions and psychopathology. Greater fear of negative and positive emotions has been reported in generalized anxiety disorder and separation anxiety disorder (Turk, Heimberg, Luterek, Mennin, & Fresco, 2005). Reduced acceptability of emotions has been shown in generalized anxiety disorder and panic disorder (Tull, 2006). Additionally, researchers have found that the Acceptance and Action Questionnaire, which assesses the degree to which one overidentifies with his or her thoughts, avoids his or her feelings, and is unable to act in the face of difficult private events, is positively correlated with self-report measures of many psychopathological symptoms, ranging from the Beck Depression Inventory (Polusny, Rosenthal, Aban, & Follette, 2004) to the Posttraumatic Stress Disorder Checklist (Tull, Gratz, Salters, & Roemer, 2004) to measures of agoraphobia (Dykstra & Follette, 1998) and anxiety about pain (McCracken, 1998).

Self-elaboration ("What does this situation mean for me?") or resisting current emotional experience ("I shouldn't be feeling this way") can recursively cause new emotional responses that theorists refer to as "secondary responses," "dirty emotions," or "negative negativity" (Greenberg & Safran, 1990; Hayes et al., 2006; Mennin & Farach, 2007; Trungpa, 1976). In this framework, a distinction is made between the primary emotion (the initial action tendency and its associated meanings for behavior; e.g., upset at losing the work project) and the secondary response (problematic reactions to primary emotions; e.g., additional upset, fear, despair, embarrassment) (Greenberg & Safran, 1990). Similarly, other theorists distinguish between clean and clear emotions and dirty or muddied emotions (Hayes et al., 2006). The Buddhist tradition has taught about these differences of natural negativity and negative negativity for thousands of years (Trungpa, 1976). Clinicians and theorists propose that the initial emotional responses to life are not too problematic, but rather it is patients' reappraisals and responses to their initial emotional reactions that exacerbate psychological suffering. It is hypothesized that a preponderance of these secondary or dirty emotions maintain psychopathology, and research is needed to draw out this distinction empirically (Greenberg & Safran, 1990; Hayes et al., 2006; Mennin & Farach, 2007; Trungpa, 1976).

To help counteract these less helpful reappraisals, one can apply adaptive cognitive reappraisals to current situations and emotional experiences. Specifically, cognitive therapy makes use of cognitive restructuring (i.e., cognitive reappraisal) to change the meaning of particular thoughts, thereby influencing the emotions that patients experience (Beck & Dempster, 1976). The premise of cognitive therapy is that it is not situations themselves that generate anxiety but rather one's thoughts about situations (Beck & Clark, 1997). The client and therapist work together on identifying automatic thoughts, which are defined as negative, often inaccurate thoughts that produce distress (Heimberg, 2002). Cognitive restructuring trains individuals to change the appraisals of their situations so that they seems less threatening, more within one's control, and less permanent. Additionally, our review of maladaptive reappraisals of self-elaboration and resistance (e.g., evaluating a situation in terms of one's self-worth or believing that one shouldn't feel a certain emotion) indicates that antagonistic reappraisals could be beneficial. This would involve not taking a situation so personally or believing it is okay to have one's current emotional experience. For example, the depressed woman whose enjoyable job is taken away could reframe it as, "This means nothing personal about me, it is just in the best interest of the company to have the most qualified person perform every job" or "It is okay for me to feel upset at the loss of something I liked."

Response Modulation

The final emotion regulatory strategy, response modulation, occurs late in the emotion-generative process, after response tendencies have been initiated. Response modulation refers to influencing experiential, behavioral, or physiological responding as directly as possible. Two of the best researched forms of response modulation are expressive suppression, which refers to efforts to inhibit ongoing emotion-expressive behavior (Gross, 1998), and experiential avoidance, which refers to efforts to inhibit the emotion experience itself (Hayes & Wilson, 1994; Kashdan, Barrios, Forsyth, & Steger, 2006; see also Boulanger et al., Chapter 5, this volume).

Gross and colleagues have documented that individuals instructed to use expressive suppression while viewing emotion-provoking films are successful in decreasing expressive behavior (Gross, 2002; Gross & Levenson, 1997). Expressive suppression decreases the subjective experience of positive emotion but has no effect on the subjective experience of negative emotion. Suppression also produces deleterious biological and cognitive effects such as increased sympathetic nervous system activation and impaired memory (Campbell-Sills, Barlow, Brown, & Hofmann, 2006). In one study, individuals who tended to naturally suppress their expressive behavior were more likely to be obsessional, anxious, and depressed (Marcks & Woods, 2005). A study comparing individuals with anxiety and mood disorders with control participants found that the former were more likely to utilize maladaptive emotion regulation strategies such as avoidant or suppressive behavior when viewing an emotion-provoking film (Campbell-Sills & Barlow, 2007). Also, individuals with panic disorder fall back on both expressive suppression and experiential avoidance in response to a carbon dioxide (CO_2) challenge, a procedure that uses CO_2-enriched air inhalation to induce the physiological sensations associated with panic (Levitt, Brown, Orsillo, & Barlow, 2004).

Overall, there is theoretical (Barlow, Allen, & Choate, 2004; Mennin, Heimberg, Turk, & Fresco, 2002), experimental (Campbell-Sills et al., 2006; Gross & John, 2003), and clinical (e.g., Fairholme et al., Chapter 12, this volume; Mennin & Fresco, Chapter 15, this volume) evidence confirming the maladaptive nature of expressive suppression for healthy adults and individuals with psychopathology. Suppression, although theoretically used in efforts to decrease emotional experiencing, appears to paradoxically increase negative emotion in healthy people (Gross & John, 2003) and people with anxiety (Amstadter, 2008). Often, a goal of emotion regulation is decreased negative emotional experience; therefore, expressive suppression is a maladaptive emotion regulation strategy because it does not decrease negative feelings and it increases one's physiological arousal. Furthermore, the habitual suppression of positive emotions can have interpersonal consequences. Suppression of positive emotional expression is maladaptive in that it decreases affiliation and closeness. Emotion-expressive behavior is essential for communicating what one wants and influencing the actions and feelings of others (Gross & Levenson, 1997).

Experiential suppression is often discussed in the literature as "experiential avoidance." Experiential avoidance may involve distraction (discussed previously), but at its heart it refers to an unwillingness to experience private events (problematic thoughts, feelings, and sensations) and to deliberate efforts to control or escape from them (Hayes, 2004; Hayes & Wilson, 1994). Researchers suggest that experiential avoidance maintains many mood and anxiety disorders (Hayes & Wilson, 1994; Kashdan et al., 2006). It is an unwillingness to have one's authentic experience and be okay with who one is. Experiential avoidance becomes a disordered process when it is applied rigidly and inflexibly such that enormous time, effort, and energy are devoted to managing, controlling, or struggling with unwanted private events.

In contrast to expressive and experiential suppression, a more adaptive stance may be "acceptance," as emphasized in acceptance and commitment therapy (Hayes, 2004). Acceptance of one's internal reactions (thoughts, feelings, impulses, and sensations) refers to allowing one's reactions to proceed without resisting them in any way. The practice of acceptance allows the rise and passage of emotions without attempts to avoid or control the experience (Roemer & Orsillo, 2005). Acceptance of internal events dissuades against maladaptive attempts at control and regulation and allows for more flexible responses and, therefore, helps with the maladaptive appraisal of judging one's internal experience to be unacceptable and to not suppress the emotional response. There is evidence that acceptance of one's internal experience is an adaptive strategy for working with one's emotional responding (Dalrymple & Herbert, 2007; Hayes et al., 2006; Turk et al., 2005; Valdivia-Salas, Sheppard, & Forsyth, Chapter 13, this volume).

Concluding Comment

Many of the psychiatric conditions described in the DSM-IV involve maladaptive emotion regulation. Research on emotion and emotion regulation processes—both in healthy and in clinical samples—promises to provide an ever more secure foundation for investigating psychopathology. In this chapter, we have described a process model of emotion regulation and used this model as a framework for considering the role of emotion regulation in the onset, maintenance, and treatment of selected forms of psychopathology.

Viewing clinical disorders within an emotion regulation framework helps us to delineate mechanisms that are common across psychological disorders (and even to subsyndromal cases). For example, the maladaptive use of distraction may be common to disorders such as generalized anxiety disorder, posttraumatic stress disorder, borderline personality disorder, bulimia nervosa, and alcohol dependence. Identifying transdiagnostic emotion regulation processing problems in psychopathology may inform interventions to effectively treat disorders. For instance, any overreliance on distraction may prove to be effectively treated with mindfulness across these disorders (e.g., Taylor & Amir, Chapter 16, this volume; Valdivia-Salas et al., Chapter 13, this volume).

Our emotion regulation framework may also be useful in specifying how different emotion regulatory mechanisms may give rise to a "single" diagnosis. For example, the woman with depression whose job was taken away may use a few maladaptive emotion regulation strategies to exacerbate her initial upset reaction into a depressed state. In an attempt to not feel upset, she may call in sick to work the next day (situation selection); complain to coworkers rather than directly communicate with her boss (situation modification); ruminate about the situation (attentional deployment); self-elaborate and resist the negative thoughts and emotions related to the situation (cognitive change); and suppress her negative feelings (response modulation). The use of these maladaptive emotion regulation strategies in tandem may not allow the upset feelings to fully arise and dissipate, but rather may contribute to the creation of "dirty emotions" that maintain a depressed mood.

As the previous example makes clear, our proposed framework urgently needs to be fleshed out by research examining emotion regulation in the context of particular disorders in individuals of varying ages and backgrounds. Such work will enable us to better understand (1) how dysfunctional patterns of emotion regulation arise, (2) the nature and extent of shared versus unique forms of emotion dysregulation in different forms of psychopathology, and (3) how these patterns of emotion dysregulation vary by age, gender, and cultural context.

References

American Psychiatric Association. (1994). *Diagnostic and statistical manual of mental disorders* (4th ed.). Washington, DC: Author.

Amstadter, A. (2008). Emotion regulation and anxiety disorders. *Journal of Anxiety Disorders, 22*(2), 211–221.

Barden, R. C., Garber, J., Leiman, B., Ford, M. E., & Masters, J. C. (1985). Factors governing the effective remediation of negative affect and its cognitive and behavioral consequences. *Journal of Personality and Social Psychology, 49,* 1040–1053.

Barlow, D. H. (2000). Unraveling the mysteries of anxiety and its disorders from the perspective of emotion theory. *American Psychologist, 55*(11), 1247–1263.

Barlow, D. H., Allen, L. B., & Choate, M. L. (2004). Toward a unified treatment for emotional disorders. *Behavior Therapy, 35*(2), 205–230.

Barrett, L. F., Gross, J. J., Christensen, T. C., & Benvenuto, M. (2001). Knowing what you're feeling and knowing what to do about it: Mapping the relation between emotion differentiation and emotion regulation. *Cognition and Emotion, 15*(6), 713–724.

Barrett, L. F., Ochsner, K. N., & Gross, J. J. (2006). *Beyond automaticity: A course correction for emotion research: Automatic processes in social thinking and behavior.* New York: Psychology Press.

Barrett, L. F., Ochsner, K. N., & Gross, J. J. (2007). On the automaticity of emotion. In J. Bargh (Ed.), *Social psychology and the unconscious: The automaticity of higher mental processes* (pp. 173–217). New York: Psychology Press.

Beck, A. T., & Clark, D. A. (1997). An information processing model of anxiety: Automatic and strategic processes. *Behaviour Research and Therapy, 35*(1), 49–58.

Beck, A. T., & Dempster, R. (1976). *Cognitive therapy and the emotional disorders.* New York: International Universities Press.

Berenbaum, H., Raghavan, C., Le, H. N., Vernon, L. L., & Gomez, J. J. (2003). A taxonomy of emotional disturbances. *Clinical Psychology: Science and Practice, 10*(2), 206–226.

Bishop, S. R., Lau, M., Shapiro, S., Carlson, L., Anderson, N. D., Carmody, J., et al. (2004). Mindfulness: A proposed operational definition. *Clinical Psychology: Science and Practice, 11*(3), 230–241.

Bonanno, G. A., Keltner, D., Holen, A., & Horowitz, M. J. (1995). When avoiding unpleasant emotions might not be such a bad thing: Verbal-autonomic response dissociation and midlife conjugal bereavement. *Journal of Personality and Social Psychology, 69*(5), 975–989.

Borkovec, T. D. (1994). The nature, functions, and origins of worry. In G. Davey & F. Tallis (Eds.), *Worrying: Perspectives on theory, assessment and treatment* (pp. 5–33). Sussex, UK: Wiley.

Borkovec, T. D., & Hu, S. (1990). The effect of worry on cardiovascular response to phobic imagery. *Behaviour Research Therapy, 28*(1), 69–73.

Bushman, B. J. (2002). Does venting anger feed or extinguish the flame?: Catharsis, rumination, distraction, anger, and aggressive responding. *Personality and Social Psychology Bulletin, 28*(6), 724–731.

Butler, E. A., & Gross, J. J. (2004). Hiding feelings in social contexts: Out of sight is not out of mind. In P. Philippot & R. S. Feldman (Eds.), *The regulation of emotion* (pp. 101–126). Mahwah, NJ: Erlbaum.

Campbell-Sills, L., & Barlow, D. H. (2007). Incorporating emotion regulation into conceptualizations and treatments of anxiety and mood disorders. In J. J. Gross (Ed.), *Handbook of emotion regulation* (pp. 542–559). New York: Guilford Press.

Campbell-Sills, L., Barlow, D. H., Brown, T. A., & Hofmann, S. G. (2006). Effects of suppression and acceptance on emotional responses of individuals with anxiety and mood disorders. *Behaviour Research and Therapy, 44*(9), 1251–1263.

Carver, C. S., & Scheier, M. F. (1981). *Attention and self-regulation: A control-theory approach to human behavior.* New York: Springer-Verlag.

Cicchetti, D., Ackerman, B. P., & Izard, C. E. (1995). Emotions and emotion regulation and developmental psychopathology. *Development and Psychopathology, 7,* 1–10.

Clark, D. M. (2001). A cognitive perspective on social phobia. In W. R. Crozier & L. E. Alden (Eds.), *International handbook of social anxiety: Concepts, research and interventions relating to the self and shyness* (pp. 405–430). Chichester, UK: Wiley.

Clark, D. M., & Wells, A. (1995). A cognitive model of social phobia. In R. G. Heimberg, M. R. Liebowitz, D. A. Hope, & F. R. Schneier (Eds.), *Social phobia: Diagnosis, assessment, and treatment* (pp. 69–93). New York: Guilford Press.

Dalrymple, K. L., & Herbert, J. D. (2007). Acceptance and commitment therapy for generalized social anxiety disorder: A pilot study. *Behavior Modification, 31*(5), 543–568.

Davidson, J. R., Krishnan, K. R., Charles, H. C., Boyko, O., Potts, N. L., Ford, S. M., et al. (1993). Magnetic resonance spectroscopy in social phobia: Preliminary findings. *Journal Clinical Psychiatry, 54*(Suppl.), 19–25.

Dykstra, T. A., & Follette, W. C. (1998). *An agoraphobia scale for assessing the clinical significance of treatment outcome.* Unpublished manuscript.

Edelmann, R. J., & Iwawaki, S. (1987). Self-reported expression and consequences of embarrassment in the United Kingdom and Japan. *Psychologia, 30*(4), 205–216.

Ekman, P., Friesen, W. V., & Ellsworth, P. (1972). *Emotion in the human face: Guidelines for research and an integration of findings.* Oxford, UK: Pergamon Press.

Ellsworth, P. C., & Scherer, K. R. (2003). Appraisal processes in emotion. In R. J. Davidson, H. Goldsmith, & K. R. Scherer (Eds.), *Handbook of affective sciences* (pp. 572–595). New York: Oxford University Press.

Farach, F. J., & Mennin, D. S. (2007). Emotion-based approaches to the anxiety disorders. In J. Rottenberg & S. L. Johnson (Eds.), *Emotion and psychopathology: Bridging affective and clinical science* (pp. 243–261). Washington, DC: American Psychological Association.

Feske, U., & Chambless, D. L. (1995). Cognitive behavioral versus exposure only treatment for social phobia: A meta-analysis. *Behavior Therapy, 26*(4), 695–720.

Frijda, N. H. (1986). *The emotions.* New York: Cambridge University Press.

Gard, D. E., Kring, A. M., Gard, M. G., Horan, W. P., & Green, M. F. (2007). Anhedonia in schizophrenia: Distinctions between anticipatory and consummatory pleasure. *Schizophrenia Research, 93*(1–3), 253–260.

Gilbert, P., & Andrews, B. (1998). *Shame: Interpersonal behavior, psychopathology, and culture.* New York: Oxford University Press.

Greenberg, L. S., & Safran, J. D. (1990). *Emotion in psychotherapy.* New York: Guilford Press.

Gross, J. J. (1998). The emerging field of emotion regulation: An integrative review. *Review of General Psychology, 2*(3), 271–299.

Gross, J. J. (2002). Emotion regulation: Affective, cognitive, and social consequences. *Psychophysiology, 39*(3), 281–291.

Gross, J. J., & John, O. P. (2003). Individual differences in two emotion regulation processes: Implications for affect, relationships, and well-being. *Journal of Personality and Social Psychology, 85*(2), 348–362.

Gross, J. J., & Levenson, R. W. (1997). Hiding feelings: The acute effects of inhibiting negative and positive emotion. *Journal of Abnormal Psychology, 106*(1), 95–103.

Gross, J. J., Richards, J. M., & John, O. P. (2006). Emotion regulation in everyday life. In D. K. Snyder, J. A. Simpson, & J. N. Hughes (Eds.), *Emotion regulation in couples and families: Pathways to dysfunction and health* (pp. 13–35). Washington, DC: American Psychological Association.

Gross, J. J., & Thompson, R. A. (2007). Emotion regulation: Conceptual foundations. In J. J. Gross (Ed.), *Handbook of emotion regulation* (pp. 3–24). New York: Guilford Press.

Hayes, S. C. (2004). Acceptance and commitment therapy, relational frame theory, and the third wave of behavioral and cognitive therapies. *Behavior Therapy, 35*(4), 639–665.

Hayes, S. C., Luoma, J. B., Bond, F. W., Masuda, A., & Lillis, J. (2006). Acceptance and commitment therapy: Model, processes and outcomes. *Behaviour Research and Therapy, 44*(1), 1–25.

Hayes, S. C., & Wilson, K. G. (1994). Acceptance and commitment therapy: Altering the verbal support for experiential avoidance. *Behavior Analyst, 17,* 289–303.

Heimberg, R. G. (2002). Cognitive-behavioral therapy for social anxiety disorder: Current status and future directions. *Biological Psychiatry, 51*(1), 101–108.

Hofmann, S. G., Gerlach, A. L., Wender, A., & Roth, W. T. (1997). Speech disturbances and gaze behavior during public speaking in subtypes of social phobia. *Journal of Anxiety Disorders, 11*(6), 573–585.

Hull, J. G., & Levy, A. S. (1979). The organizational functions of the self: An alternative to the Duval and Wicklund model of self-awareness. *Journal of Personality and Social Psychology, 37*(5), 756–768.

Hunt, M. G. (1998). The only way out is through: Emotional processing and recovery after a depressing life event. *Behaviour Research and Therapy, 36*(4), 361–384.

Jacobson, N. S., Martell, C. R., & Dimidjian, S. (2001). Behavioral activation treatment for depression: Returning to contextual roots. *Clinical Psychology: Science and Practice, 8*(3), 255–270.

John, O. P., & Gross, J. J. (2004). Healthy and unhealthy emotion regulation: Personality processes, individual differences, and life span development. *Journal of Personality*, 72(6), 1301–1334.

Kabat-Zinn, J. (2003). Mindfulness-based interventions in context: Past, present, and future. *Clinical Psychology: Science and Practice*, 10(2), 144–156.

Kashdan, T. B., Barrios, V., Forsyth, J. P., & Steger, M. F. (2006). Experiential avoidance as a generalized psychological vulnerability: Comparisons with coping and emotion regulation strategies. *Behaviour Research and Therapy*, 44(9), 1301–1320.

Kring, A. M., & Werner, K. H. (2004). Emotion regulation and psychopathology. In P. Philippot & R. S. Feldman (Eds.), *The regulation of emotion* (pp. 359–385). Hove, UK: Psychology Press.

Lazarus, R. S. (1966). *Psychological stress and the coping process.* New York: McGraw-Hill.

Lazarus, R. S., & Folkman, S. (1984). *Stress, appraisal, and coping.* New York: Springer.

Leary, M. R., Kowalski, R. M., & Campbell, C. D. (1988). Self-presentational concerns and social anxiety: The role of generalized impression expectancies. *Journal of Research in Personality*, 22(3), 308–321.

Levenson, R. W. (1994). Human emotion: A functional view. In P. Ekman & R. J. Davidson (Eds.), *The nature of emotion: Fundamental questions* (pp. 123–126). New York: Oxford University Press.

Levitt, J. T., Brown, T. A., Orsillo, S. M., & Barlow, D. H. (2004). The effects of acceptance versus suppression of emotion on subjective and psychophysiological response to carbon dioxide challenge in patients with panic disorder. *Behavior Therapy*, 35(4), 747–766.

Linehan, M. (1993). *Cognitive-behavioral treatment of borderline personality disorder.* New York: Guilford Press.

Marcks, B. A., & Woods, D. W. (2005). A comparison of thought suppression to an acceptance-based technique in the management of personal intrusive thoughts: A controlled evaluation. *Behaviour Research and Therapy*, 43(4), 433–445.

Matsumoto, D., & Ekman, P. (1989). American-Japanese cultural differences in intensity ratings of facial expressions of emotion. *Motivation and Emotion*, 13(2), 143–157.

Mauss, I. B., Levenson, R. W., McCarter, L., Wilhelm, F. H., & Gross, J. J. (2005). The tie that binds?: Coherence among emotion experience, behavior, and physiology. *Emotion*, 5(2), 175–190.

McCracken, L. M. (1998). Learning to live with the pain: Acceptance of pain predicts adjustment in persons with chronic pain. *Pain*, 74(1), 21–27.

McEwen, B. S. (2003). Mood disorders and allostatic load. *Biological Psychiatry*, 54(3), 200–207.

Mennin, D., & Farach, F. (2007). Emotion and evolving treatments for adult psychopathology. *Clinical Psychology: Science and Practice*, 14(4), 329–352.

Mennin, D. S., Heimberg, R. G., Fresco, D. M., & Turk, C. L. (2005). Preliminary evidence for an emotion dysregulation model of generalized anxiety disorder. *Behaviour Research and Therapy*, 43, 1281–1310.

Mennin, D. S., Heimberg, R. G., Turk, C. L., & Fresco, D. M. (2002). Applying an emotion regulation framework to integrative approaches to generalized anxiety disorder. *Clinical Psychology: Science and Practice*, 9(1), 85–90.

Metzger, R. L., Miller, M. L., Cohen, M., Sofka, M., & Borkovec, T. D. (1990). Worry changes decision making: The effect of negative thoughts on cognitive processing. *Journal of Clinical Psychology, 46*(1), 78–88.

Mineka, S., & Sutton, S. K. (1992). Cognitive biases and the emotional disorders. *Psychological Science, 3*(1), 65–69.

Morrow, J., & Nolen-Hoeksema, S. (1990). Effects of responses to depression on the remediation of depressive affect. *Journal of Personality and Social Psychology, 58*(3), 519–527.

Nolen-Hoeksema, S. (1993). *Sex differences in depression.* Palo Alto, CA: Stanford University Press.

Nolen-Hoeksema, S. (2000). The role of rumination in depressive disorders and mixed anxiety/depressive symptoms. *Journal of Abnormal Psychology, 109*(3), 504–511.

Northoff, G., Heinzel, A., de Greck, M., Bermpohl, F., Dobrowolny, H., & Panksepp, J. (2006). Self-referential processing in our brain—A meta-analysis of imaging studies on the self. *NeuroImage, 31*(1), 440–457.

Parrott, W. G. (1993). Beyond hedonism: Motives for inhibiting good moods and for maintaining bad moods. In D. M. Wegner & J. W. Pennebaker (Eds.), *Handbook of mental control* (pp. 278–305). Englewood Cliffs, NJ: Prentice Hall.

Polusny, M. A., Rosenthal, M. Z., Aban, I., & Follette, V. M. (2004). Experimental avoidance as a mediator of the effects of adolescent sexual victimization on negative adult outcomes. *Violence and Victims, 19*, 109.

Rapee, R. M., & Heimberg, R. G. (1997). A cognitive-behavioral model of anxiety in social phobia. *Behaviour Research and Therapy, 35*(8), 741–756.

Roemer, L., & Orsillo, S. M. (2005). An acceptance-based behavior therapy for generalized anxiety disorder. In S. M. Orsillo & L. Roemer (Eds.), *Acceptance and mindfulness-based approaches to anxiety: Conceptualization and treatment* (pp. 213–240). New York: Springer.

Rothbart, M. K., & Sheese, B. E. (2007). Temperament and emotion regulation. In J. J. Gross (Ed.), *Handbook of emotion regulation* (pp. 331–350). New York: Guilford Press.

Rottenberg, J., Gross, J. J., & Gotlib, I. H. (2005). Emotion context insensitivity in major depressive disorder. *Journal of Abnormal Psychology, 114*(4), 627.

Rottenberg, J., & Johnson, S. L. (2007). *Emotion and psychopathology: Bridging affective and clinical science.* Washington, DC: American Psychological Association.

Shaver, P. R., & Mikulincer, M. (2007). Adult attachment strategies and the regulation of emotion. In J. J. Gross (Ed.), *Handbook of emotion regulation* (pp. 446–465). New York: Guilford Press.

Smith, T. W., & Greenberg, J. (1981). Depression and self-focused attention. *Motivation and Emotion, 5*, 323–331.

Thompson, R. A. (1994). Emotion regulation: A theme in search of definition. *Monographs of the Society for Research in Child Development, 59*(2–3), 25–52.

Thompson, R. A., & Calkins, S. D. (1996). The double-edged sword: Emotional regulation for children at risk. *Development and Psychopathology, 8*, 163–182.

Trungpa, C. (1976). *The myth of freedom.* Boston: Shambhala Publications.

Tull, M. T. (2006). Extending an anxiety sensitivity model of uncued panic attack frequency and symptom severity: The role of emotion dysregulation. *Cognitive Therapy and Research, 30*(2), 177–184.

Tull, M. T., Gratz, K. L., Salters, K., & Roemer, L. (2004). The role of experiential avoidance in posttraumatic stress symptoms and symptoms of depression, anxiety, and somatization. *Journal of Nervous and Mental Disease, 192*(11), 754–761.

Turk, C. L., Heimberg, R. G., Luterek, J. A., Mennin, D. S., & Fresco, D. M. (2005). Emotion dysregulation in generalized anxiety disorder: A comparison with social anxiety disorder. *Cognitive Therapy and Research, 29*(1), 89–106.

Vassilopoulos, S. P. (2008). Social anxiety and ruminative self-focus. *Journal of Anxiety Disorders, 22*, 860–867.

Watts, F. (2007). Emotion regulation and religion. In J. J. Gross (Ed.), *Handbook of emotion regulation* (pp. 504–522). New York: Guilford Press.

Williams, J. M., Russell, I., & Russell, D. (2008). Mindfulness-based cognitive therapy: Further issues in current evidence and future research. *Journal of Consulting and Clinical Psychology, 76*(3), 524–529.

CHAPTER 2

Development of Emotion Regulation

MORE THAN MEETS THE EYE

Ross A. Thompson and Miranda Goodman

Emotion regulation has captured the interest of behavioral scientists in many disciplines, and one reason is that it addresses core scientific and practical concerns. The nature of emotion regulation—that is, the imposition of higher, rational control over lower, more basic emotion systems to accomplish adaptive goals—highlights fundamental issues in emotions theory, including the role of emotion in adaptive functioning and how to distinguish activational and regulatory influences on emotion. Emotion regulation can be studied at multiple levels of analysis, including neurobiological foundations, the cognitive construction of emotional experience, relational influences, cultural constraints, social facilitation and inhibition, and temperamental individuality, and thus poses opportunities for integrative thinking across these levels. Research on emotion regulation also has practical applications and is often motivated by these applied concerns. The association of emotion regulation with personal adjustment, social competence, and even cognitive functioning suggests that emotion regulation is a core developmental achievement with significant personal consequences. This has contributed to the conceptualization of many forms of child and adult psychopathology (including depression, anxiety disorders, conduct problems, and other internalizing and externalizing disorders) as problems of emotion dysregulation, with new therapeutic approaches to enhance capacities for emotion self-management.

Scientific enthusiasm for emotion regulation must address, however, a number of conceptual and empirical challenges. When emotion regulation is viewed in systems terms involving continuing interaction between higher and lower processes, for example, it becomes apparent that emotion regulation is a component of (rather than only a response to) emotional activation. Identifying "adaptive" and "maladaptive" emotion regulation strategies depends on context and goals, moreover, especially in conditions of psychobiological or environmental adversity, and emotion regulation thus may not always result in positive long-term outcomes even when it offers immediate benefits. Furthermore, the growth of emotion regulation derives not merely from maturation of higher neurobiological or behavioral capacities but also from more complicated development of a multifaceted network of component processes.

These are important challenges, and because they commonly arise in developmental study of emotion regulation, they are the focus of this chapter. Our goal is to profile a developmental perspective to the growth of emotion regulation and its implications for developmental psychopathology, with special attention to the challenges facing future basic and applied science in this area. Although we do not have answers for each of the dilemmas currently facing the field, we believe that they will lead researchers toward a more complex and nuanced view of the nature of emotion regulation and its functioning that will ultimately prove more useful for its practical applications. Our discussion opens by profiling some of the definitional challenges facing emotion regulation researchers, followed by a survey of some of the important developmental processes governing the growth of emotion self-management. We then consider the implications of these definitional and developmental issues for questions of emotion regulation and psychopathology before offering some concluding thoughts.

Defining Emotion Regulation

Although it is a phenomenon common to everyday experience, there is more to emotion regulation than meets the eye, and developmental researchers continue to debate the definition of emotion regulation and its core features (cf. Bridges, Denham, & Ganiban, 2004; Campos, Frankel, & Camras, 2004; Cole, Martin, & Dennis, 2004; Gross & Thompson, 2007; Thompson, 1994). Developmental scientists share in common a functionalist orientation to emotion regulation and the view that regulatory influences can create multifaceted changes in emotion (e.g., maintaining, enhancing, as well as minimizing emotional responses). However, they disagree about whether emotion and emotion regulation can be distinguished, whether emotion regulation arises from extrinsic as well as intrinsic influences, and the extent to which regulatory influences consistently advance adaptive goals. Our own definition addresses some of these definitional challenges and others:

> Emotion regulation consists of the extrinsic and intrinsic processes responsible for monitoring, evaluating, and modifying emotional reactions, especially

their intensive and temporal features, to accomplish one's goals. (Thompson, 1994, pp. 27–28)

Several features of this definition bear further comment. First, this definition implicitly distinguishes emotion from emotion regulation, although, as we later comment, this distinction is far more complex and nuanced than it might first appear. Second, regulatory processes can target positive as well as negative emotions and can create changes in both the intensity and the temporal qualities of emotional responding (such as changing the speed of onset or recovery, persistence, range, or lability of emotional responding). This is important as a corrective to the common expectation that emotion regulation is devoted to minimizing negative affect and also because many conditions of psychopathology are characterized not just by the prevalence of negative affect but also by disturbances in the intensity, persistence, or lability of negative and positive emotion. Third, emotion is managed through the extrinsic influence of other people as well as the person's own efforts. This is important to developmental analysis because emotions are primarily managed by caregivers early in life, and a child's emotional repertoire and tolerances are shaped by these experiences of extrinsic emotion regulation. This is also important to understanding emotion-related psychopathology because of how social facilitation or inhibition can contribute to managing emotion in adaptive or maladaptive ways.

Fourth, a core feature of our definition of emotion regulation is that emotion regulation is defined functionally. In other words, emotion regulation is guided by the regulator's goals in a specific emotion-eliciting context. Emphasizing the goals motivating emotion regulation and the context in which it occurs together underscores the point that strategies of emotion regulation are rarely inherently adaptive or maladaptive; such a distinction can be made only with reference to the functions of these strategies in specific contexts. This is apparent in developmental analysis. Misunderstanding children's goals for emotion management can cause adults to perceive them as emotionally dysregulated in situations where children are functioning quite well as emotional tacticians (e.g., a toddler fussing for candy, an adolescent becoming moody to elicit sympathy from friends). Multiple goals can govern emotion regulatory efforts, moreover, and different self-regulatory strategies can serve different goals in different contexts. A child who has been threatened by a peer, for example, may experience conflict between managing emotion to enlist the assistance of others (by enhancing distress and controlling anger), defending oneself and deterring aggression (by controlling fear and enhancing feelings of anger), avoiding further conflict (by controlling feelings of anger and distress), or accomplishing other goals. There may be different immediate and long-term consequences of each strategy, which makes determining their adaptiveness in this context especially difficult. The same is true of adults: A medical professional's skilled self-regulation of negative emotion in emergency situations may blunt empathic sensitivity in other contexts.

Added to this functionalist analysis are other contextual influences, such as the child's relationship with the peer and their shared culture (Nepalese children are socialized to avoid *any* expression of negative emotion; see Cole, Bruschi, & Tamang, 2002). The broader social context is also important: If the child comes from a socioeconomic setting where expressions of anger are important to self-defense and are actively encouraged by caregivers, an adaptive emotional regulatory response may be much different than in another sociocultural setting (see Miller & Sperry, 1987). Although a functionalist approach to emotion regulation introduces complexity and caution in judgments about the adaptive or maladaptive qualities of emotion regulation strategies, it enhances understanding by focusing attention on the nature of the individual's goals and the importance of contextual influences. As we discuss later, the same is true of efforts to understand psychopathology from the perspective of emotion regulation and dysregulation.

Finally, emotion regulation includes monitoring and evaluating emotional experience as well as evaluating it. In other words, emotional self-monitoring and cognitive appraisals of one's emotional experience are central to emotion regulation because these appraisals, in concert with one's emotion goals in that context, guide whether and how emotions are managed. This definitional feature is also important to developmental analysis because children's capacities for appraising their emotions change considerably from infancy through adolescence, and this has a significant influence on the growth of emotion self-regulation, as we consider next (Thompson & Lagattuta, 2006). It also recognizes that emotional appraisals are likely to be different for children who differ temperamentally, in their biological vulnerability to anxious or sad affect, or in their prior experiences of heightened emotion (such as fear), and consequently their needs for emotion regulation will be different. Indeed, one of the characteristics of children and adults who have difficulties with emotion self-management is their hypersensitivity to anticipatory cues of emotional arousal or their dysfunctional appraisal of certain emotion-eliciting situations.

Incorporating emotion appraisal into the definition of emotion regulation is important for other reasons also. It highlights that self-regulatory processes can influence emotional reactions at many points in the process of emotion activation: not just modulating emotional responses but altering cognitive appraisals and, for that matter, changing attentional deployment, context selection, and other elements of the process of emotion generation (Gross & Thompson, 2007). This multicomponent approach thus has applications to therapeutic efforts by identifying multiple approaches to enhancing self-regulatory capability.

Taken together, the purpose of definitionally unpacking the concept of emotion regulation is not just to complicate a phenomenon that otherwise seems fairly simple and straightforward. The purpose is instead to show that the complexity of emotion regulation is based on the complexity of emotion itself and the personal and social goals its expression serves. Understanding the importance of the goals for managing emotion, contextual influences, the effects of other people on emotion regulation, and the significance of the cognitive appraisals and self-monitoring is important for developmental analyses because these features change significantly from infancy through the life course. They are also important for applying the concept of emotion regulation to clinical thinking because of the complexity of the circumstances contributing to emotion-related psychopathology in children and adults.

Development of Emotion Regulation

How does emotion regulation change over the course of development? In light of the foregoing considerations, characterizing the development of emotion regulation as better management of negative emotions is incomplete (Thompson & Goodwin, 2007). The growth of emotion regulation also includes:

- The transition from emotion regulation primarily by others to increasingly self-initiated regulation as children assume responsibility for managing their own positive and negative feelings.
- Growing reliance on mentalistic strategies of emotion self-regulation (e.g., attentional redirection, cognitive reappraisal) over behavioral tactics that rely on contextual support (e.g., seeking help, avoiding emotionally arousing events).
- Increasing breadth, sophistication, and flexibility in the use of different emotion regulation strategies, including capacities to manage emotion in contextually appropriate ways, substituting more effective strategies after others have proven ineffective, and using multiple strategies when needed (e.g., simultaneously enlisting attentional and cognitive strategies to control emotion).
- Enlisting emotion-specific self-regulatory strategies (such as managing fear but not anger through encouraging self-talk) as well as emotion-general strategies (e.g., withdrawal from situations that arouse negative affect).
- Growing sophistication in the social and personal goals underlying self-regulatory efforts (e.g., enlisting emotion regulation to manage social relations, improve cognitive functioning, support self-esteem), and incorporation of cultural and subcultural norms into self-regulatory efforts.
- Development of consistent individual differences in emotion regulation goals, strategies, and general style (e.g., people as emotion suppressors, avoiders) with the development and consolidation of personality.

In this light, the development of emotion regulation involves growth in a complex network of loosely allied neurobiological, conceptual, relational, and self-referential achievements, some of which are regulatory and emotion specific but many of which are not. Many of the constituents of mature emotion self-regulation are also slowly developing. Consequently, one reason why researchers have found that early-emerging individual differences in emotion regulation are not very stable over time is because these differences are based on a changing constellation of behavioral and neurobiological capacities with different maturational timetables and origins (see Calkins, Gill, Johnson, & Smith, 1999; Grolnick, Bridges, & Connell, 1996).

In this section, we consider major advances in the development of emotion regulation in infancy, childhood and adolescence, and adulthood (see also Eisenberg & Morris, 2002; Fox & Calkins, 2003; Kopp, 1989; Thompson, 1990, 1994). We then consider the developing neurobiological correlates of these capacities and what we learn about emotion regulation from developmental neuroscience.

Infancy and Preschool

Emotion regulation begins from birth in the heroic efforts of parents and other caregivers to manage a newborn's arousal (indeed, it is arguable that emotion regulation begins *prenatally* if we consider the effects of maternal stress on fetal psychobiological stress responsivity; see Calkins & Hill, 2007). Beginning in infancy and continuing throughout much of childhood and adolescence, parents directly intervene to manage children's emotional reactions by soothing distress, engaging in exuberant play, organizing daily routines to create manageable emotional demands, providing reassurance in uncertain circumstances, and offering assistance in emotionally demanding situations (Thompson & Meyer, 2007). From a surprisingly early age, these interventions create social expectations that have emotionally regulatory effects. By 6 months of age, for example, distressed infants begin quieting in apparent anticipation of the arrival of their mother when they can hear the adult's approaching footsteps, protesting loudly if the adult approaches but does not pick them up to soothe them (Gekoski, Rovee-Collier, & Carulli-Rabinowitz, 1983; Lamb & Malkin, 1986). Together with the positive expectations and self-regulatory support provided by adults in parent–infant play (Adamson & Frick, 2003), these early experiences embed developing capacities for stress tolerance and emotion regulation in social interaction and contribute to the developing quality of the parent–child relationship.

Nascent capacities for emotion self-regulation emerge early, however. Newborns have innate approach–withdrawal responses to pleasant or aversive stimuli and are equipped with primitive self-soothing behaviors (such as sucking) that help to manage arousal. Early in the first year, the maturation of neurobiological attentional systems provides infants with greater voluntary control over looking and the ability to disengage from emotionally arousing events (Posner & Rothbart, 2000; Rothbart, Posner, & Boylan, 1990). Later in the first year, advances in motor control enable infants to be more deliberate in their efforts to manage distress by reaching toward caregivers for comfort, self-soothing (sometimes with a special toy or blanket), or avoiding or departing from unpleasant situations.

The importance of temperamental individuality further underscores the biological foundations of emotion regulation in the early years. Temperamental characteristics can affect emotion management in at least three ways (Thompson & Goodvin, 2007). First, certain qualities, particularly thresholds for the arousal of negative emotion, contribute to the intensity and persistence of emotional responses that require regulation. Toddlers who are high in emotional reactivity for fear or anger, for example, have been found to be lower in emotional self-control in independent assessments (Calkins et al., 1999; Calkins & Hill, 2007). Second, other temperamental qualities, such as effortful control, are directly associated with enhanced emotion regulation and behavioral self-control (Kochanska, Murray, & Harlan, 2000). Third, temperamental qualities may influence the development of emotion regulation through their interaction with caregiving influences: Temperament is important primarily in the context of certain qualities of care. In a study of the responses of 18-month-olds to moderate stressors, for example, Nachmias and her colleagues reported that the interaction of toddlers' inhibited temperament with an insecure parent–child relationship predicted elevations in cortisol levels (Nachmias, Gunnar, Mangelsdorf, Parritz, & Buss, 1996). Only toddlers who were both insecurely attached and highly inhibited exhibited physiological stress; for inhibited toddlers in secure relationships, the mother's presence helped to buffer the physiological effects of challenging events, and uninhibited toddlers functioned well regardless of the security of attachment. Studies such as these are important for underscoring that, although the biological foundations of emotion regulation are important, the most useful approach to understanding the growth of self-regulatory capacity is through the interaction of biological vulnerability or resiliency with social support or stress.

Childhood and Adolescence

With the growth of language in early childhood, emotions become represented mentally and better understood in relation to other events. This provides young children with greater conceptual tools for managing their feelings. By age 2, for example, they can be overheard making spontaneous comments about emotion, the causes of emotion, and even emotionally regulatory efforts (e.g., "I scared of the shark. Close my eyes" at 28 months) (see Bartsch & Wellman, 1995; Bretherton, Fritz, Zahn-Waxler,

& Ridgeway, 1986). During the preschool years, young children compre-
hend the associations between emotions and the situations that commonly
evoke them, the connections between emotions and other psychological
states (such as perceptions, desires, and expectations), the subjectivity of
emotional experience, and even the association between emotions and
mistaken beliefs (e.g., "Kato felt sad because he *thought* his mother wasn't
coming, but really she was") and memory (e.g., feeling sad because an
adult's comment reminded you of a lost pet) (see Thompson & Lagattuta,
2006, for a review). As a consequence, young children are aware that emotions can be managed by fleeing, removing, restricting their perception of,
or ignoring emotionally arousing events; they are also aware of the value
of self-comforting and seeking the assistance of caregivers for managing
their feelings (Thompson, 1990).

These conceptual advances in emotion understanding do not always
foster emotion self-regulation or socially appropriate conduct, however.
Toddlers' awareness of the association between sadness and unfulfilled
desires may cause them to become insistent on getting what they want
before they can feel better. An older preschooler's awareness of the privacy
of emotional experience (i.e., that others can be misled about how you are
feeling) can contribute to teasing and deception but also to social sensitivity, such as when a 5-year-old smiles after opening a disappointing gift in
the presence of the gift giver. Taken together, the conceptual achievements
in emotion understanding of early childhood contribute complexity to
emotional experience and enhance emotion regulation. Young children's
growing self-awareness and developing self-image also provide motivational incentives to enlist these skills to manage their feelings in ways that
will be praised by adults who matter to them.

The growth of young children's conceptual understanding of emotion also provides further opportunities for parents and other caregivers
to contribute to emotion regulation. The familiar parental maxim "Use
words to say how you feel" enlists developing language ability into emotional self-control and illustrates the growth of parental coaching of self-
regulatory strategies for young children (Thompson & Meyer, 2007). In
everyday circumstances, parents assist in emotion regulation by suggesting specific strategies that might be helpful, from cognitive reframing
("It's just a game") to problem-focused coping ("What can you do to fix
this?") to attention shifting ("Let's think of something else to do") that
enhance young children's developing self-regulatory capacities (see, e.g.,
Miller & Sperry, 1987). Their encouragement of these strategies, especially
in the context of a warm parent–child relationship, contributes to young
children's developing beliefs in the manageability of their feelings and
knowledge of what they can do. Emotion regulation is also socialized in
the context of everyday conversations in which parents and children comment about their own feelings or the emotions of others, and during which
adults provide information about emotion and its causes, convey sociocul-

tural expectations for emotion and its expression, and comment on strategies for emotion management (Thompson, Laible, & Ontai, 2003). These conversations also become a context for learning gender differences in emotion and its expression (Fivush, 1998). The growth of language-based mental representations of emotion in early childhood thus significantly expands the scope of socialization influences by which children learn to manage their feelings.

Early socialization of emotion regulation is multilayered and complex, however. It is influenced, for example, by how caregivers evaluate young children's emotional responses in sympathetic and constructive ways or instead by dismissing, denigrating, or criticizing them, particularly when children are expressing negative feelings. Considerable research indicates that children develop more constructive emotion regulatory capacities when parents respond acceptingly and supportively to their negative emotions (see Denham, Bassett, & Wyatt, 2007; Eisenberg, Cumberland, & Spinrad, 1998). However, parents sometimes misidentify children's feelings and, as a consequence, may coach emotion regulation strategies in ways that are unhelpful or irrelevant. In our lab, mothers and their 4½-year-old children participated in a frustration task and afterward separately watched a videotape of this task and were interviewed about how the children felt. Nearly 60% of the mothers reported *different* emotions from those the children self-reported, even though children's reports were confirmed by observational ratings of the frustration task. Maternal representations of emotion in their own lives (e.g., beliefs about the importance of attending to emotional experience) and the quality of the mother–child relationship were important predictors of mother–child concordance in this study.

Finally, early socialization of emotion regulation is also affected by the broader emotional climate of family life and its emotional demands, models of emotional coping, and expectations for emotional self-control. An emotionally positive home environment fosters the development of more constructive emotion regulatory capacities in children than one characterized by intrafamilial anger and hostility (Halberstadt, Crisp, & Eaton, 1999; Halberstadt & Eaton, 2003). Consistent with this view, young children with secure attachments to their caregivers are more competent at managing their negative emotions than are children with insecure attachments (see Thompson & Meyer, 2007, for a review).

With the conceptual advances of middle childhood and adolescence, emotion understanding and emotion regulation incorporate deeper insight into the mental, attitudinal, personality, and motivational qualities that also inform self-understanding (Thompson, 1990, 1994). Older children are more competently self-reflective, and as they think about their emotional experiences and those of others, they become more competently self-managing. Children's developing awareness, for example, of how emotional intensity gradually dissipates over time, how personal background and personality can yield unique emotional reactions, and how the same event can provoke mixed emotions leads to more psychologically informed strategies of emotion regulation. In middle childhood, young people recognize how emotions can be managed by internal distraction (such as thinking of happy things in difficult circumstances), redirection of thoughts (such as analyzing the technical qualities of a scary movie), cognitively reframing the situation (such as changing goals when initial objectives have been frustrated), acting in a manner that fosters a competing emotional response (such as behaving indifferently in anxious situations), altering the physiological dimensions of emotional arousal (e.g., breathing deeply), or concentrating on the benefits of managing one's feelings or their expression (Thompson, 1990). In adolescence, these self-regulatory approaches are complemented by strategies that are unique and personal, such as playing music that has special meaning to evoke desired feelings or seeking support from close friends.

One reason why older children are capable of enlisting these psychologically oriented emotion regulation strategies is because of growth in executive functions that include strategic planning, error detection and correction, and inhibitory control of initial responses (Zelazo & Cunningham, 2007). The neurobiological foundations of these executive functions (primarily in the prefrontal cortex) emerge early but have a prolonged maturational course, and the growth of executive functions in childhood and adolescence has important implications for thinking and problem solving as well as for behavioral and emotional self-control. In middle childhood, these developing capacities enable children to be more thoughtful and careful problem solvers and to respond emotionally in a less impulsive and more strategic manner.

A broadened social context also contributes to developing sophistication in emotion regulation. Peer relationships (and, to a lesser extent, sibling relationships) present children with different emotional demands, models, and incentives for emotion regulation than do parent–child relationships. Beginning in the preschool years, social competence with peers requires young children to coordinate their behavior with that of other children (who are less competent social partners than adults), manage conflict, negotiate over shared resources or interests, and assert self-interest as well as accurately perceive and respond to others' feelings and master the "feeling rules" of the peer environment. These are formidable challenges for emotion regulation, and research has shown that young children's social competence with peers is significantly affected by their emotional competence, including their skills in emotion self-regulation (Denham et al., 2003). With the increasing importance of peer relationships in middle childhood, furthermore, emotion talk between friends becomes a significant form of affective self-disclosure and a way of acquiring group norms for feeling rules as well as offering and receiving support for competent emotion self-regulation (Gottman & Parker, 1986). Peer relationships are important, therefore, because the skills of emotion regulation required in the family or other adult contexts may not generalize well to the norms and demands of the peer environment; thus, interactions with other children provide a forum for broadening a child's repertoire of self-regulatory skills as well as learning how to adapt skills to different social contexts.

Adulthood

The development of emotion regulation does not end with adolescence, and its continuing growth underscores the importance of the personal goals and social contexts governing emotional self-control. Although there are important individual differences in self-regulatory styles and biases, by early adulthood most individuals have acquired a basic repertoire of strategies for managing emotions and their social expression (John & Gross, 2007). These skills enable adults to function successfully in the employment, familial, recreational, and other social contexts that characterize their lives. In concert with personality, gender, and cultural influences on emotion regulation, these contexts guide expectations for emotional self-control and the goals for emotional management that individuals must achieve (compare, e.g., the requirements for emotional management of a judge, a medical doctor, a professional athlete, and an entertainer). To be successful, adults must refine the repertoire of self-regulatory skills needed to function in the different contexts in which they live and work, perceptive of the emotional goals that must be achieved in these contexts, and acting consistently with self-perceived personality characteristics, gender expectations, and cultural norms.

Emotion regulation also changes developmentally during the adult years in ways that are consistent with this analysis. According to socioemotional selectivity theory (Carstensen, Isaacowitz, & Charles, 1999; Charles & Carstensen, 2007), changing time perspective during the adult years alters the priority accorded different investments of time and energy. When the future time horizon is long, investment in activities with future payoffs (e.g., knowledge and skill acquisition) is emphasized, but when the future time horizon is shorter, investment in activities that are emotionally meaningful is more important. As a consequence, older adults are more concertedly self-regulatory of their emotional experiences, striving to maintain close relationships that are affirming (such as with family members), biased to appraise situations more positively, and actively modifying their circumstances to create more manageable emotional demands (such as avoiding people and contexts that create anxiety). The view that older adults engage in these strategies as part of a broadly self-regulatory approach to emotional experience emphasizes the importance of these emotional goals and context and contrasts with traditional theories of later-life emotion that emphasize either social disengagement or the association of aging with decline in neurobiological emotion systems.

Neurobiology and the Development of Emotion Regulation

Emotion fundamentally involves a dynamic relation between arousal and inhibitory systems. These neurobiological systems are active but immature at birth. Subcortical structures of the limbic system, including the amygdala and hypothalamus, function in concert with the hypothalamic–pituitary–adrenocortical (HPA) axis to activate sympathetic nervous system activity and arouse the newborn. The HPA system has an extended maturational course, and there are important declines in systemic lability during the early years that are influenced, in part, by the responsiveness of caregivers (Gunnar & Vazquez, 2006). Inhibitory systems also have a long maturational course and include multiple regions of the prefrontal cortex (PFC) (particularly the dorsolateral PFC and the orbitofrontal cortex), the anterior cingulate, and the parasympathetic nervous system (Ochsner & Gross, 2007; Porges, Doussard-Roosevelt, & Maiti, 1994; Zelazo & Cunningham, 2007). In the early years, the gradual maturation of these inhibitory systems also helps to account for developmental changes in emotionality, such as the transition from the reactive, all-or-none quality of newborn arousal to the more graded, controllable, and environmentally malleable emotions of the young child. Maturation of the prefrontal cortex later in childhood is also associated, as earlier noted, with the growth of executive functions that involve inhibitory control over impulsive reactions and the substitution of more reasoned responding, strategic planning, and error correction. These developing neurobiological capacities have significant implications for emotional regulation and also make emotional reactions more environmentally responsive and manageable through extrinsic incentives. Thus, the developmental neurobiology of emotion regulation can be regarded as the maturational unfolding of higher cortical inhibitory systems that exert regulatory control over lower limbic and neurohormonal systems governing emotional activation.

This straightforward story is, however, becoming increasingly questioned in favor of a more complex neurobiological account that emphasizes the continuing interaction between lower "activational" and higher "regulatory" emotion systems (e.g., Lewis & Todd, 2007; Ochsner & Gross, 2007; Quirk, 2007; Thompson, Lewis, & Calkins, 2009). A primary reason is the mutual influence that exists between regulatory cortical systems and limbic structures: The PFC exerts inhibitory control over the amygdala, for example, but the amygdala also constrains cortical processing according to emotional meanings that have been previously established (Lewis & Todd, 2007; Quirk, 2007). In this view, therefore, emotion regulation occurs through the interaction between higher and lower brain systems, not just the inhibitory influence of cortical systems alone.

A second reason why researchers favor a more integrative systems approach, consistent with the foregoing, is that the effects of early-emerging emotional biases may exert strong influence throughout emotion-relevant brain systems. In one study, for example, 2-year-olds who were behaviorally identified either as emotionally shy/inhibited or as uninhibited were later studied as adults, and functional magnetic resonance imaging analyses revealed heightened amygdala activation in the inhibited group when viewing novel (vs. familiar) faces but no differences in the uninhibited group (Schwartz, Wright, Shin, Kagan, & Rauch, 2003). Although more longitudinal research is needed, these findings suggest that a strong biological bias toward fearful reactions to unfamiliar events based in limbic system thresholds may color emotional processes to maturity, despite the growth of higher cortical inhibitory systems. Importantly, these early biases can be established temperamentally, experientially (such as through chronic fear activation), or by an interaction between biological predispositions and caregiving quality (Calkins & Hill, 2007). Finally, a neurobiological systems view is consistent with the recognition that emotion regulatory influences do not always follow emotional activation but may precede it. This occurs, for example, through antecedent-focused emotion regulation strategies that manage emotion through anticipatory appraisals, situation selection, and other strategies intended to avert anticipated emotional reactions before they occur (Gross & Thompson, 2007). Such antecedent-focused self-regulation strategies are likely based on a combination of lower and higher neurobiological systems.

What does this updated developmental neurobiological account mean for the development of emotion regulation? First, differences between emotion and emotion regulation cannot be directly mapped onto the distinction between antecedent activational processes and consequent inhibitory processes. Instead, emotion regulation must be viewed as a continuing component of emotion itself, with the interaction between higher and lower neurobiological systems regulating emotional reactions (Thompson et al., 2009). This does not mean that emotion regulation cannot be studied as a distinct process, but rather that the focus should be on the reciprocal influences of multiple emotion-related brain systems rather than designating some systems as exclusively "activational" and others as specifically "regulatory." Second, the developmental neurobiology of emotion regulation is not just the maturation of higher cortical inhibitory systems but also their continuing interaction with more basic emotion systems lower in the neuroaxis. As earlier suggested, this developmental systems view means that early emotional biases may have a long-standing influence on developing neurobiological emotion systems. Finally, as we discuss further next, this systems view of emotion regulation means that regulatory processes do not necessarily result in psychologically constructive or even healthy outcomes. Particularly for individuals at biological vulnerability or environmental risk, the multilevel regulation of emotion may result in emotional functioning that has potentially maladaptive outcomes owing to the growth of stable interactions between lower and higher emotion systems that contribute, for example, to depressed or anxious affect and their cognitive concomitants (Thompson et al., 2009).

Implications for Development and Psychopathology

A significant impetus to research on emotion regulation is its applications to psychopathology, including developmental psychopathology. It is not difficult to see why. Many major affective disorders (such as depression, bipolar disorder, and anxiety disorder) involve dysregulated affect, and other internalizing and externalizing disorders (such as conduct problems, posttraumatic stress disorder, and attention-deficit/hyperactivity disorder) are also characterized by emotion undercontrol. Furthermore, even young children's inability to adaptively manage their feelings can contribute to problems in social competence and emotional adjustment and potentially enhance risk for affective psychopathology. The connections between research on emotion regulation and psychopathology seem self-evident.

Emotion regulation research contributes more, of course, than merely characterizing major psychological problems as difficulties of emotion dysregulation. It is also relevant to understanding the processes leading to emotion dysregulation and its functions in clinical populations. In this chapter, for example, we have drawn attention to how parents' evaluations of children's emotions and the family emotional climate influence adaptive emotion self-regulation, which is relevant to the influence of family "expressed emotion"—parental criticism, hostility, and emotional over-involvement—in a number of clinical problems (Hirshfeld, Biederman, Brody, Faraone, & Rosenbaum, 1997). Our definition of emotion regulation includes the influence of emotion appraisals and self-monitoring, owing partly to the importance of these construals to the onset and maintenance of anxiety and mood disorders (Campbell-Sills & Barlow, 2007). With respect to assessment, Luby and Belden (2006) have used Thompson's (1994) model of emotional dynamics to characterize the emotional regulatory difficulties of children with mood disorders, describing different clinical profiles in terms of variability in not just in the intensity but also the latency, rise time, duration, and recovery of emotional reactions. These and other formulations from the emotion regulation research literature also have potential therapeutic applications.

One of the most important applications of research on emotion regulation to clinical understanding is how we characterize the emotion dysregulation of children and adults at risk. Consistent with the functionalist emphasis on emotion goals and context, it is essential to understand the circumstances in which individuals with emotional problems are striving to manage emotions and the goals that they are seeking to accomplish whenever assessing the adaptiveness or maladaptiveness of their emotion regulation strategies. In our view, the self-regulatory challenges faced by many children and adults at risk is not primarily that they are enlisting inappropriate or maladaptive strategies of emotion management, but that they are trying to cope with emotionally impossible conditions in which there may be no more adaptive manner of regulating emotion. Their self-regulatory strategies are likely to involve inherent trade-offs that purchase immediate coping at the cost of long-term difficulty and that ultimately increase rather than diminish their emotional problems (Thompson & Calkins, 1996; Thompson, Flood, & Lundquist, 1995). Because of this, emotion regulation is for them a double-edged sword: The strategies that are most adaptive for accomplishing immediate emotional goals often render individuals more vulnerable to longer term problems.

Emotion Regulation and Child Maltreatment

The importance of this approach to understanding emotion regulation is evocatively illustrated in the case of maltreated children. These children have elevated rates of a number of psychological disorders, including conduct disorder, attention-deficit/hyperactivity disorder, mood disorders, posttraumatic stress disorder, and substance abuse, so it is appropriate to view child maltreatment as a significant risk factor for psychopathology (Cicchetti & Toth, 1995). Children who experience physical or sexual abuse or chronic neglect are faced with a formidable challenge in emotion regulation: A caregiver who should be the source of support for coping is instead the source of distress. In this sense, we can view maltreated children as doubly disadvantaged: forced to manage the frequent, intense emotional trauma associated with their abuse without the assistance of caregiver support.

In this light, we would anticipate that maltreated children would be seriously deficient in skills of emotion self-regulation, but research evidence does not support this simple deficit model. Instead, a number of studies indicate that maltreated children acquire a repertoire of self-regulatory strategies that enable them to adapt to the unpredictable and potentially dangerous caregiving environment in which they live. These strategies confer some benefits to children at home but are a liability especially when these children enter other social settings, such as school or peer environments.

An important emotion regulation strategy is attention deployment: focusing on certain elements of the environment in ways that contribute to emotion management (Gross & Thompson, 2007). Several studies indicate that maltreated children are hypersensitive to adult expressions of anger, perhaps because this enables them to anticipate and prepare for abusive conduct before it begins. In one study, when pictures of adult facial expressions of emotion were progressively "morphed" from one prototypical expression (e.g., sadness) to another (e.g., anger), maltreated children were more likely to identify blended expressions as angry than were nonmaltreated children (Pollak, 2002; Pollak & Kistler, 2002). Maltreated children also exhibit a lower attentional threshold for detecting anger in the vocal expressions of their mothers (but not of an unfamiliar woman) (Shackman & Pollak, 2005) and have more difficulty attentionally disengaging from perceived angry cues (Pollak & Tolley-Schell, 2003). In a study using event-related brain potential (ERP), maltreated children showed higher ERP responses to pictures of angry facial expressions compared with nonmaltreated children, but there were no differences in their responses to pictures of happy or fearful expressions (Pollak, Klorman, Thatcher, & Cicchetti, 2001). Taken together, these findings argue that maltreated children are sensitized, not habituated, to signals of adult anger, potentially because this sensitivity manages emotion by enabling children to anticipate and prepare for aversive encounters with adults who have abused them in the past. In a sense, if one cannot avert the emotionally overwhelming attack of an abusive adult, it is helpful to be able to anticipate it and flee, avoid, or otherwise prepare for it.

Outside the home, however, their sensitivity to cues of anger and threat undermines emotion management and is more socially dysfunctional. Maltreated children are more physically and verbally aggressive toward their peers (Cicchetti & Toth, 1995) and are more likely to respond with aggression or withdrawal to peer distress (Klimes-Dougan & Kistner, 1990). In this respect, the hypersensitivity to threat that may serve as a protective factor at home is a liability at school, where the social cues of other children are more likely to be misinterpreted and imbued with hostile intent.

This double-edged sword of emotion regulation for children at risk is apparent for other conditions of developmental psychopathology. Children with anxiety disorders, some of whom are biologically vulnerable to anxious affect, exhibit heightened efforts to anticipate fearful arousal through self-regulatory strategies that include their hypervigilance to fear-provoking stimuli, active (sometimes aggressive) avoidance of these stimuli, and overattention to internal cues of physiological arousal that anticipate or accompany anxious overarousal. By enlisting these strategies, anxious children purchase immediate relief from the turmoil of encountering fear-provoking events but, at the same time, consolidate and perpetuate their pathology and undermine developmentally appropriate functioning (Thompson, 2000). Similar self-regulatory challenges arise for children who are offspring of mothers who are depressed or have bipolar disorder and who are themselves at risk of internalizing disorders because of the combination of genetic and experiential risk conferred by their caregivers (Thompson & Calkins, 1996). For these children, as for those who are maltreated, the lesson they have learned is that if their negative emotion cannot be controlled, it can at least be anticipated, but in learning to anticipate negative arousal these children become vulnerable to longer term dysfunction.

Conclusion

In characterizing emotion regulation as "more than meets the eye," our goal is to show that this familiar, everyday phenomenon is psychologically, developmentally, and neurobiologically complex, particularly when emotion regulation is applied to psychopathology. More important, what is "more than meets the eye" contributes to the developmental and clinical applications of emotion regulation research.

In developmental analysis, research findings (including our own) convince us that children's emotion self-regulation at any age is based on sophisticated emotion appraisals, goals, and contextual influences that are developmentally changing and yields responses that may be perplexing unless they are interpreted in this light. In applications to psychopathology, it is equally apparent that emotion regulation efforts are adapted to complex biological and environmental risks and the trade-offs between immediate and long-term goals that are relevant to psychological pain. In each case, we believe, greater insight into the functions of emotion regulation in typical and atypical functioning is achieved when emotion regulation is regarded not just as the imposition of higher behavioral or neurobiological control but as an interaction between higher and lower systems related to emotional activation and its management. As other chapters in this volume indicate, perspectives to emotion regulation that incorporate these complexities yield therapeutic applications that begin to address the emotion goals underlying emotion dysregulation, the appraisals and construals that perpetuate self-defeating emotion management styles, and the contextual influences that help to create the emotionally impossible environments with which distressed individuals must cope.

In a culture like ours, where emotional experience underlies the peaks and valleys of human experience, it is natural to hope that processes of emotion regulation will help to elevate the valleys and refine the peaks of that experience. The constructive—sometimes reconstructive—process by which emotion regulation accomplishes this reveals much about how deeply interconnected are emotion and its management in development and psychopathology.

References

Adamson, L., & Frick, J. (2003). The still face: A history of a shared experimental paradigm. *Infancy, 4,* 451–473.

Bartsch, K., & Wellman, H. (1995). *Children talk about the mind.* Oxford, UK: Oxford University Press.

Bretherton, I., Fritz, J., Zahn-Waxler, C., & Ridgeway, D. (1986). Learning to talk about emotions: A functionalist perspective. *Child Development, 57,* 529–548.

Bridges, L. J., Denham, S. A., & Ganiban, J. M. (2004). Definitional issues in emotion regulation research. *Child Development, 75,* 340–345.

Calkins, S. D., Gill, K. L., Johnson, M. C., & Smith, C. L. (1999). Emotional reactivity and emotional regulation strategies as predictors of social behavior with peers during toddlerhood. *Social Development, 8,* 310–334.

Calkins, S. D., & Hill, A. (2007). Caregiver influences on emerging emotion regulation: Biological and environmental transactions in early development. In J. J. Gross (Ed.), *Handbook of emotion regulation* (pp. 229–248). New York: Guilford Press.

Campbell-Sills, L., & Barlow, D. H. (2007). Incorporating emotion regulation into conceptualizations and treatments of anxiety and mood disorders. In J. J. Gross (Ed.), *Handbook of emotion regulation* (pp. 542–559). New York: Guilford Press.

Campos, J. J., Frankel, C. B., & Camras, L. (2004). On the nature of emotion regulation. *Child Development, 75,* 377–394.

Carstensen, L. L., Isaacowitz, D. M., & Charles, S. T. (1999). Taking time seriously: A theory of socioemotional selectivity. *American Psychologist, 14,* 117–121.

Charles, S. T., & Carstensen, L. L. (2007). Emotion regulation and aging. In J. J. Gross (Ed.), *Handbook of emotion regulation* (pp. 307–327). New York: Guilford Press.

Cicchetti, D., & Toth, S. L. (1995). A developmental psychopathology perspective on child abuse and neglect. *Journal of the American Academy of Child and Adolescent Psychiatry, 34*(5), 541–565.

Cole, P. M., Bruschi, C. J., & Tamang, B. L. (2002). Cultural differences in children's emotional reactions to difficult situation. *Child Development, 73,* 983–996.

Cole, P. M., Martin, S., & Dennis, T. (2004). Emotion regulation as a scientific construct: Methodological challenges and directions for child development research. *Child Development, 75,* 317–333.

Denham, S. A., Bassett, H. H., & Wyatt, T. (2007). The socialization of emotional competence. In J. E. Grusec & P. D. Hastings (Eds.), *Handbook of socialization: Theory and research* (pp. 614–637). New York: Guilford Press.

Denham, S. A., Blair, K. A., DeMulder, E., Levitas, J., Sawyer, K., Auerbach-Major, S., et al. (2003). Preschool emotional competence: Pathway to social competence? *Child Development, 74,* 238–256.

Eisenberg, N., Cumberland, A., & Spinrad, T. L. (1998). Parental socialization of emotion. *Psychological Inquiry, 9,* 241–273.

Eisenberg, N., & Morris, A. S. (2002). Children's emotion-related regulation. In R. Kail (Ed.), *Advances in child development and behavior* (Vol. 30, pp. 190–229). San Diego, CA: Academic Press.

Fivush, R. (1998). Gendered narratives: Elaboration, structure, and emotion in parent–child reminiscing across the preschool years. In C. P. Thompson & D. J. Herrmann (Eds.), *Autobiographical memory: Theoretical and applied perspectives* (pp. 79–103). Mahwah, NJ: Erlbaum.

Fox, N., & Calkins, S. (2003). The development of self-control of emotion: Intrinsic and extrinsic influences. *Motivation and Emotion, 27,* 7–26.

Gekoski, M., Rovee-Collier, C., & Carulli-Rabinowitz, V. (1983). A longitudinal analysis of inhibition of infant distress: The origins of social expectations? *Infant Behavior and Development, 6,* 339–351.

Gottman, J. M., & Parker, J. (Eds.). (1986). *Conversations of friends: Speculations on affective development.* New York: Cambridge University Press.

Grolnick, W. S., Bridges, L. J., & Connell, J. P. (1996). Emotion regulation in two-year-olds: Strategies and emotional expression in four contexts. *Child Development, 67*, 928–941.

Gross, J. J., & Thompson, R. A. (2007). Emotion regulation: Conceptual foundations. In J. J. Gross (Ed.), *Handbook of emotion regulation* (pp. 3–24). New York: Guilford Press.

Gunnar, M., & Vazquez, D. (2006). Stress neurobiology and developmental psychopathology. In D. Cicchetti & D. Cohen (Eds.), *Developmental psychopathology* (2nd ed.): *Vol. 2: Developmental neuroscience* (pp. 533–577). New York: Wiley.

Halberstadt, A. G., Crisp, V. W., & Eaton, K. L. (1999). Family expressiveness: A retrospective and new directions for research. In P. Philippot & R. S. Feldman (Eds.), *The social context of nonverbal behavior* (pp. 109–155). New York: Cambridge University Press.

Halberstadt, A. G., & Eaton, K. L. (2003). A meta-analysis of family expressiveness and children's emotion expressiveness and understanding. *Marriage and Family Review, 34*, 35–62.

Hirshfeld, D. R., Biederman, J., Brody, L., Faraone, S. V., & Rosenbaum, J. F. (1997). Associations between expressed emotion and child behavioral inhibition and psychopathology: A pilot study. *Journal of the American Academy of Child and Adolescent Psychiatry, 36*, 205–213.

John, O. P., & Gross, J. J. (2007). Individual differences in emotion regulation. In J. J. Gross (Ed.), *Handbook of emotion regulation* (pp. 351–372). New York: Guilford Press.

Klimes-Dougan, B., & Kistner, J. (1990). Physically abused preschoolers' responses to peers' distress. *Developmental Psychology, 26*, 599–602.

Kochanska, G., Murray, K. T., & Harlan, E. (2000). Effortful control in early childhood: Continuity and change, antecedents, and implications for social development. *Developmental Psychology, 26*, 220–232.

Kopp, C. B. (1989). Regulation of distress and negative emotions: A developmental review. *Developmental Psychology, 25*, 343–354.

Lamb, M., & Malkin, C. (1986). The development of social expectations in distress-relief sequences: A longitudinal study. *International Journal of Behavioral Development, 9*, 235–249.

Lewis, M. D., & Todd, R. M. (2007). The self-regulating brain: Cortical-subcortical feedback and the development of intelligent action. *Cognitive Development, 22*, 406–430.

Luby, J. L., & Belden, A. C. (2006). Mood disorders: Phenomenology and a developmental emotion reactivity model. In J. L. Luby (Ed.), *Handbook of preschool mental health: Development, disorders, and treatment* (pp. 209–230). New York: Guilford Press.

Miller, P. J., & Sperry, L. (1987). The socialization of anger and aggression. *Merrill-Palmer Quarterly, 33*, 1–31.

Nachmias, M., Gunnar, M., Mangelsdorf, S., Parritz, R. H., & Buss, K. (1996). Behavioral inhibition and stress reactivity: The moderating role of attachment security. *Child Development, 67*, 508–522.

Ochsner, K. N., & Gross, J. J. (2007). The neural architecture of emotion regulation. In J. J. Gross (Ed.), *Handbook of emotion regulation* (pp. 87–109). New York: Guilford Press.

Pollak, S.D. (2002). Effects of early experience on children's recognition of facial displays of emotion. *Developmental Psychology, 38,* 784–791.

Pollak, S. D., & Kistler, D. J. (2002). Early experience is associated with the development of categorical representations for facial expressions of emotion. *Proceedings of the National Academy Sciences, 99,* 9072–9076.

Pollak, S. D., Klorman, R., Thatcher, J. E., & Cicchetti, D. (2001). P3b reflects maltreated children's reactions to facial displays of emotion. *Psychophysiology, 38,* 267–274.

Pollak, S. D., & Tolley-Schell, S. A. (2003). Selective attention to facial emotion of physically abused children. *Journal of Abnormal Psychology, 113,* 323–338.

Porges, S. W., Doussard-Roosevelt, J. A., & Maiti, A. K. (1994). Vagal tone and the physiological regulation of emotion. *Monographs of the Society for Research in Child Development, 59*(Serial No. 240), 167–186.

Posner, M. I., & Rothbart, M. K. (2000). Developing mechanisms of self-regulation. *Development and Psychopathology, 12,* 427–441.

Quirk, G. J. (2007). Prefrontal–amygdala interactions in the regulation of fear. In J. J. Gross (Ed.), *Handbook of emotion regulation* (pp. 27–46). New York: Guilford Press.

Rothbart, M. K., Posner, M. I., & Boylan, A. (1990). Regulatory mechanisms in infant development. In J. Enns (Ed.), *The development of attention: Research and theory* (pp. 139–160). Amsterdam: Elsevier.

Schwartz, C., Wright, C., Shin, L., Kagan, J., & Rauch, S. (2003). Inhibited and uninhibited infants "grown up": Adult amygdalar response to novelty. *Science, 300,* 1952–1953.

Shackman, J. E., & Pollak, S. D. (2005). Experiential influences on multimodal perception of emotion. *Child Development, 76,* 1116–1126.

Thompson, R. A. (1990). Emotion and self-regulation. In R. A. Thompson (Ed.), *Nebraska symposium on motivation: Socioemotional development* (Vol. 36, pp. 383–483). Lincoln: University of Nebraska Press.

Thompson, R. A. (1994). Emotion regulation: A theme in search of definition. *Monographs of the Society for Research in Child Development, 59*(2–3, Serial No. 240), 25–52.

Thompson, R. A. (2000). Childhood anxiety disorders from the perspective of emotion regulation and attachment. In M. W. Vasey & M. R. Dadds (Eds.), *The developmental psychopathology of anxiety* (pp. 160–182). Oxford, UK: Oxford University Press.

Thompson, R. A., & Calkins, S. (1996). The double-edged sword: Emotional regulation for children at risk. *Development and Psychopathology, 8*(1), 163–182.

Thompson, R. A., Flood, M. F., & Lundquist, L. (1995). Emotional regulation and developmental psychopathology. In D. Cicchetti & S. Toth (Eds.), *Rochester Symposium on Developmental Psychopathology: Emotion, cognition, and representation* (Vol. 6, pp. 261–299). Rochester, NY: University of Rochester Press.

Thompson, R. A., & Goodvin, R. (2007). Taming the tempest in the teapot: Emotion regulation in toddlers. In C. A. Brownell & C. B. Kopp (Eds.), *Socioemotional development in the toddler years: Transitions and transformations* (pp. 320–341). New York: Guilford Press.

Thompson, R. A., & Lagattuta, K. (2006). Feeling and understanding: Early emotional development. In K. McCartney & D. Phillips (Eds.), *The Blackwell handbook of early childhood development* (pp. 317–337). Oxford, UK: Blackwell.

Thompson, R. A., Laible, D. J., & Ontai, L. L. (2003). Early understanding of emotion, morality, and the self: Developing a working model. In R. V. Kail (Ed.), *Advances in child development and behavior* (Vol. 31, pp. 137–171). San Diego, CA: Academic Press.

Thompson, R. A., Lewis, M. D., & Calkins, S. D. (2009). Reassessing emotion regulation. *Child Development Perspectives, 2,* 124–131.

Thompson, R. A., & Meyer, S. (2007). Socialization of emotion regulation in the family. In J. J. Gross (Ed.), *Handbook of emotion regulation* (pp. 249–268). New York: Guilford Press.

Zelazo, P. D., & Cunningham, W. A. (2007). Executive function: Mechanisms underlying emotion regulation. In J. J. Gross (Ed.), *Handbook of emotion regulation* (pp. 135–158). New York: Guilford Press.

CHAPTER 3

How We Heal
What We Don't Want to Feel

THE FUNCTIONAL NEURAL ARCHITECTURE
OF EMOTION REGULATION

**Bryan T. Denny, Jennifer A. Silvers,
and Kevin N. Ochsner**

Whether trying to mollify a fear of flying or keep one's cool in rush-hour traffic, the need to adaptively regulate emotion is ubiquitous. Perhaps because of its ubiquity, in the past decade behavioral and biological research on emotion regulation has exploded. Much of this work has sought to clarify the consequences of specific regulatory strategies and the contexts in which they are most appropriately used (Gross, 1998b). Other work has attempted to delineate the functional neural architecture underlying emotion and emotion regulation (Ochsner & Gross, 2005, 2007, 2008). This work offers an opportunity to determine what neural mechanisms allow a healthy individual to keep an even keel, to examine how the operation of these mechanisms varies across healthy individuals, and, perhaps of greatest interest for the present volume, to examine how the coordination of these neural mechanisms might falter in psychopathology.

This chapter seeks to address these questions about the neural bases of emotion and emotion regulation in four parts. In the first part, we provide a framework for understanding how emotion regulation may alter the process of generating an emotion, and focus on a particular cognitive emotion regulation strategy known as reappraisal. In the second part, we briefly review neuroimaging methods used in the field, followed by a review of evidence for a working model of the neural bases of emotion regulation. In the third part, we apply this model to understanding the typical range of variation in individual differences in emotion and its regulation. Finally, in the fourth part, we apply this model to elucidate emotion dysfunction across clinical disorders, including schizophrenia, bipolar disorder, major depressive disorder, and anxiety disorders, including posttraumatic stress disorder.

Models of Emotion and Emotion Regulation

Although there are various conceptualizations of emotion, throughout this chapter we follow appraisal theorists by treating emotion as a continuously unfolding process of assessing the significance of a stimulus to one's current goals, wants, and needs (Barrett, Ochsner, & Gross, 2007; Scherer, Schorr, & Johnstone, 2001). This appraisal process produces a set of behavioral, experiential, and physiological response tendencies appropriate for the eliciting stimulus. Emotional responses are relatively transitory and tied to a specific elicitor, in contrast to moods, which are objectless and enduring (Barrett et al., 2007; Gross, 1998a, 1998b). On this view, affect denotes a superordinate category that encompasses emotion and moods and includes any valenced response to a stimulus.

Against this backdrop, emotion regulation can be seen as any explicit or implicit process that alters which emotions an individual feels, how long they feel them, and how they express them (Gross, 1998b; Ochsner & Gross, 2005). In general, there are two classes of emotion regulation strategies. Behavioral strategies involve acting to avoid exposure to an emotion-eliciting stimulus, changing the nature of the emotion-eliciting stimulus to which one is exposed, or controlling the behavioral expression of the emotion (e.g., suppression). By contrast, cognitive strategies modify the way in which one attends to and represents the meaning of the emotional event. Each of these strategies may be used to down-regulate or up-regulate emotion, depending on one's goal.

The remainder of this chapter focuses on cognitive strategies for controlling emotion in general and on one strategy in particular, known as reappraisal (i.e., reinterpreting the meaning of a stimulus in ways that alter its emotional impact) for two reasons. First, the bulk of human neuroscience research on emotion regulation has been devoted to studying reappraisal (Ochsner & Gross, 2008). Second, behavioral work has shown that reappraisal is highly effective for enhancing positive and reducing negative emotion and promoting interpersonal relationships (Gross, 1998a; Gross & John, 2003), thus pointing to its importance as a healthy strategy to promote in psychopathology research. What's more, it does so without the negative consequences associated with some strategies, such as suppression. Relative to reappraisal, suppression impairs memory and increases physiological responding (Gross, 1998a; Richards & Gross, 2000).

A Neural Model of the Cognitive Control of Emotion

By and large, our knowledge of the neural bases of emotion and its regulation comes from human functional neuroimaging studies. In this section, we draw on this literature to build a working model of how the brain implements the appraisal processes that give rise to emotions and the cognitive control processes that enable us to regulate them. Before doing so, however, it may be useful to quickly review the two neuroimaging modalities that serve as the basis of our literature review: functional magnetic resonance imaging (fMRI) and positron emission tomography (PET).

PET and fMRI: Strengths and Weaknesses

The great advantage of both PET and fMRI is that they allow brain function to be assessed in awake, behaving participants who may or may not have some sort of clinical disorder. Both methods have limitations that should be noted, however. fMRI provides excellent spatial resolution and relatively good temporal resolution for structural and functional brain imaging, but it does not directly measure neuronal activity. Rather, fMRI measures the blood oxygen level–dependent (BOLD) response, which corresponds to the ratio of oxygenated to deoxygenated hemoglobin across multiple areas of the brain, a ratio thought to indirectly reflect the local field potential of neurons in a given region (Wager, Hernandez, Jonides, & Lindquist, 2007). One major drawback of fMRI is that, because it is sensitive to magnetic properties of the blood, noise can be introduced into its measurement by any factors that generate or alter magnetic fields, including pockets of air, as found in our sinus cavities, and fluids, as found in the ventricles and large draining veins. This means that imaging some regions critical for emotion, like the amygdala, can be difficult because they lie close to the bottom of the brain at the anterior tips of the temporal lobes, adjacent to the anterior tips of the lateral ventricles, not far from large arteries and veins in the brainstem and just behind some sinuses cavities. By contrast, PET provides a direct measurement of glucose metabolism and is not subject to magnetic susceptibility artifacts as is fMRI. The major drawbacks of PET are that it involves ionizing radiation exposure (Grubb, Raichle, Higgins, & Eichling, 1978) and has comparatively lower spatial and temporal resolution relative to fMRI (Wager et al., 2007). Whereas typical fMRI can be sensitive to changes occurring as fast as every second, PET studies average activity across time windows of 60 seconds or more.

Experimental design in fMRI and PET commonly involves the subtraction method (Posner, Petersen, Fox, & Raichle, 1988), wherein activity corresponding to the performance of a control task or behavioral state is essentially subtracted from activity corresponding to a critical task state. The result is a difference map reflecting the neural processes selectively activated during the performance of the task. Causality remains unclear, however, in such analyses because the resulting map of brain activation is only *correlated* with one task state or another. Still, many neuroimaging studies use this logic to draw inferences about differential neural systems involved in the performance of different behavioral tasks. As described later, the strength of correlations between individual differences in brain activation over a particular neural region of interest and individual differences in a behavioral measure can provide additional information about brain systems critically involved in task performance.

Neural Bases of Emotional Appraisal and Reappraisal

Although numerous studies have investigated the brain systems involved in emotional learning and response, our working model primarily derives from studies that have directly compared neural systems involved in emotion appraisal and regulation in the same paradigm. Such experiments simultaneously provide insights into the mechanisms of emotion generation and regulation. Because of space limitations, this sketch is brief, and interested readers are directed to more detailed discussions of it elsewhere (Ochsner & Gross, 2005, 2007).

Neural Bases of Emotional Appraisal

Our working model specifies roles in emotional appraisal for several brain structures that have consistently been shown to be activated during the perception of emotional stimuli and modulated during reappraisal of responses to them. We collectively refer to these brain regions as the neural bases of emotional appraisal: the amygdala, the insula, the striatum, and the medial orbitofrontal cortex. These regions are illustrated in Figure 3.1. Although this model does not include every neural region relevant to emotional appraisal, it does include the principal components based on the current literature. Critically, all components of this model were shown to be consistently activated in a comprehensive meta-analysis of 162 neuroimaging studies that examined the functional grouping of brain regions involved in emotion regardless of the specific type of emotion (e.g., fear or anger) included in each of the studies (Kober et al., 2008).

AMYGDALA

The amygdala is a pair of bilateral almond-shaped structures containing multiple nuclei located in the tip of the temporal lobe. Rodent and other small-mammal studies have noted that the lateral nucleus of the amygdala exhibits marked plasticity during the acquisition of fear conditioning; the firing rate of lateral amygdala neurons has been shown to dramatically

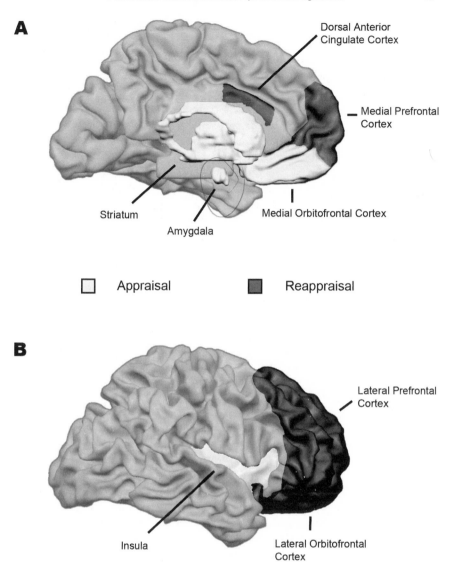

FIGURE 3.1. Overview of the working model for the functional architecture of appraisal and reappraisal. (A) Medial view of the brain showing the amygdala, striatum, and medial orbitofrontal cortex, all related to emotional appraisal. Also shown are the dorsal anterior cingulate cortex and the medial prefrontal cortex, which are important for reappraisal. (B) Lateral view of the brain showing the insula, involved in emotional appraisal, and the lateral prefrontal cortex and lateral orbitofrontal cortex, involved in reappraisal. (Color figure is available at *www.guilford.com.*)

increase during that time (Quirk, Repa, & LeDoux, 1995). However, the basolateral complex of the amygdala (consisting of the basal and lateral nuclei) has been shown to be critical for the expression of conditioned fear (Maren, Aharonov, & Fanselow, 1996). A substantial human neuroimaging literature points toward the amygdala's importance in emotional appraisal as well. In parallel with the rodent evidence, many studies have found associations between amygdala activity and the detection of rapidly (even subliminally) presented stimuli that connote the presence of potential threats, like facial expressions of fear and anger and images of threatening situations (Hariri, Tessitore, Mattay, Fera, & Weinberger, 2002; Whalen et al., 1998). Importantly, several studies have reported decreased amygdala activity during down-regulation of negative emotion via reappraisal (Goldin, McRae, Ramel, & Gross, 2008; Ochsner, Bunge, Gross, & Gabrieli, 2002; Ochsner, Ray, et al., 2004; Phan et al., 2005; van Reekum et al., 2007).

It should be noted that amygdala activation is not solely associated with fear, or even negative emotion. Indeed, several neuroimaging studies have implicated the amygdala in the appraisal of positively valenced stimuli such as sexual images, appealing animals, and appetizing food as well as high-interest, unusual images (e.g., surrealistic images) (Hamann, Ely, Hoffman, & Kilts, 2002). Furthermore, amygdala activation has been shown to not differ in processing positive and negative pictures (Garavan, Pendergrass, Ross, Stein, & Risinger, 2001). Thus, the amygdala is theorized to broadly detect whether a stimulus is emotionally salient in our working model.

INSULA

Based on its connectivity, the insula has been characterized as many things, including a visceral sensory area, a somatosensory area, a motor association area, a language area, and a "limbic" integration cortex, among others (Augustine, 1996). All of this suggests that functional neuroimaging evidence should support a role for the insula in emotional appraisal, which likely draws on all these modalities of information to assess the affective significance of a stimulus. Indeed, studies have implicated the anterior portion of the insula in particular in response to, and likely in the aversive experience of, various kinds of aversive stimuli, although lesion studies suggest it may play a special role in the perception and experience of disgust, perhaps because it receives ascending information from the viscera (Damasio et al., 2000; Lévesque et al., 2003; Phillips et al., 1997; Wager & Barrett, 2004; Wager et al., 2008; Wicker et al., 2003). Like the amygdala, the insula has shown diminished activity during the down-regulation of negative emotion via reappraisal in several studies (Goldin et al., 2008; Ochsner et al., 2002; Ochsner, Ray, et al., 2004; Phan et al., 2005).

STRIATUM

Two subcortical regions, the caudate and the putatmen, are referred to collectively as "the striatum." Both the dorsal and ventral striatum have been shown to be involved in human reward processing (O'Doherty et al., 2004). In particular, the dorsal striatum has been linked to processing reward outcomes (Delgado, Locke, Stenger, & Fiez, 2003; O'Doherty et al., 2004), while the ventral striatum, and particularly the nucleus accumbens, has been linked to processing the anticipation of reward (Knutson, Adams, Fong, & Hommer, 2001).

Furthermore, nearly 70% of neuroimaging studies involving happiness induction have reported activation in the basal ganglia, which includes the striatum, according to a meta-analysis (Phan, Wager, Taylor, & Liberzon, 2002). The striatum is not simply a "reward organ," however, and may play a more general role in mediating habitual responses (Fernandez-Ruiz, Wang, Aigner, & Mishkin, 2001). Thus, any stimulus that is relevant to learning or expressing meaningful sequences of thoughts or actions may activate the striatum, including nonrewarding but unexpected salient stimuli (Zink, Pagnoni, Martin, Dhamala, & Berns, 2003) and facial expressions of disgust (Phillips et al., 2004; Sprengelmeyer, Rausch, Eysel, & Przuntek, 1998). Striatal activity in the nucleus accumbens has been shown to be diminished during down-regulation of negative emotion via reappraisal (Phan et al., 2005). However, other researchers have shown that the dorsal striatum is engaged during reappraisal (Ochsner, Ray, et al., 2004; van Reekum et al., 2007), which could reflect either learning to regulate more effectively or the generation of positive responses to a stimulus during down-regulation of negative emotion, or both. Thus, the striatum is clearly involved in emotional appraisal, although its precise involvement in reappraisal is not clear.

MEDIAL ORBITOFRONTAL CORTEX

Brain imaging studies have implicated the medial OFC (MOFC), which has interconnections with all of the appraisal-related structures mentioned previously, in maintaining representations of the affective value of a stimulus, such as a rewarding rather than punishing monetary outcome (O'Doherty, Kringelbach, Rolls, Hornak, & Andrews, 2001) or an attractive face (O'Doherty et al., 2003), in the context of one's current goals. This means that MOFC will rapidly change its response to a stimulus that once was rewarding but now is not (Rolls, 2000). In the domain of reappraisal, attending to a negative stimulus rather than reappraising it has also been associated with activation in the MOFC (Ochsner et al., 2002). Notably, Ochsner, Ray, and colleagues (2004), in a replication and extension of Ochsner and colleagues' (2002) study, did not observe modulation of MOFC activity by reappraisal, although the authors note that this may have been due to greater instruction to attend to one's feelings in the initial study relative to an instruction to simply respond naturally in the latter study. As such, context is thought to play a large role in determining whether MOFC activation is observed during emotional appraisal.

Neural Bases of Reappraisal

Several brain structures have been implicated consistently in reappraisal studies: the lateral prefrontal cortex (LPFC), the medial PFC (MPFC), the dorsal anterior cingulate cortex (dACC), and the lateral OFC (LOFC) (see Figure 3.1). The common thread connecting these brain regions during reappraisal is likely the need to create and maintain a regulatory strategy, to integrate newly constructed top-down interpretations of stimuli and continuing bottom-up appraisals of those stimuli, and to reinterpret the meaning of internal states relevant to the stimuli being reappraised (Ochsner & Gross, 2004).

LATERAL PREFRONTAL CORTEX

Evidence from neuropsychological patients and from functional neuroimaging suggests that the dorsolateral PFC (DLPFC) is important for maintaining and manipulating information in working memory, including during reasoning and problem solving (Barcelo & Knight, 2002; Callicott et al., 1999). Especially relevant to reappraisal, which involves selecting appropriate reinterpretations of stimuli, are portions of the ventrolateral PFC (VLPFC) that have been associated specifically with selecting among competing representations of task-appropriate knowledge (Badre, Poldrack, Pare-Blagoev, Insler, & Wagner, 2005).

The lateral PFC has been consistently activated in reappraisal paradigms, potentially reflecting increased knowledge selection. Studies have implicated both the DLPFC and VLPFC during down-regulation of negative emotion via reappraisal (Goldin et al., 2008; Ochsner et al., 2002; Ochsner, Ray, et al., 2004; Phan et al., 2005). Furthermore, Ochsner, Ray, and colleagues (2004) have also reported DLPFC and VLPFC activity during up-regulation of negative emotion, strengthening its proposed role as a component of the reappraisal system.

MEDIAL PREFRONTAL CORTEX

The MPFC has been strongly implicated in making judgments about internal mental states rather than externally generated information (Lieberman, 2007; Ochsner, Knierim, et al., 2004). In addition, the MPFC has been shown to be particularly active when making self-referential judgments (Kelley et al., 2002; Ochsner, Knierim, et al., 2004) and self-focused

(rather than situation-focused) reappraisals when down-regulating negative emotion (Ochsner, Ray, et al., 2004). It has been suggested that MPFC
varies along its dorsal to ventral and caudal to rostral extents in terms of
the explicitness with which it represents affective and mental state information. On this view, increasingly rostral and dorsal portions process increasingly explicit representations about mental states (Amodio & Frith, 2006;
Gallagher & Frith, 2003; Olsson & Ochsner, 2008).

MPFC, including dorsal MPFC, has also been associated with both the
down- and up-regulation of emotion as well as selective attention to emotional states (Goldin et al., 2008; Ochsner et al., 2002; Ochsner, Hughes,
Robertson, Cooper, & Gabrieli, in press; Ochsner, Ray, et al., 2004; Phan
et al., 2005; van Reekum et al., 2007). Collectively, these studies support
a role for MPFC in generating and maintaining reappraisals in a manner
that may often involve self-reflection.

DORSAL ANTERIOR CINGULATE CORTEX

Although early reports suggested that dACC activity is more associated
with the performance of cognitive rather than emotional tasks (Bush, Luu,
& Posner, 2000), it is now clear that it is involved in monitoring conflicts
between competing responses regardless of whether they are cognitive or
affective (Botvinick, Nystrom, Fissell, Carter, & Cohen, 1999; Ochsner et
al., in press). This makes sense, given that dACC activity correlates with
self-reported affective states that likely involve conflict, such as the social
distress (Eisenberger, Lieberman, & Williams, 2003) elicited by rejection.

Conflict monitoring may be the essence of dACC activation during
reappraisal as well. dACC activity has been associated with both the down-
regulation (Ochsner, Ray, et al., 2004; Phan et al., 2005) and up-regulation
(Ochsner, Ray, et al., 2004) of negative emotion in reappraisal studies.
Activity in the dACC has also been shown to positively correlate with
reappraisal success (Ochsner et al., 2002) and to vary inversely with self-
reported intensity of negative emotion (Phan et al., 2005). These results
suggest that dACC may monitor conflict flexibly in the service of a specific
regulatory goal (if one is so instructed).

LATERAL ORBITOFRONTAL CORTEX

Prior research supports a role for OFC in flexibly selecting context-
appropriate behaviors and emotions, with LOFC showing activation, for
example, when a previously rewarded value has to be suppressed (Elliott,
Dolan, & Frith, 2000). Both structurally and functionally, LOFC is similar
to VLPFC. Several studies have implicated LOFC in down-regulating negative emotion (Goldin et al., 2008; Lévesque et al., 2003; Ochsner, Ray, et
al., 2004; Phan et al., 2005). In particular, Lévesque and colleagues (2003)
report a positive correlation between self-reported sadness and activation

of the right LOFC during emotion regulation, lending support to the idea that LOFC is important for guiding reappraisal.

Impact of Individual Differences on the Working Model

Careful study of individual differences in healthy populations may serve several purposes, particularly in the domain of emotion regulation. First, understanding stable individual differences may allow for a greater degree of experimental control that reduces noise in psychological and neuroscientific studies of emotion and emotion regulation. Second, increased investigations into basic connections between individual differences and emotional reactivity and regulation may increase opportunities for translational clinical research. This may both improve screening for individuals who may be at increased risk of developing psychopathology and help clarify connections between typical and atypical variation.

Because of space limitations and the fact that individual differences in the neural bases of emotion have been reviewed extensively elsewhere (Hamann & Canli, 2004), by way of illustration, we first briefly review two interrelated examples related to individual differences in amygdala activity. The first example concerns individual differences in trait rumination, which reflects a tendency to focus on negative emotions and negative aspects of the self (Nolen-Hoeksema, 2000). Ray and colleagues (2005) reported that greater trait rumination was correlated with greater recruitment of the amygdala when participants were asked to up-regulate their negative emotion via reappraisal and when participants were simply asked to view a negative stimulus. This suggests that the tendency to ruminate, which involves turning an event over and over again in one's mind, may depend on some of the same cognitive control systems as does reappraisal. Furthermore, it suggests that the tendency to ruminate "tunes" these systems so that they are able to more effectively down- or up-regulate the amygdala, depending on the reappraisal goal (Ray et al., 2005). These data importantly suggest that ruminators have the ability to effectively reappraise, but they may not know when to do so, or how. The second example concerns stable, trait-related individual differences in negative affect, which have been shown to be positively correlated with amygdala activation to negative pictures when participants were instructed to maintain their emotional response rather than passively view the picture (Schaefer et al., 2002). These data suggest that another factor—the tendency to experience negative affect in general—may in part be attributable to the ability to maintain activation of the amygdala during a negative event.

Another angle on individual differences is provided by the emerging field of imaging genetics, which offers insight into what lower level mechanisms might underlie differences in amygdala reactivity. Several researchers have reported an association between amygdala reactivity and a polymorphism in the human serotonin transporter gene (Munafo, Brown, & Hariri, 2008). The short allele of the serotonin transporter gene-linked polymorphic region (*5-HTTLPR*) has been associated with increased amygdala reactivity in response to fearful and angry faces (Hariri et al., 2005) and with increased diagnosable depression in response to stressful life events in a longitudinal study of a large, representative birth cohort (Caspi et al., 2003). The work reviewed in the prior paragraph suggests that these polymorphisms should also be related to the typical range of differences in factors that predispose healthy individuals to depression, such as rumination or trait negative affect. Although such relationships have yet to be examined, it is clear that genetic studies have the potential to further our understanding of how genes and environment interact to produce variance in clinical and nonclinical behavioral phenotypes.

Application of the Working Model to Psychopathology

Because characterizations of *dysfunctional* emotion regulation are only as good as the assumptions of *functional* (i.e., adaptive and effective) emotion regulation from which they are derived (Ochsner, 2008), until this point we have delayed an in-depth discussion of psychopathology. In this final section, we use our working model for the neural bases of typical emotion regulation to examine neuroimaging findings in clinical populations. In doing so, we offer broad hypotheses about brain-based abnormalities that contribute to emotional dysregulation across clinical disorders and also discuss current and future disorder-specific research endeavors. In the present review, we primarily focus on schizophrenia, bipolar disorder (BD), major depressive disorder (MDD), and anxiety disorders (AD), including posttraumatic stress disorder (PTSD). Our decision to include these four disorders was based on their prevalence in the general population, their relevance to emotional appraisal and reappraisal, and also their coverage in the neuroimaging literature.

Functional Neuroimaging in Clinical Populations

Although this section focuses primarily on functional brain differences associated with clinical disorders, it is important to acknowledge two additional factors that might influence both behavior and the results of brain imaging studies.

Implications of Brain Structure

The first factor is structural brain changes that are found in many psychopathological populations. For example, one study found that people with schizophrenia who were also violent exhibited reductions in whole brain volume (Barkataki, Kumari, Das, Taylor, & Sharma, 2006), while others showed localized abnormalities in regions associated with emotion generation and regulation. In like fashion, decreased amygdala volumes are seen in BD (Rosso et al., 2007), PTSD (Karl et al., 2006), unmedicated MDD (Hamilton, Siemer, & Gotlib, 2008), and AD (Milham et al., 2005). Diminished volumes are also noted in regions associated with emotion regulation, such as ventral and lateral portions of the PFC in BD (Adler, Levine, DelBello, & Strakowski, 2005; Lyoo et al., 2004) and the OFC and PFC in MDD (Bremner, 2005). Although the intricacies of structure–function relationships are still being worked out, for present purposes, when interpreting functional brain data, we assume that to the degree structural abnormalities exist there will be functional impairment, but that when functional abnormalities exist they may or may not arise from structural changes.

Medication and Neuroimaging

In recent years, BOLD fMRI has become an increasingly popular tool for investigating brain activity in psychopathological populations. Implicit in this work is the assumption that the BOLD signal is a reliable and constant indicator of brain activity. Although it is unclear how or whether psychotropic medications modulate the BOLD signal, other chemical agents ranging from caffeine (Laurienti et al., 2002) to opioids (Leppa et al., 2006) significantly affect BOLD responses. Additionally, common psychiatric medications like lithium (Foland et al., 2008) and neuroleptics (Lieberman et al., 2005) may alter brain morphology. Again, it is important to consider these findings when interpreting results among psychiatric patients who vary in their current or historical medication usage. Our incomplete understanding of medications' effects on neuroimaging data leads us to acknowledge that medications may impact findings, although it remains unclear the extent to which or how medications may do so.

Hypotheses and Research Questions

Earlier in this chapter, we outlined a model rooted in the reappraisal literature wherein one class of brain structures was described as sources of emotion regulatory processes (LPFC, MPFC, dACC, LOFC) and another class as appraisal regions that are targeted by those processes (amygdala, insula, striatum, MOFC). In this model, rises in emotion are correlated with enhanced activity in appraisal structures (e.g., amygdala), while the attenuation of emotion is associated with reduced activity in these structures coupled with increased activity in reappraisal structures (e.g., LPFC). Thus, by comparing patterns of hypo- and hyperactivations within and between appraisal and reappraisal systems in healthy and clinical populations, we can draw inferences about the mechanisms that might mediate dysfunction in those disorders.

By way of illustration, suppose that individuals with MDD exhibit amygdala hyperactivity during anticipation of an aversive stimulus but hypoactive ventral striatal activity during a reward-learning paradigm. Such results would suggest that individuals with MDD perhaps too readily form predictions and appraisals about negative stimuli but underrespond to positive stimuli. Now consider a scenario where both appraisal and reappraisal regions are involved. For example, if PTSD were associated with excessive amygdala activity but typical dACC responses to traumatic images, this suggests that dysfunction during appraisal rather than reappraisal contributes to abnormal emotional responses associated with the disorder. If aberrant responses were seen in both sets of brain regions (as, in fact, is the case in PTSD; Etkin & Wager, 2007), however, we might infer that enhanced activity in the amygdala was supporting a heightened tendency to perceive threat and that hypoactivity in the dACC was indicative of a reduced capacity to monitor unwanted emotional states during reappraisal.

When interpreting neuroimaging data on emotion generation and regulation in psychopathology, two additional issues should be noted. First, patients can show a range of responses to different kinds of "emotional" stimuli, with patterns of abnormal appraisal reflecting either stimulus-specific or stimulus-generic patterns of dysfunction (e.g., a person with spider phobia may respond abnormally only to spider images but not to other aversive images). Thus, it is critical to consider the "fit" of a stimulus with a given disorder. Second, in the absence of an instructed regulation condition, it is impossible to know whether any given emotional response was "unregulated" or whether participants spontaneously regulated it in idiosyncratic ways. This means that results associated with "free viewing" or uninstructed response paradigms are fundamentally ambiguous. This may be particularly relevant if there are specific regulation strategies that some clinical groups tend to use spontaneously that differ from those of healthy populations (e.g., if individuals with MDD tend to self-distract and healthy controls do not). That said, we now move forward to a review of current perspectives on the neural mechanisms of emotion regulation in various clinical disorders.

Schizophrenia

In the emotional domain, schizophrenia is characterized by reduced emotional expressivity (Kring & Moran, 2008) and an impaired ability to perceive emotions in others (Kohler & Martin, 2006). Despite these impairments in emotional expression and perception, it has been strongly suggested that individuals with schizophrenia experience typical to excessive amounts of emotion (Kring & Moran, 2008; Myin-Germeys, Delespaul, & deVries, 2000), albeit in ways that qualitatively differ from healthy controls (Cohen & Minor, in press). These affective abnormalities bring into question whether individuals with schizophrenia falter in their appraisals of emotionally evocative stimuli, their regulation of these appraisals, or both. In support of the impaired appraisal possibility, individuals with schizophrenia show reduced striatal activity compared with healthy controls in response to cues signifying potential reward (Juckel et al., 2006). Hypoactivity in the ventral striatum could underlie improper appraisals of positive stimuli and anhedonia, but it could also mean that individuals with schizophrenia fail to *anticipate* enjoying a reward but do not necessarily fail to find a reward pleasurable upon receipt (Gard, Kring, Gard, Horan, & Green, 2007). Diminished amygdala responses to negative stimuli (e.g., sad faces, aversive scenes) have also been observed in individuals with schizophrenia (Takahashi et al., 2004; Williams et al., 2004), as has reduced anterior insula activity in response to disgusted faces (Phillips et al., 1999). Thus, observations of reduced activity across appraisal regions in the brain have been associated with a failure to properly perceive, learn, and respond to positive and negative emotional stimuli in schizophrenia. Future studies may wish to investigate, however, whether such hypoactivity occurs in tasks that do not involve emotion perception (e.g., emotion induction).

Cognitive control deficits shown by individuals with schizophrenia appear linked to abnormal brain activity in regions associated with generating and maintaining reappraisals, such as the dACC, MPFC, and DLPFC (Kerns, Nuechterlein, Braver, & Barch, 2008). Interestingly, individuals with schizophrenia exhibit abnormal correlations in activity between the amygdala and the ACC/MPFC when viewing emotional faces (Das et al., 2007), which suggests dysfunctional dynamics between sources and targets of emotion regulation typically observed in reappraisal paradigms. One recent study found that individuals with schizophrenia recruit the DLPFC more strongly than controls and do not deactivate emotion generation circuitry when classifying affective stimuli in the presence of incongruent affective distracters (Park, Park, Chun, Kim, & Kim, 2008). These results were interpreted as evidence for individuals with schizophrenia exerting more cognitive effort (DLPFC hyperactivation), yet, according to behavioral results, failing to inhibit responses to task-irrelevant affective information. To date, no functional imaging studies have examined effortful emotion regulation in schizophrenia. Individuals with schizophrenia report utilizing reappraisal and suppression to regulate their emotions (Henry, Rendell, Green, McDonald, & O'Donnell, 2008), however, and a recent behavioral study found them capable of down-regulating emotional responses to amusing film clips (notably, patients failed to amplify their responses) (Henry et al., 2007). Whether individuals with schizophrenia could effectively down-regulate negative emotional responses and whether abnormal PFC activity would be observed during such regulation has yet to be explored.

Bipolar Disorder

BD is an affective disorder characterized by at least one lifetime episode of mania. Most people with BD also experience episodes of depression. Both mania and depression include symptoms of severe emotional dysregulation. With respect to the appraisal versus reappraisal equation, most of our knowledge about the neural bases of emotion regulation in BD comes from studies examining perception of emotional faces. Although faces do not elicit strong emotional responses, it is generally believed that the basic processes involved in deciding facial emotion are similar to those involved in appraising other emotional stimuli. That being said, studies of emotion perception generally suggest that individuals with BD exhibit broad impairments in appraisal processes. For example, BD is associated with deficits (e.g., slower RTs and reduced accuracy) in identifying (Malhi et al., 2007; Yurgelun-Todd et al., 2000) and recalling (Dickstein et al., 2007) emotional faces, and these tendencies may be associated with their degree of social-emotional dysfunction. Strikingly, these behavioral deficits are not accompanied by diminished activity in brain systems associated with appraisal but greater activity in them: When viewing emotional faces, individuals with BD exhibit exaggerated activity in structures typically associated with emotional identification and learning like the amygdala and striatum (Lawrence et al., 2004; Yurgelun-Todd et al., 2000).

At present, the meaning of this relative hyperactivity is not yet clear, and there are at least two questions about what it might reflect. The first is whether the hyperactivity observed is compensatory or reflects a general dysfunction of appraisal systems. In favor of compensation, it has been shown that individuals with BD show impaired overall memory for emotional faces but are more likely to recall faces that evoked relatively hyperactive dorsal striatal responses during encoding (Dickstein et al., 2007). This suggests that hyperactivity in appraisal areas may reflect attempts to compensate for overall poor performance in tasks involving emotion detection and memory by enhancing processing of, and thereby activation to, specific subsets of stimuli. In favor of general dysfunction, however, is the fact that people with BD, whether depressed or manic, exhibit elevated ventral striatum activity not just to negative emotional faces (Chen et al., 2006) but also at rest and in nonemotional attention tasks as well (Keener & Phillips, 2007).

The second question is whether heightened responses in appraisal systems relate to the cyclical shift between episodes of mania and depression that tend to recur across the lifespan for individuals with BD. Current data suggest that such variation does exist and that how it varies depends on the valence of the emotional stimulus. On one hand, individuals with BD who are currently depressed consistently show enhanced striatal and amygdala responses to positive and negative stimuli across tasks that demand differential levels of attention or cognitive processes (Chen et al., 2006; Lawrence et al., 2004; Malhi et al., 2004). On the other hand, those in the manic phase of BD show *diminished* striatal and amygdala responses to positive stimuli (Chen et al., 2006; Malhi et al., 2004) and variable amygdala responses to negative emotional stimuli. In paradigms that require individuals with mania to cognitively label a negative emotional expression or evaluate its intensity, participants often show attenuated amygdala responses (Chen et al., 2006; Lennox, Jacob, Calder, Lupson, & Bullmore, 2004), whereas those that present emotional stimuli in a task-irrelevant way or that ask participants to perform a task that does not directly relate to a stimulus's affective content (e.g., color discrimination) tend to report enhanced amgydala and insular responses (Chen et al., 2006; Elliott et al., 2004).

Taken together, these data are interesting in two respects. First, they suggest a relationship between MDD (see later discussion) and the different phases of BD: Individuals in the manic phase of BD show neural responses to positive stimuli similar to those exhibited by individuals with MDD, whereas individuals in the depressed phase of BD show responses to negative stimuli like those exhibited by individuals with MDD. This pattern could potentially be used to develop more accurate means for differentiating unipolar and bipolar depression (Keener & Phillips, 2007). Second, these data suggest that during the manic phase of BD the response of appraisal systems is more subject to cognitive modulation than it is during the depressed phase. This conclusion is limited, however, by the fact that only attentional deployment paradigms have been used to test this hypothesis.

Although no studies have directly examined reappraisal in BD, abnormal neural responses have been observed in brain regions that support reappraisal during various emotion and cognitive control tasks. For example, a number of emotion perception studies have reported individuals with BD exhibiting abnormal activity in the LPFC, MPFC, and the ACC in response to emotionally expressive faces (Chen et al., 2006; Lawrence et al., 2004). Additionally, patterns of hyperactivation across the PFC have been observed in executive function tasks in BD (Brambilla, Glahn, Balestrieri, & Soares, 2005). A handful of studies have used paradigms where participants must respond to task-relevant stimuli while exerting cognitive control to ignore task-irrelevant stimuli that may contain affective content. Findings from these studies have produced inconsistent results. On the one hand, making nonaffective assessments of affective stimuli has been shown to elicit reduced activity in lateral and medial portions of the PFC associated with regulating emotion (Lagopoulos & Malhi, 2007; Malhi,

Lagopoulos, Sachdev, Ivanovski, & Shnier, 2005) in individuals with BD. On the other hand, inhibiting responses to task-irrelevant or incompatible affective information appears to evoke enhanced activity in the LPFC and MPFC (Elliott et al., 2004) as well as a dACC region that may resolve interference between appraisals and response tendencies (Wessa et al., 2007). Future research in BD may seek to compare neural responses associated with cognitive change strategies like reappraisal to those evoked by the attentional deployment paradigms described previously. Such endeavors would clarify whether BD is marked by dysfunction in appraisal, reappraisal, or both.

Major Depressive Disorder

MDD is characterized by prolonged dysphoric mood as well as disrupted motivation, thought, and behavior. Whether tendencies among individuals with MDD to attend and respond to the negative is due to a bottom-up enhancement of negative stimuli or an impaired top-down regulatory ability is uncertain because few studies have been designed to tease apart these processes.

For example, it has been shown that individuals with MDD (1) exhibit abnormal cerebral blood flow and glucose metabolism in the amygdala, insula, striatum, and OFC as well as in the LPFC and MPFC during uninstructed "resting" conditions (Drevets, 2000); (2) show overall diminished neural activity to happy faces (Lawrence et al., 2004; Surguladze et al., 2005); (3) show enhanced striatal and amygdala responses to sad faces (Elliott et al., 2004; Surguladze et al., 2005); and (4) show sustained amygdala reactivity to emotional words (Siegle, Thompson, Carter, Steinhauer, & Thase, 2007). Although these findings suggest that negative affective information is preferentially detected and processed over positive affective information in subcortical appraisal regions in MDD, whether these observations reflect differences in reactivity or regulation is not clear. Also unclear is how amygdala reactivity to negative emotional stimuli relates to well-being; although some studies have found responsivity to positively correlate with symptom severity (Lee et al., 2007), others suggest it predicts better longitudinal outcomes (Canli et al., 2005).

Abnormal activity (particularly a lack of left lateralized activity) in the DLPFC, a brain region associated with the control processes supporting reappraisal, has also been linked to emotion dysregulation in MDD. On one hand, when healthy controls make valence judgments about emotional stimuli, they show a rise in activity in the left DLPFC that corresponds to how negative they perceive stimuli to be (Grimm et al., 2008). On the other hand, individuals with MDD exhibit hypoactivity in the left DLPFC that correlates *positively* with stimuli valence as well as hyperactivity in the right DLPFC that is associated with depression symptoms. These findings suggest that an absence of left lateralized PFC activity and the presence of right LPFC hyperactivity in response to negative emotional stimuli in MDD may be linked to inappropriate responding, ineffective spontaneous emotion regulation, or both.

At present, only two studies have examined the neural mechanisms of cognitive reappraisal in MDD. In one of these studies, healthy controls were found to only activate the left LPFC during down-regulation of negative emotion, while individuals with MDD activated bilateral LPFC (Johnstone, van Reekum, Urry, Kalin, & Davidson, 2007). This pattern of right LPFC activity during instructed regulation mirrors what was found previously during an emotion judgment task. Results from another study suggest that individuals with MDD also differ from healthy controls in that efforts to down-regulate their emotions seem to enhance, rather than diminish, amygdala and insula activity (Beauregard, Paquette, & Lévesque, 2006). This may be because left LPFC activity attenuates amygdala activity via the ventral MPFC during reappraisal in healthy controls, but in MDD this mediating effect is absent and instead the amygdala and ventral MPFC are coactivated (Johnstone et al., 2007). According to results from the Beauregard study, this activity in the amygdala and MPFC is strongly associated with the degree of difficulty experienced during down-regulation for individuals with MDD. This could mean that individuals with MDD are less successful at regulating and thus exhibit enhanced activity in areas associated with emotion perception and self-reflection. Alternatively, participants with MDD could show overall enhanced neural activity as a result of compensatory attempts at down-regulation. Future attempts to characterize voluntary emotion regulation in MDD may be enhanced by collecting in-scanner affect ratings. Doing so would build bridges between behavioral and neural responses associated with voluntary emotion regulation in MDD and would also give greater insight into whether individuals with MDD differ from healthy controls in their effectiveness at using reappraisal. MDD researchers may additionally wish to clarify how baseline reactivity to negative emotional stimuli may predict treatment outcome and how treatment might modify neural responses in voluntary emotion regulation paradigms.

Anxiety Disorders

Anxiety, as a state, may be described as agitation or arousal caused by the perception of a real or imagined threat (Amstadter, 2008). In AD, this anxious state is chronically activated by specific (e.g., social anxiety disorder [SAD], specific phobias, and PTSD) or varied (e.g., generalized anxiety disorder [GAD]) triggers. Within the context of our model of emotion regulation, AD may represent an inability to accurately appraise what is threatening, an inability to reappraise threat, or both.

In support of the appraisal possibility, the insula and amygdala consistently hyperactivate in response to negative or threatening stimuli in

SAD and specific phobias and often in PTSD as well (Etkin & Wager, 2007). These hyperactivations have been observed in response to negative emotional facial expressions (Blair et al., 2008; Evans et al., 2008) as well as a speech preparation task (Lorberbaum et al., 2004) in individuals with SAD, to trauma-themed pictures and scripts for PTSD patients (Shin et al., 2004; Whalley, Rugg, Smith, Dolan, & Brewin, 2009), and to photographs of spiders for people with spider phobia (Straube, Mentzel, & Miltner, 2006). GAD is unusual in its lack of specificity for what produces anxious feelings, and it is perhaps for this reason that some neuroimaging studies have not found anxiety or fear-inducing stimuli to activate the amygdala (Blair et al., 2008), whereas others have found it to hyperactivate the amygdala (McClure et al., 2007) in individuals with GAD. In summary, inappropriate threat appraisals in AD appear linked to abnormal activity in structures involved in perceiving, responding to, and remembering fear-inducing stimuli, such as the amygdala and insula (Etkin & Wager, 2007).

In addition to the hyperactivations observed in targets of emotion regulation described previously, a number of functional abnormalities in individuals with AD have been noted in control regions associated with emotion regulation. In contrast to healthy controls, individuals with SAD exhibit enhanced right LOFC activity—associated with the downregulation of negative emotion—in response to angry voices (Quadflieg, Mohr, Mentzel, Miltner, & Straube, 2008). SAD is also associated with enhanced rostral (Amir et al., 2005; Blair et al., 2008) and dorsal (Phan, Fitzgerald, Nathan, & Tancer, 2006) ACC activity during viewing of angry, disgusted, and fearful faces. Such ACC activity may be evidence of enhanced monitoring of negative social cues in SAD. In contrast to other negative facial expressions, fearful faces seem unique in their recruitment of lateral and medial PFC regions among individuals with SAD (Blair et al., 2008). LPFC responses to fearful face stimuli in SAD are strongly correlated with anxiety symptoms and, interestingly, are not observed in GAD, thus suggesting a functional means for differentiating the two disorders (Blair et al., 2008). Individuals with specific phobias exhibit similar hyperactivations in the LOFC (Dilger et al., 2003) as well as dorsal MPFC and dACC (Straube et al., 2006) but not typically in the LPFC when viewing phobia-related stimuli. ACC and dorsal MPFC hyperactivations in people with specific phobias are lessened by a demanding task, whereas amygdala activity is not. This suggests that fast, automatic subcortical appraisals of threat may not be attenuated by distraction but that more deliberative ones generated in the cortex may be (Straube et al., 2006). On this view, PFC hyperactivation may reflect efforts to regulate behavior when perceiving threat or elaborate processing of threatening information. Interestingly, the negative correlation in activity between these frontal regions and amygdala activity that is observed in healthy controls is dampened (Monk et al., 2008) or even positive (McClure et al., 2007) in AD, and positive correlations are linked to poorer treatment outcomes (Whalen et al., 2008).

Unlike those with other AD, individuals with PTSD exhibit hypoactivity in the dACC and ventral MPFC and an *inverse* relationship between the amygdala and MPFC regions (Etkin & Wager, 2007). MPFC hypoactivity has been implicated in reduced emotional awareness (Frewen et al., 2008) and suggests that PTSD pathology extends beyond an exaggerated fear response (Etkin & Wager, 2007).

In healthy adults, using strategies like "reality checking" to regulate state anxiety elicits enhanced activity in the LPFC, MPFC and dACC and diminished activity in the amygdala and insula (Herwig et al., 2007). Self-distraction during the anxious anticipation of shock may evoke tonic activity in the left LPFC (Kalisch, Wiech, Herrmann, & Dolan, 2006). What patterns of activity individuals with AD might elicit during voluntary emotion regulation is unclear, however. Amygdala responses to disorder-specific stimuli occur more quickly than to other types of stimuli (Larson et al., 2006) and persist even when attentional resources are low (Straube et al., 2006). For these reasons, effortful emotion regulation would be unlikely to affect initial appraisals but might successfully shape reappraisals. It would be informative to explore whether strategies like reappraisal attenuate or enhance hyperactivation in regions associated with emotion regulation during exposure to threat for individuals with AD. Knowing this might clarify whether frontal activity observed in paradigms without a regulation instruction are due to efforts at spontaneous regulation, higher level processing of threat stimuli, extended vigilance, or something else entirely.

Conclusions and Future Directions

This chapter has sought to provide an overview of neuroscientific investigations into emotion and emotion regulation, with a particular focus on describing evidence for a working model of the functional architecture of emotion regulation that can be applied to understanding mechanisms of dysfunction in clinical disorders. In so doing, we have focused on describing which neural structures have been shown to be consistently active during cognitive reappraisal in healthy individuals (i.e., LPFC, MPFC, dACC, LOFC), and have noted which neural structures implicated in emotional appraisal are often modulated during reappraisal (i.e., amygdala, insula, striatum, MOFC). In applying this model to understanding psychopathology, we found qualified support for our hypothesis that clinical disorders involve abnormal activation of emotional appraisal systems, abnormal activation of cognitive control mechanisms (e.g., reappraisal mechanisms), or both. This support is tempered by the lack of published data using true reappraisal paradigms in many forms of psychopathology.

Future research may involve investigating how patients compare with healthy controls as well as other clinical groups in reappraisal paradigms. These endeavors might be most fruitful when they involve the concurrent collection of self-reported emotional experience data, psychophysiological responses, and functional and structural brain data. This knowledge of how healthy patterns of brain activation compare with activation in psychopathology, along with increased knowledge of how salient nonclinical individual differences affect brain activation, may increase our ability to screen individuals for psychopathology and predict treatment outcomes while simultaneously furthering our understanding of the neural loci that are most crucial for emotion regulation.

Acknowledgments

We gratefully acknowledge Jochen Weber for assistance with preparation of the figure. Completion of this chapter was supported by Grant No. MH076137 from the National Institutes of Health.

References

Adler, C. M., Levine, A. D., DelBello, M. P., & Strakowski, S. M. (2005). Changes in gray matter volume in patients with bipolar disorder. *Biological Psychiatry, 58*(2), 151–157.

Amir, N., Klumpp, H., Elias, J., Bedwell, J. S., Yanasak, N., & Miller, L. S. (2005). Increased activation of the anterior cingulate cortex during processing of disgust faces in individuals with social phobia. *Biological Psychiatry, 57*(9), 975–981.

Amodio, D. M., & Frith, C. D. (2006). Meeting of minds: The medial prefrontal cortex and social cognition. *Nature Reviews Neuroscience, 7*, 268–277.

Amstadter, A. (2008). Emotion regulation and anxiety disorders. *Journal of Anxiety Disorders, 22*(2), 211–221.

Augustine, J. R. (1996). Circuitry and functional aspects of the insular lobe in primates including humans. *Brain Research Reviews, 22*(3), 229–244.

Badre, D., Poldrack, R. A., Pare-Blagoev, E. J., Insler, R. Z., & Wagner, A. D. (2005). Dissociable controlled retrieval and generalized selection mechanisms in ventrolateral prefrontal cortex. *Neuron, 47*(6), 907–918.

Barcelo, F., & Knight, R. T. (2002). Both random and perseverative errors underlie WCST deficits in prefrontal patients. *Neuropsychologia, 40*(3), 349–356.

Barkataki, I., Kumari, V., Das, M., Taylor, P., & Sharma, T. (2006). Volumetric structural brain abnormalities in men with schizophrenia or antisocial personality disorder. *Behavioural Brain Research, 169*(2), 239–247.

Barrett, L. F., Ochsner, K. N., & Gross, J. J. (2007). Automaticity and emotion. In J. Bargh (Ed.), *Social psychology and the unconscious* (pp. 173–218). New York: Psychology Press.

Beauregard, M., Paquette, V., & Lévesque, J. (2006). Dysfunction in the neural circuitry of emotional self-regulation in major depressive disorder. *NeuroReport, 17*(8), 843–846.

Blair, K., Shaywitz, J., Smith, B. W., Rhodes, R., Geraci, M., Jones, M., et al. (2008). Response to emotional expressions in generalized social phobia and generalized anxiety disorder: Evidence for separate disorders. *American Journal of Psychiatry, 165*(9), 1193–1202.

Botvinick, M., Nystrom, L. E., Fissell, K., Carter, C. S., & Cohen, J. D. (1999). Conflict monitoring versus selection-for-action in anterior cingulate cortex. *Nature, 402,* 179–181.

Brambilla, P., Glahn, D. C., Balestrieri, M., & Soares, J. C. (2005). Magnetic resonance findings in bipolar disorder. *Psychiatric Clinics of North America, 28*(2), 443–467.

Bremner, J. D. (2005). Changes in brain volume in major depression. *Depression: Mind and Body, 2*(2), 38–46.

Bush, G., Luu, P., & Posner, M. I. (2000). Cognitive and emotional influences in anterior cingulate cortex. *Trends in Cognitive Sciences, 4*(6), 215–222.

Callicott, J. H., Mattay, V. S., Bertolino, A., Finn, K., Coppola, R., Frank, J. A., et al. (1999). Physiological characteristics of capacity constraints in working memory as revealed by functional MRI. *Cerebral Cortex, 9*(1), 20–26.

Canli, T., Cooney, R. E., Goldin, P., Shah, M., Sivers, H., Thomason, M. E., et al. (2005). Amygdala reactivity to emotional faces predicts improvement in major depression. *NeuroReport, 16*(12), 1267–1270.

Caspi, A., Sugden, K., Moffitt, T. E., Taylor, A., Craig, I. W., Harrington, H., et al. (2003). Influence of life stress on depression: Moderation by a polymorphism in the 5-HTT gene. *Science, 301,* 386–389.

Chen, C. H., Lennox, B., Jacob, R., Calder, A., Lupson, V., Bisbrown-Chippendale, R., et al. (2006). Explicit and implicit facial affect recognition in manic and depressed states of bipolar disorder: A functional magnetic resonance imaging study. *Biological Psychiatry, 59*(1), 31–39.

Cohen, A. S., & Minor, K. S. (in press). Emotional experience in patients with schizophrenia revisited: Meta-analysis of laboratory studies. *Schizophrenia Bulletin.*

Damasio, A. R., Grabowski, T. J., Bechara, A., Damasio, H., Ponto, L. L., Parvizi, J., et al. (2000). Subcortical and cortical brain activity during the feeling of self-generated emotions. *Nature Neuroscience, 3*(10), 1049–1056.

Das, P., Kemp, A. H., Flynn, G., Harris, A. W., Liddell, B. J., Whitford, T. J., et al. (2007). Functional disconnections in the direct and indirect amygdala pathways for fear processing in schizophrenia. *Schizophrenia Research, 90*(1–3), 284–294.

Delgado, M. R., Locke, H. M., Stenger, V. A., & Fiez, J. A. (2003). Dorsal striatum responses to reward and punishment: Effects of valence and magnitude manipulations. *Cognitive, Affective and Behavioral Neuroscience, 3*(1), 27–38.

Dickstein, D. P., Rich, B. A., Roberson-Nay, R., Berghorst, L., Vinton, D., Pine, D. S., et al. (2007). Neural activation during encoding of emotional faces in pediatric bipolar disorder. *Bipolar Disorders, 9,* 679–692.

Dilger, S., Straube, T., Mentzel, H. J., Fitzek, C., Reichenbach, J. R., Hecht, H., et al. (2003). Brain activation to phobia-related pictures in spider phobic humans: An event-related functional magnetic resonance imaging study. *Neuroscience Letters, 348*(1), 29–32.

Drevets, W. C. (2000). Neuroimaging studies of mood disorders. *Biological Psychiatry, 48*(8), 813–829.

Eisenberger, N. I., Lieberman, M. D., & Williams, K. D. (2003). Does rejection hurt?: An fMRI study of social exclusion. *Science, 302,* 290–292.

Elliott, R., Dolan, R. J., & Frith, C. D. (2000). Dissociable functions in the medial and lateral orbitofrontal cortex: Evidence from human neuroimaging studies. *Cerebral Cortex, 10*(3), 308–317.

Elliott, R., Ogilvie, A., Rubinsztein, J. S., Calderon, G., Dolan, R. J., & Sahakian, B. J. (2004). Abnormal ventral frontal response during performance of an affective go/no go task in patients with mania. *Biological Psychiatry, 55*(12), 1163–1170.

Etkin, A., & Wager, T. D. (2007). Functional neuroimaging of anxiety: A meta-analysis of emotional processing in PTSD, social anxiety disorder, and specific phobia. *American Journal of Psychiatry, 164*(10), 1476–1488.

Evans, K. C., Wright, C. I., Wedig, M. M., Gold, A. L., Pollack, M. H., & Rauch, S. L. (2008). A functional MRI study of amygdala responses to angry schematic faces in social anxiety disorder. *Depression and Anxiety, 25*(6), 496–505.

Fernandez-Ruiz, J., Wang, J., Aigner, T. G., & Mishkin, M. (2001). Visual habit formation in monkeys with neurotoxic lesions of the ventrocaudal neostriatum. *Proceedings of the National Academy of Sciences USA, 98*(7), 4196–4201.

Foland, L. C., Altshuler, L. L., Sugar, C. A., Lee, A. D., Leow, A. D., Townsend, J., et al. (2008). Increased volume of the amygdala and hippocampus in bipolar patients treated with lithium. *NeuroReport, 19*(2), 221–224.

Frewen, P., Lane, R. D., Neufeld, R. W., Densmore, M., Stevens, T., & Lanius, R. (2008). Neural correlates of levels of emotional awareness during trauma script-imagery in posttraumatic stress disorder. *Psychosomatic Medicine, 70*(1), 27–31.

Gallagher, H. L., & Frith, C. D. (2003). Functional imaging of "theory of mind." *Trends in Cognitive Sciences, 7*(2), 77–83.

Garavan, H., Pendergrass, J. C., Ross, T. J., Stein, E. A., & Risinger, R. C. (2001). Amygdala response to both positively and negatively valenced stimuli. *NeuroReport, 12*(12), 2779–2783.

Gard, D. E., Kring, A. M., Gard, M., Horan, W. P., & Green, M. F. (2007). Anhedonia in schizophrenia: Distinctions between anticipatory and consummatory pleasure. *Schizophrenia Research, 93*(1–3), 253–260.

Goldin, P. R., McRae, K., Ramel, W., & Gross, J. J. (2008). The neural bases of emotion regulation: Reappraisal and suppression of negative emotion. *Biological Psychiatry, 63*(6), 577–586.

Grimm, S., Beck, J., Schuepbach, D., Hell, D., Boesiger, P., Bermpohl, F., et al. (2008). Imbalance between left and right dorsolateral prefrontal cortex in major depression is linked to negative emotional judgment: An fMRI study in severe major depressive disorder. *Biological Psychiatry, 63*(4), 369–376.

Gross, J. J. (1998a). Antecedent- and response-focused emotion regulation: Divergent consequences for experience, expression, and physiology. *Journal of Personality and Social Psychology, 74*(1), 224–237.

Gross, J. J. (1998b). The emerging field of emotion regulation: An integrative review. *Review of General Psychology, 2*(3), 271–299.

Gross, J. J., & John, O. P. (2003). Individual differences in two emotion regulation processes: Implications for affect, relationships, and well-being. *Journal of Personality and Social Psychology, 85*(2), 348–362.

Grubb, R. L., Jr., Raichle, M. E., Higgins, C. S., & Eichling, J. O. (1978). Measurement of regional cerebral blood volume by emission tomography. *Annals of Neurology, 4*(4), 322–328.

Hamann, S. B., & Canli, T. (2004). Individual differences in emotion processing. *Current Opinions in Neurobiology, 14*(2), 233–238.

Hamann, S. B., Ely, T. D., Hoffman, J. M., & Kilts, C. D. (2002). Ecstasy and agony: Activation of the human amygdala in positive and negative emotion. *Psychological Science, 13*(2), 135–141.

Hamilton, J. P., Siemer, M., & Gotlib, I. H. (2008). Amygdala volume in major depressive disorder: A meta-analysis of magnetic resonance imaging studies. *Molecular Psychiatry, 13*(11), 993–1000.

Hariri, A. R., Drabant, E. M., Munoz, K. E., Kolachana, B. S., Mattay, V. S., Egan, M. F., et al. (2005). A susceptibility gene for affective disorders and the response of the human amygdala. *Archives of General Psychiatry, 62*(2), 146–152.

Hariri, A. R., Tessitore, A., Mattay, V. S., Fera, F., & Weinberger, D. R. (2002). The amygdala response to emotional stimuli: A comparison of faces and scenes. *NeuroImage, 17*(1), 317–323.

Henry, J. D., Green, M. J., de Lucia, A., Restuccia, C., McDonald, S., & O'Donnell, M. (2007). Emotion dysregulation in schizophrenia: Reduced amplification of emotional expression is associated with emotional blunting. *Schizophrenia Research, 95*(1–3), 197–204.

Henry, J. D., Rendell, P. G., Green, M. J., McDonald, S., & O'Donnell, M. (2008). Emotion regulation in schizophrenia: Affective, social, and clinical correlates of suppression and reappraisal. *Journal of Abnormal Psychology, 117*(2), 473–478.

Herwig, U., Baumgartner, T., Kaffenberger, T., Bruhl, A., Kottlow, M., Schreiter-Gasser, U., et al. (2007). Modulation of anticipatory emotion and perception processing by cognitive control. *NeuroImage, 37*(2), 652–662.

Johnstone, T., van Reekum, C. M., Urry, H. L., Kalin, N. H., & Davidson, R. J. (2007). Failure to regulate: Counterproductive recruitment of top-down prefrontal-subcortical circuitry in major depression. *Journal of Neuroscience, 27*(33), 8877–8884.

Juckel, G., Schlagenhauf, F., Koslowski, M., Wustenberg, T., Villringer, A., Knutson, B., et al. (2006). Dysfunction of ventral striatal reward prediction in schizophrenia. *NeuroImage, 29*(2), 409–416.

Kalisch, R., Wiech, K., Herrmann, K., & Dolan, R. J. (2006). Neural correlates of self-distraction from anxiety and a process model of cognitive emotion regulation. *Journal of Cognitive Neuroscience, 18*(8), 1266–1276.

Karl, A., Schaefer, M., Malta, L. S., Dorfel, D., Rohleder, N., & Werner, A. (2006). A meta-analysis of structural brain abnormalities in PTSD. *Neuroscience and Biobehavioral Reviews, 30*(7), 1004–1031.

Keener, M. T., & Phillips, M. L. (2007). Neuroimaging in bipolar disorder: A critical review of current findings. *Current Psychiatry Reports, 9*(6), 512–520.

Kelley, W. M., Macrae, C. N., Wyland, C. L., Caglar, S., Inati, S., & Heatherton, T. F. (2002). Finding the self?: An event-related fMRI study. *Journal of Cognitive Neuroscience, 14*(5), 785–794.

Kerns, J. G., Nuechterlein, K. H., Braver, T. S., & Barch, D. M. (2008). Executive functioning component mechanisms and schizophrenia. *Biological Psychiatry, 64*(1), 26–33.

Knutson, B., Adams, C. M., Fong, G. W., & Hommer, D. (2001). Anticipation of increasing monetary reward selectively recruits nucleus accumbens. *Journal of Neuroscience, 21*, 1–5.

Kober, H., Barrett, L. F., Joseph, J., Bliss-Moreau, E., Lindquist, K., & Wager, T. D. (2008). Functional grouping and cortical-subcortical interactions in emotion: A meta-analysis of neuroimaging studies. *NeuroImage, 42*(2), 998–1031.

Kohler, C. G., & Martin, E. A. (2006). Emotional processing in schizophrenia. *Cognitive Neuropsychiatry, 11*(3), 250–271.

Kring, A. M., & Moran, E. K. (2008). Emotional response deficits in schizophrenia: Insights from affective science. *Schizophrenia Bulletin, 34*(5), 819–834.

Lagopoulos, J., & Malhi, G. S. (2007). A functional magnetic resonance imaging study of emotional Stroop in euthymic bipolar disorder. *NeuroReport, 18*(15), 1583–1587.

Larson, C. L., Schaefer, H. S., Siegle, G. J., Jackson, C. A., Anderle, M. J., & Davidson, R. J. (2006). Fear is fast in phobic individuals: Amygdala activation in response to fear-relevant stimuli. *Biological Psychiatry, 60*(4), 410–417.

Laurienti, P. J., Field, A. S., Burdette, J. H., Maldjian, J. A., Yen, Y. F., & Moody, D. M. (2002). Dietary caffeine consumption modulates fMRI measures. *NeuroImage, 17*(2), 751–757.

Lawrence, N. S., Williams, A. M., Surguladze, S., Giampietro, V., Brammer, M. J., Andrew, C., et al. (2004). Subcortical and ventral prefrontal cortical neural responses to facial expressions distinguish patients with bipolar disorder and major depression. *Biological Psychiatry, 55*(6), 578–587.

Lee, B. T., Seong Whi, C., Hyung Soo, K., Lee, B. C., Choi, I. G., Lyoo, I. K., et al. (2007). The neural substrates of affective processing toward positive and negative affective pictures in patients with major depressive disorder. *Progress in Neuro-Psychopharmacology and Biological Psychiatry, 31*(7), 1487–1492.

Lennox, B. R., Jacob, R., Calder, A. J., Lupson, V., & Bullmore, E. T. (2004). Behavioural and neurocognitive responses to sad facial affect are attenuated in patients with mania. *Psychological Medicine, 34*, 795–802.

Leppa, M., Korvenoja, A., Carlson, S., Timonen, P., Martinkauppi, S., Ahonen, J., et al. (2006). Acute opioid effects on human brain as revealed by functional magnetic resonance imaging. *NeuroImage, 31*(2), 661–669.

Lévesque, J., Eugene, F., Joanette, Y., Paquette, V., Mensour, B., Beaudoin, G., et al. (2003). Neural circuitry underlying voluntary suppression of sadness. *Biological Psychiatry, 53*(6), 502–510.

Lieberman, J. A., Tollefson, G. D., Charles, C., Zipursky, R., Sharma, T., Kahn, R. S., et al. (2005). Antipsychotic drug effects on brain morphology in first-episode psychosis. *Archives of General Psychiatry, 62*(4), 361–370.

Lieberman, M. D. (2007). Social cognitive neuroscience: A review of core processes. *Annual Review of Psychology, 58*, 259–289.

Lorberbaum, J. P., Kose, S., Johnson, M. R., Arana, G. W., Sullivan, L. K., Hamner, M. B., et al. (2004). Neural correlates of speech anticipatory anxiety in generalized social phobia. *NeuroReport, 15*(18), 2701–2705.

Lyoo, I. K., Kim, M. J., Stoll, A. L., Demopulos, C. M., Parow, A. M., Dager, S. R., et al. (2004). Frontal lobe gray matter density decreases in bipolar I disorder. *Biological Psychiatry, 55*(6), 648–651.

Malhi, G. S., Lagopoulos, J., Owen, A. M., Ivanovski, B., Shnier, R., & Sachdev, P. (2007). Reduced activation to implicit affect induction in euthymic bipolar patients: An fMRI study. *Journal of Affective Disorders, 97*(1–3), 109–122.

Malhi, G. S., Lagopoulos, J., Sachdev, P. S., Ivanovski, B., & Shnier, R. (2005). An emotional Stroop functional MRI study of euthymic bipolar disorder. *Bipolar Disorders, 7*(Suppl. 5), 58–69.

Malhi, G. S., Lagopoulos, J., Ward, P. B., Kumari, V., Mitchell, P. B., Parker, G. B., et al. (2004). Cognitive generation of affect in bipolar depression: An fMRI study. *European Journal of Neuroscience, 19,* 741–754.

Maren, S., Aharonov, G., & Fanselow, M. S. (1996). Retrograde abolition of conditional fear after excitotoxic lesions in the basolateral amygdala of rats: Absence of a temporal gradient. *Behavioral Neuroscience, 110*(4), 718–726.

McClure, E. B., Monk, C. S., Nelson, E. E., Parrish, J. M., Adler, A., Blair, R. J., et al. (2007). Abnormal attention modulation of fear circuit function in pediatric generalized anxiety disorder. *Archives of General Psychiatry, 64*(1), 97–106.

Milham, M. P., Nugent, A. C., Drevets, W. C., Dickstein, D. P., Leibenluft, E., Ernst, M., et al. (2005). Selective reduction in amygdala volume in pediatric anxiety disorders: A voxel-based morphometry investigation. *Biological Psychiatry, 57*(9), 961–966.

Monk, C. S., Telzer, E. H., Mogg, K., Bradley, B. P., Mai, X., Louro, H. M., et al. (2008). Amygdala and ventrolateral prefrontal cortex activation to masked angry faces in children and adolescents with generalized anxiety disorder. *Archives of General Psychiatry, 65*(5), 568–576.

Munafo, M. R., Brown, S. M., & Hariri, A. R. (2008). Serotonin transporter (5-HTTLPR) genotype and amygdala activation: A meta-analysis. *Biological Psychiatry, 63*(9), 852–857.

Myin-Germeys, I., Delespaul, P. A., & deVries, M. W. (2000). Schizophrenia patients are more emotionally active than is assumed based on their behavior. *Schizophrenia Bulletin, 26*(4), 847–854.

Nolen-Hoeksema, S. (2000). The role of rumination in depressive disorders and mixed anxiety/depressive symptoms. *Journal of Abnormal Psychology, 109*(3), 504–511.

Ochsner, K. N. (2008). The social-emotional processing stream: Five core constructs and their translational potential for schizophrenia and beyond. *Biological Psychiatry, 64*(1), 48–61.

Ochsner, K. N., Bunge, S. A., Gross, J. J., & Gabrieli, J. D. (2002). Rethinking feelings: An fMRI study of the cognitive regulation of emotion. *Journal of Cognitive Neuroscience, 14*(8), 1215–1229.

Ochsner, K. N., & Gross, J. J. (2004). Thinking makes it so: A social cognitive neuroscience approach to emotion regulation. In R. F. Baumeister & K. D. Vohs (Eds.), *Handbook of self-regulation: Research, theory, and applications* (pp. 229–255). New York: Guilford Press.

Ochsner, K. N., & Gross, J. J. (2005). The cognitive control of emotion. *Trends in Cognitive Science, 9*(5), 242–249.

Ochsner, K. N., & Gross, J. J. (2007). The neural architecture of emotion regulation. In J. J. Gross (Ed.), *Handbook of emotion regulation* (pp. 87–109). New York: Guilford Press.

Ochsner, K. N., & Gross, J. J. (2008). Cognitive emotion regulation: Insights from social cognitive and affective neuroscience. *Current Directions in Psychological Science, 17*(2), 153–158.

Ochsner, K. N., Hughes, B. L., Robertson, E., Cooper, J. C., & Gabrieli, J. (in press). Neural systems supporting the control of cognitive and affective conflict. *Journal of Cognitive Neuroscience.*

Ochsner, K. N., Knierim, K., Ludlow, D. H., Hanelin, J., Ramachandran, T., Glover, G., et al. (2004). Reflecting upon feelings: An fMRI study of neural systems supporting the attribution of emotion to self and other. *Journal of Cognitive Neuroscience, 16*(10), 1746–1772.

Ochsner, K. N., Ray, R. D., Cooper, J. C., Robertson, E. R., Chopra, S., Gabrieli, J. D., et al. (2004). For better or for worse: Neural systems supporting the cognitive down- and up-regulation of negative emotion. *NeuroImage, 23*(2), 483–499.

O'Doherty, J., Dayan, P., Schultz, J., Deichmann, R., Friston, K., & Dolan, R. J. (2004). Dissociable roles of ventral and dorsal striatum in instrumental conditioning. *Science, 304*, 452–454.

O'Doherty, J., Kringelbach, M. L., Rolls, E. T., Hornak, J., & Andrews, C. (2001). Abstract reward and punishment representations in the human orbitofrontal cortex. *Nature Neuroscience, 4*(1), 95–102.

O'Doherty, J., Winston, J., Critchley, H., Perrett, D., Burt, D. M., & Dolan, R. J. (2003). Beauty in a smile: The role of medial orbitofrontal cortex in facial attractiveness. *Neuropsychologia, 41*(2), 147–155.

Olsson, A., & Ochsner, K. N. (2008). The role of social cognition in emotion. *Trends in Cognitive Sciences, 12*(2), 65–71.

Park, I. H., Park, H. J., Chun, J. W., Kim, E. Y., & Kim, J. J. (2008). Dysfunctional modulation of emotional interference in the medial prefrontal cortex in patients with schizophrenia. *Neuroscience Letters, 440*(2), 119–124.

Phan, K. L., Fitzgerald, D. A., Nathan, P. J., Moore, G. J., Uhde, T. W., & Tancer, M. E. (2005). Neural substrates for voluntary suppression of negative affect: A functional magnetic resonance imaging study. *Biological Psychiatry, 57*(3), 210–219.

Phan, K. L., Fitzgerald, D. A., Nathan, P. J., & Tancer, M. E. (2006). Association between amygdala hyperactivity to harsh faces and severity of social anxiety in generalized social phobia. *Biological Psychiatry, 59*(5), 424–429.

Phan, K. L., Wager, T., Taylor, S. F., & Liberzon, I. (2002). Functional neuroanatomy of emotion: A meta-analysis of emotion activation studies in PET and fMRI. *NeuroImage, 16*(2), 331–348.

Phillips, M. L., Williams, L. M., Heining, M., Herba, C. M., Russell, T., Andrew, C., et al. (2004). Differential neural responses to overt and covert presentations of facial expressions of fear and disgust. *NeuroImage, 21*(4), 1484–1496.

Phillips, M. L., Williams, L. M., Senior, C., Bullmore, E. T., Brammer, M. J., Andrew, C., et al. (1999). A differential neural response to threatening and non-threatening negative facial expressions in paranoid and non-paranoid schizophrenics. *Psychiatry Research: Neuroimaging, 92*(1), 11–31.

Phillips, M. L., Young, A. W., Senior, C., Brammer, M., Andrew, C., Calder, A. J., et al. (1997). A specific neural substrate for perceiving facial expressions of disgust. *Nature, 389*, 495–498.

Posner, M. I., Petersen, S. E., Fox, P. T., & Raichle, M. E. (1988). Localization of cognitive operations in the human brain. *Science, 240*, 1627–1631.

Quadflieg, S., Mohr, A., Mentzel, H. J., Miltner, W. H., & Straube, T. (2008). Modulation of the neural network involved in the processing of anger prosody: The role of task-relevance and social phobia. *Biological Psychology, 78*(2), 129–137.

Quirk, G. J., Repa, C., & LeDoux, J. E. (1995). Fear conditioning enhances short-latency auditory responses of lateral amygdala neurons: Parallel recordings in the freely behaving rat. *Neuron, 15*(5), 1029–1039.

Ray, R. D., Ochsner, K. N., Cooper, J. C., Robertson, E. R., Gabrieli, J. D., & Gross, J. J. (2005). Individual differences in trait rumination and the neural systems supporting cognitive reappraisal. *Cognitive, Affective and Behavioral Neuroscience, 5*(2), 156–168.

Richards, J. M., & Gross, J. J. (2000). Emotion regulation and memory: The cognitive costs of keeping one's cool. *Journal of Personality and Social Psychology, 79*(3), 410–424.

Rolls, E. T. (2000). The orbitofrontal cortex and reward. *Cerebral Cortex, 10*(3), 282–294.

Rosso, I. M., Killgore, W. D., Cintron, C. M., Gruber, S. A., Tohen, M., & Yurgelun-Todd, D. A. (2007). Reduced amygdala volumes in first-episode bipolar disorder and correlation with cerebral white matter. *Biological Psychiatry, 61*(6), 743–749.

Schaefer, S. M., Jackson, D. C., Davidson, R. J., Aguirre, G. K., Kimberg, D. Y., & Thompson-Schill, S. L. (2002). Modulation of amygdalar activity by the conscious regulation of negative emotion. *Journal of Cognitive Neuroscience, 14*(6), 913–921.

Scherer, K. R., Schorr, A., & Johnstone, T. (Eds.). (2001). *Appraisal processes in emotion: Theory, methods, research.* New York: Oxford University Press.

Shin, L. M., Orr, S. P., Carson, M. A., Rauch, S. L., Macklin, M. L., Lasko, N. B., et al. (2004). Regional cerebral blood flow in the amygdala and medial prefrontal cortex during traumatic imagery in male and female Vietnam veterans with PTSD. *Archives of General Psychiatry, 61*(2), 168–176.

Siegle, G. J., Thompson, W., Carter, C. S., Steinhauer, S. R., & Thase, M. E. (2007). Increased amygdala and decreased dorsolateral prefrontal BOLD responses in unipolar depression: Related and independent features. *Biological Psychiatry, 61*(2), 198–209.

Sprengelmeyer, R., Rausch, M., Eysel, U. T., & Przuntek, H. (1998). Neural structures associated with recognition of facial expressions of basic emotions. *Proceedings of the Royal Society: B. Biological Sciences, 265,* 1927–1931.

Straube, T., Mentzel, H. J., & Miltner, W. H. (2006). Neural mechanisms of automatic and direct processing of phobogenic stimuli in specific phobia. *Biological Psychiatry, 59*(2), 162–170.

Surguladze, S., Brammer, M. J., Keedwell, P., Giampietro, V., Young, A. W., Travis, M. J., et al. (2005). A differential pattern of neural response toward sad versus happy facial expressions in major depressive disorder. *Biological Psychiatry, 57*(3), 201–209.

Takahashi, H., Koeda, M., Oda, K., Matsuda, T., Matsushima, E., Matsuura, M., et al. (2004). An fMRI study of differential neural response to affective pictures in schizophrenia. *NeuroImage, 22*(3), 1247–1254.

van Reekum, C. M., Johnstone, T., Urry, H. L., Thurow, M. E., Schaefer, H. S., Alexander, A. L., et al. (2007). Gaze fixations predict brain activation during the voluntary regulation of picture-induced negative affect. *NeuroImage, 36*(3), 1041–1055.

Wager, T. D., & Barrett, L. F. (2004). From affect to control: Functional specialization of the insula in motivation and regulation. *PsycExtra.* Retrieved May 17, 2009, from *www.columbia.edu/cu/psychology/tor/.*

Wager, T. D., Barrett, L. F., Bliss-Moreau, E., Lindquist, K. A, Duncan, S., Kober, H., et al. (2008). The neuroimaging of emotion. In M. Lewis, J. M. Haviland-Jones, & L. F. Barrett (Eds.), *Handbook of emotions* (3rd ed., pp. 249–271). New York: Guilford Press.

Wager, T. D., Hernandez, L., Jonides, J., & Lindquist, M. (2007). Elements of functional neuroimaging. In J. T. Cacioppo, L. G. Tassinary, & G. G. Berntson (Eds.), *Handbook of psychophysiology* (4th ed., pp. 19–55). Cambridge, UK: Cambridge University Press.

Wessa, M., Houenou, J., Paillere-Martinot, M. L., Berthoz, S., Artiges, E., Leboyer, M., et al. (2007). Fronto-striatal overactivation in euthymic bipolar patients during an emotional go/no go task. *American Journal of Psychiatry, 164*(4), 638–646.

Whalen, P. J., Johnstone, T., Somerville, L. H., Nitschke, J. B., Polis, S., Alexander, A. L., et al. (2008). A functional magnetic resonance imaging predictor of treatment response to venlafaxine in generalized anxiety disorder. *Biological Psychiatry, 63*(9), 858–863.

Whalen, P. J., Rauch, S. L., Etcoff, N. L., McInerney, S. C., Lee, M. B., & Jenike, M. A. (1998). Masked presentations of emotional facial expressions modulate amygdala activity without explicit knowledge. *Journal of Neuroscience, 18*(1), 411–418.

Whalley, M. G., Rugg, M. D., Smith, A. P., Dolan, R. J., & Brewin, C. R. (in press). Incidental retrieval of emotional contexts in post-traumatic stress disorder and depression: An fMRI study. *Brain and Cognition, 69*, 98–107.

Wicker, B., Keysers, C., Plailly, J., Royet, J. P., Gallese, V., & Rizzolatti, G. (2003). Both of us disgusted in My insula: The common neural basis of seeing and feeling disgust. *Neuron, 40*(3), 655–664.

Williams, L. M., Das, P., Harris, A. W., Liddell, B. B., Brammer, M. J., Olivieri, G., et al. (2004). Dysregulation of arousal and amygdala-prefrontal systems in paranoid schizophrenia. *American J of Psychiatry, 161*(3), 480–489.

Yurgelun-Todd, D. A., Gruber, S. A., Kanayama, G., Killgore, W. D., Baird, A. A., & Young, A. D. (2000). fMRI during affect discrimination in bipolar affective disorder. *Bipolar Disorders, 2*(3, Pt. 2), 237–248.

Zink, C. F., Pagnoni, G., Martin, M. E., Dhamala, M., & Berns, G. S. (2003). Human striatal response to salient nonrewarding stimuli. *Journal of Neuroscience, 23*(22), 8092–8097.

CHAPTER 4

On the Need for Conceptual and Definitional Clarity in Emotion Regulation Research on Psychopathology

Lian Bloch, Erin K. Moran, and Ann M. Kring

Every perception must lead to some nervous result. If this be the normal emotional expression, it soon expends itself, and in the natural course of things a calm succeeds. But if the normal issue be blocked from any cause, the currents may under certain circumstances invade other tracts, and there work different and worse effects. Thus vengeful brooding may replace a burst of indignation; a dry heat may consume the frame of one who fain would weep, or he may, as Dante says, turn to stone within; and then tears or a storming-fit may bring a grateful relief.
—WILLIAM JAMES (1884, pp. 198–199)

Emotion regulation may be central to understanding the cause and pathogenesis of psychopathology. Although this study has burgeoned in recent years, the field continues to be plagued by definitional ambiguity surrounding emotion regulation. In this chapter, we argue that progress in the field will advance more rapidly if greater consensus on the definition of emotion regulation is achieved. Our aim is to elucidate this challenge.

We begin by unpacking the myriad definitions of emotion and emotion regulation and how they relate to psychopathology. We then discuss the various ways in which emotion regulation has been studied within psychopathology. Finally, we suggest that a shared definition of emotion regulation across basic and applied research domains holds promise for advancing our understanding of how emotion regulation may be disrupted in psychopathology.

Defining Emotion

We eat, work, sleep, travel. Arguably, it is emotions that provide color, depth, and nuance to these life experiences. As the pioneer William James wrote, emotions live in the "aesthetic sphere of the mind, its longings, its pleasures and pains" (James, 1884, p. 188). But what exactly are these emotions? Throughout history, myriad definitions of emotions have been considered. Yet scientists still may not fully agree about what constitutes an emotion. As Joseph LeDoux once quipped, "One of the most significant things ever said about emotion may be that everyone knows what it is until they are asked to define it" (LeDoux, 1996, p. 23).

Various researchers have differentiated among the terms *emotion*, *affect*, and *mood*. Emotions, such as anger and sadness, typically are of rapid onset and short duration, lasting a matter of seconds (Ekman, 1992), and have a specific internal or external object of focus (Frijda, 1993). In contrast, moods may last hours or days (Ekman, 1992), may be objectless (Frijda, 1993), and may be composed of signals of one or many emotions (Ekman, 1999). Affect may be the superordinate category for all valenced states (Rosenberg, 1998; Scherer, 1984).

Emotions serve important functions, both intrapersonally and interpersonally (Keltner & Gross, 1999). Emotions may serve the adaptive function of translating information, even outside of awareness, into an internal experience to help identify and attain goals (e.g., Clore, 1994) and negotiate the environment (e.g., Frijda, 1994). The expressive characteristics of emotion may enable emotional communication and coordinate social interactions (e.g., Keltner & Kring, 1998; Levenson, 1994). Furthermore, emotions may serve to organize response systems (Levenson, 1994) that may (or may not) cohere across domains of subjective experience, behavior, and peripheral physiology (Barrett, 2006; Mauss, Levenson, McCarter, Wilhelm, & Gross, 2005).

Defining Emotion Regulation

Emotion regulation has been variously defined by theorists and researchers, as presented in Table 4.1. Arguably the most influential definition was by Gross (1998), who defined emotion regulation as the "processes by which individuals influence which emotions they have, when they have them, and how they experience and express these emotions" (p. 275). These processes may be automatic or controlled and conscious or unconscious. Moreover, Gross further unpacked these processes into five points in the emotion-generative process at which individuals can regulate their emotions: situation selection, situation modification, attentional deployment, cognitive change, and response modulation. The first four are referred to as antecedent-focused emotion regulation strategies, while the latter is

TABLE 4.1. Definitions of Emotion Regulation

Author	Definition
Dodge (1989, p. 340)	The process by which activation in one response domain serves to alter, titrate, or modulate activation in another response domain.
Cicchetti, Ganiban, and Barnett (1991, p. 15)	The intra- and extraorganismic factors by which emotional arousal is redirected, controlled, modulated, and modified to enable an individual to function adaptively in emotionally arousing situations.
Thompson (1994)	Emotion regulation consists of the extrinsic and intrinsic processes responsible for monitoring, evaluating, and modifying emotion reactions, especially their intensive and temporal features, to accomplish one's goals.
Gross (1998)	The processes by which individuals influence which emotions they have, when they have them, and how they experience and express these emotions.
Eisenberg and Morris (2002)	Emotion regulation is defined as the process of initiating, maintaining, modulating, or changing the occurrence, intensity, or duration of internal feeling states and emotion-related motivations and physiological processes, often in the service of accomplishing one's goals.
Cole, Martin, and Dennis (2004)	Emotion regulation refers to changes associated with activated emotions. These include changes in the emotion itself or in other psychological processes (e.g., memory, social interaction). The term *emotion regulation* can denote two types of regulatory phenomena: emotion as regulating (changes that appear to result from the activated emotion) and emotion as regulated (changes in the activated emotion).
Gratz and Roemer (2004)	Emotion regulation involves (a) awareness and understanding of emotions, (b) acceptance of emotions, (c) ability to control impulsive behaviors and behave in accordance with desired goals when experiencing negative emotions, and (d) ability to use situationally appropriate emotion regulation strategies flexibly to modulate emotional responses as desired in order to meet individual goals and situational demands.
Campos, Frankel, and Camras (2004)	Emotion regulation is the modification of any process in the system that generates emotion or its manifestation in behavior. The processes that modify emotion come from the same set of processes as the ones that are involved in emotion in the first place. Regulation takes place at all levels of the emotion process, at all times that the emotion is activated, and is evident even before an emotion is manifested.

considered a response-focused strategy. For example, averting one's gaze from a grotesque scene in a movie is a strategy to regulate feelings of disgust before they occur (i.e., attentional deployment); in contrast, suppressing facial expressions of disgust at dinner so as not to offend the chef is a strategy to regulate ongoing emotion (i.e., suppression). Emotion regulation may involve changes in duration or intensity of the various components of emotion, including experience, behavior, and physiology. Notably, Gross's definition locates emotion regulation "in the self" (i.e., within the individual).

In contrast, other definitions have placed greater emphasis on the extrinsic factors, particularly other people, which also serve emotion regulatory functions (e.g., Thompson, 1994). This is especially characteristic of researchers in developmental psychology who point out that external influences on emotion regulation are particularly salient to child development, wherein caregivers teach their children strategies for self-control of emotion (e.g., Fox & Calkins, 2003). For example, in infancy parents may directly manage their babies' emotional reactions: Baby monitors alert parents to distress, which parents may interpret as hunger and thus try to alleviate by feeding. As children mature, parents may also begin to utilize more indirect interventions to help children regulate their emotions, such as modeling effective strategies for managing anger. Others may exert emotion regulatory influence in adulthood, too. For example, a woman sitting at home feeling blue after breaking up with a romantic partner may have friends who help soothe those sad feelings by taking the woman out for an uplifting ladies' night on the town.

Gross and Thompson (2007) have elaborated a conceptualization of emotion regulation that reflects a combination of their ideas: Emotion regulation refers to the automatic or controlled, conscious or unconscious process of individuals influencing emotions in self, others, or both. Importantly, this definition integrates Thompson's (1994) emphasis on extrinsic influences on emotion regulation with Gross's (1998) process model that focused on emotion regulation in self.

It is important to situate the Gross–Thompson conceptualization within the broader panoply of emotion regulation definitions and models. Some of these definitions explicitly reference emotion regulation, whereas others define processes that are arguably close intellectual cousins to emotion regulation. In one of the early conceptualizations of emotion regulation, Dodge (1989) described emotion regulation as "the process by which activation in one response domain serves to alter, titrate, or modulate activation in another response domain" (p. 340). Similar to the Gross model of regulation, this conceptualization includes behavioral, experiential, and physiological response domains. Dodge argued that it is in understanding how a person coordinates these responses that we begin to understand emotion regulation. For example, a woman with obsessive–compulsive disorder begins to feel her heart racing at the thought of having left the oven on; then, by checking the oven repeatedly, she reduces her physiological reaction to this anxiety. It is in this step between feeling initial anxiety and reducing that anxiety via behavioral action that emotion regulation occurs. Additionally, similar to definitions proposed by Thompson (1994) and Gross and Thompson (2007), this conceptualization allows for internal and external forms of regulation.

Cole, Martin, and Dennis (2004) also explicitly acknowledge both internal and external influences on emotion regulation. In their broad definition, emotion regulation is defined as "changes associated with activated emotions." This model describes two types of regulatory processes. The first, *emotion as regulating*, refers to changes that are a result of the activated emotion. For example, a friend's sad expression makes us tell a joke in hopes of cheering her up. Ensuring that the emotion and change are linked is crucial to the definition of emotion regulation. The second type of regulatory process is *emotion as regulated*. Similar to Thompson (1994) and Gross and Thompson's (2007) conceptualizations, emotion as regulated refers to changes in the valence, intensity, or time course of emotion within the self or between people. Both processes require that the regulation be independent of the initial emotion and that an emotion state is activated (Cole et al., 2004).

Eisenberg and Spinrad (2004) raised concerns that Cole's definition was too broad and difficult to measure. They proposed a definition of emotion-related self-regulation as the process of "initiating, avoiding, inhibiting, maintaining, or modulating the occurrence, form, intensity, or duration of internal feeling states, emotion-related physiological, attentional processes, motivational states, and/or the behavioral concomitants of emotion in the service of accomplishing affect-related biological or social adaptation or achieving individual goals" (p. 338). Similar to the Gross model, Eisenberg and Spinrad's working definition acknowledges antecedent- and response-focused attempts to regulate emotion, distinguishes between regulation of self and others, and includes the modification of experience, behavior, and physiology. A point of distinction in Eisenberg's model is the notion that emotion regulation is used for biological or social adaptation and to achieve goals. They note that, although goals may not always be achieved, the motivation is a necessary component of the regulatory process (Eisenberg, Hofer, & Vaughan, 2007).

Some theorists and researchers have developed models of constructs that are conceptually similar to emotion regulation. For example, experiential avoidance has been defined by Hayes, Wilson, Gifford, Follette, and Strosahl (1996) as a time when a person "unwilling to remain in contact with particular private experiences (e.g., bodily sensations, emotions, thoughts, and memories) takes steps to alter the form or frequency of these events and the contexts that occasion them" (p. 1154). Experiential avoidance can be further parsed into cognitive avoidance and emotional avoidance (Hayes et al., 1996; see Salters-Pedneault, Steenkamp, & Litz, Chapter 6, this volume). Similar to Gross's model of emotion regulation, experiential avoidance involves suppressing or avoiding emotional experiences as the means by which to regulate emotion. However, whereas experiential avoidance focuses on the modulation of distressing emotions, Gross provides a model for the regulation of all emotions. Furthermore, experiential avoidance refers primarily to the experience component of emotion and not to other components (e.g., expression, physiology).

In contrast with experiential avoidance, mindfulness refers to the use of self-regulated attention to sit with unpleasant emotions in order to ultimately view them as less distressing (e.g., Bishop et al., 2004). This ability to attend to distressing emotions, without utilizing regulatory strategies to avoid distress, is thought to lead to a reduction in cognitive and behavioral avoidance coping mechanisms (see Valdivia-Salas, Sheppard, & Forsyth, Chapter 13, this volume). Although the role of attention is important in both Gross's model of emotion regulation and mindfulness, the two constructs view attention as a means to different ends. In mindfulness, attentional deployment is used to focus on self, emotion, and thought without distraction. In Gross's model of emotion regulation, attentional deployment can involve either distraction from an emotionally laden event or concentration toward the emotional event.

Although these varied conceptualizations of emotion regulation have all contributed to our understanding of emotion regulation in psychopathology, the field has nonetheless failed to progress in developing a clearer understanding of which aspects of emotion regulation may be central to the symptoms and even causes of different psychological disorders. One way to speed progress toward further elucidating where in the emotion generative process regulatory strategies may go awry in psychopathology is to adopt a theory and definition that identify the key processes that together form a comprehensive account of emotion regulation.

The Gross and Thompson (2007) conceptualization has two particular attributes that are helpful in this regard. First, this model systematically identifies distinct processes (situation selection, situation modification, attentional deployment, cognitive change, and response modulation) in the emotion regulation framework. This is vital to the study of psychopathology, because various disorders may be associated with the nonfunctioning of distinct emotion regulation processes. For example, emotional suppression is a form of response modulation that characterizes posttraumatic stress disorder (PTSD) (Roemer, Litz, Orsillo, & Wagner, 2001), whereas attentional deployment may be disrupted in individuals with generalized anxiety disorder (GAD) (MacLeod, Mathews, & Tata, 1986). Moreover, the identification of these distinct processes allows researchers the opportunity to vet each process completely and distinctly instead of trying to tackle a broader, perhaps less structured conceptualization of emotion regulation.

Second, this model allows for the consideration of deficits in self (e.g., difficulty controlling worry in GAD) as well as deficits related to influences by others. For example, people with a history of depression who perceive more criticism from their spouses are more likely to relapse (Hooley & Teasdale, 1989); perceived criticism may drive these individuals to amplify and deploy further attention to negative self-views, thus increasing risk of relapse. This suggests that models of emotion regulation focusing solely on the self as regulator may be missing an important aspect of emotion regulation in psychopathology. Although many disorders are indeed related to difficulties in emotion regulation, these may be complex and varied in nature. Therefore, as the prior examples illuminate, the Gross–Thompson framework may be particularly useful to identify distinct regulatory process problems in psychopathology.

Emotion Regulation and Psychopathology

In 1884, William James wrote the early description, with which we began this chapter, of the ill effect of difficulties in emotion regulation. This ill effect, or "different and worse" emotional impact, to which James refers may manifest as emotional excess or deficit and may play a key role in psychopathology. Various forms of psychological disorders have been described as disorders of emotional excess. For example, GAD involves extreme worry (e.g., Zinbarg & Barlow, 1996). Other disorders have been characterized by emotional deficits. For example, frontotemporal lobar dementia involves emotional blunting (e.g., Werner et al., 2007). These excesses and deficits may (or may not) reflect problems in the regulation of emotion. As we noted earlier, we believe that the Gross–Thompson (2007) model of emotion regulation is perhaps best suited to provide the foundation for studying emotion regulation across psychopathologies.

Indeed, emotional disturbances are prevalent in nearly all forms of psychopathology (e.g., Kring & Bachorowski, 1999). Thus, it follows that emotion regulation may be central to the cause and pathogenesis of these disorders. The literature has frequently discussed emotion regulation and psychopathology utilizing the term *emotion dysregulation*. Indeed, emotion dysregulation is implicated in more than half of the *Diagnostic and Statistical Manual of Mental Disorders* (fourth edition; American Psychiatric Association, 1994) Axis I disorders and in all of the Axis II disorders (Gross, 1998). What remains unclear is what exactly emotion dysregulation refers to and how it differs from emotion regulation.

Cicchetti, Ackerman, and Izard (1995) suggest that *emotion dysregulation* is the maladaptive implementation of emotion regulatory strategies, where the ability to implement these strategies is otherwise intact. As a separate construct, Cicchetti and colleagues propose that *problems in emotion regulation* refer to the absence of, or deficits in, regulatory strategies, where the ability to implement strategies is impaired. In our view, this perspective unnecessarily bifurcates emotion regulation in psychopathology into two constructs: emotion dysregulation and problems in emotion regulation.

By contrast, the Gross–Thompson conceptualization implicitly adopts a developmental perspective whereby it is first necessary to ascertain whether people developed emotion regulation skills and then whether they were able to use these skills in the appropriate contexts. Such inquiry requires knowledge of basic emotion regulatory processes to determine when they are being used out of context or too frequently or when they are being underutilized or are inaccessible. This emotion regulation perspective on psychopathology emphasizes the ability to not only engage in emotion regulatory strategies but also manipulate and modulate their implementation. Research has supported this perspective, suggesting that psychological adjustment may indeed depend upon the ability to flexibly enhance or suppress emotional expression in accord with situational demands (Bonanno, Papa, Lalande, Westphal, & Coifman, 2004; see also Salters-Pedneault et al., Chapter 6, this volume).

We recognize the appeal of distinguishing between regulation and dysregulation, particularly in the realm of psychopathology research, where the field has a tendency to pathologize emotion regulation by supplying the term *dysregulation*. However, we argue here that the field will move forward more productively by adopting the developmental, process-oriented approach that incorporates both components inherent to emotion regulation: adopting the relevant skill set and implementing the skill set appropriately depending upon context.

Emotion versus Emotion Regulation: Two Distinct Processes?

The debate persists over whether emotion and emotion regulation are distinct processes. Some researchers have proposed that the processes underlying emotion and emotion regulation are largely shared. For example, people often regulate their emotions even before they are generated by selecting favorable situations that will preempt negative emotions. Consequently, some researchers argue that emotion and emotion regulation cannot be meaningfully separated and that all emotion is likely regulated to some extent (e.g., Campos, Frankel, & Camras, 2004; Davidson, 2000).

However, other researchers have argued against the suggestion that all emotion is regulated emotion. This "seems akin to saying that all behavior is unconsciously motivated—it is an assertion that is essentially untestable" (Kring & Werner, 2004, p. 365). Rather, these researchers believe that differentiating between emotion and emotion regulation as separable constructs is especially vital to understanding the nature of emotion-related problems and, specifically, emotion-related disturbances in psychopathology. For example, in the case of GAD, it seems important to determine whether the excess of anxiety, worry, and irritability that characterizes the disorder results from an inability to down-regulate those emotions or whether it is simply reflective of a higher level of that emotion that remains in excess even when regulatory processes are intact. Indeed, we believe that distinguishing between emotion and emotion regulation is a vitally important process in examining emotion regulation in psychopathology.

Studies of Emotion Regulation in Psychopathology

In this section, we provide a few, brief examples of the ways that the Gross–Thompson (2007) conceptualization of emotion regulation has been studied in psychopathology in order to illustrate the promise of this approach. Research thus far has primarily investigated two processes central to this approach—suppression and reappraisal—in different mental disorders. We also illustrate the promise of other approaches, including studies of experiential avoidance, cognitive regulation, and mindfulness (all of which are more fully covered in later chapters of this volume). These latter approaches do not need to be viewed as divergent from the Gross–Thompson model. Rather, they can be understood as tests of specific processes in the broader model. Furthermore, the Gross–Thompson view does not fully capture all aspects of emotion regulation, leaving room for other approaches. Nevertheless, bonding research together by a common conceptualization will likely allow better cross-fertilization of findings across researchers and disorders.

Suppression

Perhaps the most studied regulatory strategy in psychopathology research is suppression. Suppression is a response-focused strategy that directly attempts to inhibit the expression of emotion (Gross & Thompson, 2007). Research in nonclinical samples indicates that those who report habitual use of suppression feel more negative emotions than nonsuppressors, experience fewer positive emotions, report more depressive symptoms, and feel less satisfied with life (Gross & John, 2003). In addition, in an experimental design investigating the cognitive consequences of suppression, those who were told to suppress emotional expression to a negative film clip were found to have poorer memory for the task relative to people who were not instructed to suppress or who were instructed to reappraise (Richards & Gross, 2000).

Following from evidence of the ill effects of suppression in nonclinical populations, research has focused on the role of suppression in psychological disorders. Studies have documented the greater use of suppression, among clinical populations compared with healthy controls, in a wide range of psychological disorders, including anxiety and mood disorders generally (Campbell-Sills, Barlow, Brown, & Hofmann, 2006) and panic disorder (Baker, Holloway, Thomas, Thomas, & Owens, 2004), binge-eating disorder (Milligan & Waller, 2000), and PTSD (Roemer et al., 2001) specifically.

Researchers have also worked to translate basic findings on the untoward consequences of suppression into psychosocial interventions. For example, Mennin, Heimberg, Turk, and Fresco (2002) have argued that people with GAD feel emotions more intensely, yet lack adaptive regulatory strategies to handle this intense emotional experience. In an effort to cope, GAD patients use strategies, including suppression, to decrease emotional experience, which ultimately leads to more anxiety (Mennin et al., 2002). Mennin (2004) developed an integrative, emotion-focused treatment for GAD called emotion regulation therapy (ERT). ERT first involves teaching clients to identify their own patterns of maladaptive responding to emotional experiences. Clients then learn to identify and understand their emotions as well as utilize more adaptive emotion regulatory strategies. In short, the emphasis in this treatment approach is to teach emotion regulatory strategies as well as the ability to adaptively implement these strategies in appropriate contexts. (This approach is discussed in greater detail by Mennin & Fresco, Chapter 15, this volume.)

Reappraisal

Reappraisal, an antecedent-focused regulatory strategy, is a method of changing one's thoughts about a situation so as to alter its emotional impact (Gross & Thompson, 2007). Although suppression has been found to relate to more negative outcomes, habitual use of reappraisal has been related to greater experience of positive emotion, less negative emotion, and fewer symptoms of depression (Gross & John, 2003). Henry and colleagues (2008) measured suppression and reappraisal via self-report in schizophrenia patients and controls after viewing emotionally evocative film clips. Patients and controls did not differ in their reported use of suppression or reappraisal, but greater use of reappraisal in schizophrenia patients was correlated with reduced depression. In a study with claustrophobic participants, those in an exposure-reappraisal condition showed greater levels of fear reduction than those in the exposure-only condition (Kamphuis & Telch, 2000).

Clinicians and scientists are beginning to turn their collective eye toward developing interventions that promote helpful emotion regulation strategies, such as reappraisal. For example, Campbell-Sills and Barlow (2007) developed a treatment for anxiety and mood disorders that teaches clients to utilize cognitive reappraisal through emotion regulation training. Clients are taught to recognize their maladaptive emotion-driven behaviors and are then encouraged to engage in more adaptive alternative behaviors, such as reappraisal. For example, a client with a fear of flying would be urged to identify the fearful cognitions surrounding flying. The client would then be asked to evaluate the rationality of these cognitions and taught how to reappraise the act of flying in a more realistic manner. (This approach is discussed in more detail by Fairholme, Boisseau, Ellard, Ehrenreich, & Barlow, Chapter 12, this volume.)

Difficulties in Emotion Regulation

Another approach to studying emotion regulation involves assessing emotion regulation strategies that are unhelpful. Gratz and Roemer (2004) developed the Difficulties in Emotion Regulation Scale (DERS), which measures difficulties in understanding and awareness of emotion, the ability to engage in appropriate behavior when experiencing negative emotions, and knowledge of effective emotion regulatory strategies. The DERS adopts dysfunction as its starting point. This may be useful in studying psychopathology: Researchers and clinicians want to identify what emotion regulation processes are not working well in order to intervene effectively. However, as noted earlier with respect to Cicchetti's bifurcation of emotion regulation problems and emotion dysregulation, the focus on pathology obscures an understanding of how these processes ought to ideally operate. In addition, it is important to point out that the processes central to the DERS and related questionnaires (e.g., rumination, self-blame) have been well characterized and studied in cognitive theory and research on depression and anxiety, and these may not be emotion regulatory strategies theoretically constrained by the Gross–Thompson definition.

Experiential Avoidance

Experiential avoidance focuses on the cognitive and emotional avoidance of distressing events and is arguably a concept closely related to suppression and attentional deployment in emotion regulation. From research on emotional suppression, we might expect that experiential avoidance would be related to poorer physical and mental health. Indeed, Hayes and colleagues (2004) have found that chronic attempts to engage in the experiential avoidance of negative private experiences is a strong predictor of psychopathology and is also correlated with measures of subclinical psychopathological symptomatology (see also Boulanger, Hayes, & Pistorello, Chapter 5, this volume).

Thus, experiential avoidance and suppression may be of similar nature and consequence. Indeed, the Acceptance and Action Questionnaire (AAQ; Hayes et al., 2004), a measure of experiential avoidance, is positively correlated with the Suppression subscale of the Emotion Regulation Questionnaire (Gross & John, 2003). However, the magnitude of the correlation is modest (.28), suggesting that the constructs are not entirely overlapping (Kashdan, Barrios, Forsyth, & Steger, 2006).

Mindfulness

Mindfulness involves focusing attention on all emotions rather than suppressing or avoiding an emotional event. As a relatively new area of scientific study, work is underway to both define mindfulness and develop measures suitable for assessing the construct (Baer, Smith, Hopkins, Krietemeyer, & Toney, 2006; Bishop et al., 2004). For example, Baer and colleagues (2006) examined the linkage among measures of mindfulness, emotion regulation, and experiential avoidance. When comparing measures of mindfulness with the DERS (Gratz & Roemer, 2004), ascribing to high levels of mindfulness was inversely related to difficulties in emotion regulation such as problems understanding, accepting, and using emotion regulatory strategies. Additionally, high levels of mindfulness were inversely related to experiential avoidance (as measured by the AAQ). Mindfulness has also been found to be negatively correlated with depression and anxiety symptoms and positively correlated with positive affect and subjective well-being (Brown & Ryan, 2003; Hayes & Wilson, 2003).

Current research has focused on developing and testing mindfulness interventions aimed at reducing stress and promoting psychological well-being (see Corcoran, Farb, Anderson, & Segal, Chapter 14, this volume and Valdivia-Salas et al., Chapter 13, this volume). Interventions such as mindfulness-based cognitive therapy (Segal, Williams, & Teasdale, 2002), dialectical behavior therapy (Linehan, 1993), and mindfulness-based stress reduction (Grossman, Niemann, Schmidt, & Walach, 2004) all involve mindfulness training as an aspect of intervention. Future research is needed to more clearly assess how mindfulness is used as an emotion regulation strategy constrained by the Gross–Thompson conceptualization.

Must We Unify? Can We?

The foregoing section identified just a few examples of the ways in which emotion regulation has been studied in psychopathology. Studies invariably adopt different definitions and methods for studying emotion regulation. This diversity of approaches begs the question: Do we need to agree on one definition?

Our position is yes. To encourage the communication and sharing of ideas across basic and applied research, a single, unified definition of emotion regulation will be beneficial. As evidenced by the brief review presented here, heterogeneity in approaches to studying emotion regulation results in diverse findings that are challenging to synthesize. Adopting a broad conceptualization, such as that proposed by Gross and Thompson, will make less likely the possibility that the field continues to be characterized by results that are difficult to integrate. Stated differently, we believe the field will best be served by unifying around the Gross–Thompson model, which not only will support hypothesis forming and testing in basic research but also fits well in applied research on psychopathology. This approach allows for modifications to the conceptualization as new data come in and illuminate processes that are not fully encompassed currently.

Nonetheless, adopting a shared definition is not without pitfalls. One area of difficulty is making sure the model makes room for cultural differences in emotion and emotion regulation. Norms for emotion differ across cultures (e.g., Mesquita, 2001; Tsai, Knutson, & Fung, 2006). For example, whereas independent cultures (e.g., European American) place emphasis on the individual, interdependent cultures (e.g., East Asian) place emphasis on the group and, accordingly, on forming harmonious relationships with others (Markus & Kitayama, 1991). To the extent that emotion regulation processes serve the function of aiding an individual in identifying and pursuing goals relative to maintaining and developing adaptive relationships (Thompson, 1991), then cultural differences in these emotional norms will impact emotion regulation processes. Nonetheless, adopting a broad definition, such as the definition proposed by Gross and Thompson, leaves open many entry points to the study of emotion regulation in psychopathology.

Summary

Research on emotion regulation has burgeoned in the last decade. Along with advances in basic research, there is growing interest in translational research. That is, scientists are becoming increasingly interested in the extent to which difficulties in emotion regulation may be related to the cause and pathogenesis of psychopathology. As we strive to bridge basic and applied research on emotion regulation, it becomes increasingly important to identify a broad, useful, and widely shared definition of emotion regulation. Although we may be moving toward a more unified model of emotion regulation (Gross & Thompson, 2007), the field still lacks clarity in the way it defines and studies emotion regulation across mental disorders. We acknowledge the inherent conceptual and empirical challenge in this task. For example, factors such as cross-cultural differences that may impact emotion regulation processes should be considered. These are among areas for the field to further explore. Ultimately, we believe that definitional clarity in basic and applied emotion regulation research will best promote advances in our collective understanding.

References

American Psychiatric Association. (1994). *Diagnostic and statistical manual of mental disorders* (4th ed.). Washington, DC: Author.

Baer, R. A., Smith, G. T., Hopkins, J., Krietemeyer, J., & Toney, L. (2006). Using self-report assessment methods to explore facets of mindfulness. *Assessment, 13*, 27–45.

Baker, R., Holloway, J., Thomas, P. W., Thomas, S., & Owens, M. (2004). Emotional processing and panic. *Behaviour Research and Therapy, 42*, 1271–1287.

Barrett, L. F. (2006). Solving the emotion paradox: Categorization and the experience of emotion. *Personality and Social Psychology Review, 10*, 20–46.

Bishop, S. R., Lau, M., Shapiro, S., Carlson, L., Anderson, N. D., Carmody, J., et al. (2004). Mindfulness: A proposed operational definition. *Clinical Psychology: Science and Practice, 11*, 230–241.

Bonanno, G. A., Papa, A., Lalande, K., Westphal, M., & Coifman, K. (2004). The importance of being flexible: The ability to both enhance and suppress emotional expression predicts long-term adjustment. *Psychological Science, 15*, 482–487.

Brown, K. W., & Ryan, R. M. (2003). The benefits of being present: Mindfulness and its role in psychological well-being. *Journal of Personality and Social Psychology, 84*, 822–848.

Campbell-Sills, L., & Barlow, D. H. (2007). Incorporating emotion regulation into conceptualizations and treatments of anxiety and mood disorders. In J. J. Gross (Ed.), *Handbook of emotion regulation* (pp. 542–559). New York: Guilford Press.

Campbell-Sills, L., Barlow, D. H., Brown, T. A., & Hofmann, S. G. (2006). Acceptability and suppression of negative emotion in anxiety and mood disorders. *Emotion, 6*, 587–595.

Campos, J. J., Frankel, C. B., & Camras, L. (2004). On the nature of emotion regulation. *Child Development, 75*, 377–394.

Cicchetti, D., Ackerman, B. P., & Izard, C. E. (1995). Emotions and emotion regulation in developmental psychopathology. *Development and Psychopathology, 7*, 1–10.

Cicchetti, D., Ganiban, J., & Barnett, D. (1991). Contributions from the study of high-risk populations to understanding the development of emotion regulation. In J. Garber & K. A. Dodge (Eds.), *The development of emotion regulation and dysregulation* (pp. 15–48). New York: Cambridge University Press.

Clore, G. L. (1994). Why emotions are felt. In P. Ekman & R. J. Davidson (Eds.), *The nature of emotion: Fundamental questions* (pp. 103–111). New York: Oxford University Press.

Cole, P. M., Martin, S. E., & Dennis, T. A. (2004). Emotion regulation as a scientific construct: Methodological challenges and directions for child development research. *Child Development, 75*, 317–333.

Davidson, R. J. (2000). The functional neuroanatomy of affective style. In R. D. L. L. Nadel (Ed.), *Cognitive neuroscience of emotion* (pp. 371–388). New York: Oxford University Press.

Dodge, K. A. (1989). Coordinating responses to aversive stimuli: Introduction to a special section on the development of emotion regulation. *Developmental Psychology, 25*, 339–342.

Eisenberg, N., Hofer, C., & Vaughan, J. (2007). Effortful control and its socioe-motional consequences. In J. J. Gross (Ed.), *Handbook of emotion regulation* (pp. 287–306). New York: Guilford Press.

Eisenberg, N., & Morris, A. S. (2002). Children's emotion-related regulation. In R. Kail (Ed.), *Advances in child development and behavior* (Vol. 30, pp. 190–229). Amsterdam: Academic Press.

Eisenberg, N., & Spinrad, T. L. (2004). Emotion-related regulation: Sharpening the definition. *Child Development, 75,* 334–339.

Ekman, P. (1992). An argument for basic emotions. *Cognition and Emotion, 6,* 169–200.

Ekman, P. (1999). Basic emotions. In T. Dalgleish & M. Power (Eds.), *Handbook of cognition and emotion* (pp. 45–60). Sussex, UK: Wiley.

Fox, N. A., & Calkins, S. D. (2003). The development of self-control of emotion: Intrinsic and extrinsic influences. *Motivation and Emotion, 27,* 7–26.

Frijda, N. H. (1993). Mood, emotion episodes, and emotions. In M. Lewis & J. M. Haviland-Jones (Eds.), *Handbook of emotions* (pp. 381–403). New York: Guilford Press.

Frijda, N. H. (1994). Emotions are functional, most of the time. In P. Ekman & R. J. Davidson (Eds.), *The nature of emotion: Fundamental questions* (pp. 112–122). New York: Oxford University Press.

Gratz, K. L., & Roemer, L. (2004). Multidimensional assessment of emotion regu-lation and dysregulation: Development, factor structure, and initial valida-tion of the Difficulties in Emotion Regulation Scale. *Journal of Psychopathology and Behavioral Assessment, 26,* 41–54.

Gross, J. J. (1998). Antecedent-and response-focused emotion regulation: Diver-gent consequences for experience, expression, and physiology. *Journal of Per-sonality and Social Psychology, 74,* 224–237.

Gross, J. J., & John, O. P. (2003). Individual differences in two emotion regulation processes: Implications for affect, relationships, and well-being. *Journal of Per-sonality and Social Psychology, 85,* 348–362.

Gross, J. J., & Thompson, R. A. (2007). Emotion regulation: Conceptual founda-tions. In J. J. Gross (Ed.), *Handbook of emotion regulation* (pp. 3–24). New York: Guilford Press.

Grossman, P., Niemann, L., Schmidt, S., & Walach, H. (2004). Mindfulness-based stress reduction and health benefits: A meta-analysis. *Journal of Psychosomatic Research, 57,* 35–43.

Hayes, S. C., Strosahl, K., Wilson, K. G., Bissett, R. T., Pistorello, J., Toarmino, D., et al. (2004). Measuring experiential avoidance: A preliminary test of a working model. *The Psychological Record, 54,* 553–579.

Hayes, S. C., & Wilson, K. G. (2003). Mindfulness: Method and process. *Clinical Psychology: Science and Practice, 10,* 161–165.

Hayes, S. C., Wilson, K. G., Gifford, E. V., Follette, V. M., & Strosahl, K. (1996). Experiential avoidance and behavioral disorders: A functional dimensional approach to diagnosis and treatment. *Journal of Consulting and Clinical Psychol-ogy, 64,* 1152–1168.

Henry, J. D., Rendell, P. G., Green, M. J., McDonald, S., & O'Donnell, M. (2008). Emotion regulation in schizophrenia: Affective, social, and clinical correlates of suppression and reappraisal. *Journal of Abnormal Psychology, 117,* 473–478.

Hooley, J. M., & Teasdale, J. D. (1989). Predictors of relapse in unipolar depressives: Expressed emotion, marital distress, and perceived criticism. *Journal of Abnormal Psychology, 98*, 229–235.

James, W. (1884). What is an emotion? *Mind, 9*, 188–205.

Kamphuis, J. H., & Telch, M. J. (2000). Effects of distraction and guided threat reappraisal on fear reduction during exposure-based treatments for specific fears. *Behaviour Research and Therapy, 38*, 1163–1181.

Kashdan, T. B., Barrios, V., Forsyth, J. P., & Steger, M. F. (2006). Experiential avoidance as a generalized psychological vulnerability: Comparisons with coping and emotion regulation strategies. *Behaviour Research and Therapy, 44*, 1301–1320.

Keltner, D., & Gross, J. J. (1999). Functional accounts of emotions. *Cognition and Emotion, 13*, 467–480.

Keltner, D., & Kring, A. M. (1998). Emotion, social function, and psychopathology. *Review of General Psychology, 2*, 320–342.

Kring, A. M., & Bachorowski, J. A. (1999). Emotions and psychopathology. *Cognition and Emotion, 13*, 575–599.

Kring, A. M., & Werner, K. H. (2004). Emotion regulation and psychopathology. In P. Philippot & R. S. Feldman (Eds.), *The regulation of emotion* (pp. 359–385). Hillsdale, NJ: Erlbaum.

LeDoux, J. (1996). *The emotional brain.* New York: Simon & Schuster.

Levenson, R. W. (1994). Human emotion: A functional view. In P. Ekman & R. J. Davidson (Eds.), *The nature of emotion: Fundamental questions* (pp. 123–126). New York: Oxford University Press.

Linehan, M. M. (1993). *Cognitive-behavioral treatment of borderline personality disorder.* New York: Guilford Press.

MacLeod, C., Mathews, A., & Tata, P. (1986). Attentional bias in emotional disorders. *Journal of Abnormal Psychology, 95*, 15–20.

Markus, H. R., & Kitayama, S. (1991). Culture and the self: Implications for cognition, emotion, and motivation. *Psychological Review, 98*, 224–253.

Mauss, I. B., Levenson, R. W., McCarter, L., Wilhelm, F. H., & Gross, J. J. (2005). The tie that binds?: Coherence among emotion experience, behavior, and physiology. *Emotion, 5*(2), 175–190.

Mennin, D. S. (2004). Emotion regulation therapy for generalized anxiety disorder. *Clinical Psychology and Psychotherapy, 11*, 17–29.

Mennin, D. S., Heimberg, R. G., Turk, C. L., & Fresco, D. M. (2002). Applying an emotion regulation framework to integrative approaches to generalized anxiety disorder. *Clinical Psychology: Science and Practice, 9*, 85–90.

Mesquita, B. (2001). Emotions in collectivist and individualist contexts. *Journal of Personality and Social Psychology, 80*, 68–74.

Milligan, R. J., & Waller, G. (2000). Anger and bulimic psychopathology among nonclinical women. *International Journal of Eating Disorders, 28*, 446–450.

Richards, J. M., & Gross, J. J. (2000). Emotion regulation and memory: The cognitive costs of keeping one's cool. *Journal of Personality and Social Psychology, 79*, 410–424.

Roemer, L., Litz, B. T., Orsillo, S. M., & Wagner, A. W. (2001). A preliminary investigation of the role of strategic withholding of emotions in PTSD. *Journal of Traumatic Stress, 14*, 149–156.

Rosenberg, E. L. (1998). Levels of analysis and the organization of affect. *Review of General Psychology, 2*, 247–270.

Scherer, K. R. (1984). On the nature and function of emotion: A component process approach. In K. R. Scherer & P. E. Ekman (Eds.), *Approaches to emotion* (pp. 293–317). Hillsdale, NJ: Erlbaum.

Segal, Z. V., Williams, J. M. G., & Teasdale, J. D. (2002). *Mindfulness-based cognitive therapy for depression: A new approach to preventing relapse.* New York: Guilford Press.

Thompson, R. A. (1991). Emotional regulation and emotional development. *Educational Psychology Review, 3,* 269–307.

Thompson, R. A. (1994). Emotion regulation: A theme in search of definition. *Monographs of the Society for Research in Child Development, 59,* 25–52.

Tsai, J. L., Knutson, B., & Fung, H. H. (2006). Cultural variation in affect valuation. *Journal of Personality and Social Psychology, 90,* 288–307.

Werner, K. H., Roberts, N. A., Rosen, H. J., Dean, D. L., Kramer, J. H., Weiner, M. W., et al. (2007). Emotional reactivity and emotion recognition in frontotemporal lobar degeneration. *Neurology, 69*(2), 148–155.

Zinbarg, R. E., & Barlow, D. H. (1996). Structure of anxiety and the anxiety disorders: A hierarchical model. *Journal of Abnormal Psychology, 105,* 181–193.

PART II

Problems of Emotion Regulation That Span Different Disorders

DESCRIPTIONS, MECHANISMS, COMORBIDITIES

CHAPTER 5

Experiential Avoidance as a Functional Contextual Concept

Jennifer L. Boulanger, Steven C. Hayes, and Jacqueline Pistorello

Experiential avoidance can be defined as a verbally mediated tendency to escape or avoid private psychological experiences (e.g., thoughts, emotions, sensations, memories, urges) by attempting to modify their form, frequency, intensity, or situational sensitivity even when doing so is futile or interferes with valued actions (Hayes, Wilson, Gifford, Follette, & Strosahl, 1996). Experiential avoidance often works in the short term to reduce some discomfort, but can have long-term negative effects when overextended and applied inflexibly.

Although experiential avoidance can be viewed as an emotion regulation strategy, we argue that the concept has broader implications that lead to targeted treatment interventions for a broad spectrum of psychopathology. This will be accomplished through a twofold process: a review of the empirical literature and an explication of the theoretical underpinnings of the concept. The empirical evidence reviewed later in the chapter illustrates how experiential avoidance, although typically highly correlated with known emotion regulation measures, brings added value. It is associated with decreased quality of life and functioning across both clinical and nonclinical populations; moderates the impact of treatment and other external events; mediates the impact of stressful life events and a variety of psychological variables, including many coping styles and emotion regulation strategies; and mediates the impact of acceptance and mindfulness-based treatments. The philosophical and theoretical review argues that the utility of this concept is due to the fact that experiential avoidance is designed to be a functional category, linked to manipulable and contextually embedded processes.

In more general terms, in this chapter we familiarize the reader with the evidence on the role of experiential avoidance in the development, maintenance, and treatment of various forms of psychopathology and demonstrate how experiential avoidance develops as a result of normal language processes and cultural norms that support the control of emotional and cognitive experiences. Finally, we discuss experiential avoidance as part of a transdiagnostic, functional dimensional approach to psychopathology.

The History of the Construct of Experiential Avoidance

To some degree experiential avoidance has long been recognized as an important factor in the development and maintenance of many forms of psychopathology (Hayes et al., 1996). Many systems of psychopathology or therapy have historically dealt with some aspects of the concept explicitly or implicitly. For example, psychodynamic theories pay particular attention to psychological defenses, including repression and projective identification, which function to avoid self-knowledge of painful events, thoughts, urges, and emotions (Freud, 1937). Gestalt therapists have hypothesized that psychological problems occur when emotions are blocked, suggesting that "dysfunction occurs when emotions are interrupted before they can enter awareness or go very far in organizing action" (Greenberg & Safran, 1989, p. 20). Humanistic therapies promote an openness to experience (Rogers, 1961) so that "the individual becomes more openly aware of his own feelings and attitudes as they exist in him" and "he is able to take in the evidence in a new situation, *as it is*, rather than distorting it to fit a pattern which he already holds" (p. 115). Existential psychologists focus particularly on the pathological effects of avoiding fears associated with death, "which shape character structure, and that, if maladaptive, result in clinical syndromes" (Yalom, 1980, p. 47). Cognitive-behavioral therapies also recognize the importance of avoidance of private experiences, particularly within the realm of anxiety disorders (Foa, Steketee, & Young, 1984), and the ease with which "unpleasant events are ignored, distorted, or forgotten" (p. 34).

These historical antecedents provide a foundation and context for the specific concept of experiential avoidance that has emerged in the modern era. The first reference to the term in the PsychLit database was by Hayes and Wilson (1994), and the first comprehensive review was by Hayes and colleagues (1996). As of spring 2009 there are 161 references to this concept in the PsychLit data base: seven in the first 5 years following its initial use (1994–1998), 36 in the next 5 years (1999–2003), and 113 in the last 4½ years (2004–2008). The more specific term *emotional avoidance* (e.g., Hayes & Melancon, 1989) likewise has 56 citations, most of which have also occurred in the last several years. The concept evolved from "emotional" to "experiential" avoidance to include the range of private events avoided: It is not simply emotions but also thoughts, physiological reactions, action tendencies and urges, memories, or even factual knowledge that would contradict a well-rehearsed view of oneself (see conceptualized self discussion later).

Experiential avoidance is a central theme of the so-called third-wave behavioral and cognitive therapies, which pay particular attention to the context and function of behaviors of interest, focus on second-order change, and tend to incorporate acceptance and mindfulness strategies (Hayes, 2004). This includes acceptance and commitment therapy (ACT; Hayes, Strosahl, & Wilson, 1999), which was developed specifically to target experiential avoidance as an etiological and maintaining factor in psychopathology by those who popularized the concept. There is also a clear recognition of the role of experiential avoidance in other acceptance and mindfulness-based interventions such as dialectical behavior therapy (DBT; Linehan, 1993), mindfulness-based cognitive therapy (Segal, Williams, & Teasdale, 2002), integrative behavioral couple therapy (Jacobson & Christensen, 1996), mindfulness-based stress reduction (Kabat-Zinn, 1990), and acceptance-based behavior therapy approaches (e.g., Barlow, Allen, & Choate, 2004; Roemer & Orsillo, 2009).

Experiential avoidance shares some commonalities with other concepts in the literature, such as emotion dysregulation (Gratz & Roemer, 2004), distress intolerance (Brown, Lejuez, Kahler, & Strong, 2002), intolerance of uncertainty (Dugas, Freeston, & Ladouceur, 1997), cognitive and emotional suppression (e.g., Wenzlaff & Wegner, 2000), and mindfulness, or the lack thereof (Baer, Smith, Hopkins, Krietemeyer, & Toney, 2006). A thorough discussion of how experiential avoidance differs specifically from each of these related concepts would require the thorough explication of each, which is beyond the scope of this chapter; however, the subsequent discussion highlights the distinctive features of experiential avoidance and its utility and addresses these distinctions in a global way. Other chapters in the book will address many of these similar concepts in detail. Experiential avoidance can be thought of as an emotional regulation strategy, but it is better thought of as an emotional regulation *function*. This difference is part of why experiential avoidance has distinct and unusual characteristics that provide clinical value beyond the majority of coping styles and emotion regulation strategies described and measured in the psychological literature. Thus, we first examine how it has been operationalized and consider some of the growing volume of studies we believe document its central role in human functioning. Then we consider the theoretical issues related to experiential avoidance and its utility in the understanding of psychological difficulties and human growth and development.

Operationalizing Experiential Avoidance

The most commonly used measure of experiential avoidance is the Acceptance and Action Questionnaire (AAQ; Hayes et al., 2004). The AAQ is a brief self-report measure that assesses the degree to which a person becomes entangled with difficult thoughts, avoids emotions, and is unable to act effectively in the presence of difficult private experiences. It is available in nine- to 16-item versions (Bond & Bunce, 2003; Hayes et al., 2004) as well as in a revised form that has somewhat better internal consistency in some populations (AAQ-II; Bond et al., 2008). Although it is possible to create two-factor versions that separate out experiential willingness from the ability to act in the presence of difficult thought and feelings, all available versions either include a strong latent factor or work well as a single-factor scale. The general versions of the AAQ include broad items about feelings and thoughts as well as items about anxiety and depression; they demonstrate good reliability and criterion-related, predictive, convergent, and discriminant validities. Experiential avoidance measures are also now available for children (Greco, Lambert, & Baer, 2008). These measures, like the AAQ for adults, combine items that focus on avoidance with those that focus on entanglement with distressing thoughts and feelings.

Several specific experiential avoidance measures have been developed to suit particular clinical problems. This list is rapidly growing but so far includes smoking (Gifford et al., 2004), body image (Sandoz & Wilson, 2006), weight (Lillis & Hayes, 2008), psychosis (Shawyer et al., 2007), chronic pain (McCracken, Vowles, & Eccleston, 2004; Wicksell, Renofalt, Olsson, Bond, & Melin, 2008), epilepsy (Lundgren, Dahl, & Hayes, 2008), and diabetes (Gregg, Callaghan, Hayes, & Glenn-Lawson, 2007). In the specific versions, broad items about feelings, thoughts, and actions are typically replaced with somewhat parallel items that mention domain-specific feelings, thoughts, and actions. For example, the AAQ includes the item "When I evaluate something negatively, I usually recognize that this is just a reaction, not an objective fact." The weight-specific version of the AAQ (Lillis & Hayes, 2008) includes an item that says "When I evaluate my weight or appearance negatively, I am able to recognize that this is just a reaction, not an objective fact."

As this very item shows, the general and specific versions of the AAQ measure areas that go beyond a commonsense understanding of the term *experiential avoidance*. The reasons for this extension will become clearer later in the chapter as the theory that underlies experiential avoidance is discussed, but for now it is simply worth noting that the operationalization of the concept included items on entanglement with thoughts, negative evaluations of private experience, and the ability to take action in the face of difficult thoughts and feelings in addition to items of experiential control, escape, and avoidance in a commonsense meaning of those terms.

Evidence for the Role of Experiential Avoidance in Psychopathology

A growing body of evidence demonstrates that experiential avoidance is distinct from other psychological constructs and is associated with a wide variety of psychopathology and behavioral problems (see Chawla & Ostafin, 2007 for an extensive review). A meta-analysis by Hayes, Luoma, Bond, Masuda, and Lillis (2006) showed that levels of experiential avoidance as measured by the AAQ may account for 16–28% of the variance in behavioral health problems generally. Experiential avoidance is particularly strongly correlated with depression, stress, anxiety, and general psychological distress. Well-known measures in these areas all have average correlations of .5 or above with the AAQ across clinical and nonclinical populations (Hayes et al., 2006). Experiential avoidance has also been related to substance abuse, posttraumatic stress disorder (PTSD) symptomatology and severity, deliberate self-harm, intolerance of chronic pain, internalized and externalized homophobia, trichotillomania, and phobic fear among other areas (Hayes et al., 2006).

Experiential avoidance also correlates with or moderates overt measures of distress tolerance and task persistence (Cochrane, Barnes-Holmes, Barnes-Holmes, Stewart, & Luciano, 2007; Karekla, Forsyth, & Kelly, 2004; Sloan, 2004; Spira, Zvolensky, Eifert, & Feldner, 2004; Zettle, Petersen, Hocker, & Provines, 2007), which are known to relate to a variety of behavioral health problems, including substance use (Brown et al., 2002; Daughters, Lejuez, Kahler, Strong, & Brown, 2005), problem gambling (Daughters et al., 2005), and borderline personality disorder (BPD) (Gratz, Rosenthal, Tull, Lejuez, & Gunderson, 2006).

Experiential avoidance is also negatively correlated with various quality of life indices (Hayes et al., 2004). Experiential avoidance has been related to less frequent positive events and diminished positive affect, life satisfaction, and meaning in life as well as a sense of inauthenticity or disconnection from self (Kashdan, Barrios, Forsyth, & Steger, 2006; John & Gross, 2004). Possible reasons for this relation are addressed in the present chapter.

The fact that experiential avoidance correlates so strongly with psychological symptoms across diagnostic categories suggests its usefulness in a transdiagnostic approach to psychopathology (e.g., Baer, 2007). This evidence also suggests that targeting experiential avoidance may be important in the treatment of psychological disorders characterized by an inability to persist in goal-directed behavior in the face of difficult thoughts and emotions. However, it is important to determine whether experiential avoidance is a passive correlate with negative psychological processes and outcomes or plays a more active or causal role in the development and maintenance of psychopathology. This has been examined in several ways.

Reaction to Experimentally Induced Stressors

Several researchers have considered whether experiential avoidance influences how people respond to experimentally produced stressors. For example, Karekla and colleagues (2004) examined the differences between healthy individuals who were rated as high and low experiential avoiders in response to the stress of a carbon dioxide challenge, which is used to induce symptoms of panic. Although there were no group differences in physiological arousal, the group that was high in experiential avoidance reported experiencing significantly more cognitive and physical symptoms of panic than the low experiential avoidance group. This suggests that experiential avoidance does not directly alter the physiological response to stressors so much as it alters the verbally mediated experience and psychological impact of stressful events.

A similar study gave some participants instructions to suppress their emotional responses while others were told to simply observe them (Feldner, Zvolensky, Eifert, & Spira, 2003). Participants who were higher in experiential avoidance responded with greater levels of anxiety and distress but not physiological arousal. The more avoidant group also reported greater emotional distress when asked to suppress versus observe their emotions while the less experientially avoidant group showed no such difference. This pattern seems to hold even with severe presentations such as BPD. Among a sample of women diagnosed with BPD who had had a recent hospitalization, those scoring higher on experiential avoidance were more likely than those lower in the measure to experience intrusions of an unwanted personally relevant thought when instructed to suppress the thought (Pistorello, 1998), indicating that specific emotion regulation strategies (e.g., suppression, acceptance) work differently for persons who are high or low in experiential avoidance. This supports the idea that experiential avoidance is not merely another strategy for managing emotion but actually mediates the impact of various emotion regulation strategies, a core idea that has been successfully tested in a growing number of studies (e.g., Tull & Gratz, 2008).

It is worth noting that these studies demonstrate an increase in anxiety symptomatology in healthy, nondisordered individuals, suggesting that experiential avoidance is a psychological vulnerability for, not merely a correlate or consequence of, psychopathology. This makes sense of the evidence that those high in experiential avoidance respond poorly to challenging life experiences, such as having a family member with dementia (Spira et al., 2007) or being in a war zone (Morina, 2007).

Longitudinal Studies

Another way that the possible causal role of experiential avoidance has been explored is through longitudinal studies. In longitudinal studies the presence of experiential avoidance is treated as a risk factor for later development of behavioral difficulties, which allows mere correlations to be distinguished from functionally important processes. For example, experiential avoidance predicts PTSD symptoms over a 2-month period (Marx & Sloan, 2005) and predicts deterioration of quality of life (Hayes et al., 2004), objectively assessed job errors (Bond & Bunce, 2003), number of health care center medical visits in the next 4 years among college students (Hildebrandt, Pistorello, & Hayes, 2007), and general mental health (Bond & Bunce, 2003) over a 1-year period even when controlling for other relevant variables.

Mediation of Challenges and Coping Styles

A third way to try to go beyond mere correlation is to examine the meditational role of experiential avoidance in responding to various challenges compared with other emotional regulation, coping, and psychological variables. Experiential avoidance has been shown to mediate the effects of biological stressors like physical pain or injury (McCracken et al., 2004), temperamental factors such as high emotional reactivity (Sloan, 2004), and psychosocial stressors like the violence encountered by inner-city youth (Dempsey, 2002). For example, experiential avoidance mediates the impact of anxiety sensitivity in BPD (Gratz, Tull, & Gunderson, 2008), the impact of anxiety sensitivity on depression (Tull & Gratz, 2008), and the relationship between childhood sexual abuse and psychological distress (Marx & Sloan, 2002). This mediational role suggests that specific psychological or situational challenges do not just have direct negative outcomes; rather, their negative outcomes are in part due to experientially avoidant styles of adjustment interacting with these processes and situations.

There is some evidence that experiential avoidance partially or fully mediates the impact of more formally defined emotion regulation and coping strategies. Kashdan, Elhai, and Frueh (2006) assessed the relationship between suppression or cognitive reappraisal and indices of psychological well-being and psychopathology. They found that experiential avoidance was a stronger predictor of anxiety symptomatology and emotional distress than suppression and cognitive reappraisal and a range of psychological variables, including anxiety sensitivity, uncontrollability, trait anxiety, suffocation fears, and body sensation fears. Furthermore, the relationships between alternative emotion regulation strategies and daily functioning, including positive and negative affect, life satisfaction, social anxiety, and meaning in life, were fully mediated by experiential avoidance.

These mediational data show that the presence of stressors increases the likelihood of engaging in experiential avoidance, and that the use of experientially avoidant coping further contributes to negative social, physical, and psychological effects above and beyond the direct effects of the stressor on outcome or the impact of the stressor on experiential avoidance. Stated another way, experiential avoidance is not only a core diathesis but also an actively toxic psychological process. Emotional regulation in the form of cognitive reappraisal or suppression is particularly toxic when either of these is harnessed to an experientially avoidant purpose.

Treatment Mediation and Moderation

A final way to examine experiential avoidance that goes beyond mere correlation is to look at its role as a moderator and especially as a mediator of treatment effects. Moderators predict who will respond to what treatment and mediators help to explain how a particular treatment works. Masuda and colleagues (2007) found that psychoeducation was less effective in targeting stigma toward mental illness when individuals reported higher levels of experiential avoidance. However, an ACT intervention that explicitly targets psychological flexibility was equally effective in reducing stigma regardless of participants' level of experiential avoidance. Experiential avoidance has also been shown to mediate the effects of psychological interventions explicitly aimed at reducing it, such as ACT or DBT. For example, experiential avoidance mediates the impact of ACT for diabetes (Gregg et al., 2007), smoking (Gifford et al., 2004), epilepsy (Lundgren et al., 2008), stress (Bond & Bunce, 2000), and weight control (Lillis, Hayes, Bunting, & Masuda, 2009).

A number of studies show that the AAQ and related measures have incremental validity over measures of similar constructs (Hayes et al., 2006) and indeed mediate their impact (e.g., Kashdan et al., 2006). One of the strengths of experiential avoidance is that it can be altered through psychotherapy interventions that target it in a theoretically sensible fashion, and it often mediates outcomes in these circumstances. Thus, unlike psychological variables (e.g., Big-Five personality traits) that are trait measures and relatively unresponsive to treatment, experiential avoidance is an active and modifiable treatment target.

The Theory and Philosophy Underlying Experiential Avoidance

We believe that the evidence just reviewed suggests that experiential avoidance is a particularly useful psychological concept. It correlates with most forms of psychopathology in clinical populations and with negative outcomes of all kinds in nonclinical populations; moderates the impact of treatment and other external events; mediates the impact of difficult external events, psychological variables, and a wide variety of coping styles; and mediates the impact of acceptance and mindfulness-based treatments.

In our view, the success of experiential avoidance comes from the fact that it is a concept that is deliberately designed to tap into a key cluster of inductively specified psychological processes. It is not a commonsense category, which explains why it is not measured in a commonsense way. It is an attempt to tap into core processes that reduce the psychological flexibility of people. In order to explain that idea, a deeper exploration of the approach underlying the concept is needed.

Functional Contextualism

As operationalized in the modern era, experiential avoidance is based on a behavioral analytic philosophy of science and approach to theory, which we have recently termed *contextual behavioral science* (Hayes, 2008). A contextual behavioral science adopts a functional and monistic approach to truth and meaning based on the pragmatic philosophy of functional contextualism (Hayes, 1993). This assumes that there is one, real world but many ways of successfully parsing out that world. Rather than attempting to justify the utility of our organization of the world in ontological terms, functional contextualists argue that truth is judged by the workability of analyses relative to stated goals.

Unlike the philosophies that underlie many modern psychological theories, functional contextualism looks at events holistically rather than splitting them a priori into parts, forces, and relations. All psychological events, including emotions, are considered to be the actions of whole organisms interacting with their environment in specific contexts, not simply as functions of individual systems or parts of the body. The goals of contextual behavioral science are the prediction-and-influence of psychological events with precision, scope, and depth. Precision refers to the restricted number of technical concepts that apply to a given event, scope to the ability of concepts to apply to a specified range of events, and depth to the coherence of the examination across scientific levels of analysis.

A key implication of this approach is found in the hyphens in the phrase "prediction-and-influence." In order to meet the goals of behavioral prediction *and influence* simultaneously, psychologists must provide an account that identifies manipulable contextual variables. Thus, any analysis that begins and ends in the response phase of the situated action of organisms is inherently limited. One way to say this is that what people do are always *dependent variables*. The independent variables for action will always be contextual factors because those are what can be changed directly. Emotion and cognitions are rejected as causes over other forms of psychological action not because these events do not relate in important ways, but because scientists have no means of directly altering the form or structure of a specific emotion or thought without altering contextual events (Hayes & Brownstein, 1986).

This leads to a core position that is distinctive: The goal is not to regulate or alter cognition or emotion per se but instead to alter the contexts in which cognition and emotion occur, because it is the context that accounts for the function or impact of these events. This may be one of the key differences between experiential avoidance as we conceive it currently and some common concepts in the area of emotion regulation, such as suppression, which can be linked to a variety of functions. This does not mean that emotion regulation strategies cannot be viewed functionally (e.g., Gratz & Roemer, 2004), but these concepts in general do not demand such treatment. In the case of experiential avoidance, the function is itself the concept.

Relational Frame Theory

These contexts can be understood from the point of view of traditional behavioral principles and relational frame theory (RFT; Hayes, Barnes-Holmes, & Roche, 2001). RFT is a modern behavior analytic approach to human language and cognition. Many animals can learn to relate events based on their formal properties (e.g., size, shape). For example, a child initially learns that a dime is smaller than a penny and a penny is smaller than a nickel based on physical size. Without being directly trained to do so, the child will derive other relationships based on the bidirectional (i.e., a penny is bigger than a dime and a nickel is bigger than a penny) and combinatorial (i.e., a dime is smaller than a nickel) nature of verbal relations. However, because of training by the social/verbal community (e.g., Berens & Hayes, 2007), children learn to derive such relationships based on arbitrary, nonformal stimulus properties. For example, a 4-year-old will soon learn that a dime is "bigger" than a nickel or a penny, even though it is formally smaller. The property that is being related (i.e., monetary value) is arbitrary in the sense that it is established by social convention and is not a physical aspect of the objects being related.

RFT defines verbal behavior, including higher cognition, as the action of framing events relationally. It is considered to be operant behavior that is learned through a history of multiple exemplar training (Barnes-Holmes, Barnes-Holmes, Smeets, Strand, & Friman, 2004). Relational frames develop in infancy (Lipkens, Hayes, & Hayes, 1993) based on explicit training (Luciano, Gómez, & Rodríguez, 2007) and seem to be required in order for children to develop normal language abilities (Devany, Hayes, & Nelson, 1986). There is no clear evidence that this ability can be trained in nonhumans, even in those who can use symbolic language (Hayes et al., 2001). Weakness in relational framing is associated with cognitive deficits (O'Hora, Pelaez, Barnes-Holmes, & Amesty, 2005), and training in relational framing increases higher order skills such as perspective taking and empathy (McHugh, Barnes-Holmes, & Barnes-Holmes, 2004; McHugh, Barnes-Holmes, Barnes-Holmes, & Stewart, 2006).

The meaning or psychological functions of stimuli are transformed through their participation in these relational frames. In the prior example, the dime will become more reinforcing than the nickel for a child who is looking to purchase sweets. Studies have demonstrated a range of emotional and psychological functions that transfer from one stimulus to another through relational networks. For example, if a stimulus (*B*) is repeatedly paired with an electric shock, the presentation of *B* will elicit fearful arousal and avoidance. If a person is also taught that $A < B < C$, the presentation of *C* will elicit greater physiological arousal and subjective fear, even though *C* has never been directly paired with shock (Dougher, Hamilton, Fink, & Harrington, 2007). It is this transformation of stimulus properties through relational networks that explains how objects and events can come to have powerful emotional functions even when we have no direct experience with them. Through these processes, we can fear death, loathe war, and joyfully await heaven even if we have never known these experiences directly.

Verbal and cognitive stimuli are thought to have their psychological effects through their participation in relational frames, which are regulated by both relational contextual cues that determine the nature of the relation and by functional contexts that activate the psychological functions that are relevant to an underlying derived relation (Wulfert & Hayes, 1988). The relational context (e.g., the words "bigger than" or "part of") determines how and when events are related, and the functional context (e.g., perceptual or emotional words like "taste" or "pain of") determines what functions will be transformed in terms of a relational network. For example, asking about the taste of a lemon or the pain of loss of a loved one will induce different functions than asking about the texture of a lemon or the funny memories of a person who passed. Relational responding allows humans to analyze and evaluate current situations, compare them with the past, predict potential outcomes, and generate rules for responding to a variety of novel experiences. Unfortunately, it is this very same ability that allows us to compare ourselves with other people in other situations, evaluate our efforts and outcomes as insufficient, and judge ourselves and our lives to be depressingly unsatisfactory.

Experiential avoidance thus appears on one level to be a common-sense category that is not different in kind than a wide range of terms for coping styles. However, its history and underlying theory come from a view that is focused on psychological processes and the contexts that determine their functions. This explains why the concept was operationalized as it was and why it has so readily translated into specific interventions that transcend diagnostic categories. It is designed to be a functional category, linked to manipulable and contextually embedded processes.

How Experiential Avoidance Is Learned

The bidirectional nature of language and transformation of stimulus functions means that in the right functional context knowledge of emotionally, socially, or physically painful events is itself painful. All complex organisms work to avoid or escape painful situations, but the bidirectionality of human language enormously expands that tendency for several reasons.

To begin with, painful stimulation is constantly available via relational framing. We can think about our dead loved ones anytime and anywhere. We can remember past traumas without difficulty given only happenstance cues to do so. Through relational networks, verbal events (e.g., memories, verbal reports, mental images, evaluations) related to an emotionally valenced event can take on some of the psychological functions of the event itself. Thus, a memory of combat may evoke some of the same behaviors as the actual combat experience. These behaviors may include the physiological sensations and feeling of fear, tendencies to run, hide, or attack, and the avoidance of threat cues. In this case, the remembering, feeling, and thinking about combat are themselves the threat cues.

Furthermore, sets of reactions can be drawn together by language into overarching categories. Emotions in nonverbal organisms are like adverbs: They are not things but are qualities of action that speak to what is likely to function as an important consequence in a given situation, such as when an animal who is fearful is contacting events that establish avoidance and escape as important consequences. Nonhuman animals do not fear fear as such; they fear situations. Psychologists have long known that human language and cognition changes that picture (e.g., Schachter & Singer, 1962). Verbal relations can expand such sets almost infinitely, and they can turn qualities of actions into noun-like things that can be described and avoided. Anxiety, which comes from a root word meaning difficulty in breathing, and depression, which is a construction based on a physical analogy of being squeezed down, become emotions in a new sense. This does not mean that emotions are always conscious; very often they appear to be implicit (Ruys & Stapel, 2008). However, even when they begin in an unconscious way, when they are consciously noticed, they are likely to be evaluated. Anxiety is bad. Depression is abnormal. Such evaluations lead naturally to a problem-solving mode of mind, and experiential avoidance is a name for the normal "solution" to this verbally created "problem." Unable to control pain by controlling the situation, humans naturally tend to try to control pain itself. That often requires avoidance even of positively evaluated reactions (e.g., Tull & Roemer, 2007), because what is positive could be lost, which would be negative. Eventually, *any* emotion can be a threat inside a larger pattern of experiential avoidance, and as a result even positive emotions are less likely and less welcome (Kashdan, 2007; Kashdan et al., 2006).

Language expands emotional pain and experiential avoidance still further. Humans transition from simple verbal descriptions of the internal and external world to the construction of elaborate and coherent verbal networks. Human beings tell stories, and they learn that these stories need to be internally consistent and "true" (not contradicted by "facts"). Perhaps the most elaborate story of this kind is the conceptualized self: the description of history, purpose, and results that provide a life narrative. Events that threaten the self concept can evoke strong emotions and lead to heightened experiential avoidance (Mendolia & Baker, 2008) not so much on the basis of a simple negative evaluation as on the need for consistency within the narrative. For example, joy may be avoided because a person may be entangled with the idea that previous traumas make joy impossible. Growth may be avoided because effective change would invalidate a life story. In an effort to avoid threats to the conceptualized self, ongoing knowledge of private experience (or "self-as-process") may itself be suppressed because the range of human emotion is too broad for any story or self-concept to capture, resulting in broad patterns of emotional numbing, anhedonia, alexithymia, and lack of emotional clarity (e.g., Andrew & Dulin, 2007; Kashdan, Elhai, & Frueh, 2006; Tull & Roemer, 2007).

Contexts That Support Experiential Avoidance

The capacity for experiential avoidance is built into human language and cognition and is exacerbated by specific histories and by contexts maintained by the social/verbal community. An example is a context of literality in which one treats verbal or cognitive events as if they truly are what they refer to. This context is built into many verbal interactions, and it causes people to lose sight of ongoing verbal/cognitive processes. For example, the thought "I am a failure" will be treated as if it is a representation of reality rather than an ongoing process of evaluating, comparing, and judging. When taken as the "truth," this thought may be more likely to be avoided, and relevant useful information associated with this thought (e.g., perhaps the person lost his job because he was not working collaboratively with others) may not be used to guide subsequent effective action (in this example, exploring how to work better with colleagues).

The context of reason giving also supports efforts to control and escape emotions and emotionally valenced private events. The social community demands sensible, coherent reasons for our behaviors, and private events (e.g., fatigue, social anxiety) are common acceptable reasons for why we do or do not engage in specific actions. This context of reason giving supports the notion that reasons, or verbal descriptions of events that co-occur, are, in fact, *causes* of overt behavior and are the appropriate source of behavioral regulation. Human culture uses emotional language to characterize history and context and to relate these to action. For example, we ask others what they "want." Initially, this was a crude metaphor (meaning simply that it came from the old Norse "vant," which meant "missing") that allowed the social community to access what was likely to function as a reinforcer for an individual in the absence of direct contextual and historical information. However, eventually a "want" became an "emotional state" and, furthermore, one that was causally related to action (we respond to what we want).

The trap inside this common and superficially harmless process is that if our thoughts, memories, and emotions cause our behavior, then we must logically change these in order for our behavior to change. Unfortunately, the supposedly causal private events that are entangled in "reasons" for action are often the product of our unique learning histories. The only certain way to alter them is to go back and change the past, and that is not possible. The context of experiential control is the result, in which the social/verbal community focuses on the modulation of cognitive and emotional states as a goal of successful living. In our society, being able to change one's mood or state of mind is considered to be a sign of maturity, mental health, and well-being, and a host of pills, products, and techniques are designed and sold to help us do just that.

Humans target aversive private events for change in the same ways that external events are targeted: We analyze and evaluate the situation and construct rules that specify how to act in ways that will alter the form, frequency, or intensity of these negatively evaluated events. Most of the time, efforts to solve a problem by removing harmful or unwanted aspects are quite effective. Unfortunately, the processes that allow us to evaluate a situation, predict an outcome, and generate and compare alternative responses are the same processes that make it quite unlikely that attempts to control the world inside our skin will be successful. The difficulty in distinguishing the two situations causes people to treat their own experiences as a problem to be solved. We may avoid relationships that have the potential to make us feel sad or take drugs to numb feelings of anxiety and fear, even when these efforts may prevent us from acting in ways that build valued, meaningful lives.

RFT predicts that direct attempts to regulate emotions or cognitive content are often ineffective because deliberate change involves the use of verbal rules that contain the unwanted emotions or thoughts or are based on assumptions and strategies that directly or indirectly evoke them. Checking to see whether the rule is effective necessitates contact with the aversive stimuli and thus evokes the aversive functions that were trying to be avoided. For example, the rule "Loneliness is bad and I have to get rid of it" means that I have to keep checking to see if I am feeling lonely. Because "lonely" carries some of the psychological functions of the feeling of loneliness, the very thought "Am I lonely now?" is likely to evoke the emotion I am trying to escape from. In addition, causal statements about emotionally valenced events contain stimuli that may interfere with the stated goal of the underlying rule. "I need to stop panicking or I will die" is likely to elicit anxiety, as would any event that predicts imminent death. Thus, these verbal rules can paradoxically increase the functional importance, frequency, or intensity of the very content one is trying to avoid. In some circumstances, avoidance behavior, through negative reinforcement, can further strengthen the behavior regulatory effect of the avoided private event. The avoidance behavior develops strength and is more likely to occur than other, more adaptive responses to the situation. All of these processes produce a situation in which experiential avoidance often works in the short term to reduce some discomfort but can have long-term negative effects (Baumeister, Zell, & Tice, 2007; John & Gross, 2004; Pennebaker & Chung, 2007). It must be noted that experiential avoidance in this analysis is a functional relation, not a specific form of coping or emotional regulation. Consider an emotional regulation strategy like distraction. Distraction is a form, not a function. A person who is sad could, for example, listen to a preferred song not to get rid of sadness but to appreciate the beauty of the music. When distraction had an experientially avoidant function, the present analysis would predict bad outcomes; however, when it has an appetitive function, very likely it would not. Capacity for experiential avoidance is built into human language and cognition and is exacerbated by specific histories and by contexts maintained by the social/verbal community.

Direct attempts to alter or remove cognitive or emotional content also paradoxically increase the frequency and intensity of these experiences by expanding the network of cues related to the unwanted experience. When thoughts or beliefs are suppressed in the presence of a negative emotion, a bidirectional relation is established among thought, suppression, and emotion such that the presence of one will evoke the psychological functions of the other. This results in a vicious cycle where the strategies intended to control difficult private events evoke the same aversive functions they are intended to escape from in the exact situations when it is most important to do so. Attempts to distract, soothe, or suppress are now more tightly related to the avoided emotion, thus creating more and more opportunities for the unwanted emotion to appear.

Is Experiential Avoidance Always Harmful?

Experiential avoidance, by definition, is more than simply avoiding potentially painful events or situations. Engaging in avoidance or escape behaviors when doing so is ineffective or causes additional suffering is what differentiates avoidance of aversive events from experiential avoidance. Operationalized this way, experiential avoidance as a generalized pattern is likely to be costly. However, avoidance per se may not result in these negative consequences if it is done without entanglement with rules about the necessity of removing uncomfortable events before one can behave effectively, which would lead to the overgeneralization of the strategy. In fact, avoiding negative emotions by distraction may be quite effective for some people in certain situations, and in some highly circumscribed contexts (e.g., medical paramedics' work setting) avoidance of private events may be adaptive (Mitmansgruber, Beck, & Schüssler, 2008). The trap is that this is most likely to work when the circumstances are constrained, and in many contexts it is not terribly important that the negative emotion disappear. The nature of verbal behavior seems to result in the following rule when it comes to private psychological experiences: If you're unwilling to have it, you've got it.

A key feature of experiential avoidance is that it is defined both by (1) the function of the behavior (i.e., avoidance or escape) regardless of the specific form the behavior takes and (2) the context in which the behavior occurs. Coping and regulation strategies are not effective or ineffective per se; rather, their usefulness depends on the context and flexibility with which they are used. For example, it may be quite effective or even loving to suppress one's expression of disgust when reuniting with a loved one whose body has been deformed in combat. On the other hand, avoiding social situations that evoke fears of negative evaluation may lead to isolation and loneliness, diminished positive events, and a stronger belief that one is socially inept. Problems occur when rules about how to behave reduce contact with direct environmental contingencies, making it difficult to persist or modify behavior in order to achieve long-term goals. Because language is so useful, verbal networks come to dominate over other, potentially more useful forms of behavioral control, such as direct environmental contingencies. As a result, individuals may persist in harmful or ineffective behaviors or fail to modify their actions because they are not tracking their impact on their actual environment.

The inductive, process-focused nature of this account of how experiential avoidance develops provides a set of ways of assessing, via a self-report instrument, contexts that might induce a more rigid and overextended use of experiential avoidance as an adjustment strategy. Experiential avoidance measures include cognitive fusion items, such as the one listed earlier, because these are proxies for more literal contexts that support control of psychological events. They also include evaluation items (e.g., from the AAQ: "Anxiety is bad") because they tap into the core relational processes that evoke inwardly focused problem-solving attempts; sense-making items (e.g., from the AAQ: "I often catch myself daydreaming about things I've done and what I would do differently next time") because they are proxies for contexts of reason giving and social explanation; and action items (e.g., a reverse-scored item from the AAQ: "I am able to take action on a problem even if I am uncertain what is the right thing to do") because these tap into the functional contexts that determine the impact of private events. Thus, experiential avoidance is not so much a trait as a window into the contextual features that turn the core of human language from an asset into a rigid hindrance. Indeed, the term *psychological flexibility* is now commonly used to describe the broad set of features assessed by instruments such as the AAQ (Hayes et al., 2006). Psychological flexibility is defined as the ability to fully contact the present moment and the thoughts and feelings it contains without needless defense and, depending on what the situation affords, persisting or changing in behavior in the pursuit of goals and values (Hayes et al., 2006). As can be seen, this is in essence a restatement of the concept of experiential avoidance but in terms that make it easier to see why the elements that are assessed by experiential avoidance measures are present. These differences are terminological, not substantive, which is why they have not been given a great deal of attention in this chapter, but over time psychological flexibility will undoubtedly be more important as a general label at least within the ACT community.

The evolution of the concept of experiential avoidance is consistent with evidence highlighting the importance of context, function, and flexible responding in the effectiveness of emotion regulation strategies more generally. It appears that the inflexible application of emotion regulation strategies has a greater impact on effectiveness than the strategies themselves (Bonnano, Papa, Lalande, Westphal, & Coifman, 2004), and emotionally avoidant and controlling coping strategies are more likely to be applied rigidly, independent of the current context (Folkman et al., 1986). Experientially avoidant strategies also appear to be highly resistant to extinction (Luciano et al., 2008) and so are less likely to be abandoned in favor of more workable strategies. Thus, although experiential avoidance might work in some situations, the strategy is likely to become overlearned and generalized to contexts where experiential avoidance is ineffective or even harmful.

Some forms of psychopathology have been associated with the rigid application of avoidant emotion regulation strategies. For example, depressed persons are less sensitive to emotional contexts and show less reactivity to both positive and negative emotional stimuli (Rottenberg, Gross, & Gotlib, 2005) and behavioral rigidity in tasks that require adapting one's responses to shifting contingencies (Hopkinson & Neuringer, 2003). Furthermore, the flexibility with which one applies attributions is more predictive of depressive symptoms and response to treatment than the actual content of cognitive schemas (Moore & Fresco, 2007). This kind of cognitive flexibility moderates the relationship between negative life events and depression, even after controlling for the influence of attributional style and the interaction between attributional style and negative life events (Moore & Fresco, 2007). It is possible that other forms of psychopathology may be related to the inflexible use of experiential avoidant strategies.

It is the elements themselves, not the terms, that are the key, however. The functional and contextual focus of the experiential avoidance concept helps explain from a theoretical point of view why it is distinct as a psychological concept in comparison to more topographically defined emotion regulation strategies.

Experiential Avoidance as a Transdiagnostic, Functional Dimensional Approach to Psychopathology

Psychological problems have traditionally been classified syndromally, based on collections of topographically defined co-occurring symptoms, as exemplified by the *Diagnostic and Statistical Manual of Mental Disorders* (DSM; e.g., American Psychiatric Association, 1994). It has been presumed that the identification of syndromes would lead to an understanding of a common cause, known course, and response to treatment that could guide clinicians in choosing effective assessment and treatment techniques. This system has led to a proliferation of new syndromes and techniques to manage them, but comorbidity rates remain high, and clinicians are faced with the daunting task of learning myriad new techniques and unwieldy treatment packages targeted at specific diagnoses with no basis for applying this knowledge to new situations or novel combinations of symptoms.

The report of the American Psychiatric Association planning committee for the fifth version of the DSM (Kupfer, First, & Regier, 2002) is extremely harsh in its evaluation of the current system (in all cases emphasis is added):

> The goal of validating these syndromes and discovering common causes has remained elusive. Despite many proposed candidates, *not one* laboratory marker has been found to be specific in identifying *any* of the DSM defined syndromes. (p. xviii)

> Epidemiological and clinical studies have shown extremely high rates of comorbidities among disorders, thus undermining the hypothesis that the syndromes represent distinct etiologies. Furthermore, epidemiological studies have shown a high degree of short term diagnostic instability for many disorders. With regard to treatment, lack of specificity is the rule rather than the exception. (p. xviii)

> Many, if not most, conditions and symptoms represent a somewhat arbitrarily defined pathological excess of normal behaviors and cognitive processes. This problem has led to the criticism that the system pathologizes ordinary experiences of the human condition. (p. 2)

> Researchers' *slavish* adoption of DSM-IV definitions may have *hindered* research in the etiology of mental disorders. (p. xix)

> Reification of DSM-IV entities, to the point that they are considered to be equivalent to diseases, is more likely to *obscure than to elucidate* research findings. (p. xix)

> All these limitations in the current diagnostic paradigm suggest that research exclusively focused on refining the DSM-defined syndromes may *never* be successful in uncovering their underlying etiologies. For that to happen, an as yet unknown paradigm shift may need to occur. (p. xix)

An alternative to syndromal classification is a system that inductively derives functional classes from direct observations of the phenomenon of interest and the context in which it occurs. Functional diagnostic dimensions could, in principle, have considerably more clinical utility because they identify which variables influence the behavior of interest and should be targeted for assessment and intervention. Such dimensions cut across traditional diagnostic categories, allow for the integration of data from different theoretical orientations, and identify pathological processes that inform treatment decisions (Hayes et al., 1996; Harvey, Watkins, Mansell, & Shafran, 2004). Twelve years ago we described experiential avoidance as a possible example of a functional dimension within psychopathology. At that time the evidence was quite limited. Today it is much more substantial, and so far everything indicates that experiential avoidance is indeed moving toward such a status.

Experiential avoidance is already part of the diagnostic criteria for many of the current syndromal disorders in the DSM (fourth edition, text revision; American Psychiatric Association, 2000). For example, the first criterion for BPD is "frantic efforts to avoid real *or imagined* abandonment" (American Psychiatric Association, 2000, p. 710; emphasis added) and criterion C for PTSD consists of "persistent avoidance of stimuli associated with the trauma" (p. 468). These disorders are conceptualized to be so dissimilar (e.g., one is thought of as a collection of long-standing maladaptive personality traits and the other is considered to be a response to a tragic, aversive event) that they are placed on different axes in the current syndromal classification system. From a functional dimensional perspective, these topographically distinct collections of behaviors (e.g., deliberate self-harm and suicidality in BPD; hypervigilance and dissociation in PTSD) can be seen as reasonable, though ultimately ineffective, attempts to alter, avoid, or escape from aversive private events (e.g., perceived criticism by others and fears of abandonment in BPD and traumatic memories and associated bodily sensations in PTSD). The alternative is to create therapeutic interventions that aim to decrease common core processes such as experiential avoidance (e.g., Gratz & Gunderson, 2006; Linehan, 1993). To date, every syndrome or disorder known to relate to experiential avoidance when tested has been shown to be responsive to interventions that target it (Hayes et al., 2006). That is a significant step forward in our field. Whether we will begin to speak dimensionally of "experiential avoidance disorders" is not yet known, but the existing data provide a basis to do so.

The transdiagnostic movement has a risk of perpetuating the same "topographical error" as syndromes, however. For example, we know that worry, rumination, and automatic negative thoughts are common trans-diagnostic patterns (Gruber, Eidelman, & Harvey, 2008). Although these categories can be spoken of broadly as emotion regulation strategies, they are themselves forms of action, not functions. When the *function* of worry and rumination is examined closely, it turns out that their pernicious impact depends in part on experiential avoidance as a function (e.g., Cribb, Moulds, & Carter, 2006; Santanello & Gardner, 2007).

The Relationship between Experiential Avoidance and Emotion Regulation

Throughout the chapter, we have addressed whether experiential avoidance should be viewed as simply another emotion regulation strategy. It seems superficially possible to do so, and some have explicitly made that claim (Hofmann & Asmundson, 2008), but the fit is difficult for philosophical, theoretical, and empirical reasons.

The difficulty can be illustrated by the fact that experiential avoidance can be conceptualized to involve *all* of the families of emotion regulation, as specified by Gross (1998): situation selection, situation modification, attentional deployment, cognitive change, and response modulation. Indeed, there is empirical evidence for every such relationship.

Individuals may attempt to regulate their emotions by selecting situations that are likely to induce positive emotions and avoiding situations that are likely to cause distress (e.g., engaging in a hobby for hours rather than working on a difficult writing project). One may also attempt to modify the situation in ways that minimize the likelihood of experiencing emotional distress, as when a socially anxious client insists that a supportive friend must stay by his side in order to remain at a party. Some of the action items in the AAQ are explicitly focused on situational selection and modification, and such processes are included in the definition of the concept. Overt avoidance of situations is known to correlate with measures of experiential avoidance such as the AAQ (e.g., Cribb et al., 2006).

The intrapersonal attempts to regulate emotion (e.g., attentional control, cognitive change) have received a great deal of attention in the experiential avoidance literature. As described earlier, it is often impossible for humans to select or modify distressing situations because the bidirectional nature of language allows private events (e.g., thoughts, feelings, memories, sensations) themselves to become emotionally evocative through classical conditioning and through the transformation of stimulus functions. This means that individuals must avoid awareness of any thoughts, sensations, or memories that may occasion negative emotions through distraction and inattention to events occurring in the present moment. Individuals who are unable to track the stream of ongoing cognitive and emotional responses are less able to effectively adapt their responses to an ever-changing environment. This strategy can become overlearned, resulting in problems such as anhedonia, alexithymia, and dissociation. This probably explains why such problems are empirically linked to experiential avoidance (e.g., Andrew & Dulin, 2007; Hayes et al., 2006).

Avoidant concentration is another attentional deployment strategy intended to regulate emotions and is exemplified by the excessive worry and rumination characteristic of many mood and anxiety disorders. Individuals may spend a great deal of time analyzing and replaying past events or planning and rehearsing future events in an attempt to prevent the recurrence of emotional distress. Evidence suggests that rumination and worry have effects similar to other experientially avoidant strategies, namely that they increase negative affect, decrease positive affect, and generate greater depression, which are consistent with an experiential avoidance perspective (McLaughlin, Borkovec, & Sibrava, 2007). Measures of experiential avoidance such as the AAQ correlate with worry and mediate the effect of other psychological vulnerabilities on worry (e.g., Roemer & Orsillo, 2007; Santello & Gardner, 2007).

Emotion regulation strategies intended to change our beliefs and expectations about emotions have also received a great deal of attention in the laboratory and in the therapy room. Gross and Thompson define cognitive change as "how we appraise the situation we are in to alter its emotional significance, either by changing how we think about the situation or about our capacity to manage the demands it poses" (2007, p. 14). Individuals will often attempt to suppress negative beliefs about emotions (e.g., "I can't handle another moment of this panic") and replace them with new thoughts (e.g., "It's just an emotion; it can't hurt me"). In spite of great effort to alter these thoughts, beliefs and expectancies about emotions often persist even in the face of contradictory evidence. As described previously, RFT predicts that attempts to control or suppress emotional and cognitive *content* paradoxically are likely to result in an increase in frequency and intensity of these same events, a result that has been repeatedly supported in the literature (e.g., Gross & John, 2003; Wegner, 1994).

There are healthy forms of cognitive change from the point of view of relational frame theory. For example, the flexibility to think of problems in multiple ways without having to decide necessarily which one is truth with a capital T is often helpful and indeed can be part of what is meant by cognitive reappraisal. Psychoeducation when information is truly lacking can also be helpful from this point of view. Thus, it is not surprising that cognitive change methods of emotional regulation can be mediated by experiential avoidance (Kashdan et al., 2006).

Response-focused emotional regulation strategies include the suppression or alteration of behavioral responses to an emotion. These include attempts to control verbal reports (e.g., denying that one is experiencing intense fear), affective behaviors (e.g., suppressing the urge to cry), and physiological responses (e.g., trying to hold one's hand steady when feeling anxious). Again, a variety of response-based methods of emotional regulation are known to relate to experiential avoidance (e.g., Chapman, Gratz, & Brown, 2006).

Thus, although topographically distinct, emotional regulation strategies can be, and often are, attempts to avoid, escape from, or reduce the frequency or intensity of aversive emotions. Experiential avoidance is not a *form* of emotional regulation; it is a common pathological *function* of particular emotional regulation strategies for many people in many contexts. Regardless of the method used, the empirical literature so far fits with an approach based on ACT and RFT: Whenever a given method of emotional regulation has an experiential avoidance function, that method is associated with greater psychopathology and life restriction. That same strategy, used for another function, is likely to have a different outcome. Return, for example, to the person suppressing a disgust reaction when seeing a disfigured loved one out of compassion and caring for his or her well-being. In this case, suppression is not focused on disgust as an emotion, and it is not reinforced by the removal of disgust. It is highly situated and is unlikely to generalize to other contexts in an unhealthy way. It may still be suppression, but its function is not experientially avoidant, and it is thus unlikely to have pernicious effects.

This points to a more general problem in treating functional contextual processes as if they are entities, especially entities that are described in commonsense categories. Experiential avoidance is built on a model of psychology that holds lightly all categories until they are shown to be useful in accomplishing the purpose of predicting and influencing with precision, scope, and depth the actions of whole organisms interacting in and with a context defined historically and situationally. From an RFT perspective, both for the scientist and the individual, "emotion" is not a thing but a verbal construction that is related to a set of situational aspects, bodily sensations, behavioral predispositions, states of reinforcability, thoughts, and so on. Indeed, fusion with the very idea of emotion as a causal event is part of the process that experiential avoidance views as problematic so it would be an irony to allow an ontological sense of these terms to enter into the analysis. Human "emotion" is far from the simpler set of events occurring under the label "emotion" in the nonhuman literature. Given the long history of definitional problems of emotion and the way in which emotional struggles dominate over human action inside the contexts created by human language and cognition, those who are following a contextual behavioral science approach would prefer to focus on process, function, and context.

It is probably helpful in the emotional regulation literature to define emotion as "a person-situation interaction that compels attention, has particular meaning to the individual, and gives rise to a coordinated yet flexible multisystem response to the ongoing person-situation transaction" (Gross & Thompson, 2007, p. 5). Nevertheless, it should be remembered that when we speak of emotion we are part of the very context in which attention can be compelled, in which meaning is provided, and in which action can occur. When an individual partitions an aspect of their inter-action with the world into a category as powerful as "emotion," it brings into the situation all the evaluative baggage the social/verbal community provides to such events. Experiential avoidance is part of that baggage for some individuals and even some cultures (e.g., Butler, Lee, & Gross, 2007). We cannot solve the problem by failing to speak of emotion, but neither do we solve it by reifying emotions into things.

Properly constituted, the current interest in emotion regulation could be a welcome step toward the development of a psychological science more adequate to the challenges of the human condition. The recent upsurge in research on emotion regulation (1) acknowledges the important role of motivation and of private events in human functioning, (2) focuses less on the form or type of specific emotions and more on function, (3) recognizes the role of context in determining the impact of an emotional response, and (4) looks for underlying etiological and maintaining fac-tors across different disorders. These are welcome by those in the field who advocate a functional contextual approach to conceptualizing psy-chological problems, because they are more likely to result in principle-based technologies that are more easily trained and applied to a variety of forms of psychopathology. However, a framework that focuses primarily on emotion regulation may yet have some limitations for understanding and treating the many forms of human suffering, especially if taken too literally.

A wide variety of private events—thoughts, beliefs, memories, sensa-tions, and perceptions—play an important role in the development and maintenance of psychopathology. Emotion needs to be on this list as well, but not because it is a special class of psychological event that has different sources of control and requires new theories and technologies to address these differences. Human emotions, although phenomenologically distinct from other forms of psychological events, are an amalgam of response fea-tures and should be seen through the filter of the same behavioral princi-ples and sources of control as many other types of human action. We need parsimonious theories and efficient treatments that address the impact of the full range of private and public psychological events and our attempts to regulate them.

It is even possible that therapy systems that promote the regulation of emotion as a treatment outcome may inadvertently support the context of control of private experience. For this reason, we tend not to frame treat-ment targets in terms of emotion regulation per se, although reductions in the intensity or frequency of emotional responses may indeed correlate with reductions in experiential avoidance. An approach more consistent with our philosophical and theoretical stance would be closer to that of self-regulation, such as "the ability to direct behavior toward the achieve-ment of one's goals in the presence of emotional responses."

Conclusion

In the present chapter, we have demonstrated how the capacity for experiential avoidance is built into human language and cognition and is exacerbated by specific learning histories and by contexts maintained by the social/verbal community. We have reviewed the evidence that experiential avoidance correlates with most forms of psychopathology in clinical populations and with decreased functioning and life satisfaction in nonclinical populations; moderates the impact of life events and the effectiveness of treatment; mediates the impact of stressful situations, psychological variables, and emotion regulation strategies; and mediates the impact of acceptance and mindfulness-based treatments. We have also argued that experiential avoidance is not merely an emotion regulation strategy but rather a *function* that mediates the impact of stressful life events and various forms of emotion regulation. It is this emphasis on context, function, and flexible responding that makes experiential avoidance such a useful concept in a transdiagnostic approach to psychopathology.

Experiential avoidance is arguably one of the most toxic and yet one of the most pervasive behavioral functions known in psychology. Every year the encouragement of experiential avoidance in the media and modern culture grows, and at the same time we are creating a world that is more and more filled with emotionally difficult material. Modern technology supports the idea that any discomfort is an intolerable inconvenience that can, and should, be removed. Judgment, objectification, and alienation have become "reality"-based entertainment. We are constantly bombarded through the news with horrific images of interpersonal violence and death. Together, these factors create a recipe for human suffering. We need to create modern minds better suited for health and success in the modern world, and doing so means creating a culture that is more accepting, mindful, and values based. The crude culture of feel-goodism is doing no one, whether it be our clients or ourselves, any good.

References

American Psychiatric Association. (1994). *Diagnostic and statistical manual of mental disorders* (4th ed.). Washington, DC: Author.

American Psychiatric Association. (2000). *Diagnostic and statistical manual of mental disorders* (4th ed., text rev.). Washington, DC: Author.

Andrew, D., & Dulin, P. (2007). The relationship between self-reported health and mental health problems among older adults in New Zealand: Experiential avoidance as a moderator. *Aging and Mental Health, 11*(5), 596–603.

Baer, R. A. (2007). Mindfulness, assessment, and transdiagnostic processes. *Psychological Inquiry, 18*(4), 238–271.

Baer, R. A., Smith, G. T., Hopkins, J., Krietemeyer, J., & Toney, L. (2006). Using self-report assessment methods to explore facets of mindfulness. *Assessment,* *13*(1), 27–45.

Barlow, D. H., Allen, L. B., & Choate, M. L. (2004). Toward a unified treatment for emotional disorders. *Behavior Therapy, 35,* 205–230.

Barnes-Holmes, Y., Barnes-Holmes, D., Smeets, P. M., Strand, P., & Friman, P. (2004). Establishing relational responding in accordance with more-than and less-than as generalized operant behavior in young children. *International Journal of Psychology and Psychological Therapy, 4,* 531–558.

Baumeister, R. F., Zell, A. L., & Tice, D. M. (2007). How emotions facilitate and impair self-regulation. In J. J. Gross (Ed.), *Handbook of emotion regulation* (pp. 408–426). New York: Guilford Press.

Berens, N. M., & Hayes, S. C. (2007). Arbitrarily applicable comparative relations: Experimental evidence for a relational operant. *Journal of Applied Behavior Analysis, 40,* 45–71.

Bond, F. W., & Bunce, D. (2000). Mediators of change in emotion-focused and problem-focused worksite stress management interventions. *Journal of Occupational Health Psychology, 5,* 156–163.

Bond, F. W., & Bunce, D. (2003). The role of acceptance and job control in mental health, job satisfaction, and work performance. *Journal of Applied Psychology, 88,* 1057–1067.

Bond, F. W., Hayes, S. C., Baer, R. A., Carpenter, K., Orcutt, H. K., Waltz, T., et al. (2008). *Preliminary psychometric properties of the Acceptance and Action Questionnaire-II: A revised measure of psychological flexibility and acceptance.* Manuscript submitted for publication.

Bonnano, G. A., Papa, A., Lalande, K., Westphal, M., & Coifman, K. (2004). The importance of being flexible: The ability to both enhance and suppress emotional expression predicts long-term adjustment. *Psychological Science, 15,* 482–487.

Brown, R. A., Lejuez, C. W., Kahler, C. W., & Strong, D. (2002). Distress tolerance and duration of past smoking cessation attempts. *Journal of Abnormal Psychology, 111,* 180–185.

Butler, E. A., Lee, T. L., & Gross, J. J. (2007). Emotion regulation and culture: Are the social consequences of emotion suppression culture-specific? *Emotion, 7*(1), 30–48.

Chapman, A., Gratz, K., & Brown, M. (2006). Solving the puzzle of deliberate self-harm: The experiential avoidance model. *Behaviour Research and Therapy, 44*(3), 371–394.

Chawla, N., & Ostafin, B. (2007). Experiential avoidance as a functional dimensional approach to psychopathology: An empirical review. *Journal of Clinical Psychology, 63,* 871–890.

Cochrane, A., Barnes-Holmes, D., Barnes-Holmes, Y., Stewart, I., & Luciano, C. (2007). Experiential avoidance and aversive visual images: Response delays and event related potentials on a simple matching task. *Behaviour Research and Therapy, 45,* 1379–1388.

Cribb, G., Moulds, M., & Carter, S. (2006). Rumination and experiential avoidance in depression. *Behaviour Change, 23*(3), 165–176.

Daughters, S. B., Lejuez, C. W., Kahler, C., Strong, D., & Brown, R. (2005). Psychological distress tolerance and duration of most recent abstinence attempt among residential treatment seeking substance abusers. *Psychology of Addictive Behaviors, 19*(2), 208–211.

Daughters, S. B., Lejuez, C. W., Strong, D. R., Brown, R. A., Breen, R. B., & Lesieur, H. R. (2005). The relationship among negative affect, distress tolerance, and length of gambling abstinence attempt. *Journal of Gambling Studies, 21*(4), 363–378.

Dempsey, M. (2002). Negative coping as a mediator in the relation between violence and outcomes in inner-city African American youth. *American Journal of Orthopsychiatry, 72*, 102–109.

Devany, J. M., Hayes, S. C., & Nelson, R. O. (1986). Equivalence class formation in language-able and language-disabled children. *Journal of the Experimental Analysis of Behavior, 46*, 243–257.

Dougher, M. J., Hamilton, D. A., Fink, B. C., & Harrington, J. (2007). Transformation of the discriminative and eliciting functions of generalized relational stimuli. *Journal of the Experimental Analysis of Behavior, 88*, 179–197.

Dugas, M. J., Freeston, M. H., & Ladouceur, R. (1997). Intolerance of uncertainty and problem orientation in worry. *Cognitive Therapy and Research, 21*, 593–606.

Feldner, M. T., Zvolensky, M. J., Eifert, G. H., & Spira, A. P. (2003). Emotional avoidance: An experimental test of individual differences and response suppression using biological challenge. *Behaviour Research and Therapy, 41*, 401–411.

Foa, E. B., Steketee, G., & Young, M. C. (1984). Agoraphobia: Phenomenological aspects, associated characteristics, and theoretical considerations. *Clinical Psychology Review, 4*, 431–457.

Freud, A. (1937). *The ego and the mechanisms of defense.* London: Hogarth Press.

Gifford, E. V., Kohlenberg, B. S., Hayes, S. C., Antonuccio, D. O., Piasecki, M. M., Rasmussen-Hall, M. L., et al. (2004). Acceptance theory-based treatment for smoking cessation: An initial trial of acceptance and commitment therapy. *Behavior Therapy, 35*, 689–705.

Gratz, K. L., & Gunderson, J. G. (2006). Preliminary data on acceptance-based emotion regulation group intervention for deliberate self-harm among women with borderline personality disorder. *Behavior Therapy, 37*, 25–35.

Gratz, K. L., & Roemer, L. (2004). Multidimensional assessment of emotion regulation and dysregulation: Development, factor structure, and initial validation of the Difficulties in Emotion Regulation Scale. *Journal of Psychopathology and Behavioral Assessment, 26*, 41–54.

Gratz, K. L., Rosenthal, M. Z., Tull, M. T., Lejuez, C. W., & Gunderson, J. G. (2006). An experimental investigation of emotion dysregulation in borderline personality disorder. *Journal of Abnormal Psychology, 115*(4), 850–855.

Gratz, K., Tull, M., & Gunderson, J. (2008). Preliminary data on the relationship between anxiety sensitivity and borderline personality disorder: The role of experiential avoidance. *Journal of Psychiatric Research, 42*(7), 550–559.

Greco, L., Lambert, W., & Baer, R. (2008). Psychological inflexibility in childhood and adolescence: Development and evaluation of the Avoidance and Fusion Questionnaire for Youth. *Psychological Assessment, 20*(2), 93–102.

Greenberg, L. S., & Safran J. D. (1989). Emotion in psychotherapy. *American Psychologist, 44*, 19–29.

Gregg, J. A., Callaghan, G. M., Hayes, S. C., & Glenn-Lawson, J. L. (2007). Improving diabetes self-management through acceptance, mindfulness, and values:

A randomized controlled trial. *Journal of Consulting and Clinical Psychology, 75*(2), 336–343.

Gross, J. J. (1998). The emerging field of emotion regulation: An integrative review. *Review of General Psychology, 2*, 271–299.

Gross, J. J., & John, O. P. (2003). Individual differences in two emotion regulation processes: Implications for affect, relationships, and well-being. *Journal of Personality and Social Psychology, 85*, 348–362.

Gross, J. J., & Thompson, R. A. (2007). Emotion regulation: Conceptual foundations. In J. J. Gross (Ed.), *Handbook of emotion regulation* (pp. 3–25). New York: Guilford Press.

Gruber, J., Eidelman, P., & Harvey, A. G. (2008). Transdiagnostic emotion regulation processes in bipolar disorder and insomnia. *Behaviour Research and Therapy, 46*, 1096–1100.

Harvey, A., Watkins, E., Mansell, W., & Shafran, R. (2004). *Cognitive behavioural processes across psychological disorders: A transdiagnostic approach to research and treatment.* New York: Oxford University Press.

Hayes, S. C. (1993). Analytic goals and varieties of scientific contextualism. In S. C. Hayes, L. J. Hayes, H. W. Reese, & T. R. Sarbin (Eds.), *Varieties of scientific contextualism* (pp. 11–27). Reno, NV: Context Press.

Hayes, S. C. (2004). Acceptance and commitment therapy, relational frame theory, and the third wave of behavioral and cognitive therapies. *Behavior Therapy, 35*, 639–665.

Hayes, S. C. (2008). Climbing our hills: A beginning conversation on the comparison of ACT and traditional CBT. *Clinical Psychology: Science and Practice, 15*, 286–295.

Hayes, S. C., Barnes-Holmes, D., & Roche, B. (2001). *Relational frame theory: A post-Skinnerian account of human language and cognition.* New York: Kluwer Academic/Plenum Press.

Hayes, S. C., & Brownstein, A. J. (1986). Mentalism, behavior-behavior relations and a behavior analytic view of the purposes of science. *The Behavior Analyst, 9*, 175–190.

Hayes, S. C., Luoma, J. B., Bond, F. W., Masuda, A., & Lillis, J. (2006). Acceptance and commitment therapy: Model, processes and outcomes. *Behavior Research and Therapy, 44*, 1–25.

Hayes, S. C., & Melancon, S. M. (1989). Comprehensive distancing, paradox, and the treatment of emotional avoidance. In M. Ascher (Ed.), *Paradoxical procedures in psychotherapy* (pp. 184–218). New York: Guilford Press.

Hayes, S. C., Strosahl, K., & Wilson, K. G. (1999). *Acceptance and commitment therapy: An experiential approach to behavior change.* New York: Guilford Press.

Hayes, S. C., Strosahl, K. D., Wilson, K. G., Bissett, R. T., Pistorello, J., Toarmino, D., et al. (2004). Measuring experiential avoidance: A preliminary test of a working model. *Psychological Record, 54*, 553–578.

Hayes, S. C., & Wilson, K.G. (1994). Acceptance and commitment therapy: Altering the verbal support for experiential avoidance. *The Behavior Analyst, 17*, 289–303.

Hayes, S. C., Wilson, K. G., Gifford, E. V., Follette, V. M., & Strosahl, K. (1996). Experiential avoidance and behavioral disorders: A functional dimensional approach to diagnosis and treatment. *Journal of Consulting and Clinical Psychology, 64*(6), 1152–1168.

Hildebrandt, M. J., Pistorello, J., & Hayes, S. C. (2007, May). *Predicting student attrition and healthcare utilization: Examining the role of experiential avoidance.* Paper presented at the annual meeting of the Association for Behavior Analysis, San Diego, CA.

Hofmann, S. G., & Asmundson, G. J. G. (2008). Acceptance and mindfulness-based therapy: New wave or old hat? *Clinical Psychology Review, 28,* 1–16.

Hopkinson, J., & Neuringer, A. (2003). Modifying behavioral variability in moderately depressed students. *Behavior Modification, 27,* 251–264.

Jacobson, N. S., & Christensen, A. (1996). *Integrative couple therapy: Promoting acceptance and change.* New York: Norton.

John, O. P., & Gross, J. J. (2004). Healthy and unhealthy emotion regulation: Personality processes, individual differences, and lifespan development. *Journal of Personality, 72,* 1301–1333.

Kabat-Zinn, J. (1990). *Full catastrophe living: Using the wisdom of your body and mind to face stress, pain and illness.* New York: Bantam Doubleday Dell.

Karekla, M., Forsyth, J. P., & Kelly, M. M. (2004). Emotional avoidance and panicogenic responding to a biological challenge procedure. *Behavior Therapy, 35,* 725–746.

Kashdan, T. B. (2007). Social anxiety spectrum and diminished positive experiences: Theoretical synthesis and meta-analysis. *Clinical Psychology Review, 27,* 348–365.

Kashdan, T. B., Barrios, V., Forsyth, J. P., & Steger, M. F. (2006). Experiential avoidance as a generalized psychological vulnerability: Comparisons with coping and emotion regulation strategies. *Behavior Research and Therapy, 44,* 1301–1320.

Kashdan, T. B., Elhai, J. D., & Frueh, B. C. (2006). Anhedonia and emotional numbing in combat veterans with PTSD. *Behaviour Research and Therapy, 44,* 457–467.

Kupfer, D. J., First, M. B., & Regier, D. A. (2002). *A research agenda for DSM-V.* Washington, DC: American Psychiatric Association.

Lillis, J., & Hayes, S. C. (2008). Measuring avoidance and inflexibility in weight related problems. *International Journal of Behavioral Consultation and Therapy, 4,* 30–40.

Lillis, J., Hayes, S. C., Bunting, K., & Masuda, A. (2009). Teaching acceptance and mindfulness to improve the lives of the obese: A preliminary test of a theoretical model. *Annals of Behavioral Medicine, 37*(1), 58–69.

Linehan, M. M. (1993). *Cognitive-behavioral treatment for borderline personality disorder.* New York: Guilford Press.

Lipkens, R., Hayes, S. C., & Hayes, L. J. (1993). Longitudinal study of the development of derived relations in an infant. *Journal of Experimental Child Psychology, 56,* 201–239.

Luciano, C. M., Valdivia-Salas, S., Ruiz-Jimenez, F. J., Cabello Luque, F., Barnes-Holmes, D., Dougher, M. J., et al. (2008, May). *The effect of several strategies in altering avoidance to direct and derived avoidance stimuli.* Paper presented at the 34th Annual Conference of the Association for Behavior Analysis, Chicago.

Luciano, M. C., Gómez, I., & Rodríguez, M. (2007). The role of multiple-exemplar training and naming in establishing derived equivalence in an infant. *Journal of Experimental Analysis of Behavior, 87,* 349–365.

Lundgren, T., Dahl, J., & Hayes, S. C. (2008). Evaluation of mediators of change in the treatment of epilepsy with acceptance and commitment therapy. *Journal of Behavioral Medicine, 31*, 225–235.

Marx, B. P., & Sloan, D. M. (2002). The role of emotion in the psychological functioning of adult survivors of childhood sexual abuse. *Behavior Therapy, 33*(4), 563–577.

Marx, B. P., & Sloan, D. M. (2005). Peritraumatic dissociation and experiential avoidance as predictors of posttraumatic stress symptomatology. *Behaviour Research and Therapy, 43*, 569–583.

Masuda, A., Hayes, S. C., Fletcher, L. B., Seignourel, P. J., Bunting, K., Herbst, S. A., et al. (2007). The impact of acceptance and commitment therapy versus education on stigma toward people with psychological disorders. *Behaviour Research and Therapy, 45*(11), 2764–2772.

McCracken, L. M., Vowles, K. E., & Eccleston, C. (2004). Acceptance of chronic pain: Component analysis and a revised assessment method. *Pain, 107*(1–2), 159–166.

McHugh, L., Barnes-Holmes, D., & Barnes-Holmes, Y. (2004). Perspective taking as relational responding: A developmental profile. *Psychological Record, 54*, 115–144.

McHugh, L., Barnes-Holmes, Y., Barnes-Holmes, D., & Stewart, I. (2006). Understanding false belief as generalized operant behavior. *Psychological Record, 56*, 341–364.

McLaughlin, K. A., Borkovec, T. D., & Sibrava, N. J. (2007). The effects of worry and rumination on affect states and cognitive activity. *Behavior Therapy, 38*, 23–38.

Mendolia, M., & Baker, G. A. (2008). Attentional mechanisms associated with repressive distancing. *Journal of Research in Personality, 42*, 546–563.

Mitmansgruber, H., Beck, T. , & Schüssler, G. (2008). "Mindful helpers": Experiential avoidance, meta-emotions, and emotion regulation in paramedics. *Journal of Research in Personality, 42*, 1358–1363.

Moore, M. T., & Fresco, D. M. (2007). The relationship of explanatory flexibility to explanatory style. *Behavior Therapy, 38*, 325–332.

Morina, N. (2007). The role of experiential avoidance in psychological functioning after war-related stress in Kosovar civilians. *Journal of Nervous and Mental Disease, 195*(8), 697–700.

O'Hora, D., Pelaez, M., Barnes-Holmes, D., & Amesty, L. (2005). Derived relational responding and human language: Evidence from the WAIS-III. *Psychological Record, 55*, 155–174.

Pennebaker, J. W., & Chung, C. K. (2007). Expressive writing, emotional upheavals, and health. In H. Friedman & R. Silver (Eds.), *Handbook of health psychology* (pp. 263–284). New York: Oxford University Press.

Pistorello, J. (1998). *Acceptance, suppression, and monitoring of an unwanted thought among women diagnosed with borderline personality disorder.* Unpublished doctoral dissertation, University of Nevada at Reno.

Roemer, L., & Orsillo, S. (2007). An open trial of an acceptance-based behavior therapy for generalized anxiety disorder. *Behavior Therapy, 38*(1), 72–85.

Roemer, L., & Orsillo, S. M. (2009). *Mindfulness- and acceptance-based behavioral therapies in practice.* New York: Guilford Press.

Rogers, C. A. (1961). *On becoming a person: A therapist's view of psychotherapy.* Boston: Houghton Mifflin.

Rottenberg, J., Gross, J. J., & Gotlib, I. H. (2005). Emotion context insensitivity in major depressive disorder. *Journal of Abnormal Psychology, 114*, 627–629.

Ruys, K. I., & Stapel, D. A. (2008). The secret life of emotions. *Psychological Science, 19*, 385–391.

Sandoz, E. K., & Wilson, K. G. (2006). *Assessing body image acceptance.* Unpublished manuscript, University of Mississippi.

Santanello, A., & Gardner, F. (2007). The role of experiential avoidance in the relationship between maladaptive perfectionism and worry. *Cognitive Therapy and Research, 31*(3), 319–332.

Schachter, S., & Singer, J. (1962). Cognitive, social, and physiological determinants of emotional state. *Psychological Review, 69*, 379–399.

Segal, Z. V., Williams, J. M. G., & Teasdale, J. D. (2002). *Mindfulness-based cognitive therapy for depression: A new approach to preventing relapse.* New York: Guilford Press.

Shawyer, F., Ratcliff, K., Mackinnon, A., Farhall, J., Hayes, S. C., & Copolov, D. (2007). The Voices Acceptance and Action Scale (VAAS): Pilot data. *Journal of Clinical Psychology, 63*(6), 593–606.

Sloan, D. M. (2004). Emotion regulation in action: Emotional reactivity in experiential avoidance. *Behaviour Research and Therapy, 42*, 1257–1270.

Spira, A. P., Beaudreau, S., Jimenez, D., Kierod, K., Cusing, M., Gray, H., et al. (2007). Experiential avoidance, acceptance, and depression in dementia family caregivers. *Clinical Gerontologist, 30*(4), 55–64.

Spira, A. P., Zvolensky, M. J., Eifert, G. H., & Feldner, M. T. (2004). Avoidance-oriented coping as a predictor of anxiety-based physical stress: A test using biological challenge. *Journal of Anxiety Disorders, 18*, 309–323.

Tull, M. T., & Gratz, K. L. (2008). Further examination of the relationship between anxiety sensitivity and depression: The mediating role of experiential avoidance and difficulties engaging in goal-directed behavior when distressed. *Journal of Anxiety Disorders, 22*, 199–210.

Tull, M. T., & Roemer, L. (2007). Emotion regulation difficulties associated with the experience of uncued panic attacks: Evidence of experiential avoidance, emotional nonacceptance, and decreased emotional clarity. *Behavior Therapy, 38*, 378–391.

Wegner, D. M. (1994). Ironic processes of mental control. *Psychological Review, 101*, 34–52.

Wenzlaff, R. M., & Wegner, D. M. (2000). Thought suppression. *Annual Review of Psychology, 51*, 59–91.

Wicksell, R. K., Renofalt, J., Olsson, G. L., Bond, F. W., & Melin, L. (2008). Avoidance and cognitive fusion—Central components in pain related disability?: Development and preliminary validation of the Psychological Inflexibility in Pain Scale (PIPS). *European Journal of Pain, 12*(4), 491–500.

Wulfert, E., & Hayes, S. C. (1988). Transfer of a conditional ordering response through conditional equivalence classes. *Journal of the Experimental Analysis of Behavior, 50*, 125–144.

Yalom, I.D. (1980). *Existential psychotherapy.* New York: Basic Books.

Zettle, R. D., Petersen, C. L., Hocker, T. R., & Provines, J. L. (2007). Responding to a challenging perceptual-motor task as a function of level of experiential avoidance. *Psychological Record, 57*, 49–62.

CHAPTER 6

● —————— ● —————— ●

Suppression

**Kristalyn Salters-Pedneault, Maria Steenkamp,
and Brett T. Litz**

A large part of our brain has been selected to scan the environment for threats and to secure our survival in the face of threat. As a result, our physiology is biased toward producing, and responding to, defensive emotional reactions, which trigger elaborate routines in service of returning to homeostasis. In the modern world, negative emotions can arise nonfunctionally, at least with respect to the survival mandate, and they can be expressed swiftly and automatically, which can result in the aversive experience of noncontrol and intrusiveness. As a result, people develop and deploy repertoires to manage or control their emotional reactions when they occur in an unbidden fashion or are experienced as unhelpful or otherwise aversive experientially. Although this is generally a functional process, attempts to control emotional reactions may also have unintended negative consequences. Frequent, intensive, and habitual avoidance of inner experience and triggering contexts is a central tenet of most models of psychopathology (e.g., Breuer & Freud, 1966; Foa & Kozak, 1986; Greenburg & Safran, 1987; Hayes, Wilson, Gifford, Follette, & Strosahl, 1996).

Recently, investigators have examined the effects of one very specific form of emotional avoidance: suppression. Suppression is an emotion modulation strategy intended to reduce unwanted emotional experiences. The thesis is that suppression interferes with recovery from distressing provocations and, if habitual, reflects problems with emotion regulation. Suppression has been defined in a variety of ways. For the purposes of this chapter, we use a broad definition that includes direct attempts to remove any component of an emotional response from conscious experience, including suppression of the experienced feeling of the emotion, expressive inhibition of the expressive components of emotion (Richards

& Gross, 2006), and inhibition of thoughts associated with emotional reactions. By direct, we mean that suppression attempts act directly on the emotional response. For example, one can attempt to remove an emotion from conscious experience by using substances or by attending instead to positively valenced material, but these are not examples of suppression. Suppression is an attempt to act directly on a response to put it "out of mind" or to push it away. Thus, we do not discuss indirect means to circumvent unwanted emotions, such as worry (see Borkovec, Alcaine, & Behar, 2004), distraction, thought replacement, or cognitive reappraisal. Although we review research related to diverse forms of suppression (e.g., suppression of emotional thoughts, emotional expressions, experienced feelings), we also acknowledge that these different forms may represent very distinct emotion modulation strategies (Valentiner, Hood, & Hawkins, 2006).

Framework and Definitions

As a heuristic framework for this chapter, we use Lang's (1979) bioinformational conceptualization of emotion. Lang characterized emotions as "action tendencies" that reside within a network of associated information. Relevant aspects of this emotional network include the stimulus (and any closely related stimuli that become associated by way of higher order conditioning and stimulus generalization), the emotional response itself, and any other information that may be related to the stimulus–response association, such as context or meaning information. In this model, *emotional response* is defined quite broadly and includes behavioral (e.g., expressive), subjective, physiological, and cognitive components. Lang's conceptualization of emotion is situated within an evolutionary functional framework; the various components of emotion entail the coordinated activation and inhibition of various basic brain functions serving hedonic or defensive needs, which ultimately promote decision making, social inclusion, problem solving, and communication (and other survival functions; for a more complete discussion, see Cosmides & Tooby, 2000; Keltner & Kring, 1998).

In our view, emotion regulation is a meta-emotional phenomenon. That is, there is a primary emotional response, and emotion regulation is a set of processes that involve how one perceives, interprets, and reacts to that response. This may include attempts to modulate (enhance or attenuate) the response (e.g., Gross, 1998b), although the choice not to modulate a response may also be a component of emotion regulation (e.g., Gratz & Roemer, 2004). Emotional regulation occurs automatically and unconsciously as well as deliberately and strategically and may occur at any point in the response sequence, including during attentional processes related to the emotional stimulus or long after the primary emotional response (Gross, 1998b).

In this chapter, we depart from the traditional definition of emotion regulation. Most have defined emotion regulation as the effective control or management (i.e., modulation) of emotional experiences (e.g., Gross, 1998b; Kopp, 1989). For example, Gross (1998b) defines emotion regulation as "the processes by which individuals influence which emotions they have, when they have them, and how they experience and express these emotions" (p. 275). In this definition, regulation is synonymous with modulation; emotion regulation is seen as a process by which various components of the emotional response are up- or down-regulated either early or late in the response sequence. For our purposes, however, our use of the term *emotion regulation* incorporates both Gross's definition and additional elements as outlined by Gratz and Roemer (2004), who define optimal emotion regulation as the ability to employ modulation strategies to up- or down-regulate emotional responses when appropriate (like Gross, 1998b) but also include awareness, understanding, and acceptance of emotions; ability to control emotionally motivated impulsive behaviors; and ability to engage in goal-directed behaviors when distressed. Thus, when we refer to emotion regulation, we are referring to this broader conceptualization laid out by Gratz and Roemer. We use the terms *emotion modulation* and *emotion control* to refer to attempts to modify any domain of the emotional response.

Our conceptualization makes a clear distinction between emotion and emotion regulation. The emotion of fear includes experienced feelings of fearfulness, physiological arousal, facial expressions of fearfulness, an urge to behaviorally avoid or escape, and thoughts such as "I am afraid," and "I need to get (or stay) away." Emotion regulation of fear can occur on various levels. Elements of the emotion regulation process include (1) awareness that the response is fear (specificity); (2) a functional causal awareness (attribution), that is, clarity about why the emotion is occurring (e.g., stimulus–response contingency awareness, contextual factors, i.e., "I am afraid because *X* stimulus [or my interpretation of *X* stimulus] is frightening to me"); (3) priming of strategies that would allow the individual to modify the experience of fear where appropriate or necessary (schemas); and (4) useful meta-reactions to the fear response (acceptance).

Suppression, then, is an emotion modulation strategy with implications for the broader domain of emotion regulation. We view suppression as a process that is applicable to all aspects of human experience and all maladaptive repertoires of behavior and formal psychological disorders. Because any form of psychopathology involves painful, conflictual, or unbidden internal events, including thoughts, feelings, behaviors, and physical sensations, all disorders produce experiences that people struggle to manage, keep at bay, avoid, or suppress. However, suppression of emotional experience has only been studied in a few conditions to date (e.g., see Purdon, 1999).

Although suppression falls under the umbrella of "experiential avoid-ance" (e.g., Hayes et al., 1996) in that it is done with the purpose of avoiding or escaping unpleasant internal experiences, it is a special form of experiential avoidance that has some unique properties and consequences. For example, although experiential avoidance may occur at any point in the unfolding of an emotional response, suppression refers to a very specific way of terminating an emotional response that has already begun, whereas other forms of experiential avoidance may serve to avoid an emotion before it develops. We review the consequences of suppression here, with the recognition that many of the concepts addressed in Chapter 5, this volume, likely also apply.

The Relationship between Suppression and Emotion Regulation

Some have argued that psychological disorders are partly caused by excessive or unnecessary emotion modulation (e.g., Campbell-Sills & Barlow, 2007), a position that has been supported by correlational research. Chronic suppression has been associated with posttraumatic stress disorder, obsessive–compulsive disorder, depression, generalized anxiety disorder, and specific phobia (for reviews, see Beevers, Wenzlaff, Hayes, & Scott, 1999; Purdon, 1999). In addition, emotional suppression can be seen as an individual difference characteristic, and those with this tendency often endorse difficulties with specific domains of emotion regulation, including diminished positive and enhanced negative emotional experience (Gross & John, 2003), diminished emotional clarity and ability to modulate emotion (Fernández-Berrocal, Alcaide, Extremera, & Pizarro, 2006), and difficulties with controlling impulsive behaviors, such as aggression (Nagtegaal & Rassin, 2004) and deliberate self-harm and suicide attempts (Najmi, Wegner, & Nock, 2007). On the surface, these relationships seem straightforward: People who have intense and impairing emotional reactions are more likely to attempt to suppress those responses. However, a growing experimental literature suggests that suppression might lead to emotion dysregulation and psychopathology.

The study of the psychological consequences of suppression was in large part started with Wegner and colleagues' seminal "white bear" experiment (Wegner, Schneider, Carter, & White, 1987) on thought suppression. The premise of the study was simple: Do people who are initially instructed to suppress thoughts about a white bear subsequently experience more thoughts of the bear than those who are initially allowed free expression of white bear thoughts? Wegner's study demonstrated the paradoxical rebound effect of thought suppression: Suppressing neutral target thoughts leads to a subsequent increase in the frequency of target thought occurrence. The finding spurred a flurry of research on the effects of thought suppression, with dozens of studies conducted to date, many demonstrating an immediate (Lavy & van den Hout, 1994; Salkovskis & Campbell, 1994) or delayed (Clark, Ball, & Pape, 1991; Clark, Winton, & Thynn, 1993) paradoxical effect of thought suppression on target thought frequency. A meta-analysis of more than 40 experimental studies of thought suppression found a small to moderate rebound effect of thought suppression, with some variation in the effect size dependent on the methodological characteristics of the study (Abramowitz, Tolin, & Street, 2001). These findings led researchers to speculate that suppression of other types of material, including emotional thoughts and components of emotional responses, may have similar paradoxical effects.

The consequences of suppression are now known to extend far beyond the effect on thought frequency rebound. In addition to investigating different types of suppression (i.e., suppression of various domains of the emotional response) and suppression of various forms of emotional content (e.g., personally relevant thoughts [Salkovskis & Campbell, 1994]; threat-related material [Kircanski, Craske, & Bjork, 2008]; stressful memories [Klein & Bratton, 2007]; embarrassment [Harris, 2001]; disgust [Gross & Levenson, 1993]), a variety of outcomes have been explored. Experimental studies have now addressed the consequences of suppression on emotional experiences, physiology, cognitive processes, behavior, learning, and social interaction. Next, we highlight some of the demonstrated outcomes of suppression that have implications for emotion regulation and psychopathology. For more comprehensive reviews, see Wenzlaff and Wegner (2000), Beevers and colleagues (1999), and Purdon (1999); for a meta-analysis and thoughtful discussion of methodological variations between studies, see Abramowitz and colleagues (2001).

Cognition

Suppression has an impact on cognitive and emotional systems as they interact and determine the course and outcome of emotional processing and regulation (e.g., Clore et al., 1994). Cognitive events such as thoughts, beliefs, or attentional or memory processes may increase the duration of emotional reactions, impact mood, or alter interpretations of various events in the chain of emotional responding. These cognitive processes may also increase the likelihood of certain emotional reactions and put specific demands on the emotion regulation system. In addition to these interactions, optimal emotion regulation is arguably dependent on beliefs that one has the ability to understand and modulate one's emotional experiences. Thus, experiences that decrease an individual's expectation that they can modulate internal events presages suboptimal emotion regulation.

Studies using the modified Stroop paradigm (e.g., Lavy & van den Hout, 1994) or the dot probe task (Fawzy, Hecker, & Clark, 2006) have demonstrated that suppression of thoughts leads to a paradoxical or unintended attentional bias toward target-related thoughts, as predicted by Wegner and colleagues (1987). As evidence of the sustained impact of suppression on accessibility, Wegner, Wenzlaff, and Kozak (2004) have demonstrated that instructions to suppress thoughts of a target person lead to increased dreaming about that person relative to control instructions. The impact of suppression on attention is important because attention and intention are necessary components of emotion regulation. If one's attention is consistently biased toward negative target-related material, resources needed for adaptive interaction with the environment may be depleted.

In addition, suppression may affect memory. For example, Richards and Gross (2006) found that greater spontaneous expressive suppression during an aversive film depicting a surgical procedure was associated with worse memory for details of the film. In an experimental extension of this study, participants instructed to suppress their expressive-motor emotional behavior during a film depicting an interpersonal conflict had less memory for the film than controls and comparable memory as individuals instructed to distract themselves from the film's content. However, although memory for events occurring during suppression may be disrupted, suppression may paradoxically heighten memory for target-related material. In anxious individuals, instructions to suppress thoughts of threat-related material under conditions of cognitive load lead to an explicit memory bias for the threat-related material (Kircanski et al., 2008). Memory disruptions created by suppression appear to impact emotion regulation by disrupting adaptive interaction with the environment (because necessary details are not remembered). Alternatively, memory bias toward threatening material appears to create an internal environment more prone toward negatively valenced emotion.

Suppression may also deplete resources available for performance on other tasks. Baumeister, Bratslavsky, Muraven, and Tice (1998) found that instructions to engage in expressive suppression and suppression of emotional responses led to diminished performance on cognitive tasks. Klein and Bratton (2007) found that suppression of emotional memories resulted in delayed response times in a concurrent sentence verification task. This suggests a mechanism for the untoward influence of suppression on emotion regulation: If suppression is an activity that competes for attentional capacity and working memory (e.g., Conway & Engle, 1994), it may consume available resources for emotion regulation (and other adaptive behaviors).

An area that has been less studied but that likely holds great significance for emotion regulation is the effect of suppression on attitudes and beliefs. For example, Borton, Markowitz, and Dieterich (2005) demonstrated that suppression may impact self-evaluation. Participants who were instructed to suppress negative self-referent thoughts endorsed lower state self-esteem than monitor-only controls. Although the effect may have been due to greater accessibility of the self-referent thoughts or a function of internal attributions about suppression failures (e.g., "What is wrong with me? Why can't I just put this out of my mind?"), either process could have implications for emotion regulation. Individuals who experience themselves as being unable to modulate internal events when necessary may become fearful of thoughts and emotions.

Experienced Emotion

Attempts to suppress elements of the emotional response may have the paradoxical effect of producing a stronger experience of emotion. Experimental instructions to suppress thoughts about emotional material lead to increases in both anxiety (Roemer & Borkovec, 1994) and discomfort (Purdon & Clark, 2001) related to the emotional material. Similar effects have been found in studies in which participants were instructed to suppress emotions (as opposed to emotional thoughts). Campbell-Sills, Barlow, Brown, and Hofmann (2006b) assigned individuals with mood and anxiety disorders to engage in either suppression or acceptance of emotional responses to an evocative film clip. Suppression was both ineffective in diminishing experiences of negative emotional responses and associated with slower mood recovery. Tull, Jakupcak, and Roemer (2008) also found that, although instructions to accept emotional responses to a distressing film led to a decrease in negative emotional responses after a context change, individuals who were instructed to suppress did not report a diminished emotional response after the context change. Suppression was also associated with more general distress than acceptance during a later recovery phase. Effects on mood have also been observed; Borton and colleagues (2005) found that individuals instructed to suppress negative self-referent thoughts reported more anxious and depressed mood than control participants instructed to monitor thoughts.

Some studies have failed to replicate the subjective effects of suppression. For example, Gross and colleagues' studies of expressive suppression have not demonstrated an effect on emotional experience despite effects on other channels of emotional responding (e.g., physiology) (Goldin, McRae, Ramel, & Gross, 2008; Gross, 1998a; Gross & Levenson, 1993, 1997). This suggests that more work is needed to elucidate the moderators of the specific effects of suppression on experienced emotion.

Physiology

Studies of suppression of thoughts (e.g., Merckelbach, Muris, van den Hout, & de Jong, 1991; Wegner, Shortt, Blake, & Page, 1990) and other components of the emotional response (e.g., Gross & Levenson, 1993, 1997; Richards & Gross, 2006) have demonstrated that suppression also affects psychophysiology. Gross and Levenson (1993) found that instructions to engage in expressive suppression led to increases in several markers of sympathetic activation (skin conductance, more pronounced shortening of finger pulse transmission times, and greater decreases in finger pulse amplitude) during and after a disgust-eliciting film clip relative to a just-watch control condition (although expressive suppression was also associated with lower heart rate). In a second study, Gross and Levenson (1997) found that expressive suppression led to greater sympathetic activation (but decreased heart rate) during an amusement film and greater skin conductance, sympathetic activation, and respiratory activity during a sadness film, than just-watch instructions. In a third study, Gross (1998a) replicated the paradoxical effects of expressive suppression on sympathetic activation during a disgust-eliciting film clip compared with both a just-watch and a cognitive reappraisal control condition.

Other groups have also found effects of suppression on psychophysiology using stimuli evoking different emotional content and examining suppression of other emotional channels. For example, expressive suppression of embarrassment (compared with no suppression instructions) has been shown to increase blood pressure but not heart rate (Harris, 2001). Suppressing discussion of a personally relevant emotional topic (vs. expression) has been shown to increase cardiovascular threat reactivity across contexts (Mendes, Reis, Seery, & Blascovich, 2003). Also, Campbell-Sills and colleagues (2006b) found that suppression of emotional responses to distressing stimuli led to greater heart rate increases for suppression versus acceptance condition participants with mood and anxiety disorders. Another study found that participants instructed to suppress emotional responses to a carbon dioxide (CO_2) challenge evidence higher heart rate during a recovery period than those instructed to simply observe their emotional responses (Feldner, Zvolensky, Stickle, Bonn-Miller, & Leen-Feldner, 2006). The neural correlates of this effect were explored by Goldin and colleagues (2008), who compared instructions to reappraise with instructions to engage in expressive suppression in response to emotions generated by a disgusting film. Relative to the reappraisal condition, individuals in the suppression condition evidenced lower ratings of negative emotion but sustained elevated amygdalar and insular responses.

There are also examples of failures to replicate the paradoxical psychophysiological effects of suppression. For example, Eifert and Heffner (2003) instructed high anxiety sensitivity participants to suppress or accept internal experiences (or gave no instructions) during a CO_2 challenge and found no differences between conditions on measures of arousal. In addition, the effect of emotion suppression on physiology may not be unique to emotion; a study of attempts to suppress another biologically prepared response, the acoustic startle response, found that suppression resulted in increased autonomic arousal (Hagemann, Levenson, & Gross, 2006). This finding suggests that effects of suppression on arousal may occur just by virtue of demand on the organism's resources. Thus, more work is needed to clarify the relationship between suppression and physiology.

Behavior

There is a small but growing literature examining the impact of suppression on behavior. An examination of suppression and expressive-motor behavior outcomes found that attempts to suppress emotional experience to evocative images resulted in decreased eyeblink startle magnitude and corrugator activity (an expressive-motor measure of negative affect) compared with "enhance" or no-instruction controls (Jackson, Malmstadt, Larson, & Davidson, 2000). In addition to expression of emotion, the act of suppression may alter behavioral routines. For example, two studies found that individuals in an acceptance condition were more willing to approach emotionally evocative tasks than those in a suppression condition (Eifert & Heffner, 2003; Levitt, Brown, Orsillo, & Barlow, 2004). Muraven, Tice, and Baumeister (1998) found that suppression was associated with quicker disengagement from frustrating or distressing tasks. Increased avoidant behavior may impact overall emotion regulation by leading to less adaptive behavior generally and interfering with the natural occurrence of extinction or habituation of the emotional response.

Social–Interpersonal Behaviors

In addition to the intraindividual consequences of suppression, there is experimental evidence that suppression can have interpersonal consequences. For example, Butler and colleagues (2003) found that instructions to engage in expressive suppression interferes with successful social interactions by reducing rapport and relationship formation, while increasing negative arousal in the suppressor and their dyadic partner. Interestingly, the interpersonal effects of suppression may be mediated by cultural influences (e.g., Butler, Lee, & Gross, 2007).

Summary

To fully appreciate the ways that suppression may impact emotion regulation, the dynamic, complex nature of the emotional system needs to be understood. Emotions are evolutionarily prepared action tendencies that reside within a dense store of information that includes behavioral, psychophysiological, stimulus, and cognitive representations (Lang, 1979). If any one aspect of this system is derailed (and particularly if it is derailed frequently and across contexts), the system may begin to break down. Learning is interrupted and behavioral responses fail to match environmental demands. Downstream consequences such as an increasingly confusing internal and external environment emerge, leading to yet stronger and less comprehensible emotional experiences.

In this framework, the consequences of suppression may have complex and interacting effects on emotion regulation. First, suppression may reduce the individual's awareness of his or her primary emotional response. If suppression is initially successful in reducing the emotional response, as is suggested by findings of delayed paradoxical effects, an individual may not be aware that an emotional response has occurred (particularly if suppression is habitual and automatic). Being unaware of an emotional response essentially negates the purpose of emotion: to provide information about relationship of the current relevant stimuli to the goals of the individual and to motivate appropriate action.

When the potential paradoxical effects of suppression do emerge, many (e.g., increased intrusion of suppressed material, physiological arousal, experienced negative emotion and mood, and more negative beliefs) may tax the emotion regulatory system just by nature of the individual having more emotional reactivity to manage. However, these paradoxical effects may also diminish clarity about emotional experiences. If aspects of the emotional response are artificially heightened (or diminished in the case of positive emotion, although this has rarely been explored; for an exception, see Nezlek & Kuppens, 2008) and temporally disconnected from the evoking stimulus, the individual's understanding of his or her response may be reduced. The effects of suppression on mood are also implicated here; negative mood may lead to stronger corresponding emotional responses, and negatively valenced mood may also diminish the clarity of emotional responses.

Suppression may also alter beliefs about the self or about one's ability to alter internal events when necessary, which may increase fear or judgment of emotion and diminish attempts to use effective modulation strategies. Furthermore, the possibly increased cognitive load, diminished cognitive performance, and disrupted memory and attention created by suppression may both deplete working memory resources necessary for the successful implementation of the emotion regulatory system and interfere with general adaptive responding (leaving the individual to experience the world as increasingly confusing and frustrating, thereby increasing negatively valenced emotionality). Some have proposed that suppression may interfere with emotional acceptance by reinforcing the idea that negative emotions or thoughts are dangerous or damaging (Cheavens et al., 2005).

Why Do People Suppress?

The experimental research reviewed previously suggests that suppression is, at best, a relatively ineffective way to modulate emotional experiences.

At worst, suppression produces paradoxical effects that heighten negative affectivity and drain resources. There are a variety of reasons for these suppression failures. Behavioral theory suggests that any activity that results in avoidance of any component of the emotional response may interfere with the natural course of extinction/habituation (e.g., Foa & Kozak, 1986) and thereby maintain nonfunctional emotional responses. Wegner's (1994) ironic process theory, which was originally formulated to explain the rebound effect of thought suppression but may hold broadly to other forms and consequences of suppression, extends this. Wegner proposed that suppression requires two mechanisms: (1) an intentional operating process that searches for internal experiences that are not consistent with the to-be-suppressed material and (2) an automatic monitoring process that searches for instances of the suppressed material. Wegner proposed that if the intentional operating process is compromised in any way (e.g., cognitive load), the automatic monitoring system will be unmodulated and will result in increased accessibility of the suppressed target.

If suppression is an inherently flawed emotion modulation strategy, why do people use it (how can it be reinforcing)? Several factors may motivate suppression, but few have been tested empirically. First, the individual's beliefs about the acceptability of his or her emotions appear to play an important role. Individuals who deem certain emotions to be aversive and unacceptable may engage in suppression as a way of avoiding or modulating the emotion (Amstadter, 2008). There is some experimental evidence that nonacceptance of emotion is particularly associated with avoidance-based regulation strategies in individuals with psychological disorders. In a laboratory study using emotion-eliciting films, patients with anxiety and mood disorders viewed their emotions as less acceptable and endorsed greater use of emotion suppression than nondisordered controls (Campbell-Sills, Barlow, Brown, & Hofmann, 2006a). Appraising negative emotions as unacceptable mediated the relationship between emotional intensity and the use of suppression in these participants.

Beliefs about the unacceptability and aversiveness of emotion may be acquired developmentally (Matsumoto, Yoo, & Nakagawa, 2008). Parents' reaction to emotional expression in their children has been shown to have long-term implications and predict children's later emotional experiences, beliefs about emotion, and use of emotion regulation strategies. Specifically, several studies have linked the use of emotional suppression in adulthood to emotional abuse and invalidation in childhood (e.g., Gratz, Bornovalova, Delany-Brumsey, & Lejuez, 2007). Parental punishment, minimization of emotion, and, in particular, parental distress when faced with the children's emotional displays are associated with children's overreliance on avoidant regulatory strategies such as emotion and thought suppression (Krause, Mendelson, & Lynch, 2003). Moreover, the relationship between childhood emotional invalidation and later psychological maladjustment in nonclinical samples has been shown to be fully mediated by emotional inhibition, including emotion and thought suppression (Krause et al., 2003). A similar line of research has examined the relationship between attachment style and emotion regulation (Cassidy, 1994), with evidence of attachment-related variations of thought suppression (Mikulincer, Dolev, & Shaver, 2004).

A broader perspective points to cultural factors playing an important role in shaping individuals' beliefs about how and when emotions should be expressed and felt and serve to create and enforce norms concerning emotion regulation (Matsumoto et al., 2008; Soto, Levenson, & Ebling, 2005). Recent cross-cultural research on emotion regulation has shown different use of reappraisal and suppression across different countries, with higher use of suppression in countries that value power and status differentials and emphasize propriety and restraint and greater use of reappraisal in countries that value more individualistic goals, such as the independent pursuit of well-being (Matsumoto et al., 2008).

Finally, several other learning explanations of suppression may account for its use. Research demonstrating a delayed rebound effect suggests that people who use suppression may find that it is actually quite effective in the short term (Wenzlaff & Wegner, 2000), which negatively reinforces the behavior. In the moment, individuals may either not care about the long-term consequences of their attempts to suppress, or they may simply be unaware of these consequences because of the temporal disconnect. Hayes, Strosahl, and Wilson (1999) have suggested that people use ineffective control-oriented emotion modulation strategies because efforts to control other experiences (e.g., behavior) are effective and lead people to generalize control strategies to domains where they are ineffective (e.g., internal events). Also, people may suppress because they either have not learned or cannot implement more effective emotion modulation strategies (e.g., cognitive reappraisal) (Gross, 2001). Many individuals may have either observational or verbal learning histories that support the use of suppression (i.e., observing parents using suppression or receiving messages about suppressing emotions) (Wenzlaff & Eisenberg, 1998).

Suppression in Context:
Are There Always Negative Consequences?

Although the research reviewed previously suggests that many forms of suppression are ineffective in the long term, does this mean that suppression is always bad? There is very little research that addresses this question in depth, but we might speculate that for many people suppression is a fairly harmless and infrequently used modulation strategy. When used occasionally, suppression likely has few clinically relevant consequences. However, if an individual begins to rely on this strategy more frequently (which is negatively reinforced), over time the use of suppression may become rigid, chronic, and automatic.

It may be that the ability to use a variety of modulation strategies and to match the strategy to the context is more important for emotional health than the particular strategies used (Bonanno, Papa, Lalande, Westphal, & Coifman, 2004). Cheng (2001) proposed that inconsistencies in findings about the role of coping on adaptation could be addressed by examining the flexibility of coping rather than continuing to focus on the use of specific strategies within one context. Bonanno and colleagues (2004) extended this idea to the realm of emotion, suggesting that optimal emotion regulation would include the ability to both express and suppress emotion depending on situational demands. They found that college students who were better able to enhance and suppress their expression of emotion reported less distress 1 year later. Indeed, research suggests that expressing emotion may be harmful to emotional health under some circumstances (e.g., conjugal bereavement) (Bonanno & Keltner, 1997).

In what contexts, then, is suppression most likely to create harmful consequences? Ironic process theory suggests that suppression will be least effective during times of stress (Wegner, 1994). This is supported by research examining suppression under cognitive load (see Wenzlaff & Wegner, 2000). Suppression may also be particularly ineffective when the target material is more emotionally intense (Davies & Clark, 1998; Roemer & Borkovec, 1994). Unfortunately, this means that suppression has particularly negative consequences when people are most in need of an effective strategy.

Finally, there may be individual differences in suppression success. For example, individuals with greater working memory may be more successful at suppression (Brewin & Beaton, 2002; Brewin & Smart, 2005). So some individuals may be able to suppress without ever experiencing negative consequences, whereas others may experience consequences after even minimal suppression attempts.

Clinical Implications

Research on emotional processes and emotional regulation is increasingly informing clinical treatment (Moses & Barlow, 2006). Individual differences in emotion regulation have been linked to vulnerability and resilience to psychological disorders, and maladaptive attempts at modulating distressing emotions and thoughts appear to play an important role in the development and maintenance of these disorders (Campbell-Sills & Barlow, 2007; Hayes et al., 1996). Suppression appears to be widely used among patients (Campbell-Sills et al., 2006a; Purdon, 1999) and may serve to maintain symptoms (Moses & Barlow, 2006; Salters-Pedneault, Tull, &

Roemer, 2004), suggesting that individuals may benefit from treatments incorporating emotion regulation skills.

Recent cognitive-behavioral therapies have placed greater emphasis on the healthy regulation of emotion, such as dialectical behavior therapy (Linehan, 1993), acceptance and commitment therapy (Hayes, Strohsahl, & Wilson, 1999; see Valdivia-Salas, Sheppard, & Forsyth, Chapter 13, this volume), and the unified protocol for emotional disorders (Barlow, Allen, & Choate, 2004; see Fairholme, Boisseau, Ellard, Ehrenreich, & Barlow, Chapter 12, this volume). A central tenet of these treatments is that psychopathology in part stems from efforts to avoid painful emotional experiences through counterproductive attempts at overcontrol (Amstadter, 2008). The aim is for patients to attain greater awareness and clarity regarding their emotional reactions but simultaneously to accept these emotions without judgments or attempts to alter or avoid the emotion. Results from treatment outcome studies point to the clinical value of these interventions (e.g., Bach & Hayes, 2002; Linehan et al., 2006).

It appears that treatments should not consider all forms of suppression as negative. Rather, treatments should promote flexibility and breadth of regulation repertoires (Salters-Pedneault et al., 2004). James Gross's experimental work (Gross, 1998a; Gross & Levenson, 1993, 1997) with healthy controls suggests a specific alternative emotion modulation strategy to suppression that may be incorporated into emotion regulation skills training: reappraisal (or altering thoughts or interpretations of the emotional stimulus so as to reduce the emotional response to that stimulus) (e.g., Gross, 1998a). Experimental studies show that reappraisal, as compared with suppression, seems to promote more adaptive outcomes. Whereas habitual use of suppression has been shown to result in diminished control over emotion and poorer interpersonal functioning, memory, and well-being (Gross & John, 2003), reappraisal has been associated with enhanced interpersonal functioning, effective emotion modulation (with fewer intrusive thoughts), and better psychological and physical functioning. Reappraisal may also increase insight and a sense of meaning as well as foster the individual's access to supportive relationships and a sense of intimacy (Butler et al., 2003; Gross & John, 2003).

Teaching patients strategies to modulate their emotions before the emotion is fully elicited through reappraisal may prevent feelings of distress and preempt engagement in maladaptive behavioral and cognitive attempts at avoiding the emotion (Amstadter, 2008). However, although research suggests that adding cognitive reappraisal to therapy may be beneficial, the clinical literature is mixed in this regard. It is unclear whether cognitive restructuring techniques such as reappraisal are necessary for therapeutic change to occur (e.g., Anholt et al., 2007) or whether combining cognitive therapy and exposure provides an additive benefit over exposure therapy alone (Norton & Price, 2007). It may be that targeting suppression directly through approach-based emotional engagement strategies such as exposures is sufficient to reduce symptoms.

In addition, recent experimental research suggests that, compared with suppression, focused distraction and concentrating on an alternative task may be more effective short-term techniques, leading to fewer intrusive thoughts and lower anxiety (Lin & Wicker, 2007). However, clinical research regarding the usefulness of incorporating alternative emotional avoidance strategies into treatment has also been mixed (Amstadter, 2008). For example, dismantling studies of panic disorder treatments suggest that cognitive-behavioral therapy (CBT), including breathing retraining, which can be understood as a technique aimed at avoidance of emotion, is associated with poorer outcome (less complete recovery and heightened risk for relapse) than CBT without breathing retraining (Schmidt, Woolaway-Bickel, & Trakowski, 2000).

Conclusion

There are a variety of documented effects of suppression that may have significant negative consequences for the emotion regulatory system, including increased emotional and physiological reactivity, attentional bias toward and enhanced memory of suppressed material, more negative self-referent beliefs, diminished task performance, more avoidant behavior, and less adaptive social interaction. Many of these effects have been explored in relationship to a range of internal events within normal, analogue, and clinical populations, and thus the literature reviewed here likely has wide applicability to a variety of forms of psychopathology. Because the literature in suppression is so large, there are many contradictory findings, likely because of differences in methodological characteristics of studies, although in a meta-analysis some of these findings have emerged as reliable despite some replication failures (e.g., Abramowitz et al., 2001). More experimental work, with clear precision in terms of operational definitions, is needed to fully understand the complex consequences of suppression.

Despite the evidence for an impact of suppression on emotion regulatory function, it is important to note that most people periodically use suppression with few practical consequences. When used occasionally, flexibly, and in appropriate contexts, it is unlikely that suppression is actually a maladaptive modulation regulation strategy. However, when used rigidly, chronically, and across situations, suppression may have a significant detrimental impact on the emotional system, particularly if suppression becomes automatic and nonconscious. Future research should investigate the nature of suppression efforts over time and within and across contexts, the mechanisms by which these efforts may fail, and the factors that predict poor outcome of suppression.

References

Abramowitz, J. S., Tolin, D. F., & Street, G. P. (2001). Paradoxical effects of thought suppression: A meta-analysis of controlled studies. *Clinical Psychology Review*, *21*, 683–703.

Amstadter, A. (2008). Emotion regulation and anxiety disorders. *Journal of Anxiety Disorders*, *22*, 211–221.

Anholt, G. E., Kempe, P., de Haan, E., van Oppen, P., Cath, D. C., Smit, J. H., et al. (2007). Cognitive versus behavior therapy: Processes of change in the treatment of obsessive-compulsive disorder. *Psychotherapy and Psychosomatics*, *77*, 38–42.

Bach, P., & Hayes, S. C. (2002). The use of acceptance and commitment therapy to prevent the rehospitalization of psychotic patients: A randomized controlled trial. *Journal of Consulting and Clinical Psychology*, *70*, 1129–1139.

Barlow, D. H., Allen, L. B., & Choate, M. L. (2004). Toward a unified treatment for emotional disorders. *Behavior Therapy*, *35*, 205–230.

Baumeister, R. F., Bratslavsky, E., Muraven, M., & Tice, D. M. (1998). Ego depletion: Is the active self a limited resource? *Journal of Personality and Social Psychology*, *74*, 1252–1265.

Beevers, C. G., Wenzlaff, R. M., Hayes, A. M., & Scott, W. D. (1999). Depression and the ironic effects of thought suppression: Therapeutic strategies for improving mental control. *Clinical Psychology: Science and Practice*, *6*, 133–148.

Bonanno, G. A., & Keltner, D. (1997). Facial expressions of emotion and the course of conjugal bereavement. *Journal of Abnormal Psychology*, *106*, 126–137.

Bonanno, G. A., Papa, A., Lalande, K., Westphal, M., & Coifman, K. (2004). The importance of being flexible: The ability to both enhance and suppress emotional expression predicts long-term adjustment. *Psychological Science*, *15*, 482–487.

Borkovec, T. D., Alcaine, O., & Behar, E. (2004). Avoidance theory of worry. In R. G. Heimberg, C. L. Turk, & D. S. Mennin (Eds.), *Generalized anxiety disorder: Advances in research and practice* (pp. 77–108). New York: Guilford Press.

Borton, J. L. S., Markowitz, L. J., & Dieterich, J. (2005). Effects of suppressing negative self-referent thoughts on mood and self-esteem. *Journal of Social and Clinical Psychology*, *24*, 172–190.

Breuer, J., & Freud, S. (1966). *Studies on hysteria*. New York: Avon. (Original work published 1895)

Brewin, C. R., & Beaton, A. (2002). Thought suppression, intelligence, and working memory capacity. *Behaviour Research and Therapy*, *40*, 923–930.

Brewin, C. R., & Smart, L. (2005). Working memory capacity and suppression of intrusive thoughts. *Journal of Behavior Therapy and Experimental Psychiatry*, *36*, 61–68.

Butler, E. A., Egloff, B., Wilhelm, F. H., Smith, N. C., Erickson, E. A., & Gross, J. J. (2003). The social consequences of expressive suppression. *Emotion*, *3*, 48–67.

Butler, E. A., Lee, T. L., & Gross, J. J. (2007). Emotion regulation and culture: Are the social consequences of emotion suppression culture-specific? *Emotion*, *7*, 30–48.

Campbell-Sills, L., & Barlow, D. H. (2007). Incorporating emotion regulation into conceptualizations and treatments of anxiety and mood disorders. In J. J.

Gross (Ed.), *Handbook of emotion regulation* (pp. 542–559). New York: Guilford Press.

Campbell-Sills, L., Barlow, D. H., Brown, T. A., & Hofmann, S. G. (2006a). Acceptability and suppression of negative emotion in anxiety and mood disorders. *Emotion, 6,* 587–595.

Campbell-Sills, L., Barlow, D. H., Brown, T. A., & Hofmann, S. G. (2006b). Effects of suppression and acceptance on emotional responses of individuals with anxiety and mood disorders. *Behaviour Research and Therapy, 44,* 1251–1263.

Cassidy, J. (1994). Emotion regulation: Influences of attachment relationships. *Monographs of The Society for Research in Child Development, 59,* 228–283.

Cheavens, J. S., Rosenthal, M. Z., Daughters, S. B., Nowak, J., Kosson, D., Lynch, T. R., et al. (2005). An analogue investigation of the relationships among perceived parental criticism, negative affect, and borderline personality disorder features: The role of thought suppression. *Behaviour Research and Therapy, 43,* 257–268.

Cheng, C. (2001). Assessing coping flexibility in real-life and laboratory settings: A multimethod approach. *Journal of Personality and Social Psychology, 80,* 814–833.

Clark, D. M., Ball, S., & Pape, D. (1991). An experimental investigation of thought suppression. *Behaviour Research and Therapy, 29,* 253–257.

Clark, D. M., Winton, E., & Thynn, L. (1993). A further experimental investigation of thought suppression. *Behaviour Research and Therapy, 31,* 207–210.

Clore, G. L., Ellsworth, P. C., Frijda, N. H., Izard, C. E., Lazarus, R., LeDoux, J. E., et al. (1994). What are the minimal cognitive prerequisites for emotion? In P. Ekman & R. J. Davidson (Eds.), *The nature of emotion: Fundamental questions* (pp. 179–234). New York: Oxford University Press.

Conway, A. R. A., & Engle, R. W. (1994). Working memory and retrieval: A resource-dependent inhibition model. *Journal of Experimental Psychology: General, 123,* 354–373.

Cosmides, L., & Tooby, J. (2000). Evolutionary psychology and the emotions. In M. Lewis & J. M. Haviland-Jones (Eds.), *Handbook of emotions* (pp. 91–115). New York: Guilford Press.

Davies, M. I., & Clark, D. M. (1998). Predictors of analogue posttraumatic intrusive cognitions. *Behavioural and Cognitive Psychotherapy, 26,* 303–314.

Eifert, G. H., & Heffner, M. (2003). The effects of acceptance versus control contexts on avoidance of panic-related symptoms. *Journal of Behavior Therapy and Experimental Psychiatry, 34,* 293–312.

Fawzy, T. I., Hecker, J. E., & Clark, J. (2006). The relationship between cognitive avoidance and attentional bias for snake-related thoughts. *Journal of Anxiety Disorders, 20,* 1103–1117.

Feldner, M. T., Zvolensky, M. J., Stickle, T. R., Bonn-Miller, M. O., & Leen-Feldner, E. W. (2006). Anxiety sensitivity-physical concerns as a moderator of the emotional consequences of emotion suppression during biological challenge: An experimental test using individual growth curve analysis. *Behaviour Research and Therapy, 44,* 249–272.

Fernández-Berrocal, P., Alcaide, R., Extremera, N., & Pizarro, D. (2006). The role of emotional intelligence in anxiety and depression among adolescents. *Individual Differences Research, 4,* 16–27.

Foa, E. B., & Kozak, M. J. (1986). Emotional processing of fear: Exposure to corrective information. *Psychological Bulletin, 99*, 20–35.

Goldin, P. R., McRae, K., Ramel, W., & Gross, J. J. (2008). The neural bases of emotion regulation: Reappraisal and suppression of negative emotion. *Biological Psychiatry, 63*, 577–586.

Gratz, K., Bornovalova, M. A., Delany-Brumsey, A., & Lejuez, C. W. (2007). A laboratory-based study of the relationship between childhood abuse and experiential avoidance among inner-city substance users: The role of emotional nonacceptance. *Behavior Therapy, 38*, 256–268.

Gratz, K. L., & Roemer, L. (2004). Multidimensional assessment of emotion regulation and dysregulation: Development, factor structure, and initial validation of the difficulties in Emotion Regulation Scale. *Journal of Psychopathology and Behavioral Assessment, 26*, 41–54.

Greenburg, L. S., & Safran, J. D. (1987). *Emotion in psychotherapy.* New York: Guilford Press.

Gross, J. J. (1998a). Antecedent- and response-focused emotion regulation: Divergent consequences for experience, expression, and physiology. *Journal of Personality and Social Psychology, 74*, 224–237.

Gross, J. J. (1998b). The emerging field of emotion regulation: An integrative review. *Review of General Psychology, 2*, 271–299.

Gross, J. J. (2001). Emotion regulation in adulthood: Timing is everything. *Current Directions in Psychological Science, 10*, 214–219.

Gross, J. J., & John, O. P. (2003). Individual differences in two emotion regulation processes: Implications for affect, relationships, and well-being. *Journal of Personality and Social Psychology, 85*, 348–362.

Gross, J. J., & Levenson, R. W. (1993). Emotional suppression: Physiology, self-report, and expressive behavior. *Journal of Personality and Social Psychology, 64*, 970–986.

Gross, J. J., & Levenson, R. W. (1997). Hiding feelings: The acute effects of inhibiting negative and positive emotion. *Journal of Abnormal Psychology, 106*, 95–103.

Hagemann, T., Levenson, R. W., & Gross, J. J. (2006). Expressive suppression during an acoustic startle. *Psychophysiology, 43*, 104–112.

Harris, C. R. (2001). Cardiovascular responses of embarrassment and effects of emotional suppression in a social setting. *Journal of Personality and Social Psychology, 81*, 886–897.

Hayes, S. C., Strosahl, K. D., & Wilson, K. G. (1999). *Acceptance and commitment therapy: An experiential approach to behavior change.* New York: Guilford Press.

Hayes, S. C., Wilson, K. G., Gifford, E. V., Follette, V. M., & Strosahl, K. (1996). Experiential avoidance and behavioral disorders: A functional dimensional approach to diagnosis and treatment. *Journal of Consulting and Clinical Psychology, 64*, 1152–1168.

Jackson, D. C., Malmstadt, J. R., Larson, C. L., & Davidson, R. J. (2000). Suppression and enhancement of emotional responses to unpleasant pictures. *Psychophysiology, 37*, 515–522.

Keltner, D., & Kring, A. M. (1998). Emotion, social function, and psychopathology. *Review of General Psychology, 2*, 320–342.

Kircanski, K., Craske, M. G., & Bjork, R. A. (2008). Thought suppression enhances memory bias for threat material. *Behaviour Research and Therapy, 46*, 462–476.

Klein, K., & Bratton, K. (2007). The costs of suppressing stressful memories. *Cognition and Emotion, 21,* 1496–1512.

Kopp, C. B. (1989). Regulation of distress and negative emotions: A developmental view. *Developmental Psychology, 25,* 343–354.

Krause, E. D., Mendelson, T., & Lynch, T. R. (2003). Childhood emotional invalidation and adult psychological distress: The mediating role of emotional inhibition. *Child Abuse and Neglect, 27,* 199–213.

Lang, P. J. (1979). A bio-informational theory of emotional imagery. *Psychophysiology, 16,* 495–512.

Lavy, E. H., & van den Hout, M. A. (1994). Cognitive avoidance and attentional bias: Causal relationships. *Cognitive Therapy and Research, 18,* 179–191.

Levitt, J. T., Brown, T. A., Orsillo, S. M., & Barlow, D. H. (2004). The effects of acceptance versus suppression of emotion on subjective and psychophysiological response to carbon dioxide challenge in patients with panic disorder. *Behavior Therapy, 35,* 747–766.

Lin, Y-J., & Wicker, F. W. (2007). A comparison of the effects of thought suppression, distraction, and concentration. *Behaviour Research and Therapy, 45,* 2924–2937.

Linehan, M. M. (1993). *Skills training manual for treating borderline personality disorder.* New York: Guilford Press.

Linehan, M. M., Comtois, K. A., Murray, A. M., Brown, M. Z., Gallop, R. J., Heard, H. L., et al. (2006). Two-year randomized controlled trial and follow-up of dialectical behavior therapy vs therapy by experts for suicidal behaviors and borderline personality disorder. *Archives of General Psychiatry, 63,* 757–766.

Matsumoto, D., Yoo, S. H., & Nakagawa, S. (2008). Culture, emotion regulation, and adjustment. *Journal of Personality and Social Psychology, 94,* 925–937.

Mendes, W. B., Reis, H. T., Seery, M. D., & Blascovich, J. (2003). Cardiovascular correlates of emotional expression and suppression: Do content and gender context matter? *Journal of Personality and Social Psychology, 84,* 771–792.

Merckelbach, H., Muris, P., van den Hout, M., & de Jong, P. (1991). Rebound effects of thought suppression: Instruction-dependent? *Behavioural Psychotherapy, 19,* 225–238.

Mikulincer, M., Dolev, T., & Shaver, P. R. (2004). Attachment-related strategies during thought suppression: Ironic rebounds and vulnerable self-representations. *Journal of Personality and Social Psychology, 87,* 940–956.

Moses, E. B., & Barlow, D. H. (2006). A new unified treatment approach for emotional disorders based on emotion science. *Current Directions in Psychological Science, 15,* 146–150.

Muraven, M., Tice, D. M., & Baumeister, R. F. (1998). Self-control as a limited resource: Regulatory depletion patterns. *Journal of Personality and Social Psychology, 74,* 774–789.

Nagtegaal, M. H., & Rassin, E. (2004). The usefulness of the thought suppression paradigm in explaining impulsivity and aggression. *Personality and Individual Differences, 37,* 1233–1244.

Najmi, S., Wegner, D. M., & Nock, M. K. (2007). Thought suppression and self-injurious thoughts and behaviors. *Behaviour Research and Therapy, 45,* 1957–1965.

Nezlek, J. B., & Kuppens, P. (2008). Regulating positive and negative emotions in daily life. *Journal of Personality, 76,* 561–579.

Norton, P. J., & Price, E. C. (2007). A meta analytic review of adult cognitive-behavioral treatment outcome across the anxiety disorders. *Journal of Nervous and Mental Disease, 195*, 521–531.

Purdon, C. (1999). Thought suppression and psychopathology. *Behaviour Research and Therapy, 37*, 1029–1054.

Purdon, C., & Clark, D. A. (2001). Suppression of obsession-like thoughts in non-clinical individuals: Impact on thought frequency, appraisal and mood state. *Behaviour Research and Therapy, 39*, 1163–1181.

Richards, J. M., & Gross, J. J. (2006). Personality and emotional memory: How regulating emotion impairs memory for emotional events. *Journal of Research in Personality, 40*, 631–651.

Roemer, L., & Borkovec, T. D. (1994). Effects of suppressing thoughts about emotional material. *Journal of Abnormal Psychology, 103*, 467–474.

Salkovskis, P. M., & Campbell, P. (1994). Thought suppression induces intrusion in naturally occurring negative intrusive thoughts. *Behaviour Research and Therapy, 32*, 1–8.

Salters-Pedneault, K., Tull, M. T., & Roemer, L. (2004). The role of avoidance of emotional material in the anxiety disorders. *Applied and Preventive Psychology, 11*, 95–114.

Schmidt, N. B., Woolaway-Bickel, K., & Trakowski, J. (2000). Dismantling cognitive-behavioral treatment for panic disorder: Questioning the validity of breathing retraining. *Journal of Consulting and Clinical Psychology, 68*, 417–424.

Soto, J. A., Levenson, R. W., & Ebling, R. (2005). Cultures of moderation and expression: Emotional experience, behavior, and physiology in Chinese American and Mexican Americans. *Emotion, 5*, 154–165.

Tull, M. T., Jakupcak, M., & Roemer, L. (2008). *Emotional suppression: A preliminary experimental investigation of immediate effects and subsequent reactivity to new stimuli.* Manuscript submitted for publication.

Valentiner, D. P., Hood, J. T., & Hawkins, A. (2006). Differentiating thought suppression and the suppression of emotional expression. *Cognition and Emotion, 20*, 729–735.

Wegner, D. M. (1994). Ironic processes of mental control. *Psychological Review, 101*, 34–52.

Wegner, D. M., Schneider, D. J., Carter, S. R., & White, T. L. (1987). Paradoxical effects of thought suppression. *Journal of Personality and Social Psychology, 53*, 5–13.

Wegner, D. M., Shortt, J. W., Blake, A. W., & Page, M. S. (1990). The suppression of exciting thoughts. *Journal of Personality and Social Psychology, 58*, 409–418.

Wegner, D. M., Wenzlaff, R. M., & Kozak, M. (2004). Dream rebound: The return of suppressed thoughts in dreams. *Psychological Science, 15*, 232–236.

Wenzlaff, R. M., & Eisenberg, E. R. (1998). Parental restrictiveness of negative emotion: Sowing the seeds of thought suppression. *Psychological Inquiry, 9*, 310–313.

Wenzlaff, R. M., & Wegner, D. M. (2000). Thought suppression. *Annual Review of Psychology, 51*, 59–91.

CHAPTER 7

Emotion Context Sensitivity in Adaptation and Recovery

Karin G. Coifman and George A. Bonanno

Human uniqueness lies in the flexibility of what our brain can do . . .
I think it probable that natural selection acted to maximize the flexibility
of our behavior. What would be more adaptive for a learning and
thinking animal: genes selected for aggression, spite, and xenophobia; or
selection for learning rules that can generate aggression in appropriate
circumstances and peacefulness in others?
— STEPHEN J. GOULD (1996, p. 361)

Why do we have emotions? Although the possible answers to this seemingly
simple question are as varied as the seasons, over the past several decades
a single dominant view has emerged: Emotions help people respond adaptively to environmental demands and opportunities (Frijda, 1988; Levenson, 1994; Nesse, 1990). The adaptive function of emotions is evident in
the face of everyday stressors as well as ongoing challenges, stressful transitions, and acute crises. However, the functional usefulness of emotions is
not limitless. Rather, emotions are context bound (Bonanno, Colak, et al.,
2007; Cole, Michel, & Teti, 1994). That is, emotions are most effective and,
by extension, most likely to promote adaptation when they are enacted in
the situational contexts for which they most likely evolved.

Anger, for example, is thought to have become part of the human
emotional repertoire because it facilitates adaptation to situations in
which a goal is frustrated or blocked and there is an obvious, blamewor-
thy person or thing that can be assigned responsibility. The experience of
anger is adaptive because it motivates the mobilization of resources and

the focus of energies on an effective response. The expression of anger is adaptive because it communicates the willingness and the ability to defend the self.

Research on anger supports this contextualized function. For example, Lerner, Gonzalez, Dahl, Hariri, and Taylor (2005) had a group of participants complete a series of simple but challenging mental tasks. To make the tasks goal relevant, they told participants that their task performance was diagnostic of their level of intelligence, and that they intended to compare the performance of all the participants in the study so that they could identify the most intelligent people. However, the study also included a "harassing experimenter" whose job was to inform the participants each time they made an error and to continually urge them to work faster. The harassing experimenter, of course, was likely to be experienced as blocking participants' performance goals and likely to be the target of their anger.

Consistent with this assumed contextualized function, participants who expressed greater indignation (a combination of anger and disgust) in their faces during the stressful task phase had a reduced cardiovascular response to the task and also lower levels of the stress hormone cortisol. By contrast, participants who showed greater facial expressions of a different negative emotion—fear—had the opposite response; fear was related to a more prolonged cardiovascular response and to higher levels of cortisol.

The logical explanation for this divergent pattern of results is that the anger response was most appropriate to the situational context and, therefore, most adaptive. Fear, on the other hand, was not a well-matched response to a harassing experimenter, and as a result fear in this context was less adaptive. Fear is generally thought to have evolved for situations that involve high levels of uncertainty and dread. However, because the harassing experimenter presented a threat that was relatively localized and manageable, fear was an inappropriate response and did little to relieve stress.

Despite this kind of inherent contextual assumption, there has been surprisingly little research on the possible role of context in emotional responding. This chapter aims to zero in more closely on the idea of context in emotion. We begin by exploring the general principles of contextualized functioning in emotion. Later, we explore individual differences in context sensitivity in emotional responding, the relationship to psychopathology, and how this might inform adaptation to adversity and clinical treatment.

The Nature and Function of Emotions

Whereas early philosophical perspectives tended to view emotion as a disruptive force that is inferior to reason (Salomon, 2000), the tide turned in the early 1980s to a more functional conception of emotion as an essentially adaptive, genetically endowed set of mechanisms. This view is encapsulated in Levenson's definition of emotions as "short-lived psychological–physiological phenomena that represent efficient modes of adaptation to changing environmental demands" (Levenson, 1994, p. 123). As evolutionary theorists have argued, biologically based emotions are vital to human survival because they help prepare and trigger rapid motor responses to potential threats. Emotions foster adaptation in other ways as well. They facilitate decision making (Isen, 2000; Isen, Daubman, & Nowicki, 1987) and promote learning (Stein, Trabasso, & Liwag, 2000). They also alert us to relevant mismatches between our goals and the environment (Schwarz & Clore, 1983).

Perhaps most important, emotions are crucial to human social behavior. This is evident even in the earliest moments of life. Emotion expression serves important ontogenetic functions, for example, by helping the infant maintain proximity to and receive nurturing from caregivers and by providing a channel for social learning (Izard & Ackerman, 2000). The expression of emotions continues to structure interactions throughout adulthood (Averill, 1980) and helps maintain social cohesion by influencing judgments about other people and by providing information about their needs, desires, and behavioral intentions (Keltner, 1995; Rozin, Lowery, Imada, & Haidt, 1999). As Campos, Campos, and Barrett put it, emotions are "processes of establishing, maintaining, or disrupting the relations between the person and the internal or external environment, when such relations are significant to the individual" (1989, p. 395).

An important feature of most functional accounts of emotion is that they are multicomponential dynamic systems that organize and couple biological and psychological subsystems (Levenson, 1994; Mayne & Ramsey, 2001). There is some divergence among contemporary emotion theorists, however, on the structure and necessary components of emotion (Mayne & Ramsey, 2001). On the one end of the spectrum are those who view emotions as a constructed set of social categories that are culturally relative (Averill, 1980; Shweder, 1994). At the other end are those who insist on the existence of discrete, innate, and universal emotions with unique experiential, behavioral, and physiological attributes. For example, Ekman and colleagues have proposed that facial actions produce emotion-specific patterns of autonomic nervous system activity that shape the quality of emotional experiences (e.g., Ekman, 1984; Ekman, Levenson, & Friesen 1983). Yet other investigators prefer to view emotions in terms of dimensions of affect that are located on orthogonal continua of positive to negative valence and low to high arousal (e.g., Barrett, 1995; for a review of these issues, see Barrett, 2006).

One way to understand differences in the way theorists conceptualize emotion is that different researchers have studied emotion from different levels of analysis (Ochsner & Barrett, 2001; Westphal & Bonanno, 2004). Investigators who focus on the experiential data of emotion or subjective "affect," which is typically obtained through self-report questionnaires or affect checklists, would tend toward a dimensional or continuous understanding of emotion. By contrast, explorations of the physiognomic configurations in the face associated with the expression of emotions such as anger or joy would tend toward a more episodic or discrete emotions perspective.

Despite this variability, most investigators nonetheless abide by the evolutionary premise that emotions serve to facilitate adaptation to a changing environment and allow us to meet the demands of daily living and survival (Keltner & Haidt, 2001; Tooby & Cosmides, 1990). A loosely coupled system (Bonanno & Keltner, 2004) that includes behavioral (e.g., facial expressions), physiological (e.g., autonomic activity), and experiential (e.g., feeling) components, emotions are maximally responsive to both interpersonal and *intra*personal demands (Frijida, 1986; Keltner & Kring, 1998; Levenson, 1994). For example, positive emotions, such as joy, are thought to have evolved when environmental threats are low but social demands are high. They are characterized by relationship-building expressions (e.g., genuine smiles), a broadening of cognitive awareness so as to allow for a building of resources (i.e., relationships and plans) for the future (Fredrickson, 1998, 2001) as well as a means to regulate negative emotional experience meeting a critical intrapersonal need (Fredrickson & Joiner, 2002; Fredrickson & Levenson, 1998; Fredrickson, Mancuso, Branigan, & Tugade, 2000).

Despite the conception that emotions evolved in response to a balance of both contextual and internal demands, the majority of lines of inquiry over past decades have focused on determining the utility or quality of specific emotions for the individual (e.g., Ekman, 1992; Levenson, 1998). Often the purpose of this work has been to seek evidence for a universality of emotions (e.g., Ekman, 1992; Ekman et al., 1983; Levenson, Ekman, Heider, & Friesen, 1992). Although some efforts have proven quite fruitful, the body of evidence this approach has generated has been criticized for its inconsistency (Barrett, 2006). In fact, some have argued that the challenges to isolating universal patterns of response may be due to the frequent failure to consider contextual influences (e.g., Stemmler, 1989). For example, there is now sufficient evidence demonstrating strong cultural differences in behavioral expressions of emotion (e.g., Matsumoto & Kudoh, 1993; for a review, see also Russell, 1995) such that certain emotions are both exhibited and interpreted differently across cultures.

Moreover, despite numerous attempts to establish the autonomic specificity of certain emotions, recent work indicates that context is a primary component in the emotion response system and that neglecting contextual differences can have confounding effects. For example, in an investigation focused on the autonomic specificity of fear and anger, Stemmler, Heldmann, Pauls, and Scherer (2001) demonstrated that both emotions were exhibited with striking differences when the context was varied from real life to imagined.

Emotions in Context

The conceptual and empirical relevance of context in emotional responding is impossible to ignore. Context-sensitive emotion responses can be thought of as a form of emotion regulation. However, the construct of emotion context sensitivity appears to extend beyond a particular regulatory strategy (e.g., reappraisal or expressive suppression, see Goldin, McRae, Ramel, & Gross, 2008). Instead, emotion context sensitivity describes a broad ability that may encompass individual differences in neuroanatomy or function (e.g., rapid time to recovery from emotional episodes; see Davidson, 1998) as well as cognitive processes related to emotional intelligence (see Mayer, Salovey, & Caruso, 2008) or regulation (see Gross, 2008), As such, context sensitivity has relevance extending well beyond the field of emotion and can be linked to the etiology or persistence of pathology. Some argue that ways of defining dysfunctional emotion responses are those that occur outside their "typical incentive contexts" (Goldsmith & Davidson, 2004, p. 363), such that the response extends beyond the demands of the situation or, alternatively, is insufficient or inappropriate to the current conditions. This kind of emotion dysregulation or context *in*sensitivity has often been tied closely to the development of psychopathology (Cole et al., 1994), most notably in mood and anxiety disorders.

One needn't reach far for compelling instances of context-inappropriate or context-insensitive responses in day-to-day life. For example, imagine your reaction to a product that breaks just after the warranty expires. Most individuals, responding with anger and feelings of indignation, would contact customer service with the goal of either replacing the product or receiving some appropriate compensation. If, during the negotiation with the service representative, you express too much anger, you may lose the ability to negotiate effectively and potentially frustrate the service representative, thereby decreasing the chances that your goal will be met. If, however, you express too little anger, you may fail to convince the representative of your cause, and the same may also be true. Alternatively, imagine your reaction if an individual laughs to signal his or her discomfort, perhaps during a somber or distressing event such as a funeral. In this context, laughter is an inappropriate response and, rather than engendering sympathy or compassion from others, it might result in ostracizing behavior or even provoke anger from others present.

Despite the potential frequency of these instances, only a handful of empirical investigations have focused on demonstrating the critical role of context in assessing adaptive versus maladaptive emotion responding.

One important example is an investigation of fear across conditions in very young children. In this study, Buss, Davidson, Kalin, and Goldsmith (2004) demonstrated the utility of shifting context in evaluating fear-related behaviors as well as sympathetic and neuroendocrine reactivity. The investigation focused specifically on the degree of emotion (i.e., fear) relative to the conditions. Results indicated that only children who exhibited excessive fear reactions (i.e., freezing behavior) within less threatening conditions were at significantly higher risk of developing psychiatric and behavioral disorders in the future. By contrast, children who demonstrated contextually sensitive responses (i.e., stronger fear reaction to high-threat conditions and lower fear reaction to less threatening conditions) were not at greater risk of later developing psychopathology and behavior disorders (Buss et al., 2004).

Other recent work has focused on the use of shifting context to demonstrate the consequences of emotion responses mismatched or inappropriate to the conditions. For example, Arsenio, Cooperman, and Lover (2000) examined the emotional behavior of preschoolers during aggressive interactions. They found that children showing positive emotion, or displays of happiness, during aggressive contact with peers had significant social costs and that those children showed overall poor social adjustment. In contrast, however, displays of anger, an emotion appropriate and well matched to the context response, were not related to poor social adjustment (Arsenio et al., 2000). In both of these investigations, the use of shifting contexts brought to light key dysfunction in the emotion response systems of these children: either the inability to modulate responses in accordance with conditions (Buss et al., 2004) or the inability to match responses appropriately with conditions (Arsenio et al., 2000).

More recently, in a study of an adult sample, Papa and Bonanno (2008) measured genuinely positive or "Duchenne" emotional displays in a group of New York City students who had begun college just days before the 2001 terrorist attacks. In this study, the students viewed either a sad or amusing film and then spoke uninterrupted for 5 minutes to an interviewer about their experiences since the 9/11 attacks. Videotapes of the interviews were subsequently coded for Duchenne smiles (i.e., smile involving activity of the orbicularis oculi muscles surrounding the eye and indicative of genuine positive emotion; see Duchenne de Bologne, 1862; see also Ekman & Friesen, 1982; Keltner & Bonanno, 1997). Finally, the students were followed over a 2-year period and assessed at the end of the study for their level of psychological distress. Although Duchenne smiles in general predicted reduced distress 2 years later, there were also important context effects. Specifically, the association of smiling with reduced long-term distress interacted with film context. For participants who viewed the amusing film, Duchenne smiling was unrelated to long-term outcome. However, for participants who viewed the sad film, Duchenne smiling predicted reduced long-term distress. In other words, smiling after an amusing experience can be pleasurable and may be related in some general sense to overall adjustment. However, only the ability to smile during adverse conditions had a lasting positive impact on long-term adjustment.

This study also produced two important mediating effects that help illuminate the contextualized functions of smiling. The interaction effect of smiling and film context was mediated by both the reduction in negative affect during the interview and the size of the participant's social network. In essence, these effects showed that smiling in the face of adversity fosters long-term adjustment because it helps people regulate or undo negative affect (Fredrickson, 1998, 2001) and because it promotes a broader and more usable network of social resources.

Emotion, Context Sensitivity, and Psychopathology

As the previous evidence indicates, adaptive and maladaptive emotion responses can be identified by varying conditions or contextual demands. As such, there is potentially an important transdiagnostic link between emotion context insensitivity and psychopathology. In fact, a growing body of evidence has consistently demonstrated deficits in emotion context sensitivity in mental illness (e.g., Gehricke & Shapiro, 2000; Rottenberg & Gotlib, 2004; Rottenberg, Gross, & Gotlib, 2005; Shestyuk, Deldin, Brand, & Deveney, 2005). Most evidence has been garnered through investigations of depressive disorders. For example, Rottenberg, Kasch, Gross, and Gotlib (2002) found consistent evidence of unresponsive or insensitive affective responding to both negative and positive emotional stimuli in individuals diagnosed with major depressive disorder (MDD). This "inflexible" responding (Rottenberg et al., 2002, p. 136) may be part of a broad pattern of unresponsiveness, such that the depressed individual cannot shift emotion responses appropriately by changing context or conditions. Other investigations have suggested that similar deficits may be present in anxiety disorders (e.g., relatively stronger experience of negative emotion irrespective of context in generalized anxiety disorder) (Mennin, Heimburg, Turk, & Fresco, 2005) as well as personality disorders (e.g., borderline personality disorder) (for a review, see Johnson, Hurley, Benkelfat, Herpertz, & Taber, 2003). Together, this body of work suggests a need to organize psychopathology based on broad emotion deficits that cut across current diagnostic categories (see Kring, 2008, for review). The construct of emotion context sensitivity may prove to be a useful heuristic when evaluating emotion processes common to many diagnoses.

One reason for the link between context-insensitive emotion responses and psychopathology, particularly mood and anxiety disorders, may be related to the biases of attention, memory, and ideation common to these disorders. In a review of this literature, Mathews and MacLeod (2005) summarized findings demonstrating consistent cognitive biases in depression and anxiety that result in contextually insensitive responses. For example, depressed individuals typically demonstrate attentional bias toward emotionally negative information, thus making it far more difficult for them to respond with positive emotion when conditions demand. In contrast, individuals with anxiety disorders typically show attentional biases toward threatening conditions; therefore, they are more likely to respond with higher levels of fear in less threatening contexts. Moreover, biases of memory and interpretation are also quite common to mood and anxiety disorders and consequently could contribute strongly to challenges with emotion-sensitive responses (see also Joorman, Yoon, & Siemer, Chapter 8, and Taylor & Amir, Chapter 16, this volume).

Evidence from neuroimaging studies also suggests a link between emotion context insensitivity and particular neurological deficits or dysfunction. For example, there is now evidence to suggest that contextual sensitivity may be dependent on functioning in the prefrontal cortex and hippocampus (for a review, see Davidson, Pizzagalli, Nitschke, & Kalin, 2003). Impairments of both areas may be due to their sensitivity to prolonged exposure to elevated glucocorticoids as a result of stressful life experiences (McEwen, 1998; Sapolsky, 2000). However, much work remains to be done in deciphering this link (see Goldsmith & Davidson, 2004).

Emotion Context Sensitivity: Implications for Recovery

Overall, there is compelling evidence demonstrating the critical role of emotion context sensitivity in adaptive or healthy responses. However, the construct of emotion context sensitivity also has important implications for understanding the recovery process. According to the *Diagnostic and Statistical Manual of Mental Disorders* (fourth edition, text revision), recovery from a particular mental disorder involves the alleviation of signs and symptoms of that disorder (American Psychiatric Association, 2000, p. 2). However, the concept of recovery can be understood in a variety of ways. A growing body of empirical work has demonstrated that recovery is complex, particularly when considering responses to stressful or potentially traumatic events, events that are thought to trigger psychopathology in some people.

Reviews of the available literature on patterns of adjustment from stressful life events has suggested three dominant prototypical responses: a stable trajectory of healthy functioning or resilience, a more gradual return to baseline or recovery, and severe and chronic persistence in psychological and physiological disturbances (Bonanno, 2004, 2005). Only in the past decade has there been sufficient empirical evidence to differentiate between these three distinct trajectories. For example, there is now compelling evidence demonstrating that most individuals follow the resilient trajectory, responding with little to no disruption in functioning despite experiencing initial distress in the weeks after the event (e.g., Bonanno et al., 2002, 2005). In contrast, others show clear signs of initial dysfunction, including elevated distress and threshold levels of psychopathology in the early months. Of this group, some individuals return to normal levels of functioning within 1 to 2 years, characterizing a "recovery trajectory" (Bonanno, 2004). However, other individuals experience persistent symptoms and ultimately chronic disturbances in functioning over the long term that can include the development of diagnosable pathology, in a "chronic trajectory" (Bonanno, 2004; Figure 7.1).

The distinction between the recovery and chronic trajectories may be of particular relevance to the issue of emotion context sensitivity. Unlike resilience, in which individuals typically only experience "transient perturbations in normal functioning" (Bonanno, 2004, p. 21), a key feature of recovery is that it is characterized by the presence of symptoms in the early months following the event. Therefore, differentiating between those individuals whose pattern of initial symptomatology will dissipate over a relatively brief time period versus those whose symptomatology becomes pervasive and a chronic pattern of maladaptive functioning suggests potentially important public health implications. In particular, the determination of variables that might inform the divergence of these paths would hold important clues to possible early intervention (Bonanno, Galea, Bucciarelli, & Vhahov, 2007).

As described earlier, emotion context sensitivity is a useful heuristic in assessing adaptive versus potentially pathological emotion responding.

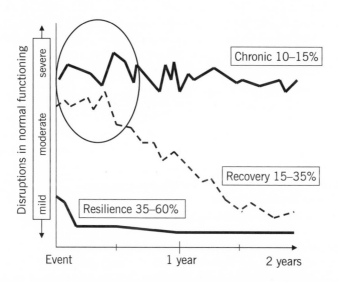

FIGURE 7.1. Prototypical outcome trajectories. From Bonanno (2004). Copyright 2004 by the American Psychological Association. Adapted by permission.

Within the context of recovery, emotion context sensitivity may be key in determining who may or may not return to normal levels of functioning. Several investigations demonstrate the usefulness of this idea. For example, work by Rottenberg and colleagues (2002) established the importance of context-sensitive emotion responses in predicting recovery in individuals with clinically significant symptoms of depression. Their investigation showed that participants who were less emotionally responsive to both sad and amusing contexts showed the *least* relief from symptoms 6 months later. Moreover, in a follow-up investigation, Rottenberg and colleagues (2005) demonstrated that, when comparing emotion context sensitivity in samples of individuals currently meeting criteria for MDD and those whose MDD symptoms had remitted as well as healthy controls, individuals who had recovered from MDD closely resembled healthy controls in their ability to respond appropriately to shifting emotional contexts. By contrast, the sample currently diagnosed with MDD had clear difficulties responding sensitively to changing conditions. These two investigations together suggest not only that emotion context insensitivity may be a marker of depressive disorders, but that the ability to maintain or adjust one's emotional responses so that they are contextually sensitive may be a hallmark of recovery.

Recent work by Bonanno, Colak, and colleagues (2007) involving individuals who suffered childhood sexual abuse (CSA) demonstrates a similar link between emotion context sensitivity and recovery. In this study, Bonanno et al. interviewed participants with documented histories of CSA, measured their expressions of positive emotion (i.e., Duchenne and non-Duchenne smiling and laughter) during the interview, and then followed the participants' level of adjustment over a 2-year period. One of the questions this study asked was whether the context of disclosing a past abuse experience would moderate the functional consequences of the positive displays, a question rendered especially intriguing because of the potential social stigma associated with childhood abuse. Although there is a large body of evidence demonstrating the salutary benefits of positive emotion (e.g., Bonanno & Keltner, 1997; Folkman & Moskowitz, 2000; Fredrickson, 1998, 2001; Levenson, 1988), very little work has examined the potential maladaptive consequences of such displays in such socially stigmatizing contexts. In an attempt to understand how stigma might come into play, Bonanno, Colak, and colleagues looked to a social capital model (Kurzban & Leary, 2001; Tooby & Cosmides, 1996). In such a model, cooperative relationships require that each person be able to judge the other person's goals and values, which in turn fosters each person's ability to reliably predict the others' actions based on inferences about their intentions. Individuals whose intentions cannot be easily predicted or whose behavior characteristically violates societal norms and expectations are primary candidates for social exclusion. When seen from this perspective, CSA survivors who exhibit positive emotional displays while disclosing a potentially highly evocative abuse experience may confuse observers or, worse, may instill in observers a reluctance to invest their limited social resources in the person.

Overwhelmingly, the evidence suggested that general displays of positive emotion were associated with better social adjustment 2 years later. However, consistent with the social capital model, there were markedly different effects for participants who displayed genuine positive emotional expressions while discussing their abuse experience in particular. These individuals showed poorer long-term social adjustment, indicating a strong link between contextually insensitive responses and long-term recovery from CSA (Bonanno, Colak, et al., 2007).

Finally, Coifman and Bonanno (2009) examined the role of emotion context sensitivity in recovery from the untimely loss of a loved one in a sample of recently bereaved participants. In this investigation, the authors sought to examine how emotion responses across negative and positive contexts were related to long-term adjustment. In particular, the focus was on individuals showing clear signs of distress and depressive symptoms in the early months following the loss (i.e., nonresilient individuals; see Bonanno, 2004, 2005) in the interest of differentiating between those who recovered with the next 12 to 14 months and those who showed chronic disturbances of functioning. Consistent with the three investigations described previously, context-sensitive emotion responses were linked with recovery and the alleviation of symptoms by 18 months after the loss. However, this investigation was unique in that it demonstrated specifically that context-sensitive emotion responding was able to differentiate between those participants who did and those who did *not* recover from their loss.

Of particular note in Coifman and Bonanno's (2009) work was the methodology, which focused on emotion responses unrelated to the loss itself. The authors sought to measure the ability of participants to disengage from the loss emotions in order to respond appropriately to both negative and positive events in their daily lives, shedding some light on the function of emotion context sensitivity in adaptation to stressful life events. As described, psychopathology associated with emotion context insensitivity (e.g., depressive disorders) appears to involve a degree of inflexibility in responses, making it difficult for individuals to shift responses to changing conditions. Yet appropriate and contextually sensitive emotion responses are required in daily life, whether in casual social contexts (e.g., laughing with a coworker) or in more demanding circumstances (e.g., comforting a sick child). If individuals are unable to engage appropriately and sensitively in emotional interactions or emotional events, their ability to function is quite impaired. Hence, there is a clear link between emotion context insensitivity and significant mental illness such as MDD. However, as Coifman and Bonanno demonstrate, if, in the context of significant emotional disruption (e.g., the loss of a spouse or child), individuals are still able to engage emotionally in an appropriate and sensitive manner to unrelated emotional events, they are more likely to return to higher levels of functioning and to recover.

Emotion Context Sensitivity in Clinical Treatment

The implications of a more thorough understanding of emotion context sensitivity extend into many areas, most notably into the development of effective treatment protocols and other clinical interventions. As the prior evidence suggests, the maintenance or restitution of emotion context-sensitive responses has been linked to recovery from psychopathology (e.g., MDD) as well as from potentially traumatic events (e.g., bereavement). As such, there is a great need for treatment interventions that effectively incorporate context-sensitive emotion responding into their goals and objectives.

Although the numbers are still limited, several recently developed treatment interventions have begun to incorporate methodologies that address this need. For example, there are two new protocols for the treatment of complicated grief that seem to incorporate the maintenance or development of emotion context sensitivity in their methodology. Individuals with complicated grief demonstrate persistent and significant symptomatology (typically encompassing a combination of grief, depression, and trauma symptoms) as well as chronic disruptions in functioning that are distinct from depression or anxiety disorders (Bonanno, Neria, et al., 2007; Prigerson & Jacobs, 2001). Most notably, these individuals struggle with getting back to the business of living following the loss and often have difficulty reengaging in their daily lives. As evidenced previously (i.e., Coifman & Bonanno, 2009), the ability to engage emotionally in a contextually sensitive manner to events outside of a trauma (e.g., daily life activities) is linked to recovery from the event. As such, two recent targeted interventions for chronic or complicated grief (Boelen, Keijser, van den Hout, & van den Bout, 2007; Shear, Frank, Houck, & Reynolds, 2005) focus, in part, on multiple aspects of coping with loss: emphasizing the importance of adjustment to the loss as well as restoration of other aspects of life. For example, these interventions focus on managing maladaptive reactions to the loss itself (using techniques such as imaginal exposure therapy) as well as on improving emotion modulation during other aspects of life through the use of such treatment approaches as behavioral activation (see Syzdek, Addis, & Martell, Chapter 17, this volume). Although these interventions are breaking new ground, there is still room for greater use of this construct. For example, evaluating emotion responses across contexts might aid in diagnosis and treatment planning for any number of emotion disorders. Moreover, regular evaluations of patients' emotion responses, across contexts and over time, could allow for clinicians to assess treatment progress and prognosis. As such, there is clearly still much work to be done to further our understanding of emotion context sensitivity and its implications for improving the effectiveness of clinical interventions.

Conclusion

Contextually sensitive emotion responses are an integral part of our adaptation to the environment and to daily life. As such, dysfunctional or insensitive responses can be linked to lasting psychopathology and poor prognosis following potentially traumatic events. Moreover, the construct of emotion context sensitivity is a useful heuristic for furthering our understanding of emotion processes and for evaluating adaptive versus maladaptive responses and has great potential to assist in assessing prognosis and outcomes in clinical treatment. It is our hope that the small but compelling body of work in this area will continue to develop and influence the study of emotion as well as its applications in clinical treatment.

References

American Psychiatric Association. (2000). *Diagnostic and statistical manual of mental disorders* (4th ed., text rev.). Washington, DC: Author.

Arsenio, W. F., Cooperman, S., & Lover, A. (2000). Affective predictors of preschoolers' aggression and peer acceptance: Direct and indirect effects. *Developmental Psychology, 36*(4), 438–448.

Averill, J. R. (1980). A constructivist view of emotion. In R. Plutchik & H. Kellerman (Eds.), *Emotion: Theory, research, and experience* (pp. 305–339). Orlando, FL: Academic Press.

Barrett, L. F. (1995). Valence focus and arousal focus: Individual differences in the structure of affective experience. *Journal of Personality and Social Psychology, 69*, 153–166.

Barrett, L. F. (2006). Are emotions natural kinds? *Perspectives on Psychological Science, 1*, 28–58.

Boelen, P. A., Keijser, J., van den Hout, M. A., & van den Bout, J. (2007). Treatment of complicated grief: A comparison between cognitive-behavioral therapy and supportive counseling. *Journal of Consulting and Clinical Psychology, 75*(2), 277–284.

Bonanno, G. A. (2004). Loss, trauma, and human resilience: Have we underestimated the human capacity to thrive after extremely aversive events? *American Psychologist, 59*, 20–29.

Bonanno, G. A. (2005). Resilience in the face of potential trauma. *Current Directions in Psychological Science, 14*, 135–138.

Bonanno, G. A., Colak, D. M., Keltner, D., Shiota, M. N., Papa, A., Noll, J. G., et al. (2007). Context matters: The benefits and costs of expressing positive emotion among survivors of childhood sexual abuse. *Emotion, 7*(4), 824–837.

Bonanno, G. A., Galea, S., Bucciarelli, A., & Vlahov, D. (2007). What predicts psychological resilience after disaster?: The role of demographics, resources, and life stress. *Journal of Consulting and Clinical Psychology, 75*, 671–682.

Bonanno, G. A., & Keltner, D. (1997). Facial expression of emotion in the course of conjugal bereavement. *Journal of Abnormal Psychology, 106,* 126–137.

Bonanno, G. A., & Keltner, D. (2004). The coherence of emotion systems: Comparing "online" measures of appraisal and facial expressions, and self-report. *Cognition and Emotion, 18*(3), 431–444.

Bonanno, G. A., Moskowitz, J. T., Papa, A., & Folkman, S. (2005). Resilience to loss in bereaved spouses, bereaved parents and bereaved gay men. *Journal of Personality and Social Psychology, 88*(5), 827–843.

Bonanno, G. A., Neria, Y., Mancini, A., Coifman, K. G., Litz, B., & Insel, B. (2007). Is there more to complicated grief than depression and posttraumatic stress disorder? A test of incremental validity. *Journal of Abnormal Psychology, 116*(2), 342–351.

Bonanno, G. A., Wortman, C. B., Lehman, D. R., Tweed, R. G., Haring, M., Sonnega, J., et al. (2002). Resilience to loss and chronic grief: A prospective study from pre-loss to 18 months post-loss. *Journal of Personality and Social Psychology, 83,* 1150–1164.

Buss, K. A., Davidson, R. J., Kalin, N. H., & Goldsmith, H. H. (2004). Context-specific freezing and associated physiological reactivity as a dysregulated fear response. *Developmental Psychology, 40*(4), 583–594.

Campos, J. J., Campos, R. G., & Barrett, K. C. (1989). Emergent themes in the study of emotional development and emotion regulation. *Developmental Psychology, 25,* 394–402.

Coifman, K. G., & Bonanno, G. A. (2009). *When distress isn't depression: Emotion context sensitivity and recovery from bereavement.* Unpublished manuscript.

Cole, P. M., Michel, M. K., & Teti, L. O. (1994). The development of emotion regulation and dysregulation: A clinical perspective. *Monographs of the Society for Research in Child Development, 59*(2–3, Serial No. 240), 73–100.

Davidson, R. J. (1998). Affective style and affective disorders: Perspectives from affective neuroscience. *Cognition and Emotion, 12,* 307–330.

Davidson, R. J., Pizzagalli, D., Nitschke, J. B., & Kalin, N. H. (2003). Parsing the subcomponents of emotion and disorders of emotion: Perspectives from affective neuroscience. In R. J. Davidson, K. Scherer, & H.H. Goldsmith (Eds.), *Handbook of affective sciences* (pp. 8–24). New York: Oxford University Press.

Duchenne de Bologne, G. B. (1862). *The mechanism of human facial expression* (R. A. Cuthbertson, Trans.). New York: Cambridge University Press.

Ekman, P. (1984). Expression and the nature of emotion. In K. Scherer & P. Ekman (Eds.), *Approaches to emotion* (pp. 319–344). Hillsdale, NJ: Erlbaum.

Ekman, P. (1992). Are there basic emotions? *Psychological Review, 99*(3), 550–553.

Ekman, P., & Friesen, W. V. (1982). Felt, false, and miserable smiles. *Journal of Nonverbal Behavior, 6,* 238–252.

Ekman, P., Levenson, R. W., & Friesen, W. V. (1983). Autonomic nervous system activity distinguishes among emotions. *Science, 221,* 1208–1210.

Folkman, S., & Moskowitz, J. T. (2000). Positive affect and the other side of coping. *American Psychologist, 55,* 647–654.

Fredrickson, B. L. (1998). What good are positive emotions? *Review of General Psychology, 2,* 300–319.

Fredrickson, B. L. (2001). The role of positive emotions in positive psychology: The broaden-and-build theory of positive emotions. *American Psychologist, 56,* 218–226.

Fredrickson, B. L., & Joiner, T. (2002). Positive emotions trigger upward spirals toward emotional well-being. *Psychological Science, 13*, 172–175.

Fredrickson, B. L., & Levenson, R. W. (1998). Positive emotions speed recovery from the cardiovascular sequelae of negative emotions. *Cognition and Emotion, 12*(2), 191–220.

Fredrickson, B. L., Mancuso, R. A., Branigan, C., & Tugade, M. M. (2000). The undoing effect of positive emotions. *Motivation and Emotion, 24*(4), 237–258.

Frijda, N. H. (1986). *The emotions: Studies in emotion and social interaction.* Cambridge, UK: Cambridge University Press.

Frijda, N. H. (1988). The laws of emotion. *American Psychologist, 43*, 349–358.

Gehricke, J., & Shapiro, D. (2000). Reduced facial expression and social context in major depression: Discrepancies between facial muscle activity and self-reported emotion. *Psychiatry Research, 95*, 157–167.

Goldin, P. R., McRae, K., Ramel, W., & Gross, J. J. (2008). The neural basis of emotion regulation: Reappraisal and suppression of negative emotion. *Biological Psychiatry, 63*, 577–586.

Goldsmith, H. H., & Davidson, R. J. (2004). Disambiguating the components of emotion regulation. *Child Development, 75*(2), 361–365.

Gould, S. J. (1996). *The mismeasure of man.* New York: Norton.

Gross, J.J. (2008). Emotion regulation. In M. Lewis, J. M. Haviland-Jones, & L. F. Barrett (Eds.), *Handbook of emotions* (3rd ed., pp. 497–512). New York: Guilford Press.

Isen, A. M. (2000). Positive affect and decision making. In M. Lewis & J. M. Haviland-Jones (Eds.), *Handbook of emotions* (pp.417–435). New York: Guilford Press.

Isen, A. M., Daubman, K. A., & Nowicki, G. P. (1987). Positive affect facilitates creative problem solving. *Journal of Personality and Social Psychology, 47*, 1206–1217.

Izard, C. E., & Ackerman, B. P. (2000). Motivational, organizational, and regulatory functions of discrete emotions. In M. Lewis & J. M. Haviland-Jones (Eds.), *Handbook of emotions* (pp. 253–264). New York: Guilford Press.

Johnson, P. A., Hurley, R. A., Benkelfat, C., Herpertz, S. C., & Taber, K. H. (2003). Understanding emotion regulation in borderline personality disorder: Contributions of neuroimaging. *Journal of Neuropsychiatry and Clinical Neuroscience, 15*(4), 397–402.

Keltner, D. (1995). Signs of appeasement: Evidence for the distinct displays of embarrassment, amusement, and shame. *Journal of Personality and Social Psychology, 68*, 441–454.

Keltner, D., & Bonanno, G. A. (1997). A study of laughter and dissociation: Distinct correlates of laughter and smiling during bereavement. *Journal of Personality and Social Psychology, 73*, 687–702.

Keltner, D., & Haidt, J. (2001). Social functions of emotions. In T. J. Mayne & G. A. Bonanno (Eds.), *Emotions: Current issues and future directions* (pp. 192–213). New York: Guilford Press.

Keltner, D., & Kring, A. M. (1998). Emotion, social function, and psychopathology. *Review of General Psychiatry, 2*, 230–342.

Kring, A. M. (2008) Emotion disturbances as transdiagnostic processes in psychopathology. In M. Lewis, J. M. Haviland-Jones, & L. F. Barrett (Eds.), *Handbook of emotions* (3rd ed., pp. 691–705). New York: Guilford Press.

Kurzban, R., & Leary, M. R. (2001). Evolutionary origins of stigmatization: The functions of social exclusion. *Psychological Bulletin, 127*, 187–208.

Larson, C. L., Nitschke, J. B., & Davidson, R. J. (2007) Common and distinct patterns of affective response in dimensions of anxiety and depression. *Emotion, 7*(1), 182–191.

Lerner, J. S., Gonzalez, R. M., Dahl, R. E., Hariri, A. R., & Taylor, S. E. (2005). Facial expressions of emotion reveal neuroendocrine and cardiovascular stress response. *Biological Psychiatry, 58*, 743–750.

Levenson, R. W. (1994). Human emotion: A functional view. In P. Ekman & R. J. Davidson (Eds.), *The nature of emotion* (pp. 123–126). New York: Oxford University Press.

Levenson, R. W. (1998). Emotion and the autonomic nervous system: A prospectus for research on autonomic specificity. In H. L. Wagner (Ed.), *Social psychophysiology and emotion: Theory and clinical applications* (pp. 17–42). London: Wiley.

Levenson, R. W., Ekman, P., Heider, K., & Friesen, W. V. (1992). Emotion and autonomic nervous system activity in the Minangkabau of West Sumatra. *Journal of Personality and Social Psychology, 62*, 972–988.

Mathews, A., & MacLeod, C. (2005). Cognitive vulnerability to emotional disorders. *Annual Review of Clinical Psychology, 1*, 167–195.

Matsumoto, D., & Kudoh, T. (1993). American–Japanese cultural differences in attributions of personality based on smiles. *Journal of Nonverbal Behavior, 17*, 231–243.

Mayer, J. D., Salovey, P., & Caruso, D. R. (2008). Emotional intelligence: New ability or eclectic traits? *American Psychologist, 63*(6), 503–517.

Mayne, T. J., & Ramsey, J. (2001). The structure of emotion: A nonlinear dynamic systems approach. In T. J. Mayne & G. A. Bonanno (Eds.), *Emotions: Current issues and future directions* (pp. 1–37). New York: Guilford Press.

McEwen, B. S. (1998). Protective and damaging effects of stress mediators. *New England Journal of Medicine, 338*, 171–179.

Mennin, D. S., Heimberg, R. G., Turk, C. L., & Fresco, D. M. (2005). Preliminary evidence for an emotion dysregulation model for generalized anxiety disorder. *Behaviour Research and Therapy, 43*(10), 1281–1310.

Nesse, R. (1990). Evolutionary explanations of emotions. *Human Nature, 1*, 261–289.

Ochsner, K. N., & Barrett, L. F. (2001). A multiprocess perspective on the neuroscience of emotion. In T. J. Mayne & G. A. Bonanno (Eds.), *Emotions: Current issues and future directions* (pp. 38–81). New York: Guilford Press.

Papa, A., & Bonanno, G. A. (2008). Smiling in the face of adversity: The interpersonal and intrapersonal functions of smiling. *Emotion, 8*(1), 1–12.

Prigerson, H. G., & Jacobs, S. C. (2001). Traumatic grief as a distinct disorder: A rationale, consensus criteria, and a preliminary empirical test. In M. S. Stroebe, R. O. Hansson, W. Stroebe, & H. A. W. Schut (Eds.), *Handbook of bereavement research: Consequences, coping, and care* (pp. 613–647). Washington, DC: American Psychological Association.

Rottenberg, J., & Gotlib, I. H. (2004). Socioemotional functioning in depression. In M. Power (Ed.), *Mood disorders: A handbook of science and practice* (pp. 61–77). New York: Wiley.

Rottenberg, J., Gross, J. J., & Gotlib, I.H. (2005). Emotion context insensitivity in major depressive disorder. *Journal of Abnormal Psychology, 114*, 627–639.

Rottenberg, J., Kasch, K. L., Gross, J. J., & Gotlib, I. H. (2002). Sadness and amusement reactivity differentially predict concurrent and prospective functioning in major depressive disorder. *Emotion, 2*(2), 135–146.

Rozin, P., Lowery, L., Imada, S., & Haidt, J. (1999). The CAD triad hypothesis: A mapping between three moral emotions (contempt, anger, disgust) and three moral codes (community, autonomy, divinity). *Journal of Personality and Social Psychology, 76*, 574–586.

Russell, J. A. (1995). Facial expressions of emotion: What lies beyond minimal universality? *Psychological Bulletin, 118*(3), 379–391.

Salomon, R. C. (2000). The philosophy of emotions. In M. Lewis & J. M. Haviland-Jones (Eds.), *Handbook of emotions* (pp. 3–15). New York: Guilford Press.

Sapolsky, R. M. (2000). Glucocorticoids and hippocampal atrophy in neuropsychiatric disorders. *Archives of General Psychiatry, 57*, 925–935.

Schwarz, N., & Clore, G. L. (1983). Mood, misattribution, and judgments of well-being: Informative and directive functions of affective states. *Journal of Personality and Social Psychology, 45*, 513–523.

Shear, K., Frank, E., Houck, P. R., & Reynolds, C. F. (2005). Treatment of complicated grief: A randomized controlled trial. *Journal of the American Medical Association, 293*(21), 2601–2608.

Shestyuk, A. Y., Deldin, P. J., Brand, J. E., & Deveney, C. M. (2005). Reduced sustained brain activity during processing of positive emotional stimuli in major depression. *Biological Psychiatry, 57*, 1089–1096.

Shweder, R. (1994). "You're not sick, you're just in love": Emotion as an interpretive system. In P. Ekman & R. J. Davidson (Eds.), *The nature of emotion: Fundamental questions* (pp. 32–44). New York: Oxford University Press.

Stein, N. L., Trabasso, T., & Liwag, M. D. (2000). A goal appraisal theory of emotional understanding: Implications for development and learning. In M. Lewis & J. M. Haviland-Jones (Eds.), *Handbook of emotions* (pp. 436–457). New York: Guilford Press.

Stemmler, G. (1989). The autonomic differentiation of emotions revisited: Convergent and discriminant validation. *Psychophysiology, 26*, 617–632.

Stemmler, G., Heldmann, M., Pauls, C. A., & Scherer, T. (2001). Constraints for emotion specificity in fear and anger: The context counts. *Psychophysiology, 38*, 275–291.

Tooby, J., & Cosmides, L. (1990). The past explains the present: Emotional adaptations and the structure of ancestral environments. *Ethology and Sociobiology, 11*, 375–424.

Tooby, J., & Cosmides, L. (1996). Friendship and the banker's paradox: Other pathways to the evolution of adaptive altruism. *Proceedings of the British Academy, 88*, 119–143.

Westphal, M., & Bonanno, G. A. (2004). Emotion self-regulation. In M. Beauregard (Ed.), *Consciousness, emotional self-regulation, and the brain* (pp. 1–34). Philadelphia: Benjamins.

CHAPTER 8

• — • — • — •

Cognition and Emotion Regulation

Jutta Joormann, K. Lira Yoon, and Matthias Siemer

Cognition plays a critical role in human emotion. According to cognitive theories of emotion, cognitive appraisals determine whether an emotion is experienced and which emotion is experienced. Accordingly, cognition is the primary route through which emotions are regulated. Consider, for example, a recent incident that involved traveling on a plane when sudden turbulence made the plane shake and fall in seemingly uncontrollable ways. As you can imagine, almost everyone on the plane responded with fear. A mother, however, started to talk to her scared-looking son in a calm, collected voice, telling him how much fun it is that the plane goes up and down and how it reminded her of their recent roller-coaster ride at Disney World. The boy smiled, and it seemed that he was starting to enjoy the experience. Why did this simple intervention work? The mother helped her son reinterpret the shaking and falling of the plane in a nonthreatening way, guided the boy's attention toward the fun aspects of the experience, and helped him recall a similar event from the past that was associated with an emotion (joy) incongruent with the primary emotion (fear) elicited by the current situation. Admittedly, the success of cognitive interventions in this specific situation may be limited to 5-year-olds with little exposure to plane disaster movies, but similar situations are encountered frequently in everyday life. Changing cognition to change emotion is also a critical part of many of our most successful therapeutic interventions. Exposure therapy, for example, is an intense experience for both therapists and patients that results in novel interpretations and appraisals, modifications in attention processes, and the encoding of new memories that associate the feared situation with a sense of mastery instead of helplessness.

In this chapter, we investigate the relation between cognition and emotion regulation by first discussing theories of emotion that explain why and how cognition influences the emotion experience. We further discuss how emotion regulation can be conceptualized in these models and why it may be easier said than done to use cognition to change the trajectory or quality of an emotional response. We then discuss in depth specific cognitive processes such as interpretation and attention that help and hinder emotion regulation. Finally, we investigate individual differences in these cognitive processes and link them to clinical disorders. We review empirical evidence of the importance of investigating cognitive processes to increase our understanding of emotion regulation in psychopathology and end with a short presentation of future directions of what we believe is a very important line of work.

Cognition, Emotion, and Emotion Regulation

There is no doubt that cognition plays an important role in the emotion experience. Appraisal theories of emotion, for example, state that the cognitive appraisal of a situation, not the situation itself, determines the quality and intensity of the emotional response (Ellsworth & Scherer, 2003; Scherer, 2001; Siemer, Mauss, & Gross, 2007). Appraisal theories propose that emotional events are interpreted along a number of appraisal dimensions, including importance, expectedness, responsibility, and degree of controllability (Lazarus, 1991; Ortony, Clore, & Collins, 1988). There is a long history of discussion, however, about the question of whether cognition is a necessary component of the conditions that need to be present for an emotion to occur (e.g., Parkinson, 2007; Siemer & Reisenzein, 2007). Specifically, theories differ in their claim of whether cognitive appraisals are merely sufficient causes of emotional responses or are also necessary causes of the quality and intensity of an emotion (Siemer et al., 2007). If appraisals are truly necessary, no factors other than the cognitive appraisals determine why people respond to the same situation with different emotions or indeed any emotion at all. This proposition has been challenged by many authors who argue that noncognitive factors such as drugs, hunger, or pain can cause emotions and that appraisals are not necessary under these circumstances (Berkowitz & Harmon-Jones, 2004; Izard, 1993). Appraisal theorists, however, have pointed out that these other factors only elicit specific emotional responses if they trigger (at least simple automatic or schematic) appraisals (Clore & Centerbar, 2004; Smith & Kirby, 2004). The long-lasting nature of this debate demonstrates that attention, interpretation, attributions, and memories are intricately related to the emotion experience and that it is difficult to separate cognition and emotion. Indeed, many emotion researchers have pointed out that cognition is such an integral part of the emotion response that separating cognition from emotion is artificial (e.g., Lazarus, 1991). Emotions also influence cognition. It has been argued that emotional states facilitate the activation of mood-congruent memories (Bower, 1981) and that emotional states can be considered a disposition to make certain types of appraisals (e.g., Lerner & Keltner, 2000), thereby increasing the probability that people will experience specific emotions (Siemer, 2005b).

Given the difficulties in defining the relation between cognition and emotion, it is not surprising that defining the relation between emotion and emotion regulation is even more complicated. Some authors have begun to formulate core features of these concepts (Gross, 2002). Emotions are seen as a response to a specific situation (internal or external) or as a person–situation transaction (Lazarus, 1991; Scherer, 1984). Emotions change over time in response to changing demands of the situation and the coping attempts of the person. Situational demands or changes compel the person to attend, and this attention is linked to specific appraisals, which lead to an emotional response to the situation that is caused by and corresponds to the appraisal pattern. This sequence is seen as a recursive loop that can be entered at any point. It is possible, for example, that the situation did not change but that the person suddenly pays attention to it or that the appraisal of the situation is otherwise modified. It is also possible that the emotional response itself changes the appraisal of the situation, for example, by changing attentional deployment to different aspects of the situation. Emotional response tendencies may also change the situation, which then changes appraisals of the situation and so forth. It is furthermore possible that a situation is already entered with a preexisting emotional state, which affects the appraisal of the situation (Lerner & Keltner, 2000; Siemer, 2001).

It is critical to keep the recursive nature of the emotion generation and regulation process in mind because it means that there are numerous entry points at which people can intervene to change their emotional responses. In the example we provided at the beginning of the chapter, the boy started responding with fear, which led his mother to intervene by changing attention to the situation and the appraisal of the situation as dangerous, which led to a change in the child's emotional responding. Accordingly, Gross (2002) has presented a model in which emotion regulation can take place at any point in the emotion generation sequence. Situation selection and modification lead to changes in the situation that was attended to and elicited the appraisal. Attentional deployment influences the appraisal of a situation and determines whether the situation will be appraised in an emotion-generating fashion. Cognitive change modifies appraisals directly, and response modulation changes the response to the appraisal. This brief discussion of the emotion generation sequence and the steps at which emotion regulation takes place clearly reveals the central importance of cognition. At least two steps in the sequence, attentional deployment and appraisals, make it necessary to pay close attention to processes such as attention, interpretation, and memory. Indeed, studies have demonstrated that voluntary changes in the appraisals of a situation can change the intensity of an emotional reaction (Gross, 1998; Ochsner, Bunge, Gross, & Gabrieli, 2002; Ochsner et al., 2004). Moreover, it is noteworthy that noncognitive emotion regulation strategies, such as inhibition of emotion expressions, have been consistently found to be less effective than strategies that influence cognition (Gross, 1998; Gross & Levenson, 1997). Given that appraisals are such a core feature of the emotion generation and regulation process, it seems critical to gain a better understanding of factors that determine appraisals.

Before discussing this in more detail, we should point out, however, that most of the processes we have discussed so far can be initiated strategically or can occur automatically. Given the crucial role of automatic processes in cognition and emotion, emotion generation and regulation can occur at a much faster pace and less accessible to conscious thought than the just-mentioned examples suggest. Automaticity of the involved (cognitive) processes can make it difficult to separate the components of the described sequence and also complicates the separation of emotion generation from emotion regulation. Indeed, emotion regulation may often require that an automatic (i.e., fast and unconscious) appraisal of a situation be replaced with a more controlled evaluation of the circumstance, meaning, and consequences of the event (Siemer & Reisenzein, 2007). Whereas emotion regulation is often strategically initiated, it can also take place without the person's knowledge or intention, which further adds to the difficulties in differentiating emotion generation and emotion regulation (Mauss, Cook, & Gross, 2007)

Differentiating emotion and emotion regulation can be difficult. Empirical research addressing these concepts requires delivering one of the following two patterns of evidence. Researchers can demonstrate that an emotional response was present in the first place that was somehow changed, truncated, or terminated as a result of emotion regulation. Emotion regulation, however, can sometimes be used so early in the emotion generation sequence that the emotional response is effectively prevented from occurring (anticipatory emotion regulation). Similarly, automatic emotion regulation processes can be so fast and efficient that an emotional response cannot be detected. In these cases, researchers have to demonstrate that if the person had behaved differently (i.e., not regulated the emotion or had used a different strategy), an emotional response would have occurred. Clearly, researchers cannot attribute the absence of (or differences in) emotional reactions to emotion regulation without this additional evidence. Even though the occurrence of anticipatory or automatic emotion regulation may be difficult to prove in individual cases, differentiating emotion generation and regulation clearly is critical if we want to investigate these processes in an empirically meaningful way. If simply having an emotional response is taken as an indicator of (the lack of) emotion regulation but not having an emotional response is also taken as an indicator of emotion regulation, this concept becomes meaningless and research becomes tautological.

Given that some disorders are characterized by dysfunctional emotional responses whereas others may better be thought of as mood disorders, it is also important to differentiate between different affective states. Specifically, whereas emotions are responses to acute changes in the environment, mood states are often described as diffuse and nonintentional (e.g., Siemer, 2009). Thus, emotions, as opposed to moods, are typically the result of appraisals of the current situation, which provide them with focus and direction. As a result, some strategies (e.g., reappraisal) may work particularly well when trying to modify an emotion, whereas others may work particularly well when trying to modify a mood (e.g., distraction). Differentiating between mood and emotion regulation may thus be critical when investigating psychological disorders, and we return to this point later in this chapter.

Another complication is the issue of how emotion and the change in emotion as a result of emotion regulation are assessed. Emotional responses are multicomponent phenomena that are associated with bodily symptoms, subjective experiences, cognitive changes, and action tendencies (e.g., Levenson, 1994; Scherer, 1984). Evidence suggests that changes in these levels occur in a less coherent or synchronized way than was previously assumed (Mauss, Levenson, McCarter, Wilhelm, & Gross, 2005; Reisenzein, Bordgen, Holtbernd, & Matz, 2006). As a result, emotion regulation does not necessarily lead to changes on all of these levels. It is, therefore, debatable whether demonstrating that any one of these components is present or modified is sufficient to indicate that emotion regulation has taken place. If we present positive and negative pictures to participants who are taking part in a functional magnetic resonance imaging (fMRI) experiment and demonstrate increased blood flow in their amygdala whenever a gruesome picture is presented or if someone's heart rate rises when they watch a sad video, is this sufficient to state that an emotional response was observed? Indeed, research on amygdala function suggests that, although emotion regulation may alter amygdala response to emotional stimuli (Ochsner et al., 2002), activation in this structure is not identical to emotion generation (Phelps, 2006; Tranel, Gullickson, Koch, & Adolphs, 2006).

In any case, it seems difficult to answer these questions without consulting experience ratings, but what about cases in which the experience is not synchronized with the bodily changes or the cognitions? If other indicators (such as changes in cognition or physiological changes) are used, especially in the absence of self-reported emotional experience, researchers need to present an explicit theory of how emotion and emotion regulation are operationalized. We believe that it is necessary to keep these issues in mind when discussing cognition and emotion regulation in the next parts of our chapter. There is an unfortunate tendency, for example, to assume that attentional allocation to emotional faces will induce affect and that reallocation of attention to neutral material will regulate this affect without actually measuring whether changes in emotion have occurred or without demonstrating that an emotional response would have occurred (e.g., with a control condition) in the absence of attentional reallocation. The emotion generation sequence discussed earlier, however, suggests that simply attending to a potentially emotion-eliciting stimulus may not be sufficient to induce or change emotion as long as attention deployment is not followed by changes in appraisals. Investigating the role of cognition in emotion regulation requires the simultaneous assessment of cognition and emotion.

Finally, it has been discussed in previous research that emotion regulation is not to be confused with the down-regulation of negative affect or with the avoidance of unpleasant feelings (Gross, 2002). Selecting the company of friends who make you feel good, avoiding negative feedback to maintain a positive mood state after success, and recalling a failed exam when you feel that a negative mood helps you study for the next one are only some examples that demonstrate that positive and negative emotions can be increased or decreased depending on that person's goals, motivation, and expectations. Attention, memory, and interpretation play an important role in all these instances of emotion regulation, but we focus primarily on the down-regulation of negative emotions given that this is the area most pertinent to emotional disorders (of course, there are exceptions, like mania).

Given that cognition is such an intricate part of the emotion experience, it is interesting to note the relative scarcity of research that investigates the relation of cognition and emotion regulation in emotional disorders. Even though research on cognitive aspects of disorders has increased dramatically over the past years, rarely do studies investigate whether cognitive processes are causal in generating difficulties in emotion regulation. We know, for example, that depression is associated with biased processing of negative information, but very few studies have tried to link research on cognitive biases in this disorder to the hallmark feature of depression, which is sustained negative affect. Similarly, we know that anxiety is associated with an orienting bias toward threat-relevant stimuli, but few studies are available to show whether these biases impair the regulation of anxiety. Simply studying whether people who are diagnosed with emotional disorders differ from control samples in their cognition is no proof that cognition is causing emotion dysregulation. Making explicit the link between cognitive processes and emotional experience in psychological disorders will, therefore, be a main aim of this chapter but will often remain speculative given the lack of empirical studies that target both cognition and emotion at the same time.

Individual differences in cognition impact emotion regulation in two important ways. Reappraisal and attentional deployment, for example, can

directly modify emotions and are, therefore, considered emotion regulation strategies. People may be more or less able or motivated to use these
strategies to change the intensity or quality of their emotions. Other cognitive processes, however, do not directly change emotions but make it easier
or harder to use certain emotion regulation strategies. Cognitive inflexibility, for example, can affect a person's ability to reappraise. Cognitive
biases in perception and attention may lead to inflexible, automatic, and
unconscious appraisals that make it difficult to regulate emotions by using
deliberate reappraisal of the situation (Siemer & Reisenzein, 2007). Individual differences in these processes can also lead to the use of strategies
that do not fit the situation. Implicit memory for traumatic events may alert
the individual and lead to situation selection or situation modification,
even though the situation is not dangerous and may not elicit the degree
of fear that is expected. Given that these processes do not affect emotion
directly, cognitive flexibility and cognitive biases would not be considered
emotion regulation strategies. It is still important to investigate their role
in emotion regulation because they can affect the selection and the effectiveness of strategies. It is probably not the case that emotional disorders
are associated with the use of emotion regulation strategies that differ dramatically from strategies used by other people. It is more likely that the
inflexible use of certain strategies, the poor fit of the regulation strategy
with the situation, and differences in the ability to implement effective
strategies are important in psychopathology. Individual differences in cognition can help us understand how these difficulties are associated with
emotional disorders.

Perception and Attention

The easiest and probably most effective (but not necessarily the most adaptive) way to regulate emotions is to avoid the emotion-eliciting situation, to
ignore the cues that elicit the emotion, or to attend to the situation initially
but to quickly disengage from it and redirect attention. These strategies
are so effective that it may be difficult to evaluate whether emotion regulation did indeed occur. A passenger on the plane who uses headphones and
concentrates on the movie while turbulences occur may not be an obvious example of someone who is regulating fear; he might just be a person
enjoying the movie. From the outside, it is difficult to distinguish between
someone enjoying the movie and someone regulating fear through distraction because neither person experiences fear or has experienced fear at
any point during the flight. We need to know whether the person chose
to put on headphones and chose to concentrate on the movie after feeling the turbulence (or in anticipation that turbulence may occur during
the flight) and did so with the intention of distracting himself from this
fear-eliciting situation if and when it arose. If this is the case, this person

may be a good example of someone using attention redirection effectively. Individual differences in perception and attention, however, can also influence the selection and effectiveness of other emotion regulation strategies such as situation selection and modification. A person with flight phobia, for example, may attend to the weather forecast and choose to cancel the flight anticipating the turbulences. Another person who is scared of flying may attend to the weather forecast and stock up on sleep medication before boarding the plane. In both cases, the emotion of fear is avoided, and we can be fairly certain that had these people not attended to the weather forecast they would have experienced unpleasant emotions. Thus, attention aids the implementation of emotion regulation strategies such as situation selection and modification. Further complicating matters, attention and perception in these cases may operate on an automatic level, leading people to avoid or modify situations unintentionally and without proper evaluation of the situation and of the probability that it will indeed elicit the emotion one strives to avoid.

Not surprisingly, there is ample evidence that individual differences in perception of emotion-eliciting stimuli and in attention to these stimuli are associated with different forms of psychopathology. Disorders differ in whether automatic processing biases and early perception of stimuli are an issue, whether people demonstrate attentional biases toward emotion-eliciting material, or whether they have difficulties disengaging from this material. All of these difficulties may affect emotion regulation in one way or another. Enhanced perception of emotion-relevant stimuli will frequently elicit the use of anticipatory emotion regulation strategies such as situation selection and modification. Automatic processing biases that lead to the early detection of potentially relevant stimuli and guide attention toward the processing of these stimuli will make it difficult to disengage attention or may result in cognitive avoidance. Problems in disengaging attention from certain stimuli may hinder people's use of attentional deployment as an important emotion regulation strategy. These processes, in turn, increase the probability that certain appraisals will follow.

The question of whether emotional disorders are associated with enhanced perception of emotion-relevant stimuli has been investigated in studies using either subliminal material or material with low degrees of emotional intensity or very fast presentation times. Some of the most compelling support for unconscious processing of threat-relevant material in anxiety disorders comes from Öhman and his colleagues (e.g., Öhman & Soares, 1993, 1998), who, for example, demonstrated that snake-fearful participants show heightened fear responses without being aware that a picture of a snake had been presented. Similar observations of the processing of subliminally presented anxiety-provoking stimuli have been reported in anxiety disorders with a number of tasks (see Mathews & MacLeod, 2005, for a review). These results suggest that anxiety disorders are associated with automatic processes that are involved in easy perception and initial orienting of attention toward threatening stimuli (e.g., McNally, 1995; Mogg & Bradley, 2005), which can affect the selection and effectiveness of emotion regulation strategies. Importantly, the effect of these processes on emotion generation and regulation may be outside of people's awareness.

Strikingly, no study to date has found similar biases in clinically depressed participants when depression-relevant (or other) stimuli have been masked in order to investigate unconscious processing (see Mathews & MacLeod, 2005, for a review). Based on such findings, Williams, Watts, MacLeod, and Mathews (1997) proposed that anxiety-congruent biases are observed in tasks that assess the early, orienting stage of processing before awareness. In contrast, depressive biases are observed in strategic elaboration and make it difficult for depressed people to disengage from negative material.

As described previously, early perception of emotion-eliciting stimuli may make it more difficult to use emotion regulation strategies that adequately match the situation. Similarly, if attention is biased toward emotion-eliciting cues, attention redirection may be difficult. There is mounting evidence that individuals with anxiety disorders attend to threat stimuli (see Bar-Haim, Lamy, Pergamin, Bakermans-Kranenburg, & van IJzendoorn, 2007; Mathews & MacLeod, 2005; Zinbarg & Yoon, 2008, for reviews). Most studies in this area of research have used either the modified Stroop task or an attention allocation paradigm, like the dot-probe task. In the dot-probe task, a pair of stimuli (words or faces) is presented simultaneously: One stimulus is neutral and the other is emotional. Participants are asked to respond to a probe that replaces the neutral or the emotional stimulus. Allocation of attention to the spatial position of the stimuli is determined from response latencies to the probes. In the emotional Stroop task, individuals with anxiety disorders typically take longer to respond to threat words compared with neutral words, suggesting that their attention was "grabbed" by the content of the threat words (e.g., Ehlers, Margraf, Davies, & Roth, 1988, for panic disorder; Mathews & MacLeod, 1985, for generalized anxiety disorder [GAD]; Mattia, Heimberg, & Hope, 1993, for social anxiety disorder [SAD]). Furthermore, these Stroop effects were specific to the domain of their concern. Patients with posttraumatic stress disorder (PTSD), for example, exhibited Stroop interference only for the PTSD words and not for the obsessive–compulsive disorder (OCD)–related words (McNally, Kaspi, Riemann, & Zeitlin, 1990).

Studies using the dot-probe paradigm also consistently demonstrate that individuals with anxiety disorder attend to threat words that are relevant to the specific concerns related to the anxiety disorder (e.g., Asmundson, Sandler, Wilson, & Walker, 1992, for panic disorder; Asmundson & Stein, 1994, for SAD; Bryant & Harvey, 1997, for PTSD). Attentional biases in anxiety disorders have also been observed in response to facial expressions of emotion (e.g., Bradley, Mogg, White, Groom, & De Bono, 1999). Interestingly, studies in anxiety disorders suggest that the initial vigilance toward threatening material that is observed when stimuli are presented shortly is replaced with attentional avoidance when stimuli are presented for an extended period of time (vigilance–avoidance hypotheses; Mogg, Bradley, Miles, & Dixon, 2004). This suggests that in anxiety disorders initial vigilance is followed by attentional redirection, an effective emotion regulation strategy. Given the observation that anxiety is characterized by attentional biases toward subliminally and supraliminally presented material (see Mathews & MacLeod, 2005, for a review), attentional deployment may be used inflexibly and involuntarily without a proper analysis of the situation.

Biases in perception and attention are not limited to anxiety disorders. The Stroop task is by far the most commonly used paradigm to examine addiction-related attentional biases (see Cox, Fadardi, & Pothos, 2006, for a review on alcohol- and smoking-related Stroop). Similar to the findings in the anxiety literature, Stroop interference effects for alcohol-related stimuli in individuals with alcohol dependence are frequently reported (e.g., Johnsen, Laberg, Cox, Vaksdal, & Hughdal, 1994; Lusher, Chandler, & Ball, 2004). Attentional biases for disorder-related material were also observed in individuals with other substance use disorders (e.g., Franken, Kroon, Wiers, & Jansen, 2000, for opiate dependence; Hester, Dixon, & Garavan, 2006, for cocaine dependence).

Studies have further investigated whether eating disorders are characterized by attentional biases and demonstrated that individuals diagnosed with bulimia nervosa generally demonstrate Stroop interference effects for both food and body shape–related words (see Dobson & Dozois, 2004; Lee & Shafran, 2004, for a review). In their meta-analysis, Dobson and Dozois obtained moderate effect sizes for the Stroop interference effects for food and body shape–related words in bulimic patients. For the anorexia nervosa group, they found a moderate effect size for the body shape–related words only. These results suggest that attentional biases in individuals with anorexia are specifically related to body size. To the best of our knowledge, only two studies to date have investigated attentional biases in clinically diagnosed eating disorder using the dot-probe task. The results generally indicate that individuals with eating disorder exhibit attentional biases for body weight–related stimuli (e.g., Shafran, Lee, Cooper, Palmer, & Fairburn, 2007). A recent study focused on differentiating the engagement versus disengagement aspect of attentional biases in eating disorder using a visual search paradigm (Smeets, Roefs, van Furth, & Jansen, 2008). In this study, a group of patients with eating disorders exhibited speeded detection of body-related stimuli and increased distraction by food-related stimuli.

Given the observation that such diverse disorders as anxiety, substance abuse, and eating disorders are characterized by biases in attention, it seems surprising that numerous studies have failed to find similar biases in depression (e.g., Mogg, Bradley, Williams, & Mathews, 1993). Most studies using the Stroop task do not find differences between depressed participants and controls (e.g., Mogg et al., 1993). Bradley, Mogg, Millar, and White (1995), for example, found that depression was not associated with increased Stroop interference, and the well-replicated interference effect in anxiety was not present in patients with GAD who were comorbid with depression. Several investigators have used the dot-probe task, and here, too, results have not been encouraging (e.g., Mogg, Bradley, & Williams, 1995).

It may be premature, however, to conclude that depression is not characterized by attentional biases. Studies using the dot-probe task, for example, have reported selective attention in depression but only under conditions of long stimuli exposures (Bradley, Mogg, & Lee, 1997; Joormann & Gotlib, 2007). In two studies, these findings were replicated in samples of remitted depressed adults (Joormann & Gotlib, 2007) and nondisordered girls at high risk for depression because of their mothers' psychopathology (Joormann, Talbot, & Gotlib, 2007). These findings suggest that attentional biases are not simply a symptom of depression or a "scar" of a previous depressive episode but may play an important role in vulnerability to depression. Indeed, Beevers and Carver (2003) demonstrated that changes in attentional bias for negative but not positive words following a negative mood induction interacted with life stress to predict onset of depressive symptoms in college students.

Overall, these results suggest that depressed individuals do not direct their attention to negative information more frequently than control participants, but once it captures their attention they exhibit difficulties disengaging from it. Similar difficulties in disengaging attention from negative material have been demonstrated in other tasks. Rinck and Becker (2005), for example, reported that depressed participants did not show enhanced detection of depression-related words in a visual search task but were more easily distracted by negative words. Eizenman and colleagues (2003) used eye-tracking technology to continuously monitor point of gaze. Depressed individuals spent significantly more time looking at pictures featuring sadness and loss than nondepressed controls.

We discussed previously that simply showing that emotional disorders are associated with biased cognitive processes provides only indirect evidence that these processes play a role in emotion regulation. More direct proof for the role of cognitive biases in emotion regulation would require evidence that changes in the processes are related to changes in emotional states. The only set of studies that provide such direct evidence comes from recent work on cognitive bias modification. These studies demonstrate that training highly anxious people to disengage their attention from threat material leads to changes in mood and reduced reactivity to stressful events. In a typical training paradigm, the dot probe is presented more consistently after the non-threat-relevant stimuli (rather than equally following threat and nonthreat stimuli), so that participants learn to attend to neutral stimuli. Using this approach, MacLeod, Rutherford, Campbell,

Ebsworthy, and Holker (2002) first established that attentional biases could be modified by working with participants who scored in the middle third of the distribution on the State–Trait Anxiety Inventory (STAI; Spielberger, Gorusch, & Lushene, 1971). They found that following attentional training away from threat, participants reported reduced negative affect to a standardized stress manipulation. In a subsequent study, Mathews and MacLeod (2002) established that the attentional training was effective at reducing anxiety among a sample of high-STAI scorers during the month before a school examination. On the basis of these findings, researchers have begun to examine attentional training with clinical samples (see also Taylor & Amir, Chapter 16, this volume).

What are the implications of biases in perception and attention for emotion regulation in these different disorders? In individuals with anxiety disorders, high sensitivity toward the detection of emotion-eliciting stimuli may result in anticipatory emotion regulation characterized by avoidance behavior (situation selection) and the use of safety strategies (situation modification). Given that biases are often automatic, avoidance behavior and the adoption of safety strategy may be unintentional and may occur without a careful analysis of the specifics of the situation. This may result in an inflexible and frequent use of these emotion regulation strategies that quickly generalizes to related situations. Depression, in contrast, is mostly associated with difficulties in using attentional disengagement. Difficulties disengaging from negative stimuli may preclude depressed people from using highly effective emotion regulation strategies such as distraction and may result in the sustained processing of emotion-eliciting stimuli, leading to sustained negative affect.

Interpretation and Appraisal

Most situations that evoke emotions are ambiguous. How cues in these situations are initially interpreted and appraised determines the emotional response and whether this response is appropriate in this situation or not. Does the frowning face in the audience mean that the presentation was a failure? Is the weird sound coming from the engine a sign that the plane is in trouble? Did the person in front of me intentionally step on my foot? Reinterpretation and reappraisal are potent emotion regulation strategies because they allow flexible emotional responding without changing the situation and without ignoring the emotion-eliciting cues. Interpretation and appraisal processes, however, can be biased. Biases in interpretation, especially when they are automatic and unconscious, can be difficult to change and can lead to inflexible and inappropriate responding because of difficulties in emotion regulation (Siemer & Reisenzein, 2007).

Interpretation biases and automatic appraisal processes are at the core of various emotional disorders, making it challenging for people to use cognitive reappraisal, a very effective emotion regulation strategy. There is consensus that anxious individuals, for example, favor negative interpretations of ambiguous stimuli and often do so in tasks that suggest that these biases operate on an automatic level (see Mathews & MacLeod, 2005; Zinbarg & Yoon, 2008, for reviews). Individuals with panic disorder, for example, interpret descriptions of physical sensations as symptoms of catastrophic disease (e.g., Clark 1988), and individuals with social phobia overestimate the likelihood of negative social events and the negative consequences of events (e.g., Foa, Franklin, Perry, & Herber, 1996). Results from earlier studies, however, might be confounded with response bias or demand because these studies relied heavily on the self-report of the interpretation (MacLeod & Cohen, 1993). To overcome these limitations, researchers have developed alternative techniques, mainly based on priming paradigms, to assess interpretive bias without asking participants to emit or endorse alternative response options. These recent studies confirmed the presence of negative interpretive biases (e.g., MacLeod & Cohen, 1993; Yoon & Zinbarg, 2008) or the absence of positive interpretive biases (e.g., Hirsch & Mathews, 2000) in anxious participants.

As outlined previously, identifying cognitive biases in emotional disorders is not in itself compelling evidence that these biases are indeed related to problems in emotion regulation as long as no measures of affective states are included. Researchers have, therefore, begun to modify interpretive biases in anxiety in hopes of modifying emotional responding. Mathews and Mackintosh (2000) used ambiguous scenarios to train individuals to make either positive (nonanxious) or negative (anxious) interpretations of ambiguous text. The authors used the STAI-State to compare state levels of anxiety before and after the training and reported that participants in the negative training condition displayed elevated levels of anxiety and those in the positive training condition decreased symptoms of anxiety, supporting the hypothesis that interpretive biases play a causal role in affecting anxiety levels. Yiend, Mackintosh, and Mathews (2005) demonstrated that the effects of interpretive training on anxiety were still present after a 24-hour delay between the training and a subsequent test. In a different study, participants who received interpretive training using ambiguous homophones were subsequently presented four distressing television clips of real-life emergency rescue situations (Wilson, MacLeod, Mathews, & Rutherford, 2006). Participants who were trained to interpret ambiguity in a nonthreatening manner had an attenuated anxiety reaction to the subsequent video stressor (see also Mackintosh, Mathews, Yiend, Ridgeway, & Cook, 2006). These results suggest that changes in interpretation biases can indeed lead to changes in emotional responding.

Results have been mixed with regard to whether depression is characterized by similar automatic interpretation biases (Lawson, MacLeod, & Hammond, 2002). Butler and Mathews (1983), for example, presented clinically depressed participants with ambiguous scenarios and found that, compared with nondepressed participants, depressed individuals ranked negative interpretations higher than other possible interpretations. In a study assessing biases using response latencies to target words that were presented after ambiguous sentences, no interpretation bias was found (Lawson & MacLeod, 1999). Lawson and colleagues (2002) also examined startle magnitude during imagery elicited by emotionally ambiguous text. Using this measure, these authors reported evidence for more negative interpretations in their depressed sample and concluded that the failure to find a bias in previous studies was due to the use of response latencies. Rude, Wenzlaff, Gibbs, Vane, and Whitney (2002) demonstrated that a measure of interpretation bias, the Scrambled Sentences Test, predicted increases in depressive symptoms after 4 to 6 weeks in a large sample of undergraduate students, especially when administered under cognitive load. Clearly, further studies are needed that investigate interpretive biases in depression.

Although automatic interpretive biases may not play a central role in depression, studies using self-report measures of attribution have reported numerous findings that depression is associated with dysfunctional attitudes and a specific attributional style that may lead to the interpretation of specific situations in depression-relevant ways and may make it difficult to reinterpret and reappraise. Researchers investigating the role of dysfunctional attitudes and attributional style have relied almost exclusively on self-report measures, specifically the Dysfunctional Attitude Scale (DAS) and the Cognitive Styles Questionnaire (CSQ). The DAS assesses maladaptive cognitions like perfectionist standards and concerns about being evaluated by others (Weissman & Beck, 1978). The CSQ assesses the tendency to respond to positive and negative events with internal, stable, and global attributions (Alloy et al., 2000). Numerous studies in which these and other questionnaires were administered to depressed and nondepressed participants have reported associations among dysfunctional attitudes, attributional styles, and other negative cognitions in currently depressed adults (Alloy, Abramson, & Francis, 1999; Fresco, Alloy, & Reilly-Harrington, 2006), adolescents, and children (for a review, see Ingram, Nelson, Steidtmann, & Bistricky, 2007). In addition, research on cognitive reactivity has used mood inductions before assessing dysfunctional cognitions in remitted participants. This research is interesting because it suggests that changes in cognition once a mood state is experienced may be critical in our understanding of emotional disorders (for a review, see Scher, Ingram, & Segal, 2005). Gemar, Segal, Sagrati, and Kennedy (2001), for example, reported that, compared with never-depressed participants, formerly depressed participants demonstrated a greater change in dysfunctional attitudes after a negative mood induction (see also Miranda, Persons, & Byers, 1990). This finding suggests that negative mood states may induce biases in interpretation and appraisal in depression that interfere with an effective regulation of this emotion.

To summarize, these studies suggest that emotional disorders are characterized by biases in interpretation and appraisals. These biases are associated with automatic appraisals of emotion-eliciting situations and make it difficult to regulate emotions by deliberately reappraising the situation. The evidence so far suggests that only patients with anxiety disorders exhibit automatic biases but that depression is characterized by a specific style of attribution. The depression findings also suggest that cognitive processes that hinder emotion regulation may only become obvious after people have been exposed to a negative mood state. Unfortunately, research on individual differences in interpretation and appraisal so far seems limited to depression and anxiety. It will be important to investigate the role of these processes in other disorders.

Memory

Memories affect emotion regulation in important ways. Memory biases, for example, may determine people's perception of a specific situation, change their appraisals, and guide their attention toward specific aspects of that situation. Biased recall can have important consequences, particularly if it depends on implicit memory. Implicit memory for stimuli that were present during a traumatic event may, for example, lead to unintentional situation selection and modification and to the appraisal of harmless situations as life-threatening experiences, as frequently seen in PTSD (McNally, 1997). Individual differences in the (strategic or automatic) accessibility of material in memory may determine emotional responses and interfere with the selection and use of effective emotion regulation strategies. If the shaking plane brings up memories of news reports depicting plane crashes instead of memories of roller-coaster rides on a sunny vacation day, emotional responding will be different and emotion regulation may be affected. Implicit associations between a red traffic light and memories of a traumatic accident can make it impossible to use voluntary reappraisal to overcome fear of driving. Memory processes can help or hinder the use of emotion regulation strategies, but memory itself can also be a potent means of regulating emotions. If it is easy to concentrate on the roller-coaster ride or to replace the plane crash pictures with the pictures of the sunny vacation day, or if memories of happy times become easily accessible when someone feels sad, recall can easily change emotion experience. Research has indeed demonstrated that memories of unpleasant, versus pleasant, events fade faster and that this differential fading is associated with happiness (Walker, Skowronski, & Thompson, 2003); that recalling positive autobiographical memories can repair an induced negative mood state (Joormann & Siemer, 2004); and that remembering positive events and forgetting negative events are associated with increased well-being over the lifespan (Charles, Mather, & Carstensen, 2003). Selective recall, therefore, can affect other emotion regulation strategies (e.g., situation selection or attention), but it is also an effective strategy for directly changing emotions and mood states. Although the strong association between memory and emotion usually works in our favor, enhanced memory for traumatic events and the role of biased recall in maintaining emotional disorders demonstrate that it can come at a cost.

In contrast to strong evidence of memory biases in depression, evidence regarding memory biases in anxiety disorders is mixed at best (for reviews, see Coles & Heimberg, 2002; Mathews & MacLeod, 2005). Most studies on explicit memory bias in anxiety disorders failed to find such biases in SAD (see Hirsch & Clark, 2004, for a review), GAD (e.g., Mogg, Mathews, & Weinman, 1987), and specific phobia (Watts & Dalgleish, 1991). One notable exception is panic disorder. Results from various studies indicate enhanced recall of threat-relevant material in panic disorder, especially when the encoding task encourages deep processing of the materials (see Coles & Heimberg, 2002, for a review). As for implicit memory biases, the results are mixed also. Some studies demonstrated biases in individuals with panic disorder (Amir, McNally, Riemann, & Clements, 1996), SAD (e.g., Lundh & Öst, 1996), GAD (Mathews, Mogg, May, & Eysenck, 1989), and PTSD (Amir, McNally, & Wiegartz, 1996), whereas other studies demonstrated no such biases in individuals with anxiety disorders (e.g., Amir, Foa, & Coles, 2000; Paunovic, Lundh, & Öst, 2002).

Based on the notion that more realistic and relevant stimuli might elicit memory biases better, pictorial stimuli were used to examine memory biases in anxiety disorders. Individuals with SAD were better at remembering faces that they had previously judged to be critical (Coles & Heimberg, 2005; Lundh & Öst, 1996), whereas individuals with panic disorder were better at remembering faces judged to be safe (Lundh, Thulin, Czyzykow, & Öst, 1998). Similarly, crime victims with acute PTSD exhibited enhanced memory for faces they perceived as hostile compared with nonhostile faces, whereas memory in controls did not vary according to perceived hostility (Paunovic, Lundh, & Öst, 2003).

Only a handful of studies investigated memory biases in eating disorders (see Lee & Shafran, 2004, for a review). In general, individuals with eating disorders seem to show enhanced memory for words related to their concern (e.g., "fatness"-related words) on an explicit memory task (e.g., Hermans, Pieters, & Eelen, 1998). Explicit memory biases for eating disorder-related words are not specific to clinical populations. That is, restrained eaters and obese females (King, Polivy, & Herman, 1991) and females with high levels of body dysphoria (Baker, Williamson, & Sylve, 1995) also exhibited such biases.

Preferential recall of negative compared with positive material is one of the most robust findings in the depression literature (Mathews & MacLeod, 2005; Matt, Vazquez, & Campbell, 1992). In a meta-analysis of studies assessing recall performance, Matt and colleagues found that people with major depression remember 10% more negative words than positive words. Nondepressed controls, in contrast, demonstrated a memory bias for positive information in 20 of 25 studies. It should be noted, however, that memory biases are found most consistently in free-recall tasks and may also be restricted to explicit memory. Results using recognition or implicit memory measures have been much less conclusive. In his review of the implicit memory literature, Watkins (2002; see also Barry, Naus, & Lynn, 2004) reports that across studies no bias is found in depressed participants when the encoding or the recall of the emotional material depends purely on perceptual processing. For example, if depressed participants are asked to count the letters in emotional words at encoding and to complete word stems or word fragments at recall, no evidence of an implicit memory bias is obtained (Watkins, Martin, & Stern, 2000). If, however, participants are asked to rate the recency of their experience with the word or to imagine themselves in a scene involving the word at encoding and are asked to freely associate to a cue word or to provide a word that fits a given definition, implicit memory biases are obtained more consistently. Encoding and recall in these latter studies are conceptual instead of perceptual. This suggests that depressive deficits are mostly due to differences in the elaboration of emotional material between depressed individuals and their nondepressed counterparts.

Memory biases may affect emotion regulation, but as discussed previously simply demonstrating that a disorder is associated with a bias provides no evidence of a causal relationship between cognition and emotion regulation. We also discussed that few studies have investigated the association between cognition and emotion regulation in emotional disorders. A rare exception is a series of studies investigating mood-incongruent recall in depression. Literature on mood regulation suggests that mood-incongruent recall is often used as a mood-repair strategy in response to a negative mood induction (e.g., Rusting & DeHart, 2000). Studies investigating the use and effectiveness of mood regulation strategies in depression suggest that, in contrast to nondepressed persons, depressed individuals are unable to use positive autobiographical memories to regulate induced negative mood states (Joormann & Siemer, 2004; Joormann, Siemer, & Gotlib, 2007). In two studies, we examined the formulation that dysphoria and rumination are critical factors in determining whether mood-congruent memory retrieval, as opposed to mood-repair processes, occurs (Joormann & Siemer, 2004). Nondysphoric participants' mood ratings improved under distraction as well as under mood-incongruent recall instructions. In contrast, dysphoric participants did not benefit from the recall of positive memories, although distraction alleviated their sad mood. We replicated these findings in a sample of currently depressed participants (Joormann et al., 2007). Interestingly, previously depressed participants exhibited similar difficulties to repair their negative mood with positive memories. Overall, the results are largely consistent with the literature on mood regulation (McFarland & Buehler, 1998; Rusting & DeHart, 2000) and support the notion that mood-incongruent recall is used as a mood-repair strategy in response to a negative mood induction. These results suggest that depression is associated with problems in using an important emotion regulation strategy.

Depression is associated not only with enhanced recall of negative events but also with the recall of rather generic memories despite instructions to recall specific events (i.e., overgeneral memory; see Williams et al., 2007, for a review). The tendency to retrieve overgeneral memories is also found in individuals diagnosed with PTSD (e.g., McNally, Lasko, Macklin, & Pitman, 1995) and eating disorders (e.g., Dalgleish et al., 2003). Furthermore, the extent to which an individual retrieves overgeneral memories predicted worse symptom outcome in a longitudinal study of motor vehicle accident victims (Harvey, Bryant, & Dang, 1998) and delayed recovery from affective disorders (e.g., Dalgleish, Spinks, Yiend, & Kuyken, 2001). Williams (1996) proposed that overgeneral memory is an emotion regulation strategy. That is, individuals attempt to minimize negative affect attached to distressing memories by blocking access to details of such memories or by retrieving these memories in a less specific way. Understanding overgeneral memory in the context of emotion regulation in disorders may, therefore, be an important goal for future research. In sum, memory biases may play a role in anxiety and eating disorders but are definitely important to consider in depression. Depression is associated not only with increased accessibility of negative material but also with difficulties in using an effective emotion regulation strategy (i.e., the recall of mood-incongruent material).

Cognitive Control, Working Memory, and Inhibition

Reappraisal is an important emotion regulation strategy. We already discussed different biases in cognition (attentional biases, memory biases) that may affect a person's ability to use this strategy effectively. A critical cognitive process that affects individual differences in the ability to reappraise is cognitive control. Overriding prepotent responses and inhibiting the processing of irrelevant material that captures our attention are core abilities that allow us to respond flexibly and to adjust our behavior and our emotional responses to changing situations. Cognitive control is related to the functioning of executive control processes such as inhibition in working memory (Hasher & Zacks, 1988; Hasher, Zacks, & May, 1999). Working memory is a limited-capacity system that provides temporary access to a select set of representations in the service of current cognitive processes (Cowan, 1999; Miyake & Shah, 1999). Thus, working memory reflects the focus of attention and the temporary activation of representations that are the contents of awareness. Given the capacity limitation of this system, it is important that the contents of working memory be updated efficiently, a task controlled by executive processes (e.g., Friedman & Miyake, 2004; Hasher et al., 1999). Executive processes must selectively gate access to working memory, shielding it from intrusion from irrelevant material, as well as discard information that is no longer relevant. In this context, individual differences in the experience and resolution of interference are likely to affect cognitive and emotional functioning. The occurrence of intrusive thoughts might be one consequence of poor interference resolution. Indeed, increased interference from irrelevant representations has been proposed as a source of low working memory capacity (Engle, Kane, & Tuholski, 1999) and has been found in various populations, including older adults (Hasher, Stoltzfus, Zacks, & Rypma, 1991), children with attention-deficit disorder (Bjorklund & Harnishfeger, 1990), patients with OCD (Enright & Beech, 1990), and patients with schizophrenia (e.g., Frith, 1979). Several researchers have also suggested that rumination and depression are associated with deficits in cognitive control (Hertel, 1997; Joormann, 2005).

Deficits in controlling the contents of working memory may affect emotion regulation. The experience of a mood state or an emotion is generally associated with the activation of mood-congruent representations in working memory (e.g., Siemer, 2005a). The ability to control the contents of working memory might, therefore, play an important role in emotion regulation. Thus, an inability to appropriately expel mood-congruent items from working memory as they become irrelevant would lead to difficulties attending to and processing new information and might also result in rumination and the use of other maladaptive emotion regulation strategies. Difficulties inhibiting salient but irrelevant thoughts and memories would also discourage the use of more effective emotion regulation strategies, such as reappraisal.

There is emerging evidence that depression is characterized by deficits in the inhibition of mood-congruent material. These deficits could result in prolonged processing of negative, goal-irrelevant aspects of presented information, thereby hindering recovery from negative mood and leading to the sustained negative affect that characterizes depressive episodes. Indeed, it has been suggested that deficits in cognitive inhibition lie at the heart of memory and attention biases in depression and set the stage for ruminative responses to negative events and negative mood states (Hertel, 1997; Joormann, 2005). Over the last 15 to 20 years, a number of experimental methodologies have emerged that have the potential to test inhibition models (Anderson & Bjork, 1994).

Using a negative priming task, Joormann (2004) found that dysphoric participants and participants with a history of depressive episodes exhibited reduced inhibition of negative material. Thus, these participants responded faster when a negative target was presented after a to-be-ignored negative distractor on the previous trial. As predicted, no group difference was found for the positive adjectives. In a related study, participants who scored high on a self-report measure of rumination exhibited a reduced ability to inhibit the processing of emotional distractors, a finding that remained significant even after controlling for level of depressive symptoms (Joormann, 2006). Importantly, these findings were replicated using a negative priming task with emotional faces (Goeleven, DeRaedt, Baert, & Koster, 2006).

Although these studies suggest that depression and probably also rumination involve difficulties keeping irrelevant emotional information from *entering* working memory, few studies have examined whether depression and rumination are also associated with difficulties *removing* previously relevant negative material from working memory. Difficulties inhibiting the processing of negative material that was, but is no longer, relevant might explain why people respond to negative mood states and negative life events with recurring, uncontrollable, and unintentional negative thoughts. To test this hypothesis, Joormann and Gotlib (2008) used a modified Sternberg task that combines a short-term recognition task with instructions to ignore a previously memorized list of words to assess inhibition of irrelevant positive and negative stimuli. They found that participants diagnosed with major depression exhibited difficulties removing irrelevant negative material from working memory. Specifically, compared with never-depressed controls, depressed individuals exhibited longer decision latencies to an intrusion probe (i.e., a probe from the irrelevant list) than to a new probe (i.e., a completely new word), reflecting the strength of the residual activation of the contents of working memory that were declared to be no longer relevant. Importantly, this pattern was not found for positive material. Difficulty removing negative irrelevant words from working memory was highly correlated with self-reported rumination, even after controlling for level of depressive symptoms. In sum, therefore, these findings indicate that depression and rumination are associated with inhibitory impairments in the processing of emotional material, specifically with difficulties removing irrelevant negative material from working memory. More research on these processes in other disorders is needed.

Summary and Future Directions

In this chapter, we examined whether individual differences in cognitive processes may affect emotion regulation and, therefore, play an important role in the onset and maintenance of disorders. It is unlikely that people diagnosed with disorders differ from others in that they use dramatically different regulation strategies. It is, therefore, difficult to differentiate adaptive from maladaptive emotion regulation per se. Flexibility in the use of strategies, selection of strategies that fit the situation, and differences in the ability to implement effective strategies are important aspects to explore in research on psychopathology. One might argue, for example, that some anxiety disorders are characterized by emotion regulation that is too effective. Individuals with social anxiety, for example, often can avoid fear associated with social situations by staying at home and avoiding contact with other people. Avoidance is a highly effective emotion regulation strategy that is not necessarily maladaptive but leads to many problems if used inflexibly and in the wrong situations. As outlined previously, cognitive biases and automatic appraisals may increase the probability of inflexible use and inadequate selection. Exposure therapy may play a critical role in changing these automatic appraisals and in helping people select more adequate regulation strategies. Also, reflecting on the situation that led to sadness is not necessarily maladaptive, but if people have a difficult time disengaging from this reflection it may lead them into maladaptive forms of rumination such as brooding, which may sustain the negative mood (Nolen-Hoeksema, Wisco, & Lyubomirsky, 2008). Individual differences in cognitive control may be important in determining how easy it is for people to disengage and distract themselves when necessary.

Even though all of the disorders we discussed are associated with some form of maladaptive emotion regulation, disorders seem to differ in the specific strategies that are most frequently used and in why these strategies are maladaptive. Again, flexibility seems to be the key. We also identified, however, that some strategies do not seem to work in some disorders. Depressed people, for example, cannot use mood-incongruent recall to repair their mood state, a strategy that works well in nondepressed participants. Individuals with anxiety disorders such as PTSD may find it difficult to use reappraisal of the emotion-eliciting cues because of strong implicit associations of these cues with life-threatening danger. Alternatively, if reappraisal is used in these disorders, often the wrong aspects of the situation may be reappraised. Patients with panic disorder, for example, may interpret everyday situations such as sitting on a bus as not dangerous only if they carry a cell phone with which they can call for help at any time. Differences among disorders may be due to the fact that some disorders require the regulation of emotions whereas others require the regulation of mood states. As described previously, emotions differ from mood states in that mood states are more diffuse and are not closely associated with an eliciting situation or with action tendencies. Emotional responses are easily regulated by avoiding or changing the eliciting situation or by reappraising that situation. A main problem for people with anxiety disorders may be that emotional responses and automatic appraisals of the situation get triggered too easily and avoidance, therefore, generalizes to novel situations. Mood states, however, have no clear elicitor, and avoidance and reappraisal may, therefore, be more difficult to accomplish or may be ineffective. Cognitive avoidance strategies, distraction, and mood-incongruent recall may be more effective strategies to regulate mood states. Depressed individuals' difficulties disengaging from negative material and using mood-incongruent recall may, therefore, play an important role in sustaining negative mood. Further exploration of the differences in emotional responding and regulation among psychological disorders is definitely warranted.

Importantly, future research should directly investigate cognitive processes and emotional states in disorders and should examine the causal impact of cognitive biases on difficulties in emotion regulation. Our brief review of the literature demonstrates that previous research has identified cognitive processes that cut across different disorders (see also Harvey, Watkins, Mansell, & Shafran, 2004). This brief overview, however, also showed that research has concentrated largely on anxiety and mood disorders and that studies that investigate these processes in other disorders are lacking. As outlined previously, however, demonstrating that people diagnosed with depression differ from nondepressed controls in perception, attention, and memory is important but is not, by itself, answering the question of whether biases affect the selection or effectiveness of emotion regulation strategies. Studies need to include measures of cognition and emotion within the same design and need to explore whether changes in cognition change emotion. There are very few examples of studies that have begun to examine these processes. Studies on cognitive bias modification, for example, demonstrate that changes in selective attention and automatic interpretation biases in anxiety disorders can affect people's emotional responses when exposed to stressors. Few studies have investigated such manipulations in depression or other disorders. Whereas researchers have examined whether cognitive processes are related to rumination in depression and to people's tendencies to engage in thought suppression, no studies have investigated reappraisal in emotional disorders. Why do people prefer certain emotion regulation strategies? Are certain strategies effective for some people but not others, and if so, why? Are individual differences in attention, interpretation, memory, and cognitive control indeed related to the selection and effectiveness of regulation strategies? How do people learn to use these strategies and how can we help them unlearn? These and other questions should be the main focus of future studies in this exciting area of research.

References

Alloy, L. B., Abramson, L. Y., & Francis, E. L. (1999). Do negative cognitive styles confer vulnerability to depression? *Current Directions in Psychological Science, 8,* 128–132.

Alloy, L. B., Abramson, L. Y., Hogan, M. E., Whitehouse, W. G., Rose, D. T., Robinson, M. S., et al. (2000). The Temple-Wisconsin Cognitive Vulnerability to Depression Project: Lifetime history of axis I psychopathology in individuals at high and low cognitive risk for depression. *Journal of Abnormal Psychology, 109,* 403–418.

Amir, N., Foa, E. B., & Coles, M. E. (2000). Implicit memory bias for threat-relevant information in generalized social phobia. *Journal of Abnormal Psychology, 109*, 713–720.

Amir, N., McNally, R. J., Riemann, B. C., & Clements, C. (1996). Implicit memory bias for threat in panic disorder: Application of the white noise paradigm. *Behaviour Research and Therapy, 34*, 157–162.

Amir, N., McNally, R. J., & Wiegartz, P. S. (1996). Implicit memory bias for threat in panic disorder: Application of the "white noise" paradigm. *Behaviour Research and Therapy, 34*, 157–162.

Anderson, M. C., & Bjork, R. A. (1994). Mechanisms of inhibition in long-term memory: A new taxonomy. In D. Dagenbach & T. Carr (Eds.), *Inhibitory processes in attention, memory, and language* (pp. 265–325). San Diego, CA: Academic Press.

Asmundson, G. J. G., Sandler, L. S., Wilson, K. G., & Walker, J. R. (1992). Selective attention toward physical threat in patients with panic disorder. *Journal of Anxiety Disorders, 6*, 295–303.

Asmundson, G. J. G., & Stein, M. B. (1994). Selective processing of social threat in patients with generalized social phobia: Evaluation using a dot-probe paradigm. *Journal of Anxiety Disorders, 8*, 107–117.

Baker, J. D., Williamson, D. A., & Sylve, C. (1995). Body-image disturbance, memory bias and body dysphoria: Effects of a negative mood induction. *Behavior Therapy, 26*, 747–759.

Bar-Haim, Y., Lamy, D., Pergamin, L., Bakermans-Kranenburg, M. J., & van IJzendoorn, M. H. (2007). Threat-related attentional bias in anxious and nonanxious individuals: A meta-analytic study. *Psychological Bulletin, 133*, 1–24.

Barry, E. S., Naus, M. J., & Lynn P. R. (2004). Depression and implicit memory: Understanding mood congruent memory bias. *Cognitive Therapy and Research, 28*, 387–414.

Beevers, C. G., & Carver, C. S. (2003). Attentional bias and mood persistence as prospective predictors of dysphoria. *Cognitive Therapy and Research, 27*, 619–637.

Berkowitz, L., & Harmon-Jones, E. (2004). Toward an understanding of the determinants of anger. *Emotion, 4*(2), 107–130.

Bjorklund, D. F., & Harnishfeger, K. K. (1990). Children's strategies: Their definitions and origins. In D. F. Bjorklund (Ed.), *Children's strategies: Contemporary views of cognitive development* (pp. 309–323). Hillsdale, NJ: Erlbaum.

Bower, G. H. (1981). Mood and memory. *American Psychologist, 36*, 129–148.

Bradley, B. P., Mogg, K., & Lee, S. C. (1997). Attentional biases for negative information in induced and naturally occurring dysphoria. *Behaviour Research and Therapy, 35*, 911–927.

Bradley, B. P., Mogg, K., Millar, N., & White, J. (1995). Selective processing of negative information: Effects of clinical anxiety, concurrent depression, and awareness. *Journal of Abnormal Psychology, 104*, 532–536.

Bradley, B. P., Mogg, K., White, J., Groom, C., & De Bono, J. (1999). Attentional bias for emotional faces in generalized anxiety disorder. *British Journal of Clinical Psychology, 38*, 267–278.

Bryant, R. A., & Harvey, A. G. (1997). Processing threatening information in posttraumatic stress disorder. *Journal of Abnormal Psychology, 104*, 537–541.

Butler, G., & Mathews, A. (1983). Cognitive processes in anxiety. *Advances in Behaviour Research and Therapy, 5,* 51–62.

Charles, S. T., Mather, M., & Carstensen, L. L. (2003). Aging and emotional memory: The forgettable nature of negative images for older adults. *Journal of Experimental Psychology: General, 132,* 310–324.

Clark, D. M. (1988). A cognitive model of panic attacks. In S. Rachman & J. D. Maser (Eds.), *Panic: Psychological perspectives* (pp. 71–89). Hillsdale, NJ: Erlbaum.

Clore, G. L., & Centerbar, D. B. (2004). Analyzing anger: How to make people mad. *Emotion, 4*(2), 139–144.

Coles, M. E., & Heimberg, R. G. (2002). Memory biases in the anxiety disorders: Current status. *Clinical Psychology Review, 22,* 587–627.

Coles, M. E., & Heimberg, R. G. (2005). Recognition bias for critical faces in social phobia: A replication and extension. *Behaviour Research and Therapy, 43,* 109–120.

Cowan, N. (1999). An embedded-processes model of working memory. In A. Miyake & P. Shah (Eds.), *Models of working memory: Mechanisms of active maintenance and executive control* (pp. 62–101). New York: Cambridge University Press.

Cox, W. M., Fadardi, J. S., & Pothos, E. M. (2006). The Addiction-Stroop test: Theoretical considerations and procedural recommendations. *Psychological Bulletin, 132,* 443–476.

Dalgleish, T., Spinks, H., Yiend, J., & Kuyken, W. (2001). Autobiographical memory style in seasonal affective disorder and its relationship to future symptom remission. *Journal of Abnormal Psychology, 110,* 335–340.

Dalgleish, T., Tchanturia, K., Serpell, L., Hems, S., Yiend, J., de Silva, P., et al. (2003). Self-reported parental abuse relates to autobiographical memory style in patients with eating disorders. *Emotion, 3,* 211–222.

Dobson, K., & Dozois, D. J. A. (2004). Attentional biases in eating disorders: A meta-analytic review of Stroop performance. *Clinical Psychology Review, 23,* 1001–1022.

Ehlers, A., Margraf, J., Davies, S., & Roth, W. T. (1988). Selective processing of threat cues in subjects with panic attacks. *Cognition and Emotion, 2,* 201–220.

Eizenman, M., Yu, L. H., Grupp, L., Eizenman, E., Ellenbogen, M., Gemar, M., et al. (2003). A naturalistic visual scanning approach to assess selective attention in major depressive disorder. *Psychiatry Research, 118,* 117–128.

Ellsworth, P. C., & Scherer, K. R. (2003). Appraisal processes in emotion. In R. J. Davidson, H. H. Goldsmith, & K. R. Scherer (Eds.), *Handbook of affective sciences* (pp. 572–595). New York: Oxford University Press.

Engle, R. W., Kane, M. J., & Tuholski, S. W. (1999). Individual differences in working memory capacity and what they tell us about controlled attention, general fluid intelligence, and functions of the prefrontal cortex. In A. Miyake & P. Shah (Eds.), *Models of working memory: Mechanisms of active maintenance and executive control* (pp. 102–134). New York: Cambridge University Press.

Enright, S. J., & Beech, A. R. (1990). Obsessional states: Anxiety disorders or schizotypes?: An information processing and personality assessment. *Psychological Medicine, 20,* 621–627.

Foa, E. B., Franklin, M. E., Perry, K. J., & Herber, J. D. (1996). Cognitive biases in generalized social phobia. *Journal of Abnormal Psychology, 105,* 433–439.

Franken, I. H., Kroon, L. Y., Wiers, R. W., & Jansen, A. (2000). Selective cognitive processing of drug cues in heroin dependence. *Journal of Psychopharmacology*, *14*, 395–400.

Fresco, D. M., Alloy, L. B., & Reilly-Harrington, N. (2006). Association of attributional style for negative and positive events and the occurrence of life events with depression and anxiety. *Journal of Social and Clinical Psychology*, *25*, 1140–1159.

Friedman, N. P., & Miyake, A. (2004). The relations among inhibition and interference control functions: A latent-variable analysis. *Journal of Experimental Psychology: General*, *133*, 101–135.

Frith, C. D. (1979). Consciousness, information processing and schizophrenia. *British Journal of Psychiatry*, *134*, 225–235.

Gemar, M. C., Segal, Z. V., Sagrati, S., & Kennedy, S. J. (2001). Mood-induced changes on the Implicit Association Test in recovered depressed patients. *Journal of Abnormal Psychology*, *110*, 282–289.

Goeleven, E., DeRaedt, R., Baert, S., & Koster, E. H. W. (2006). Deficient inhibition of emotional information in depression. *Journal of Affective Disorders*, *93*, 149–152.

Gross, J. J. (1998). Antecedent- and response-focused emotion regulation: Divergent consequences for experience, expression, and physiology. *Journal of Personality and Social Psychology*, *74*, 224–237.

Gross, J. J. (2002). Emotion regulation: Affective, cognitive, and social consequences. *Psychophysiology*, *39*, 281–291.

Gross, J. J., & Levenson, R. W. (1997). Hiding feelings: The acute effects of inhibiting negative and positive emotion. *Journal of Abnormal Psychology*, *106*, 95–103.

Harvey, A. G., Bryant, R. A., & Dang, S. T. (1998). Autobiographical memory in acute stress disorder. *Journal of Consulting and Clinical Psychology*, *66*, 500–506.

Harvey, A. G., Watkins, E., Mansell, W., & Shafran, R. (2004). *Cognitive behavioural processes across psychological disorders: A transdiagnostic approach to research and treatment*. Oxford, UK: Oxford University Press.

Hasher, L., Stoltzfus, E. R., Zacks, R. T., & Rypma, B. (1991). Age and inhibition. *Journal of Experimental Psychology: Learning, Memory, and Cognition*, *17*, 163–169.

Hasher, L., & Zacks, R. T. (1988). Working memory, comprehension, and aging: A review and a new view. In G. H. Bower (Ed.), *The psychology of learning and motivation* (Vol. 22, pp. 193–225). San Diego, CA: Academic Press.

Hasher, L., Zacks, R. T., & May, C. P. (1999). Inhibitory control, circadian arousal, and age. In D. Gopher & A. Koriat (Eds.), *Attention and performance XVII: Cognitive regulation of performance: Interaction of theory and application* (pp. 653–675). Cambridge, MA: MIT Press.

Hermans, D., Pieters, G., & Eelen, P. (1998). Implicit and explicit memory for shape, body weight and food-related words in patients with anorexia and non-dieting controls. *Journal of Abnormal Psychology*, *107*, 193–202.

Hertel, P. T. (1997). On the contributions of deficient cognitive control to memory impairments in depression. *Cognition and Emotion*, *11*, 569–584.

Hester, R., Dixon, V., & Garavan, H. (2006). A consistent attentional bias for drug-related material in active cocaine users across word and picture versions of the emotional Stroop task. *Drug and Alcohol Dependence, 81,* 251–257.

Hirsch, C. R., & Clark, D. M. (2004). Information-processing bias in social phobia. *Clinical Psychology Review, 24,* 799–825.

Hirsch, C. R., & Mathews, A. (2000). Impaired positive inferential bias in social phobia. *Journal of Abnormal Psychology, 109,* 705–712.

Ingram, R. E., Nelson, T., Steidtmann, D. K., & Bistricky, S. L. (2007). Comparative data on child and adolescent cognitive measures associated with depression. *Journal of Consulting and Clinical Psychology, 75,* 390–403.

Izard, C. E. (1993). Four systems for emotion activation: Cognitive and noncognitive processes. *Psychological Bulletin, 100,* 68–90.

Johnsen, B. H., Laberg, J. C., Cox, W. M., Vaksdal, A., & Hugdahl, K. (1994). Alcoholic subjects' attentional bias in the processing of alcohol-related words. *Psychology of Addictive Behaviors, 8,* 111–115.

Joormann, J. (2004). Attentional bias in dysphoria: The role of inhibitory processes. *Cognition and Emotion, 18,* 125–147.

Joormann, J. (2005). Inhibition, rumination, and mood regulation in depression. In R. W. Engle, G. Sedek, U. von Hecker, & D. N. McIntosh (Eds.), *Cognitive limitations in aging and psychopathology: Attention, working memory, and executive functions* (pp. 275–312). New York: Cambridge University Press.

Joormann, J. (2006). The relation of rumination and inhibition: Evidence from a negative priming task. *Cognitive Therapy and Research, 30,* 149–160.

Joormann, J., & Gotlib, I. H. (2007). Selective attention to emotional faces following recovery from depression. *Journal of Abnormal Psychology, 116,* 80–85.

Joormann, J., & Gotlib, I. H. (2008). Updating the contents of working memory in depression: Interference from irrelevant negative material. *Journal of Abnormal Psychology, 117,* 182–192.

Joormann, J., & Siemer, M. (2004). Memory accessibility, mood regulation, and dysphoria: Difficulties in repairing sad mood with happy memories? *Journal of Abnormal Psychology, 113,* 179–188.

Joormann, J., Siemer, M., & Gotlib, I. H. (2007). Mood regulation in depression: Differential effects of distraction and recall of happy memories on sad mood. *Journal of Abnormal Psychology, 116,* 484–490.

Joormann, J., Talbot, L., & Gotlib, I. H. (2007). Biased processing of emotional information in girls at risk for depression. *Journal of Abnormal Psychology, 116,* 135–143.

King, G. A., Polivy, J., & Herman, C. P. (1991). Cognitive aspects of dietary restraint: Effects on person memory. *International Journal of Eating Disorders, 10,* 313–321.

Lawson, C., & MacLeod, C. (1999). Depression and the interpretation of ambiguity. *Behaviour Research and Therapy, 37,* 463–474.

Lawson, C., MacLeod, C., & Hammond, G. (2002). Interpretation revealed in the blink of an eye: Depressive bias in the resolution of ambiguity. *Journal of Abnormal Psychology, 111,* 321–328.

Lazarus, R. S. (1991). *Emotion and adaptation.* Oxford, UK: Oxford University Press.

Lee, M., & Shafran, R. (2004). Information processing biases in eating disorders. *Clinical Psychology Review, 24,* 215–238.

Lerner, J. S., & Keltner, D. (2000). Beyond valence: Toward a model of emotion-specific influences on judgment and choice. *Cognition and Emotion, 14*, 473–494.

Levenson, R. W. (1994). Human emotions: A functional view. In P. Ekman & R. J. Davidson (Eds.), *The nature of emotion. Fundamental questions* (pp. 123–126). New York: Oxford University Press.

Lundh, L.-G., & Öst, L.-G. (1996). Recognition bias for critical faces in social phobics. *Behaviour Research and Therapy, 34*, 787–794.

Lundh, L.-G., Thulin, U., Czyzykow, S., & Öst, L.-G. (1998). Recognition bias for safe faces in panic disorder with agoraphobia. *Behaviour Research and Therapy, 36*, 323–337.

Lusher, J., Chandler, C., & Ball, D. (2004). Alcohol dependence and the alcohol Stroop paradigm: Evidence and issues. *Drug and Alcohol Dependence, 75*, 225–231.

Mackintosh, B., Mathews, A., Yiend, J., Ridgeway, V., & Cook, E. (2006). Induced biases in emotional interpretation influence stress vulnerability and endure despite changes in context. *Behavior Therapy, 37*, 209–222.

MacLeod, C., & Cohen, I. (1993). Anxiety and the interpretation of ambiguity: A test comprehension study. *Journal of Abnormal Psychology, 102*, 238–247.

MacLeod, C., Rutherford, E., Campbell, L., Ebsworthy, G., & Holker, L. (2002). Selective attention and emotional vulnerability: Assessing the causal basis of their association through the experimental manipulation of attentional bias. *Journal of Abnormal Psychology, 111*, 107–123.

Mathews, A., & Mackintosh, B. (2000). Induced emotional interpretation bias and anxiety. *Journal of Abnormal Psychology, 109*, 602–615.

Mathews, A., & MacLeod, C. (1985). Selective processing of threat cues in anxiety states. *Behaviour Research and Therapy, 23*, 563–569.

Mathews, A., & MacLeod, C. (2002). Induced processing biases have causal effects on anxiety. *Cognition and Emotion, 16*, 331–354.

Mathews, A., & MacLeod, C. (2005). Cognitive vulnerability to emotional disorders. *Annual Review of Clinical Psychology, 1*, 167–195.

Mathews, A., Mogg, K., May, J., & Eysenck, M. (1989). Implicit and explicit memory bias in anxiety. *Journal of Abnormal Psychology, 98*, 236–240.

Matt, G. E., Vazquez, C., & Campbell, W. K. (1992). Mood-congruent recall of affectively toned stimuli: A meta-analytic review. *Clinical Psychology Review, 12*, 227–255.

Mattia, J. I., Heimberg, R. G., & Hope, D. A. (1993). The revised Stroop color-naming task in social phobics. *Behaviour Research and Therapy, 31*, 305–313.

Mauss, I. B., Cook, C. L., & Gross, J. J. (2007). Automatic emotion regulation during anger provocation. *Journal of Experimental Social Psychology, 43*(5), 698–711.

Mauss, I. B., Levenson, R. W., McCarter, L., Wilhelm, F. H., & Gross, J. J. (2005). The tie that binds?: Coherence among emotion experience, behavior, and physiology. *Emotion, 5*(2), 175–190.

McFarland, C., & Buehler, R. (1998). The impact of negative affect on autobiographical memory: The role of self-focused attention to moods. *Journal of Personality and Social Psychology, 75*(6), 1424–1440.

McNally, R. J. (1995). Automaticity and the anxiety disorders. *Behaviour Research and Therapy, 33*, 747–754.

McNally, R. J. (1997). Implicit and explicit memory for trauma-related information in PTSD. In R. Yehuda & A. C. McFarlane (Eds.), *Psychobiology of posttraumatic stress disorder* (pp. 219–224). New York: New York Academy of Sciences.

McNally, R. J., Kaspi, S. P., Riemann, B. C., & Zeitlin, S. B. (1990). Selective processing of threat cues in posttraumatic stress disorder. *Journal of Abnormal Psychology, 99*, 398–402.

McNally, R. J., Lasko, N. B., Macklin, M. L., & Pitman, R. K. (1995). Autobiographical memory disturbance in combat-related posttraumatic stress disorder. *Behaviour Research and Therapy, 33*, 619–630.

Miranda, J., Persons, J. B., & Byers, C. N. (1990). Endorsement of dysfunctional beliefs depends on current mood state. *Journal of Abnormal Psychology, 99*, 237–241.

Miyake, A., & Shah, P. (1999). *Models of working memory: Mechanisms of active maintenance and executive control*. New York: Cambridge University Press.

Mogg, K., & Bradley, B. P. (2005). Attentional bias in generalized anxiety disorder versus depressive disorder. *Cognitive Therapy and Research, 29*, 29–45.

Mogg, K., Bradley, B. P., Miles, F., & Dixon, R. (2004). Time course of attentional bias for threat scenes: Testing the vigilance-avoidance hypothesis. *Cognition and Emotion, 18*, 689–700.

Mogg, K., Bradley, B. P., & Williams, R. (1995). Attentional bias in anxiety and depression: The role of awareness. *British Journal of Clinical Psychology, 34*, 17–36.

Mogg, K., Bradley, B. P., Williams, R., & Mathews, A. (1993). Subliminal processing of emotional information in anxiety and depression. *Journal of Abnormal Psychology, 102*, 304–311.

Mogg, K., Mathews, A., & Weinman, J. (1987). Selective processing of threat cues in anxiety states: A replication. *Behaviour Research and Therapy, 27*, 317–323.

Nolen-Hoeksema, S., Wisco, B. E., & Lyubomirsky, S. (2008). Rethinking rumination. *Perspectives on Psychological Science, 3*, 400–424.

Ochsner, K. N., Bunge, S. A., Gross, J. J., & Gabrieli, J. D. E. (2002). Rethinking feelings: An fMRI study of the cognitive regulation of emotion. *Journal of Cognitive Neuroscience, 14*, 1215–1229.

Ochsner, K. N., Knierim, K., Ludlow, D. H., Hanelin, J., Ramachandran, T., Glover, G., et al. (2004). Reflecting upon feelings: An fMRI study of neural systems supporting the attribution of emotion to self and other. *Journal of Cognitive Neuroscience, 16*, 1746–1772.

Öhman, A., & Soares, J. J. F. (1993). On the automatic nature of phobic fear: Conditioned electrodermal responses to masked fear-relevant stimuli. *Journal of Abnormal Psychology, 102*, 121–132.

Öhman, A., & Soares, J. J. F. (1998). Emotional conditioning to masked stimuli: Expectancies for aversive outcomes following nonrecognized fear-relevant stimuli. *Journal of Experimental Psychology: General, 127*, 69–82.

Ortony, A., Clore, G. L., & Collins, A. (1988). *The cognitive structure of emotions*. Cambridge, UK: Cambridge University Press.

Parkinson, B. (2007). From situations to emotions: Appraisals and other paths. *Emotion, 7*, 21–25.

Paunovic, N., Lundh, L.-G., & Öst, L.-G. (2002). Attentional and memory bias for emotional information in crime victims with acute posttraumatic stress disorder. *Journal of Anxiety Disorders, 16*, 675–692.

Paunovic, N., Lundh, L.-G., & Öst, L.-G. (2003). Memory bias for faces that are perceived as hostile by crime victims with acute posttraumatic stress disorder. *Cognitive Behaviour Therapy, 32*, 203–214.

Phelps, E. A. (2006). Emotion and cognition: Insights from studies of the human amygdala. *Annual Review of Psychology, 57*, 27–53.

Reisenzein, R., Bordgen, S., Holtbernd, T., & Matz, D. (2006). Evidence for strong dissociation between emotion and facial displays: The case of surprise. *Journal of Personality and Social Psychology, 91*(2), 295–315.

Rinck, M., & Becker, E. S. (2005). A comparison of attentional biases and memory biases in women with social phobia and major depression. *Journal of Abnormal Psychology, 114*, 62–74.

Rude, S. S., Wenzlaff, R. M., Gibbs, B., Vane, J., & Whitney, T. (2002). Negative processing biases predict subsequent depressive symptoms. *Cognition and Emotion, 16*, 423–440.

Rusting, C. L., & DeHart, T. (2000). Retrieving positive memories to regulate negative mood: Consequences for mood-congruent memory. *Journal of Personality and Social Psychology, 78*(4), 737–752.

Scher, C. D., Ingram, R. E., & Segal, Z. V. (2005). Cognitive reactivity and vulnerability: Empirical evaluation of construct activation and cognitive diatheses in unipolar depression. *Clinical Psychology Review, 25*, 487–510.

Scherer, K. R. (1984). On the nature and function of emotion: A component process model. In K. R. Scherer & P. Ekman (Eds.), *Approaches to emotion* (pp. 293–318). Hillsdale, NJ: Erlbaum.

Scherer, K. R. (2001). Appraisal considered as a process of multilevel sequential checking. In K. R. Scherer, A. Schorr, & T. Johnstone (Eds.), *Appraisal processes in emotion: Theory, methods, research. Series in affective science* (pp. 92–120). New York: Oxford University Press.

Shafran, R., Lee, M., Cooper, Z., Palmer, R. L., & Fairburn, C. G. (2007). Attentional bias in eating disorders. *International Journal of Eating Disorders, 40*, 369–380.

Siemer, M. (2001). Mood-specific effects on appraisal and emotion judgments. *Cognition and Emotion, 15*, 453–485.

Siemer, M. (2005a). Mood-congruent cognitions constitute mood experience. *Emotion, 5*, 296–308.

Siemer, M. (2005b). Moods as multiple-object directed and as objectless affective states: An examination of the dispositional theory of moods. *Cognition and Emotion, 19*, 815–845.

Siemer, M. (2009). Mood experience: Implications of a dispositional theory of moods. *Emotion Review, 1*, 253–260.

Siemer, M., Mauss, I., & Gross, J. J. (2007). Same situation—Different emotions: How appraisals shape our emotions. *Emotion, 7*(3), 592–600.

Siemer, M., & Reisenzein, R. (2007). Appraisals and emotions: Can you have one without the other? *Emotion, 7*, 26–29.

Smeets, E., Roefs, A., van Furth, E., & Jansen, A. (2008). Attentional bias for body and food in eating disorders: Increased distraction, speeded detection, or both? *Behaviour Research and Therapy, 46*, 229–238.

Smith, C. A., & Kirby, L. D. (2004). Appraisal as a pervasive determinant of anger. *Emotion, 4*, 133–138.

Spielberger, C. D., Gorusch, R. L., & Lushene, R. E. (1971). *State-Trait Anxiety Inventory*. Palo Alto, CA: Consulting Psychologists Press.

Tranel, D., Gullickson, G., Koch, M., & Adolphs, R. (2006). Altered experience of emotion following bilateral amygdala damage. *Cognitive Neuropsychiatry*, *11*(3), 219–232.

Walker, W. R., Skowronski, J. J., & Thompson, C. P. (2003). Life is pleasant—And memory helps to keep it that way! *Review of General Psychology*, *7*, 203–210.

Watkins, P. C. (2002). Implicit memory bias in depression. *Cognition and Emotion*, *16*, 381–402.

Watkins, P. C., Martin, C. K., & Stern, L. D. (2000). Unconscious memory bias in depression: Perceptual and conceptual processes. *Journal of Abnormal Psychology*, *109*, 282–289.

Watts, F., & Dalgleish, T. (1991). Memory for phobia-related words in spider phobics. *Cognition and Emotion*, *5*, 313–329.

Weissman, A. N., & Beck, A. T. (1978, March). *Development and validation of the Dysfunctional Attitude Scale: A preliminary investigation*. Paper presented at the annual meeting of the American Educational Research Association, Toronto, Ontario, Canada.

Williams, J. M. G. (1996). Depression and the specificity of autobiographical memory. In D. C. Rubin (Ed.), *Remembering our past: Studies in autobiographical memory* (pp. 244–267). Cambridge, UK: Cambridge University Press.

Williams, J. M. G., Barnhofer, T., Crane, C., Hermans, D., Raes, F., Watkins, E., et al. (2007). Autobiographical memory specificity and emotional disorders. *Psychological Bulletin*, *133*, 122–148.

Williams, J. M. G., Watts, F., MacLeod, C., & Mathews, A. (1997). *Cognitive psychology and emotional disorders* (2nd ed.). Chichester, UK: Wiley.

Wilson, E. J., MacLeod, C., Mathews, A., & Rutherford, E. M. (2006). The causal role of interpretive bias in anxiety reactivity. *Journal of Abnormal Psychology*, *115*, 103–111.

Yiend, J., Mackintosh, B., & Mathews, A. (2005). Enduring consequences of experimentally induced biases in interpretation. *Behaviour Research and Therapy*, *43*, 779–797.

Yoon, K. L., & Zinbarg, R. E. (2008). Interpreting neutral faces as threatening: A default mode for social anxiety. *Journal of Abnormal Psychology*, *117*, 680–685.

Zinbarg, R. E., & Yoon, K. L. (2008). RST and clinical disorders: Anxiety and depression. In P. J. Corr (Ed.), *The reinforcement sensitivity theory of personality* (pp. 360–397). Cambridge, UK: Cambridge University Press.

CHAPTER 9

Goal Dysregulation in the Affective Disorders

Sheri L. Johnson, Charles S. Carver, and Daniel Fulford

This chapter addresses goal dysregulation in depression and mania. It begins with an overview of some of the processes involved in normal goal regulation. To help illustrate why a discussion of goal regulation belongs in a book about emotion regulation, we first focus on how goal regulation processes relate to affect and how they are influenced, in turn, by that affect. We also point to some ways in which goal regulation can go awry. The second section examines evidence of goal regulation problems in depression and mania. We then briefly note some of the ways in which goal dysregulation might operate in other disorders, with a focus on transdiagnostic processes that share commonalities with mania and depression. We then turn to clinical approaches that draw on goal regulation findings. A final section raises some unaddressed issues and future directions.

We note at the outset that this chapter differs from others in this volume in focusing on goal-directed efforts and the affective experiences that surround those efforts rather than on strategic attempts to regulate affect. The view we take here assumes that the normal processes of goal striving influence the creation and regulation of normative affects, and that failures in some of those processes result in affective extremes. Our focus here is on processes of goal regulation and how dysfunctions in them appear to be involved in affective disorders. We use the term *goal regulation* here rather than the more encompassing self-regulation because our focus is more on the management of goals than on the strategic management of affect.

Basic Processes in Goal Regulation

We begin with the goal concept. Goals are mental representations of states a person is trying to attain (Austin & Vancouver, 1996; Pervin, 1989). A goal is a point of reference for evaluating one's present state and a guidepost to use in energizing and directing current and future behavior.

People hold many diverse goals at once. Goal regulation in human behavior thus presents a complex problem in multitasking. People typically shift from one goal to another—to make progress toward most or all of them—although sometimes people are able to attain multiple goals in a single activity. Given this shifting, awareness of a given goal fluctuates from moment to moment. The single goal that is represented in consciousness at any given time has the most resources being directed to its attainment. Yet it is clear that goals can influence behavior even when they are not represented in consciousness (e.g., Gollwitzer & Bargh, 2005).

Although the term *goal* has a rather static feel, many goals are quite dynamic. The goal of taking a vacation isn't to be sitting in your driveway at the end of 2 weeks but to experience the range of events that have been planned for the vacation. The goal of having a professional career isn't entirely a matter of at some point being "established"; it's the pathway of steps involved in getting there. Most goals can be reached in many ways, leading to the potential for vast complexity in the organization of action.

Variations among Goals

Goals vary in many ways. One basic distinction is that some are values to move toward, whereas others are values to avoid or move away from. Differentiating approach from avoidance is not a new idea, but this distinction has become newly prominent in a family of theories with roots in neuropsychology, animal conditioning, and psychopharmacology (see also Elliot, 2008). Theories of this family (e.g., Cloninger, 1987; Davidson, 1998; Depue & Collins, 1999; Fowles, 1980; Gray, 1994) hold that approach and avoidance are managed by partially independent neurobiological systems.

Sometimes approach and avoidance goals are both in place, such that a person tries to avoid a punishing situation by approaching a rewarding one. This conceptual structure seems to characterize what Higgins (1987) refers to as an "ought" self, defined as a quality that one feels compelled to embody in order to avoid social disapproval. It similarly characterizes what Ryan and colleagues (e.g., Ryan & Deci, 2000) refer to as introjected behavior: behaving in particular ways in order to avoid self-criticism. It also seems implicit in what Crocker and colleagues (e.g., Crocker & Wolfe, 2001) refer to as contingent self-esteem, in which self-acceptance is contingent upon attainment of certain standards; although this concept is usually framed in terms of approach, there is a heavy undercurrent of avoidance of disapproval for failing to meet the contingency.

Goal Regulation, Emotion, and Affect

Another important element in the pursuit of goals is affect, or emotion. Life is partly about actions and partly about emotions that accompany actions. How does goal regulation relate to feelings? There is fairly general agreement that feelings often pertain to goals. There is less agreement, however, about precisely what the relationship is and where the feelings come from. This chapter adopts one particular viewpoint on those questions.

Before continuing, a few words about terminology are in order. The terms *affect* and *emotion* sometimes are treated as interchangeable (e.g., Isen, 2000) and sometimes are distinguished from each other (e.g., Fredrickson, 2001; Russell & Barrett, 1999). The word *affect* connotes a hedonic experience, a subjective sense of positive or negative, as does the word *emotion*. Many use the word *emotions* to indicate specific feelings that share a hedonic tone, such as joy and contentedness. Others reserve the word *emotion* to refer to a broader complex of elements that include, among other things, physiological changes. Because the empirical literature on depression and mania relies mostly on self-report measures of feelings, we use the word *affect* in describing most of the findings.

This chapter takes a view in which emotions and affects are closely linked to goal regulation processes. More specifically, we adopt Carver and Scheier's (1998) argument that affect is created by a feedback loop that tracks and controls the rate of progress of goal attainment efforts. If perceived progress toward a goal (or away from a threat) is lower than a criterion (usually an expected or intended rate of progress), negative affect arises; this negative affect prompts efforts to do better (to try harder). If perceived progress toward a goal (or away from a threat) is higher than the criterion, positive affect arises; this positive affect is a sign that you could relax a bit with respect to that goal. In essence, in this view, feelings mark how well or how poorly you are doing with respect to a goal.

Doing well versus doing poorly is part of the story, but there is also more complexity. These complexities help us to understand how goal regulation relates to more specific emotions. Following Higgins (1987), Carver and Scheier (1998) held that the existence of two motivational systems with divergent aims—one to approach incentives, the other to avoid threats—suggests differences in the precise nature of the emotions that arise from the two systems. Each motivational system can create both positive and negative affective valence, depending on how well the system is doing. However, the positives are a little different from each other and the negatives are a little different from each other. The approach system, doing well, yields eagerness, joy, and delight; doing poorly, it yields frustration, anger, sadness, and depression (Carver, 2004). The avoidance system, doing well, yields relief and contentment (Carver, 2009); doing poorly, it yields anxiety, fear, and probably depression as well.

This view on affect shares features with several other theories, including those of Higgins (1987), Roseman (1991), and Rolls (2005), although there are also differences. A more detailed description of similarities and differences between this and other views is beyond the scope of this discussion (for a more complete treatment, see, e.g., Carver & Harmon-Jones, 2009). For now, we simply adopt the Carver–Scheier viewpoint.

Struggle versus Giving Up, Pursuit versus Coasting

The foregoing description suggests two bipolar dimensions of affect. That is, rate of progress toward a goal (or away from a threat) is a dimension. However, different emotions emerge at different regions of high and low progress. For example, this view treats both anger and depression as potential consequences of doing poorly in approach. Which feeling occurs, however, is presumed to depend on whether the incentive seems ultimately attainable (see also Klinger, 1975; Wortman & Brehm, 1975). Figure 9.1 portrays this issue with respect to approach (Carver, 2004; Carver & Scheier, 2008). Progress somewhat below expectation yields frustration and anger. Progress so far below expectation that the goal seems unattainable yields sadness, dejection, and despondency.

These two kinds of negative feelings are also presumed to have two very different effects on ongoing actions. When the person falls behind but the goal is not seen as lost, the feelings of frustration and anger accompany an increase in effort, a struggle to gain the incentive despite setbacks. This struggle is adaptive (thus, the affect is adaptive) because the struggle fosters goal attainment (Duckworth, Peterson, Matthews, & Kelly, 2007).

When effort appears futile, sadness and despondency imply that things cannot be set right, that further effort is pointless, and these feelings accompany *reduction* of effort. Reduction of effort when goals are unattainable can also be adaptive. It serves to conserve energy rather than waste it futilely pursuing the unattainable (Nesse, 2000). Furthermore, withdrawing effort can diminish commitment to the goal (Klinger, 1975). This eventually readies the person to take up pursuit of other incentives in place of this one. This works, however, *only if the person can relinquish the goal.* Continued commitment to an unattainable goal yields continued distress. Indeed, this combination has been suggested as the underlying root of depression (Carver & Scheier, 1998; Pyszczynski & Greenberg, 1992).

The left side of Figure 9.1 also displays a discontinuity, although one that is less obvious. When approach is proceeding well enough but only as well as it has to or is expected to, the valence experienced is neutral. As that value is exceeded, positive valence arises: a sense of eagerness or enthusiasm. The function of this sort of affect is to sustain the effort at goal pursuit. If the criterion is exceeded substantially enough, however,

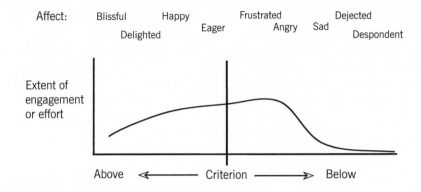

FIGURE 9.1. Hypothesized approach-related affects as a function of doing well versus doing poorly compared with a criterion velocity. A second (vertical) dimension indicates the degree of behavioral engagement posited to be associated with affects at different degrees of departure from neutral. From Carver (2004). Copyright 2004 by the American Psychological Association. Adapted by permission.

eagerness gives way to pleasure and joy. The Carver–Scheier (1998, 2008; Carver, 2003) argument is that positive affect normally induces a tendency to bask in the feeling, to withdraw some effort, to coast (see also Louro, Pieters, & Zeelenberg, 2007). This response would conserve resources, and it would permit the person to consider other goals that might need attention more than this one does. It has been argued that this arrangement would foster the capacity to multitask, to shift among simultaneously active goals (for discussion, see Carver, 2003).

Affect and Behavior as Interwoven

In this view of goal regulation, affect regulation is tethered to goal regulation. The emergence of affect is accompanied by (or promotes) shifts in behavior. Thus, action and affect are always intertwined: two systems working in concert. It is of interest for understanding affect regulation that the behavioral responses linked to the affects also lead to reduction of the affects. We thus suggest that the affect system is, in a very basic sense, self-regulating (cf. Campos, Frankel, & Camras, 2004). It is undeniable that people also engage in voluntary efforts to regulate emotions. Nonetheless, if the affect system is functioning normally, it does a good deal of affect regulation on its own. Long-lasting extremes of affect (ecstasy, depression) occur when the system is not doing an effective job of self-regulating.

That is, in theory, both extreme cases—depressed affect and elation—are maintained only if the person remains engaged with that goal and progress remains at that very low or very high level. In normal functioning, depressed affect promotes disengagement. Disengagement from the goal causes the sad affect to fade. In normal functioning, elation promotes coasting. With coasting, the rate of progress tends to slow and the elation fades. Thus, the responses normally cued by both affects contribute to the eventual reduction of the affects.

An important longer term consequence of very high or very low rates of progress is change in the criterion value for rate (Carver & Scheier, 2000). A person who frequently outperforms his or her expectations will begin to adjust those expectations upward. One who chronically under-performs will begin to adjust those expectations downward. In general, this recalibration process is believed to occur more slowly than the contextual reduction in affect that was just described.

To be clear, there are many different ways that people engage in affect regulation. However, it is also the case that problems in goal regulation will promote affective disturbances. In the same way, corrections in goal setting and goal engagement can promote healthier affective regulation.

Goal Dysregulation and Mood Disorders

We turn now to information that suggests mood disorders involve some aspects of goal dysregulation. Our interest is in phenomena that have been found to differentiate depression and mania from healthy samples. We consider depression and mania separately. Where studies of diagnosed samples are available, we focus on those rather than analog samples. In many domains, though, research is limited to analog samples, and we include this research (labeled as such) as a way of pointing toward future directions.

For both depression and mania, we begin by describing literature on motivational sensitivity to threat and reward. Then we consider goal setting, reactions to high and low goal progress, and goal disengagement. Although much of the literature is cross-sectional, we also consider available evidence on whether various patterns can be documented after remission and whether they predict the course of disorder.

Goal Dysregulation in Depression

The experience of depression typically incorporates several elements that can be linked to the goal regulation view outlined earlier in the chapter. Depression involves hopelessness about being able to move toward desired endpoints. Perhaps for that reason there often is a blunted motivational responsiveness to incentives. In contrast, depression may frequently entail oversensitivity to threats. Often the goals to which depressed people are committed are imposed by people outside the self, and an inability to disengage seems bound up in the need for acceptance from those people. It generally seems not to be the case that the goals are extremely high (thus making them unattainable) but rather that they reflect contingencies of self-worth. The focus on the inability to move forward in depression is also reflected in negative generalizations about the self when failures occur and an inability to enjoy positive experiences when they occur. There may also be an inability to disengage and turn to more promising goals.

Sensitivity to Incentives and Threats in Depression

For several decades, theory has suggested that depression is related to low incentive sensitivity and high threat sensitivity (Depue, Krauss, & Spoont, 1987; Fowles, 1980). Several self-report measures assess such sensitivities, including the Behavioral Inhibition and Behavioral Activation Scales (BIS/BAS; Carver & White, 1994). These scales assess individual differences in the experience of excitement and energy in response to incentives and goal attainment and of anxiety in response to threat. Electroencephalogram (EEG) frontal asymmetry has also been used as an index of relative approach versus avoidance motivation (and has been related to the BIS/BAS scales; Sutton & Davidson, 1997). Laboratory tasks that manipulate reinforcement and punishment contingencies also have been used to study sensitivity to reward and punishment.

There is some evidence of high threat sensitivity associated with current major depressive disorder (MDD) (Pinto-Meza et al., 2006), even when controlling for anxiety diagnoses (Johnson, Turner, & Iwata, 2003). Two studies have found that people with MDD show greater decrements in performance after failure than healthy controls do (Elliott, Sahakian, McKay, & Herrod, 1996; Holmes & Pizzagalli, 2008), suggesting elevated responsiveness to punishment. One study, though, found no difference in behavioral choices after punishment (loss of money; Henriques & Davidson, 2000).

On the other hand, a recent review has suggested that in laboratory studies, persons with MDD have blunted affective and psychophysiological reactivity to negative emotion stimuli, such as film clips or negative pictures, compared with healthy controls (Bylsma, Morris, & Rottenberg, 2008). In parallel, blunted activity in the medial prefrontal cortex in response to negative stimuli has been observed in one study comparing participants with MDD with healthy controls (Steele, Kumar, & Ebmeier, 2007). Hence, participants with MDD do not show reactivity to negative stimuli in general; indeed, they may be less reactive to photos or film clips of others' negative experiences. In two of three studies, though, they do seem to be more sensitive to punishment.

Evidence is more complex regarding incentive sensitivity and depression (see Dillon & Pizzagalli, Chapter 10, this volume). One major study found that people with remitted MDD do not differ from healthy controls on self-reported incentive sensitivity (Johnson et al., 2003). Another study found that formerly depressed persons exhibited less left frontal brain

activity in response to emotionally salient film clips than did healthy controls (Henriques & Davidson, 1991). Hence, it is difficult to draw firm conclusions about whether a history of MDD is related to a trait-like deficit in
incentive sensitivity.

Among persons with current MDD, on the other hand, many studies
have found evidence of blunted approach. Deficits include less self-reported
incentive sensitivity (Pinto-Meza et al., 2006), fewer behavioral responses
to opportunities to win money (Henriques & Davidson, 2000), lower EEG
in left prefrontal areas associated with approach motivation (Henriques
& Davidson, 1991), and less psychophysiological and affective reactivity to
positive cues (Bylsma et al., 2008). There is also evidence of lower activity
in brain regions such as the nucleus accumbens (Forbes et al., 2006) and
the ventral striatum (Epstein et al., 2006; Steele et al., 2007) during functional magnetic resonance imaging tasks involving reward, despite at least
one nonreplication (Knutson, Bhanji, Cooney, Atlas, & Gotlib, 2008).

Hence, though the data are not entirely uniform during remission
(Johnson et al., 2003), the depression experience appears to involve a drop
in the sensitivity to incentives. Perhaps most intriguing, low incentive sensitivity is related to severity within current depression (Kasch, Rottenberg,
Arnow, & Gotlib, 2002; McFarland, Shankman, Tenke, Bruder, & Klein,
2006), earlier age of onset (Shankman, Klein, Tenke, & Bruder, 2007), and
slower recovery over a 6-month period among persons with MDD (Kasch
et al., 2002). Thus, although low incentive sensitivity may not be a vulnerability feature, it co-occurs with depressive symptoms, and it may have an
important bearing on the course of disorder. Self-reported threat sensitivity appears to be a more trait-like feature of depression, but results are
clearer for punishment than for other types of stimuli.

Consistent with the overall evidence concerning incentive sensitivity
and threat sensitivity levels, depressive symptoms are related to a greater
propensity to set avoidance goals than approach goals. In one study (Dickson & MacLeod, 2006), adolescents had 75 seconds to describe goals that
were important to achieve and another 75 seconds to describe goals that
were important to avoid. Adolescents experiencing moderate to severe
depression generated more avoidance goals and fewer approach goals than
did healthy controls.

Goal Setting in Depression

There are good reasons to expect depression to be associated with high
goal setting. That is, higher goals are harder to attain; failure to attain
goals should promote negative affect. Many aspects of goal setting, however, do not differentiate people with MDD from other people. For example, a history of MDD does not appear related to holding unrealistically
high ambitions (Johnson, Eisner, & Carver, 2009) nor to holding oneself
to high standards (e.g., Carver, La Voie, Kuhl, & Ganellen, 1988; Eisner,

Johnson, & Carver, 2009). The tendency to overvalue achievement-related goals (which has been called autonomy) does not predict depression in response to achievement-related stress (Fresco, Sampson, Craighead, & Koons, 2001; Nietzel & Harris, 1990). It does not seem that high standards per se characterize depressed persons.

There are, however, aspects of goal setting that do appear to be linked to depression. One problem in depression seems to be the contingency aspect of goal attainment. In a review of goal regulation and depression, Street (2002) proposed that depression may be related to the belief that happiness occurs only through the attainment of goals (cf. Crocker & Wolfe, 2001). Results of several studies are consistent with this idea (e.g., Lam & Power, 1991).

Related to the idea that people with MDD may overvalue the importance of goal attainment, several researchers have studied perfectionism. In studies of the construct of perfectionism, Flett, Besser, Hewitt, and Davis (2007) have linked depression principally to one particular aspect of perfectionism: socially prescribed perfectionism, or the belief that others have extremely high standards for oneself and will be satisfied only if these standards are constantly met (e.g., "My family expects me to be perfect"). This sets the stage for depression in the face of any minor failing. Thus, depression may be related to inappropriately linking the sense of self-worth to living up to others' expectations.

Consistent with this view is evidence on one related topic. Sociotropy, defined by a tendency to overvalue interpersonal goals, predicted greater risk of depression, particularly in the face of interpersonal losses (Nietzel & Harris, 1990). That is, sociotropy seems to reflect a contingency held for self-worth. Failing to meet that contingency can trigger depression.

In sum, depression does appear to be related to some specific difficulties pertaining to goal setting. Whereas the disorder is not related to overly high life ambitions or broadly high standards, it is related to the idea that goals must be achieved to have self-worth and to be valued by others. In this way, then, pressures in meeting goals may have implications for mood.

Perceptions of Inadequate Goal Progress in Depression

Several studies suggest that people with depression see their goal-directed efforts as going poorly. People with depressive symptoms rate their goals as more uncertain, more stressful, and more difficult to attain than those lower in depressive symptoms (Beevers & Meyer, 2002; Lecci, Karoly, Briggs, & Kuhn, 1994; Meyer, Beevers, & Johnson, 2004; Salmela-Aro & Nurmi, 1996a). Among adolescents, depressive symptoms correlate with lower expectancies for doing well on laboratory tasks (Dickson & MacLeod, 2006). In a study of patients hospitalized for heart attacks, goal disturbance (defined as the inability to achieve important higher order goals) was correlated with depressive symptoms, even after controlling for demographics and medical characteristics, as well as prior lifestyle (Boersma, Maes, & Joekes, 2005).

Consistent with the idea that people with depression perceive poor goal progress, MDD appears to relate to discrepancies between ideal and actual selves (Scott & O'Hara, 1993; Strauman, 1989). The magnitudes of these self-ideal discrepancies appear to be stable over time (Strauman, 1996). Thus, depression relates to larger perceived distance between where one is (actual self) and where one wants to be (ideal self).

Two studies suggest that difficulties attaining goals predict the course of depression. A 2-year longitudinal study of undergraduates found that negative perceptions of goal progress correlated with baseline symptoms of depression and predicted increases in depressive symptoms over time (Salmela-Aro & Nurmi, 1996b). Depressive symptoms have also been predicted by reports of "having to hold back from doing what one wanted to do" in a longitudinal community study of married persons (Folkman & Lazarus, 1986).

Reactivity to Goal Progress in Depression

How do people react when their goals are actually being achieved? Dysphoric symptoms relate to less self-reported ability to savor goal attainment and good outcomes (Bryant, 2003; Carver & Johnson, in press). Other research has found that depressive symptoms relate to a relative inability to take pride in, or satisfaction with, goal attainment (Grant & Higgins, 2003). Such findings are consistent with the depression symptom of anhedonia, or lacking the capacity for enjoyment.

There is also substantial literature on how people respond when goals are *not* achieved. A tendency to generalize from specific failures to the overall sense of self-worth has been related to diagnoses of MDD (Carver et al., 1988). Moreover, negative generalization predicts unique variance in depressive symptoms, even after controlling for self-criticism, high standards, attributions for failure, and other negative cognitive tendencies (Carver, Ganellen, & Behar-Mitrani, 1985). Negative generalization also relates to depression history in bipolar disorder, even when controlling for current depressive symptoms (Eisner et al., 2009) and has predicted increases in depressive symptoms in interaction with negative events over time (Carver, 1998; Hayes, Harris, & Carver, 2004).

Inability to Disengage in Depression

Most people encounter unattainable goals during their lifetime. It is important to be able to step away from such goals and turn to something else. Is the inability to disengage related to depression? Less is known about this question than might be expected, but there is some research. In one study, the self-reported ability to disengage from goals was strongly related to lower levels of depressive symptoms among parents of children diagnosed with cancer (Wrosch, Scheier, Miller, Schulz, & Carver, 2003). In another study of disabled older adults, dwelling on unattainable health-related goals was related to depression (Schulz, Wrosch, Yee, Heckhausen, & Whitmer, 1998).

Wrosch, Bauer, and Scheier (2005) have described regret as a signal that a person has not been able to disengage from unattained goals. They developed a measure of regret that captures the intensity of negative feelings and the intrusiveness of thoughts about the unattained goal. This measure was correlated with depressive symptoms. Early findings, then, are supportive of the idea that depression is related to difficulties in disengaging from unattainable goals.

Summary for Depression

In sum, depression appears characterized by chronically elevated threat sensitivity and, at least as depression symptoms emerge, blunted reward sensitivity. People who are depressed tend to believe that their self-worth and their acceptance by others depend on displaying perfection. Against this backdrop, depressed people also perceive greater difficulty in attaining goals, and failures to achieve small goals often take on broader meaning for the overall sense of self-worth.

Goal Dysregulation in Mania

How does the experience of mania fit the goal regulation viewpoint? We suggest that mania is linked to an oversensitive incentive system. This may lead to the setting of extremely high goals and an overconfidence about achieving them, especially after initial success. For these people, success leads not to coasting but to immediate escalation of aspirations. There is distractibility, as would be expected if positive affect induces multitasking, but also a sharper ramping upward of goal setting than normally expected after goal progress.

Sensitivity to Reward and Threat in Bipolar Disorder

Several tests of the reward sensitivity model have used the Carver and White (1994) BAS scales. Across studies, higher BAS scores were found among persons with remitted bipolar I disorder compared with healthy controls (Gruber & Johnson, 2009; Meyer, Johnson, & Winters, 2001; Salavert et al., 2007) as well as among students diagnosed with bipolar-spectrum disorder (Alloy et al., 2008). BAS levels also have been found to predict increases in manic symptoms over time (Alloy et al., 2008; Meyer, Johnson, & Winters, 2001). Consistent with the idea that bipolar disorder relates to greater incentive sensitivity, Jones, Shams, and Liversidge (2007) examined approach-oriented goals in relation to the Hypomanic Personality Scale (HPS; Eckblad & Chapman, 1986; Kwapil et al., 2000). The HPS is a measure of subsyndromal fluctuations in manic symptoms that has been found to robustly predict the onset of manic episodes over a 13-year follow-up (Kwapil et al., 2000). Jones and colleagues found in two samples that undergraduates with higher scores on the HPS endorsed more pursuit of approach-oriented goals.

Although there are many positive findings, two studies have failed to replicate the pattern of higher incentive sensitivity related to mania (Hofmann & Meyer, 2006; Jones, Tai, Evershed, Knowles, & Bentall, 2006). Hayden and colleagues (2008) also failed to find elevated BAS scores in people with bipolar disorder compared with healthy controls, but they did find that those with bipolar disorder were behaviorally more responsive to a reward task.

BAS self-reports in mania may depend on more complex issues. There is evidence from a longitudinal study of people with bipolar disorder that BAS scores tend to fall as depressive symptoms increase (Meyer et al., 2001). Hence, it may be important to consider current symptom state in studying BAS sensitivity in bipolar disorder.

In parallel, there is evidence that BIS, or threat sensitivity, increases as depressive symptoms increase (Meyer et al., 2001). Threat sensitivity does not appear to be particularly elevated among persons with bipolar disorder during states of remission (Meyer et al., 2001). Indeed, HPS scores have been found to be inversely associated with BIS scores in at least two samples (Carver & Johnson, in press).

In sum, a body of research suggests that mania is related to increases in reward sensitivity and approach goals. One caveat, though, is the importance of considering the ways in which current symptoms shape both threat and reward sensitivity.

Goal Setting in Bipolar Disorder

Apart from general incentive motivation, people diagnosed with bipolar disorder are also more likely to take up the pursuit of extremely ambitious goals. Johnson and Carver (2006) developed a measure of extreme life ambitions in diverse areas. Higher ambitions for goals such as popular fame and great wealth have been found among students diagnosed with bipolar disorder compared with those with MDD and those with no mood disorder (Johnson et al., 2009), even after controlling for current mood symptoms. Similar results have come from several analog samples (Gruber & Johnson, 2009; Johnson & Carver, 2006).

Consistent with this pattern, several researchers have found that people diagnosed with bipolar disorder are more likely than those with no mood disorder to endorse items on the Dysfunctional Attitudes Scale (Weissman & Beck, 1978) pertaining to the importance of achievement-oriented goals (Lam, Wright, & Smith, 2004; Scott, Stanton, Garland, & Ferrier, 2000). Items on this scale include "A person should do well on everything he undertakes" and "If I try hard enough, I should be able to excel at anything I attempt." Similarly, persons with remitted bipolar disorder endorsed valuing achievement more so than healthy controls on a brief self-report measure (Spielberger, Parker, & Becker, 1963). Overvaluing achievement goals does not appear to be mood-state dependent (Wright, Lam, & Newsom-Davis, 2005). In sum, several studies suggest that people with bipolar disorder and those at risk for the disorder are characterized by high goal setting.

Goal Appraisals in Mania

People at risk for mania, as defined by high scores on the HPS, appear to display elevated confidence about their goal-directed efforts as well. Several aspects of goal appraisals were assessed in one study of college students (Meyer et al., 2004). Participants with elevated hypomania construed their goals as more likely to be attained, more enjoyable, and more controllable, after controlling for current mood state. Meyer and Krumm-Merabet (2003) also found that persons at risk for bipolar disorder, defined by high scores on the HPS, were more confident about their chances of great academic and occupational success than were those with low scores on the HPS.

Although less directly relevant, findings of several studies are consistent with the idea that people with bipolar disorder may be overly positive about their current efforts. For example, Ernst and colleagues (2004) found that children and adolescents diagnosed with juvenile bipolar disorder reported greater confidence about the outcomes of a gambling task. Similarly, Murphy and colleagues (2001) found that participants diagnosed with bipolar disorder were more willing to pursue potential large rewards without regard to the costs during a gambling task. Taken together, there seems to be evidence that people with bipolar disorder can be overly confident about their goal progress.

There is also some indication that the confidence associated with mania is suppressed by depression (Meyer et al., 2004). Similarly, research suggests that self discrepancies fluctuate with mood episodes. For example, patients with current manic symptoms tend to perceive their actual selves as close to achieving their ideal self goals (Bentall, Kinderman, & Manson, 2005). It appears that as depression increases, self-evaluations are harsher, whereas self-evaluations are more positive during mania.

Reactivity to Goal Progress in Mania

How do people at risk for mania react to success? Several analog studies suggest that when they experience one success they respond with a burst of confidence for other goals. For example, Stern and Berrenberg (1979) asked undergraduates the odds of their successfully guessing a coin toss after false success feedback. Those with a history of hypomanic symptoms were inappropriately confident about their ability to guess but only after success feedback. These findings were replicated in a study asking undergraduates to choose the difficulty level for an upcoming task after receiving success feedback (Johnson, Ruggero, & Carver, 2005). Those at higher risk of mania chose more difficult tasks after false success feedback.

Drawing on this pattern of findings, Eisner and colleagues (2009) created a measure of overly confident reactions to success in the form of overgeneralization. Factor analysis yielded three scales, reflecting tendencies to overgeneralize in three ways. HPS scores correlated with higher scores on all three scales, particularly with the scale measuring overgeneralization to loftier goals in the same domain. Hence, hypomania risk appeared to be robustly related to the tendency to become more confident about achieving larger goals after a small success.

Inability to Disengage in Mania

The combination of ambition and confidence might be expected to yield greater persistence as tasks become difficult. There is evidence that this is so. To examine task persistence, Harmon-Jones and colleagues (2008) had participants complete a task in which blocks became progressively more difficult. Left frontal EEG cortical activation was used as an index of task engagement (approach orientation). Although the healthy control participants showed a decrease in left frontal cortical activation as tasks became harder (suggesting a reduction in approach effort), people diagnosed with bipolar I disorder continued to show increases in activation in this area.

If people prone to mania have trouble disengaging, do they become more frustrated when their approach goals are thwarted? Apparently so. Wright, Lam, and Brown (2008) found that people with bipolar I disorder reported more emotional reactivity to goal frustration and also took more days to recover from negative moods after goal frustration events. Taken together, there is a suggestion that people with bipolar disorder are likely to respond with more robust psychophysiological activity and more frustration when goal pursuit is challenged.

Summary of Findings Regarding Mania

People with diagnosed bipolar disorder and those at risk for mania seem to have high levels of reward sensitivity and to set very high goals. Likewise, people diagnosed with bipolar disorder as well as those at risk for the disorder have high levels of confidence. Analog studies suggest that students at risk for bipolar disorder feel more of a surge of confidence when goal pursuit is going well. There is also evidence that people at risk for mania are likely to be more psychophysiologically reactive and more frustrated than other people when goals are thwarted.

Overall Summary

As indicated by evidence described in the previous sections, several elements of goal dysregulation appear to be associated with mood disorders. The specific patterns that emerge for depression and for mania are quite different in their content. Yet there is a striking commonality in some of the functional properties (see also Carver & Johnson, in press). On the depression side, the observed correlates appear to coalesce around failure in goal pursuit and the perception of inability to progress normally toward goal pursuit. Being sensitive to threat, being relatively insensitive to reward, generalizing from failure to the broad sense of self-worth all seem to reflect an ineffective goal-seeking system. There also is evidence of a contingency-based mindset in depression: the sense that happiness comes from satisfying other people's expectations, which often feel far out of reach.

On the manic side, the observed correlates appear to coalesce around high engagement in goal pursuit. Highly engaged goal pursuit benefits from strong motivation to approach incentives, from setting of high goals, and from responding to success experiences with a generalized sense of confidence about diverse life domains. These tendencies seem to suggest a person who is ultra–goal engaged (Johnson, 2005).

Although the specifics are quite different for depression compared with mania, there is also a certain conceptual parallel in the correlates of the two syndromes. Both deviate from nonclinical samples in their sensitivities to the possibility of attaining rewards, albeit in opposite directions. Both relate to reported tendencies to generalize cognitively after events with the valence that is salient in that syndrome (failure for depression and positive events for mania). In brief, both seem to reflect normal processes of goal regulation gone awry.

Transdiagnostic Implications of Goal Dysregulation

Although we have focused specifically on mania and depression in this chapter, many aspects of goal dysregulation appear involved in a much broader range of psychopathologies. For example, many of the aspects of goal regulation that relate to depression appear to be involved in anxiety disorders as well. Anxiety disorders have been related to high levels of BIS sensitivity (Johnson et al., 2003), a relative dominance of avoidance goals over approach goals (cf. Dickson & MacLeod, 2004b; Rodebaugh, 2007), and overinvestment in the importance of achieving goals (Pomerantz, Saxon, & Oishi, 2000). Low expectancy of achieving important goals appears to be a feature of anxiety disorders (Doerfler & Aron, 1995) and can predict increases in anxiety symptoms (Boersma, Maes, & van Elderen, 2005; Nordin, Wasteson, Hoffman, Glimelius, & Sjoden, 2001).

As goal dysregulation deficits are documented across a range of disorders, we hope that researchers will begin to study the common and specific facets of these deficits across different psychopathologies. Anxiety and depression are strongly correlated, and most studies do not use samples selected to be exclusively anxious or exclusively depressed. Indeed, this issue is also important in the literature we reviewed on depression. It is not clear, for example, whether some of the similarities in the anxiety literature are products of comorbid depression. Neither are we sure whether the findings in the depression literature are products of comorbid anxiety. So far, purely anxious samples have been differentiated from purely depressed samples by a greater focus on avoidance goals (Dickson & MacLeod, 2004a) and higher actual–ought self discrepancy scores (Scott & O'Hara, 1993).

Researchers have also described goal regulation deficits in other disorders that appear similar to those observed in mania. For example, alcohol and drug abuse appear related to high incentive sensitivity and low threat sensitivity (Johnson et al., 2003). Narcissistic traits relate to setting overly ambitious goals and being highly reactive to goal progress (Fulford, Johnson, & Carver, 2008). Few have considered, however, how these other disorders might relate to the affective disorders. In sum, goal regulation models may represent a transdiagnostic perspective that is useful in many areas.

Treatment Implications

Several treatment programs have been developed to address deficits in goal regulation. One of the issues in depression is the failure to engage successfully in the pursuit of approach-relevant goals. Major trials suggest that behavioral activation treatments for depression, designed simply to engage people in reinforcing activities that are achievable, provide as much relief as more comprehensive cognitive therapy treatments (Jacobson et al., 1996; Jacobson, Martell, & Dimidjian, 2001; see also Syzdek, Addis, & Martell, Chapter 17, this volume). Beyond enhancing general goal engagement, Strauman and colleagues (2006) have developed self-system therapy (SST), a depression treatment designed to enhance the pursuit of approach, or promotion, goals. In a randomized controlled trial of 45 patients with depression, the authors found that SST was as efficacious as cognitive therapy. SST was particularly effective for those participants lacking an emphasis on promotion goals before treatment.

We have also briefly noted the preponderance of avoidance goals compared with approach goals among persons diagnosed with anxiety disorders. It is intriguing to note that exposure therapy, the most well-validated treatment for addressing many anxiety disorders (Deacon & Abramowitz, 2004), promotes approach-related behavior to change avoidance behavior. That is, a person is coached to stop avoiding feared stimuli as a way to conquer anxiety and to regain freedom to pursue important life goals. Although goal regulation is not often discussed as the framework for such work, it might be helpful to consider such principles in refining the therapy rationale offered for clients.

With regard to mania, Johnson has developed an intervention designed to address goal dysregulation. Offered as an adjunct to medication, the program teaches clients to recognize their heightened reward sensitivity and ambitions and to become more adept at monitoring and regulating changes in confidence and symptoms during periods of rapid goal progress. Early data indicate that the program led to reductions in unrealistic ambitions and manic symptoms in a small sample of persons with bipolar I disorder (Johnson & Fulford, 2009).

Across several disorders, then, there is evidence that goal regulation models can enhance and guide treatment efforts. Goal dysregulation conceptualizations have been applied in different ways across the psychopathologies, but generally provide a rich framework for considering therapeutic rationales and providing more specific treatment targets and interventions.

Future Directions

Evidence suggests that both mania and depression are related to goal dysregulation. There is certainly a need for replication and extension. It is also important to note that findings have been mixed in some domains, such as studies of incentive sensitivity. It appears that symptom status, severity of clinical history, and treatment status may influence various aspects of goal regulation, but these confounds are often not controlled. Little is understood about how developmental processes across the lifespan, including the ongoing barriers to successful goal attainment erected by serious episodes, change goal regulation. Perhaps most importantly, much of the research has been cross-sectional. Although it is clear that deficits can be observed among persons with mood disorders, there is a need for prospective studies beyond those that have been conducted on incentive and threat sensitivity.

One more issue should be addressed regarding normal goal regulation. A number of theories have been proposed in which people are assumed to simultaneously process experience in two different modes. A basic, and evolutionarily more primitive, mode of processing has been referred to with terms such as *implicit, reflexive, impulsive, automatic, experiential,* and *"hot"*; a second, evolutionarily recent, mode has been referred to with such terms as *explicit, reflective, rational, planful, "cool," effortful,* and *deliberative* (e.g., Epstein, 1994; Lieberman, Gaunt, Gilbert, & Trope, 2002; Metcalfe & Mischel, 1999). The two modes have different operating characteristics, and they sometimes are in competition to determine behavior. Theories of this sort are now common in psychology.

It is generally assumed that the basic mode incorporates approach and avoidance functions and guides these sensitivities (e.g., Derryberry &

Rothbart, 1997; Eisenberg et al., 2004; Rothbart, Ellis, Rueda, & Posner, 2003). In contrast, qualities of constraint, or effortful control, are seen as being managed by the explicit processing system. This system is superordinate to approach and avoidance temperaments. It can override those temperaments as long as it has the processing resources available to do so.

In the absence of effortful control, whichever basic goal-related tendency (approach or avoidance) engages a stronger reaction to the current circumstance (desire vs. fear) dominates current behavior. Effortful control, however, can counter the automatic tendency. If enough effortful control capacity is available, the impulsive grabbing of incentives that arises from a sensitive approach system can be restrained (Kochanska & Knaack, 2003). The impulsive avoidance from a sensitive threat system can be countered. The person who is not motivated to do something he knows he should do can force himself to engage in that action. Effortful control, therefore, has an important role in goal-directed behavior.

Although these ideas are becoming influential across psychology, they have only fairly recently been applied to understanding disorders. It has been suggested, however, that a relative deficit of effortful control is an important influence in experiences such as depression, impulsive aggression, and perhaps anxiety and mania (Carver, Johnson, & Joormann, 2008; Strakowski et al., 2005). Deficits in effortful control, however, have not yet been integrated into studies of goal regulation within these psychopathologies.

In sum, a large theoretical and basic research base has been developed for understanding goal regulation processes in healthy individuals. This literature is being increasingly applied to understanding mood disorders, and the findings to date are promising. Early strides are being made in applying these ideas to treatment development. There is a need for more methodologically careful studies, for studies comparing goal regulation processes across disorders, and for studies integrating goal regulation with emergent understanding of deficits in effortful control. We hope this chapter provides a concise window into those findings and provokes a new set of ideas about gaps to fill.

References

Alloy, L. B., Abramson, L. Y., Walshaw, P. D., Cogswell, A., Grandin, L. D., Hughes, M. E., et al. (2008). Behavioral approach system and behavioral inhibition system sensitivities and bipolar spectrum disorders: Prospective prediction of bipolar mood episodes. *Bipolar Disorders, 10,* 310–322.

Austin, J. T., & Vancouver, J. B. (1996). Goal constructs in psychology: Structure, process, and content. *Psychological Bulletin, 120,* 338–375.

Beevers, C. G., & Meyer, B. (2002). Lack of positive experiences and positive expectancies mediate the relationship between BAS responsiveness and depression. *Cognition and Emotion, 16,* 549–564.

Bentall, R. P., Kinderman, P., & Manson, K. (2005). Self-discrepancies in bipolar disorder: Comparison of manic, depressed, remitted and normal participants. *British Journal of Clinical Psychology, 44,* 457–473.

Boersma, S. N., Maes, S., & Joekes, K. (2005). Goal disturbance in relation to anxiety, depression, and health-related quality of life after myocardial infarction. *Quality of Life Research, 14,* 2265–2275.

Boersma, S. N., Maes, S., & van Elderen, T. (2005). Goal disturbance predicts health-related quality of life and depression 4 months after myocardial infarction. *British Journal of Health Psychology, 10,* 615–630.

Bryant, F. B. (2003). Savoring Beliefs Inventory (SBI): A scale for measuring beliefs about savouring. *Journal of Mental Health, 12,* 175–196.

Bylsma, L. M., Morris, B. H., & Rottenberg, J. (2008). A meta-analysis of emotional reactivity in major depressive disorder. *Clinical Psychology Review, 28,* 676–691.

Campos, J. J., Frankel, C. B., & Camras, L. (2004). On the nature of emotion regulation. *Child Development, 75,* 377–394.

Carver, C. S. (1998). Generalization, adverse events, and development of depressive symptoms. *Journal of Personality, 66,* 607–619.

Carver, C. S. (2003). Pleasure as a sign you can attend to something else: Placing positive feelings within a general model of affect. *Cognition and Emotion, 17,* 241–261.

Carver, C. S. (2004). Negative affects deriving from the behavioral approach system. *Emotion, 4,* 3–22.

Carver, C. S., Ganellen, R. J., & Behar-Mitrani, V. (1985). Depression and cognitive style: Comparisons between measures. *Journal of Personality and Social Psychology, 49,* 722–728.

Carver, C. S., & Harmon-Jones, E. (2009). Anger is an approach-related affect: Evidence and implications. *Psychological Bulletin, 135,* 183–204.

Carver, C. S., & Johnson, S. L. (in press). Tendencies toward mania and tendencies toward depression have distinct motivational, affective, and cognitive correlates. *Cognitive Therapy and Research.*

Carver, C. S., Johnson, S. L., & Joormann, J. (2008). Serotonergic function, two-mode models of self-regulation, and vulnerability to depression: What depression has in common with impulsive aggression. *Psychological Bulletin, 134,* 912–943.

Carver, C. S., La Voie, L., Kuhl, J., & Ganellen, R. J. (1988). Cognitive concomitants of depression: A further examination of the roles of generalization, high standards, and self-criticism. *Journal of Social and Clinical Psychology, 7,* 350–365.

Carver, C. S., & Scheier, M. F. (1998). *On the self-regulation of behavior.* New York: Cambridge University Press.

Carver, C. S., & Scheier, M. F. (2000). Scaling back goals and recalibration of the affect system are processes in normal adaptive self-regulation: Understanding "response shift" phenomena. *Social Science and Medicine, 50,* 1715–1722.

Carver, C. S., & Scheier, M. F. (2008). Feedback processes in the simultaneous regulation of action and affect. In J. Y. Shah & W. L. Gardner (Eds.), *Handbook of motivation science* (pp. 308–324). New York: Guilford Press.

Carver, C. S., & White, T. L. (1994). Behavioral inhibition, behavioral activation, and affective responses to impending reward and punishment: The BIS/BAS scales. *Journal of Personality and Social Psychology, 67,* 319–333.

Cloninger, C. R. (1987). A systematic method of clinical description and classification of personality variants: A proposal. *Archives of General Psychiatry, 44,* 573–588.

Crocker, J., & Wolfe, C. T. (2001). Contingencies of self-worth. *Psychological Review, 108,* 593–623.

Davidson, R. J. (1998). Anterior electrophysiological asymmetries, emotion, and depression: Conceptual and methodological conundrums. *Psychophysiology, 35,* 607–614.

Deacon, B. J., & Abramowitz, J. S. (2004). Cognitive and behavioral treatments for anxiety disorders: A review of meta-analytic findings. *Journal of Clinical Psychology, 60,* 429–441.

Depue, R. A., & Collins, P. F. (1999). Neurobiology of the structure of personality: Dopamine, facilitation of incentive motivation, and extraversion. *Behavioral and Brain Sciences, 22,* 491–517.

Depue, R. A., Krauss, S. P., & Spoont, M. R. (1987). A two-dimensional threshold model of seasonal bipolar affective disorder. In D. Magnusson & A. Oehman (Eds.), *Psychopathology: An interactional perspective. Personality, psychopathology, and psychotherapy* (pp. 95–123). Orlando, FL: Academic Press.

Derryberry, D., & Rothbart, M. K. (1997). Reactive and effortful processes in the organization of temperament. *Development and Psychopathology, 9,* 633–652.

Dickson, J. M., & MacLeod, A. K. (2004a). Anxiety, depression and approach and avoidance goals. *Cognition and Emotion, 18,* 423–430.

Dickson, J. M., & MacLeod, A. K. (2004b). Approach and avoidance goals and plans: Their relationship to anxiety and depression. *Cognitive Therapy and Research, 28,* 415–432.

Dickson, J. M., & MacLeod, A. K. (2006). Dysphoric adolescents' causal explanations and expectancies for approach and avoidance goals. *Journal of Adolescence, 29,* 177–191.

Doerfler, L. A., & Aron, J. (1995). Relationship of goal setting, self-efficacy, and self-evaluation in dysphoric and socially anxious women. *Cognitive Therapy and Research, 19,* 725–738.

Duckworth, A. L., Peterson, C., Matthews, M. D., & Kelly, D. R. (2007). Grit: Perseverance and passion for long-term goals. *Journal of Personality and Social Psychology, 92,* 1087–1101.

Eckblad, M., & Chapman, L. J. (1986). Development and validation of a scale for hypomanic personality. *Journal of Abnormal Psychology, 95,* 214–222.

Eisenberg, N., Spinrad, T. L., Fabes, R. A., Reiser, M., Cumberland, A., Shepard, S. A., et al. (2004). The relations of effortful control and impulsivity to children's resiliency and adjustment. *Child Development, 75,* 25–46.

Eisner, L., Johnson, S. L., & Carver, C. S. (2008). Cognitive responses to failure and success relate uniquely to bipolar depression versus mania. *Journal of Abnormal Psychology, 117,* 154–163.

Elliot, A. J. (Ed.). (2008). *Handbook of approach and avoidance motivation.* Mahwah, NJ: Erlbaum.

Elliott, R., Sahakian, B. J., McKay, A. P., & Herrod, J. J. (1996). Neuropsychological impairments in unipolar depression: The influence of perceived failure on subsequent performance. *Psychological Medicine, 26,* 975–989.

Epstein, J., Pan, H., Kocsis, J. H., Yang, Y., Butler, T., Chusid, J., et al. (2006). Lack of ventral striatal response to positive stimuli in depressed versus normal subjects. *American Journal of Psychiatry, 163,* 1784–1790.

Epstein, S. (1994). Integration of the cognitive and the psychodynamic uncon-
   scious. *American Psychologist, 49,* 709–724.
Ernst, M., Dickstein, D., Munson, S., Eshel, N., Pradella, A., Jazbec, S., et al. (2004).
   Reward-related processes in pediatric bipolar disorder: A pilot study. *Journal
   of Affective Disorders, 82,* S89–S101.
Flett, G. L., Besser, A., Hewitt, P. L., & Davis, R. A. (2007). Perfectionism, silencing
   the self, and depression. *Personality and Individual Differences, 43,* 1211–1222.
Folkman, S., & Lazarus, R. S. (1986). Stress processes and depressive symptomatol-
   ogy. *Journal of Abnormal Psychology, 95,* 107–113.
Forbes, E. E., May, J. C., Siegle, G. J., Ladouceur, C. D., Ryan, N. D., Carter, C. S.,
   et al. (2006). Reward-related decision-making in pediatric major depressive
   disorder: An fMRI study *Journal of Child Psychology and Psychiatry, and Allied
   Disciplines, 47,* 1031–1040.
Fowles, D. C. (1980). The three arousal model: Implications of Gray's two-factor
   learning theory for heart rate, electrodermal activity, and psychopathy. *Psychophysiology, 17,* 87–104.
Fredrickson, B. L. (2001). The role of positive emotions in positive psychology:
   The broaden-and-build theory of positive emotions. *American Psychologist, 56,*
   218–226.
Fresco, D. M., Sampson, W. S., Craighead, L. W., & Koons, A. N. (2001). The rela-
   tionship of sociotropy and autonomy to symptoms of depression and anxiety.
   Journal of Cognitive Psychotherapy, 15, 17–31.
Fulford, D., Johnson, S. L., & Carver, C. S. (2008). Commonalities and differ-
   ences in characteristics of persons at risk for narcissism and mania. *Journal of
   Research in Personality, 42,* 1427–1438.
Gollwitzer, P. M., & Bargh, J. A. (2005). Automaticity in goal pursuit. In A. J. Elliot
   & C. S. Dweck (Eds.), *Handbook of competence and motivation* (pp. 624–646).
   New York: Guilford Press.
Grant, H., & Higgins, E. T. (2003). Optimism, promotion pride, and prevention
   pride as predictors of quality of life. *Personality and Social Psychology Bulletin,
   29,* 1521–1532.
Gray, J. A. (1994). Three fundamental emotion systems. In P. Ekman & R. J. David-
   son (Eds.), *The nature of emotion: Fundamental questions* (pp. 243–247). New
   York: Oxford University Press.
Gruber, J., & Johnson, S. L. (2009). Positive emotional traits and ambitious goals
   among people at risk for bipolar disorder: The need for specificity. *International Journal of Cognitive Therapy, 2,* 176–187.
Harmon-Jones, E., Abramson, L. Y., Nusslock, R., Sigelman, J. D., Urosevic, S., Turonie, L. D., et al. (2008). Effect of bipolar disorder on left frontal cortical
   responses to goals differing in valence and task difficulty. *Biological Psychiatry,
   63,* 693–698.
Hayden, E. P., Bodkins, M., Brenner, C., Shekhar, A., Nurnberger, J. I. Jr., O'Donnell,
   B., et al. (2008). A multimethod investigation of the behavioral activation
   system in bipolar disorder. *Journal of Abnormal Psychology, 117,* 164–170.
Hayes, A. M., Harris, M. S., & Carver, C. S. (2004). Predictors of self-esteem variability. *Cognitive Therapy and Research, 28,* 369–385.
Henriques, J. B., & Davidson, R. J. (1991). Left frontal hypoactivation in depression. *Journal of Abnormal Psychology, 100,* 535–545.
Henriques, J. B., & Davidson, R. J. (2000). Decreased responsiveness to reward in
   depression. *Cognition and Emotion, 14,* 711–724.

Higgins, E. T. (1987). Self-discrepancy: A theory relating self and affect. *Psychological Review, 94,* 319–340.

Hofmann, B. U., & Meyer, T. D. (2006). Mood fluctuations in people putatively at risk for bipolar disorders. *British Journal of Clinical Psychology, 45,* 105–110.

Holmes, A. J., & Pizzagalli, D. A. (2008). Spatiotemporal dynamics of error processing dysfunctions in major depressive disorder. *Archives of General Psychiatry, 65,* 179–188.

Isen, A. M. (2000). Positive affect and decision making. In M. Lewis & J. M. Haviland-Jones (Eds.), *Handbook of emotions* (2nd ed., pp. 417–435). New York: Guilford Press.

Jacobson, N. S., Dobson, K. S., Truax, P. A., Addis, M. E., Koerner, K., Gollan, J. K., et al. (1996). A component analysis of cognitive-behavioral treatment for depression. *Journal of Consulting and Clinical Psychology, 64,* 295–304.

Jacobson, N. S., Martell, C. R., & Dimidjian, S. (2001). Behavioral activation treatment for depression: Returning to contextual roots. *Clinical Psychology: Science and Practice, 8,* 255–270.

Johnson, S. L. (2005). Mania and dysregulation in goal pursuit. *Clinical Psychology Review, 25,* 241–262.

Johnson, S. L., & Carver, C. (2006). Extreme goal setting and vulnerability to mania among undiagnosed young adults. *Cognitive Therapy and Research, 30,* 377–395.

Johnson, S. L., Eisner, L. R., & Carver, C. S. (2009). Elevated expectations among persons diagnosed with bipolar disorder. *British Journal of Clinical Psychology, 48,* 217–222.

Johnson, S. L., & Fulford, D. (2009). Preventing mania: A preliminary examination of the GOALS program. *Behavior Therapy, 40,* 103–113.

Johnson, S. L., Ruggero, C. J., & Carver, C. S. (2005). Cognitive, behavioral, and affective responses to reward: Links with hypomanic symptoms. *Journal of Social and Clinical Psychology, 24,* 894–906.

Johnson, S. L., Turner, R. J., & Iwata, N. (2003). BIS/BAS levels and psychiatric disorder: An epidemiological study. *Journal of Psychopathology and Behavioral Assessment, 25,* 25–36.

Jones, S. H., Shams, M., & Liversidge, T. (2007). Approach goals, behavioural activation and risk of hypomania. *Personality and Individual Differences, 43,* 1366–1375.

Jones, S. H., Tai, S., Evershed, K., Knowles, R., & Bentall, R. (2006). Early detection of bipolar disorder: A pilot familial high-risk study of parents with bipolar disorder and their adolescent children. *Bipolar Disorders, 8,* 362–372.

Kasch, K. L., Rottenberg, J., Arnow, B. A., & Gotlib, I. H. (2002). Behavioral activation and inhibition systems and the severity and course of depression. *Journal of Abnormal Psychology, 111,* 589–597.

Klinger, E. (1975). Consequences of commitment to and disengagement from incentives. *Psychological Review, 82,* 1–25.

Knutson, B., Bhanji, J. P., Cooney, R. E., Atlas, L. Y., & Gotlib, I. H. (2008). Neural responses to monetary incentives in major depression. *Biological Psychiatry, 63,* 686–692.

Kochanska, G., & Knaack, A. (2003). Effortful control as a personality characteristic of young children: Antecedents, correlates, and consequences. *Journal of Personality, 71,* 1087–1112.

Kwapil, T. R., Miller, M. B., Zinser, M. C., Chapman, L. J., Chapman, J., & Eckblad,

M. (2000). A longitudinal study of high scorers on the Hypomanic Personality Scale. *Journal of Abnormal Psychology, 109,* 222–226.

Lam, D. H., & Power, M. J. (1991). A questionnaire designed to assess roles and goals: A preliminary study. *British Journal of Medical Psychology, 64,* 359–373.

Lam, D. H., Wright, K., & Smith, N. (2004). Dysfunctional assumptions in bipolar disorder. *Journal of Affective Disorders, 79,* 193–199.

Lecci, L., Karoly, P., Briggs, C., & Kuhn, K. (1994). Specificity and generality of motivational components of depression: A personal projects analysis. *Journal of Abnormal Psychology, 103,* 403–408.

Lieberman, M. D., Gaunt, R., Gilbert, D. T., & Trope, Y. (2002). Reflection and reflexion: A social cognitive neuroscience approach to attributional inference. *Advances in Experimental Social Psychology, 34,* 199–249.

Louro, M. J., Pieters, R., & Zeelenberg, M. (2007). Dynamics of multiple-goal pursuit. *Journal of Personality and Social Psychology, 93,* 174–193.

McFarland, B. R., Shankman, S. A., Tenke, C. E., Bruder, G. E., & Klein, D. N. (2006). Behavioral activation system deficits predict the six-month course of depression. *Journal of Affective Disorders, 91*(2–3), 229–234.

Metcalfe, J., & Mischel, W. (1999). A hot/cool-system analysis of delay of gratification: Dynamics of willpower. *Psychological Review, 106,* 3–19.

Meyer, B., Beevers, C. G., & Johnson, S. L. (2004). Goal appraisals and vulnerability to bipolar disorder: A personal projects analysis. *Cognitive Therapy and Research, 28,* 173–182.

Meyer, B., Johnson, S. L., & Winters, R. (2001). Responsiveness to threat and incentive in bipolar disorder: Relations of the BIS/BAS scales with symptoms. *Journal of Psychopathology and Behavioral Assessment, 23,* 133–143.

Meyer, T. D., & Krumm-Merabet, C. (2003). Academic performance and expectations for the future in relation to a vulnerability marker for bipolar disorders: The hypomanic temperament. *Personality and Individual Differences, 35,* 785–796.

Murphy, F. C., Rubinsztein, J. S., Michael, A., Rogers, R. D., Robbins, T. W., Paykel, E. S., et al. (2001). Decision-making cognition in mania and depression. *Psychological Medicine, 31,* 679–693.

Nesse, R. M. (2000). Is depression an adaptation? *Archives of General Psychiatry, 57,* 14–20.

Nietzel, M. T., & Harris, M. J. (1990). Relationship of dependency and achievement/autonomy to depression. *Clinical Psychology Review, 10,* 279–297.

Nordin, K., Wasteson, E., Hoffman, K., Glimelius, B., & Sjoden, P. (2001). Discrepancies between attainment and importance of life values and anxiety and depression in gastrointestinal cancer patients and their spouses. *Psycho-Oncology, 10*(6), 479–489.

Pervin, L. A. (1989). *Goal concepts in personality and social psychology.* Hillsdale, NJ: Erlbaum.

Pinto-Meza, A., Caseras, X., Soler, J., Puigdemont, D., Perez, V., & Torrubia, R. (2006). Behavioural inhibition and behavioural activation systems in current and recovered major depression participants. *Personality and Individual Differences, 40,* 215–226.

Pomerantz, E. M., Saxon, J. L., & Oishi, S. (2000). The psychological trade-offs of goal investment. *Journal of Personality and Social Psychology, 79,* 617–630.

Pyszczynski, T., & Greenberg, J. (1992). *Hanging on and letting go: Understanding the onset, progression, and remission of depression.* New York: Springer-Verlag.

Rodebaugh, T. L. (2007). The effects of different types of goal pursuit on experience and performance during a stressful social task. *Behaviour Research and Therapy, 45*, 951–963.

Rolls, E. T. (2005). *Emotion explained*. Oxford, UK: Oxford University Press.

Roseman, I. J. (1991). Appraisal determinants of discrete emotions. *Cognition and Emotion, 5*, 161–200.

Rothbart, M. K., Ellis, L. K., Rueda, M. R., & Posner, M. I. (2003). Developing mechanisms of temperamental effortful control. *Journal of Personality, 71*, 1113–1144.

Russell, J. A., & Barrett, L. F. (1999). Core affect, prototypical emotional episodes, and other things called emotion: Dissecting the elephant. *Journal of Personality and Social Psychology, 76*, 805–819.

Ryan, R. M., & Deci, E. L. (2000). Self-determination theory and the facilitation of intrinsic motivation, social development, and well-being. *American Psychologist, 55*, 68–78.

Salavert, J., Caseras, X., Torrubia, R., Furest, S., Arranz, B., Duenas, R., et al. (2007). The functioning of the behavioral activation and inhibition systems in bipolar I euthymic patients and its influence in subsequent episodes over an eighteen-month period. *Personality and Individual Differences, 42*, 1323–1331.

Salmela-Aro, K., & Nurmi, J. (1996a). Depressive symptoms and personal project appraisals: A cross-lagged longitudinal study. *Personality and Individual Differences, 21*, 373–381.

Salmela-Aro, K., & Nurmi, J. (1996b). Uncertainty and confidence in interpersonal projects: Consequences for social relationships and well-being. *Journal of Social and Personal Relationships, 13*, 109–122.

Schulz, R., Wrosch, C., Yee, J. L., Heckhausen, J., & Whitmer, R. (1998, June). *Avoiding depression in late life. Using selective and compensatory control processes to manage physical illness and disability*. Paper presented at the 15th biennial meeting of the International Society of the Study of Behavioral Development, Bern, Switzerland.

Scott, J., Stanton, B., Garland, A., & Ferrier, I. N. (2000). Cognitive vulnerability in patients with bipolar disorder. *Psychological Medicine, 30*, 467–472.

Scott, L., & O'Hara, M. W. (1993). Self-discrepancies in clinically anxious and depressed university students. *Journal of Abnormal Psychology, 102*, 282–287.

Shankman, S. A., Klein, D. N., Tenke, C. E., & Bruder, G. E. (2007). Reward sensitivity in depression: A biobehavioral study. *Journal of Abnormal Psychology, 116*, 95–104.

Spielberger, C. D., Parker, J. B., & Becker, J. (1963). Conformity and achievement in remitted manic-depressive patients. *Journal of Nervous and Mental Disease, 137*, 162–172.

Steele, J. D., Kumar, P., & Ebmeier, K. P. (2007). Blunted response to feedback information in depressive illness. *Brain, 130*, 2367–2374.

Stern, G. S., & Berrenberg, J. L. (1979). Skill-set, success outcome, and mania as determinants of the illusion of control. *Journal of Research in Personality, 13*, 206–220.

Strakowski, S. M., Adler, C. M., Holland, S. K., Mills, N. P., DelBello, M. P., & Eliassen, J. C. (2005). Abnormal fMRI brain activation in euthymic bipolar disorder patients during a counting Stroop interference task. *American Journal of Psychiatry, 162*, 1697–1705.

Strauman, T. J. (1989). Self-discrepancies in clinical depression and social phobia:

Cognitive structures that underlie emotional disorders. *Journal of Abnormal Psychology, 98,* 14–22.

Strauman, T. J. (1996). Stability within the self: A longitudinal study of the structural implications of self-discrepancy theory. *Journal of Personality and Social Psychology, 71,* 1142–1153.

Strauman, T. J., Vieth, A. Z., Merrill, K. A., Kolden, G. G., Woods, T. E., Klein, M. H., et al. (2006). Self-system therapy as an intervention for self-regulatory dysfunction in depression: A randomized comparison with cognitive therapy. *Journal of Consulting and Clinical Psychology, 74,* 367–376.

Street, H. (2002). Exploring relationships between goal setting, goal pursuit and depression: A review. *Australian Psychologist, 37,* 95–103.

Sutton, S. K., & Davidson, R. J. (1997). A biological substrate of the behavioral approach and inhibition systems. *Psychological Science, 8,* 204–210.

Weissman, A. N., & Beck, A. T. (1978, March). *Development and validation of the Dysfunctional Attitudes Scale: A preliminary investigation.* Paper presented at the annual meeting of the American Educational Research Association, Toronto, Ontario, Canada.

Wortman, C. B., & Brehm, J. W. (1975). Responses to uncontrollable outcomes: An integration of reactance theory and the learned helplessness model. In L. Berkowitz (Ed.), *Advances in experimental social psychology* (Vol. 8, pp. 277–336). New York: Academic Press.

Wright, K. A., Lam, D., & Brown, R. G. (2008). Dysregulation of the behavioral activation system in remitted bipolar I disorder. *Journal of Abnormal Psychology, 117,* 838–848.

Wright, K. A., Lam, D., & Newsom-Davis, I. (2005). Induced mood change and dysfunctional attitudes in remitted bipolar I affective disorder. *Journal of Abnormal Psychology, 114,* 689–696.

Wrosch, C., Bauer, I., & Scheier, M. F. (2005). Regret and quality of life across the adult life span: The influence of disengagement and available future goals. *Psychology and Aging, 20,* 657–670.

Wrosch, C., Scheier, M. F., Miller, G. E., Schulz, R., & Carver, C. S. (2003). Adaptive self-regulation of unattainable goals: Goal disengagement, goal reengagement, and subjective well-being. *Personality and Social Psychology Bulletin, 29,* 1494–1508.

CHAPTER 10

• —— • —— • —— •

Maximizing Positive Emotions

A TRANSLATIONAL, TRANSDIAGNOSTIC LOOK
AT POSITIVE EMOTION REGULATION

Daniel G. Dillon and Diego A. Pizzagalli

Emotional dysfunction and emotion regulation impairments are hallmark features of many forms of psychopathology (American Psychiatric Association, 2000; Taylor & Liberzon, 2007). Although theoretical arguments and abundant empirical evidence indicate that several psychiatric disorders are characterized by dysfunctions involving negative emotion (e.g., Brown & Barlow, 1992; Watson, 2005), the present chapter considers how difficulties related to positive emotion contribute to psychopathology. The chapter is divided into four sections. In the first section, we discuss what the terms *emotion* and *emotion regulation* mean with reference to positive emotion, emphasizing that positive emotions can both regulate negative emotions and be the targets of regulation attempts. In the second section, we briefly review the neural systems that support the experience and regulation of positive emotion, with an emphasis on reward processing. In the third section, the prevalence and nature of problems related to positive emotion and regulation of positive emotion across various forms of psychopathology are reviewed. We conclude with some brief suggestions for future research on positive emotion regulation.

Positive Emotion and Regulation of Positive Emotion

Pinning down the term *emotion* is difficult, but in recent years affective scientists have reached a consensus definition. Specifically, emotions are usually defined as temporally brief, loosely coordinated response tendencies that cut across cognition, behavior, and physiology in order to mobilize action in the face of stimuli that have been appraised as offering a personally important challenge or opportunity (Fredrickson, 2001; Gross, 1998; Lang, 1995). With its focus on action, this definition is motivational in nature, consistent with a substantial body of research that organizes emotions in terms of large-scale neural systems that support approach and withdrawal (e.g., Davidson, 1998; Lang, 1995) as well as in terms of valence (ranging from unpleasant to pleasant) and arousal (ranging from calm to excited) (Russell, 1979). In this context, positive emotions can by defined operationally: They are associated with activation of the brain's approach systems and are characterized by reports of pleasant valence and moderate to high levels of arousal (Lang, 1995).

This position is supported by many psychophysiological studies that have compared responses to negative, neutral, and positive stimuli (e.g., Bradley, Codispoti, Cuthbert, & Lang, 2001). Although many findings from these studies covary with emotional arousal and are insensitive to valence, several results are specific to positive emotions. For example, whereas startle responses are reliably potentiated in arousing negative contexts, they are attenuated in arousing positive contexts, an effect referred to as pleasure attenuation (Bradley et al., 2001; Lang, 1995). This finding supports the hypothesis that positive emotions not only prime approach behaviors but also concurrently inhibit defensive reactions, including the startle reflex (Lang, 1995). Intriguingly, pleasure-attenuated startle appears to depend on the integrity of mesolimbic dopamine (DA) circuitry, because lesions of the nucleus accumbens in rodents eliminate this effect (Koch, Schmid, & Schnitzler, 1996). Consistent with the existence of dissociable neural systems for negative and positive emotion, the same study showed that lesions of the amygdala, which disrupt cue-driven fear-potentiated startle (Hitchcock & Davis, 1987), do not affect pleasure-attenuated startle.

As a second example, positive and negative emotions are associated with different patterns of activity in the resting electroencephalogram (EEG), with approach-related positive emotions eliciting relatively increased activity over left versus right prefrontal scalp sites and withdrawal-related negative emotions generally eliciting the opposite pattern (e.g., Davidson, Ekman, Saron, Senulis, & Friesen, 1990; for review, see Coan & Allen, 2004; Davidson, 1998). Stable individual differences in resting left versus right EEG asymmetry over anterior sites have been tied to a number of important phenomena, including depression vulnerability (Henriques & Davidson, 1990, 1991), emotion regulation abilities (Jackson et al., 2003), and overall psychological well-being (Urry et al., 2004). In each case, a relative leftward shift in activity is associated with more beneficial outcomes.

Finally, emotionally positive states and stimuli, particularly unexpected rewards and reward-predicting cues, elicit activity in midbrain DA neurons that extend to several projection sites, including the basal ganglia, orbitofrontal cortex (OFC), and anterior cingulate cortex (ACC) (Ashby, Isen, & Turken, 1999; Schultz, 1998, 2000). Although DA is not as closely tied to positive emotional experience as was once supposed (Berridge & Robinson, 1998), phasic bursts of midbrain DA neurons play a key role in reward-related learning and serve to guide motivated behavior (Berridge & Robinson, 1998; Rangel, Camerer, & Montague, 2008). By supporting incentive motivation in this way, DA contributes to approach and is linked to positive emotion (Berridge & Robinson, 1998). The neuroscience of reward is explored in more detail in the second section.

The foregoing examples have emerged from a perspective on positive emotion that puts the focus squarely on approach motivation. However, other lines of research have advanced the domain by focusing on the consummatory or goal attainment phase of incentive processing (Davidson, 1998; Gard, Gard, Kring, & John, 2006). Notably, Fredrickson's *broaden-and-build* theory proposes that many positive emotions associated with goal attainment, such as contentment, joy, and pride, do not have an obvious motivational quality (Fredrickson, 2000). Instead, these emotions encourage reflection and widen the scope of an individual's attention, in direct opposition to the stereotyped action tendencies and focused attention elicited by prominent negative emotions such as fear or anger (Fredrickson, 2001). Via this mechanism, positive emotions elicit creativity and promote a flexible approach to problem solving, ultimately helping individuals to stockpile durable personal and social resources that can be drawn on in the future (Fredrickson, 2000; Fredrickson, Cohn, Coffey, Pek, & Finkel, 2008). Considering all these data, positive emotions may be defined as states characterized by pleasant valence that are reliably evoked by stimuli that elicit approach but that may also occur following goal attainment.

Positive Emotions Regulate Negative Emotions

Having characterized positive emotions, a reasonable question is, what are they good for? A corollary of the broaden-and-build theory provides an answer: Namely, Fredrickson's "undoing" hypothesis proposes that positive emotions serve to regulate negative emotions (Fredrickson, 2000, 2001; Fredrickson & Levenson, 1998). Whereas negative emotions place constraints on an individual's options in the service of survival (e.g., fear narrows attention, focuses cognition on a few key computations, and mobilizes the body for fight or flight), positive emotions undo these by reducing activity in the sympathetic nervous system, widening the scope of attention, and prompting the individual to consider a wider range of cognitive and behavioral possibilities. These changes increase the individual's chances of solving problems and building relationships, which serve to promote survival over the long haul.

In support of this hypothesis, a series of experiments demonstrated that following an arousal-eliciting negative stimulus (either a fear-evoking film or a public speaking task), films provoking either contentment or happiness prompted a faster return to baseline cardiovascular activity than films that elicited either no emotion or sadness (Fredrickson & Levenson, 1998; Fredrickson, Mancuso, Branigan, & Tugade, 2000). Importantly, these results do not appear to simply reflect replacement of a highly arousing negative state with an especially low arousing positive state, because the positive and neutral films elicited indistinguishable levels of sympathetic nervous system activity when viewed alone, yet responses to the positive films drove a significantly faster return to baseline than the neutral film (Fredrickson et al., 2000).

On a similar note, individual difference studies have revealed that increased positive emotion, particularly in negative emotional contexts, is related to long-term adjustment (Papa & Bonanno, 2008) and resilience (Tugade & Fredrickson, 2004). For example, in a naturalistic study of students, Papa and Bonanno (2008) found that the number and intensity of Duchenne smiles (i.e., smiles associated with positive emotional experience) following a negative mood induction was associated with less psychological distress over the first 2 years of college. Consistent with the undoing hypothesis, this effect was mediated by (1) the extent to which smiling reduced the subjective experience of negative emotion elicited by the mood induction and (2) a positive association between smiling and social integration. Approaching the relationship between adjustment and positive emotion from the opposite direction, Tugade and Fredrickson (2004) showed that highly resilient individuals, as defined by self-report, experienced more happiness and interest during an anxiety-inducing speech task than less resilient individuals. Furthermore, highly resilient individuals showed more rapid cardiovascular recovery from the task, especially when it was described as threatening. Again in support of the undoing hypothesis, this finding was mediated by self-reported experience of positive emotion, suggesting that positive emotion helped highly resilient individuals to quickly resolve task-induced negative emotion.

Regulation of Positive Emotion

Although positive emotions can undo the effects of negative emotions, it is sometimes necessary to direct regulation attempts at positive emotions themselves. For example, one might purposefully attempt to reduce a positive emotion in order to avoid embarrassment (e.g., squelching inappropriate laughter during an important meeting) or attempt to amplify positive emotions in order to heighten a pleasant experience (e.g., deliberately focusing on all the positive outcomes associated with beginning a new job). Unfortunately, although it is clear that certain strategies for regulating negative emotions are differentially associated with psychological health, with reappraisal generally leading to better outcomes than expressive suppression (Gross & John, 2003), few studies speak directly to regulation of positive emotions (Tugade & Fredrickson, 2007). The handful of psychophysiological and neuroimaging experiments that have studied reappraisal of positive emotional stimuli are reviewed in the next section (Beauregard, Lévesque, & Bourgouin, 2001; Delgado, Gillis, & Phelps, 2008; Dillon & LaBar, 2005; Kim & Hamann, 2007; Krompinger, Moser, & Simons, 2008). Here we consider two studies that have provided initial evidence for the regulation of positive emotions in daily life.

Nezlek and Kuppens (2008) collected 3 weeks of daily reports on the extent to which undergraduates used reappraisal or expressive suppression to regulate positive or negative emotions. Of the four strategy/ emotion combinations investigated—2 strategies (reappraisal, suppression) × 2 valences (positive, negative)—reappraisal of positive emotion was reported most frequently and suppression of positive emotion was reported least frequently. Consistent with research on negative emotions (Gross & John, 2003), these two combinations had divergent consequences: Reappraisal of positive emotions was associated with increased positive affect, self-esteem, and psychological adjustment, whereas suppression of positive emotions was negatively correlated with these outcomes and positively correlated with increased negative affect. However, the conclusions that can be drawn from this study about reappraisal of positive emotions are limited by the fact that the item used to probe positive reappraisal— "When I wanted to feel a more positive emotion (such as happiness or amusement), I changed what I was thinking about"—may have also elicited information about instances when reappraisal was used to change a negative emotion for the better rather than being directed at an ongoing positive emotion.

Gross, Richards, and John (2006) used interview and survey methods to examine regulation attempts directed at positive and negative emotions during daily life in a healthy sample. Critically, they clearly distinguished between emotion regulation attempts intended to modulate positive emotions versus those intended to improve negative emotions. For example, to illustrate regulation directed at a positive emotion, they cited a respondent's attempt to disguise facial expressions of pleasure at receiving a good grade on an assignment in front of his roommate, who had received a poor grade. Perhaps not surprisingly, the authors found that regulation attempts were more frequently directed at negative than positive emotions, with even the least frequently regulated negative emotion (disgust) being regulated more often than the most frequently regulated positive emotion (pride). Nonetheless, the interview method revealed that 9% of regulation attempts were directed at positive emotions. Thus, these two studies confirm that individuals do try to regulate positive emotions in daily life, although this appears to happen less frequently than attempts to regulate negative emotions.

Neural Correlates of Reward Processing and Regulation of Positive Emotion

Understanding of positive emotion and positive emotion regulation has received a boost from the fact that these topics have attracted considerable interest from neuroscientists in recent years, with many studies focusing specifically on reward processing (Berridge & Robinson, 1998; Rangel et al., 2008; Schultz, 2000). Although clearly limited in scope, reward processing offers several advantages for researchers interested in positive emotions. First, although it is difficult to directly assess positive emotion in nonhuman animals, the fact that all organisms are motivated by rewards permits cross-species analysis of reward-related behavior and relevant neural systems (Berridge & Kringelbach, 2008). Second, the neural systems implicated in reward processing generally respond to a wide variety of specific reinforcers (e.g., food, money, drugs of abuse); thus, insights into these systems apply at a relatively general level of analysis (Berridge & Kringelbach, 2008). Third, reward processing can be divided into anticipatory and consummatory components, which are dissociable at psychological (e.g., Gard et al., 2006), neural (e.g., Knutson, Adams, Fong, & Hommer, 2001; Knutson, Fong, Bennett, Adams, & Hommer, 2003), and neurochemical (e.g., Berridge & Robinson, 1998) levels. This dissociation offers the opportunity to determine whether deficits in reward processing reflect problems in reward anticipation, consummation, or both and also maps nicely onto the distinction between approach-related versus consummatory positive emotions described earlier. Finally, dysfunctional reward processing has been consistently tied to anhedonia (e.g., Bogdan & Pizzagalli, 2006; Pizzagalli, Iosifescu, Hallett, Ratner, & Fava, 2009; Pizzagalli, Jahn, & O'Shea, 2005), which refers to decreased capacity to experience pleasure and is a core component of multiple forms of psychopathology, including major depressive disorder (MDD) and schizophrenia (American Psychiatric Association, 2000). Thus, understanding the neural mechanisms of reward processing ultimately promises to provide insight into anhedonia. For all these reasons, this section briefly reviews key findings from the neuroscientific study of reward processing as a window into the neuroscience of positive emotions more broadly.

Neural Mechanisms of Reward Processing

The neuroscientific study of reward processing has a long history (e.g., Olds & Milner, 1954), but it received strong impetus from studies of reward-related activity in midbrain DA neurons (Hollerman & Schultz, 1998; Schultz, 1998; Schultz, Dayan, & Montague, 1997). Working with nonhuman primates, Schultz and colleagues showed that these neurons code a reward-related temporal prediction error (Hollerman & Schultz, 1998). In appetitive conditioning paradigms, DA neurons initially fired strongly to unexpected rewards, but as learning progressed the activity in DA neurons ultimately shifted away from the rewards and came to be elicited by reward-predicting cues. Furthermore, dips below the basal firing rate were observed when an expected reward was omitted (Hollerman & Schultz, 1998; Schultz et al., 1997). This pattern of results highlights a mechanism by which cue–reward associations are coded in the brain. More importantly, the shift of DA activity from rewards to cues and the dip in DA activity in response to omitted rewards reveal that this system learns to predict *when* a reward will be presented and can also signal when these predictions need to be updated. These mechanisms are assumed to guide complex reward-related learning and adaptive behavior (Schultz et al., 1997).

These seminal findings have been strengthened by two subsequent developments. First, neuroimaging has revealed that similar mechanisms are at work in the human brain, demonstrating that reward-predicting cues elicit activation in downstream targets of DA neurons, including the ventral striatum (Knutson, Adams, et al., 2001; for a review, see Knutson & Cooper, 2005). Second, the new domain of neuroeconomics has begun to elucidate how a variety of brain regions compute complex components of reward-related decision making such as expected utility and risk (Glimcher & Rustichini, 2004; Platt & Huettel, 2008; Rangel et al., 2008). An early finding from this line of work was the observation that the neural systems implicated in reward anticipation and consummation are partly dissociable, at least when reward delivery is predictable (Knutson, Fong, Adams, Varner, & Hommer, 2001). In studies using cue–outcome paradigms, reward anticipation usually elicits robust activity in the basal ganglia, particularly in ventral regions such as the nucleus accumbens but often extending to the caudate and putamen depending on the motor demands of the paradigm (Knutson & Cooper, 2005; O'Doherty et al., 2004). By contrast, reward delivery more frequently activates the mesial prefrontal cortex (PFC) and OFC (Dillon et al., 2008; Knutson, Fong, et al., 2001; Knutson et al., 2003; O'Doherty, Kringelbach, Rolls, Hornak, & Andrews, 2001), although robust basal ganglia responses to rewards are observed in certain designs (e.g., Tricomi, Delgado, & Fiez, 2004).

Considering brain regions besides the midbrain and basal ganglia, the contributions made by the OFC and ACC to reward-related processing are perhaps best understood (Frank & Claus, 2006; Kennerley, Walton, Behrens, Buckley, & Rushworth, 2006; Rushworth, Behrens, Rudebeck, & Walton, 2007). Although a detailed review of relevant studies is beyond the scope of this chapter, the key difference between the contributions made by these structures is that the OFC—by virtue of its connections to the ventral striatum, amygdala, and temporal lobe—plays a critical role in maintaining and updating stimulus–reward representations, whereas the ACC—by virtue of its connections to the ventral striatum and motor cortex—appears to be more important for action–reward representations

(Rushworth et al., 2007). Thus, bilateral OFC lesions disrupt the ability to perform reward-based reversal learning tasks that involve using one action to choose among different visual stimuli (Hornak et al., 2004), whereas lesions of the ACC disrupt the ability to choose among multiple possible actions based on the history of reward–action associations (Kennerley et al., 2006).

This thumbnail sketch provides just a glimpse of the growing literature on the neural substrates of reward processing, but it is sufficient to illustrate two points. First, reward encoding and reward-related decision making depend heavily on DA circuitry that extends from the midbrain to the basal ganglia and several regions of frontal cortex. Second, this fact implies that deficits in reward processing, such as anhedonia, could reflect structural or functional changes in at least five brain regions: the midbrain, basal ganglia, OFC, ACC, and mesial PFC. Because these regions support different reward-related functions, an important goal for psychiatric neuroimaging will be to parse anhedonia into separate components that can be aligned with dysfunction in different brain regions.

Neural Mechanisms of Regulation of Positive Emotions

Compared with the neuroscience of reward processing, understanding of the neural mechanisms implicated in regulation of positive emotions is in its infancy, because most research has focused on regulation of negative emotion (e.g., Eippert et al., 2007; Hajcak & Nieuwenhuis, 2006; Kalisch et al., 2005; Ochsner, Bunge, Gross, & Gabrieli, 2002; Ochsner et al., 2004; Urry et al., 2006). Two psychophysiological studies have examined regulation of positive emotions and found essentially no differences vis-à-vis regulation of negative emotion. Dillon and LaBar (2005) presented positive, negative, and neutral pictures and instructed participants to *enhance*, *maintain*, or *suppress* (i.e., decrease by reappraising) any emotions elicited by the pictures. There were no effects of reappraisal instruction on neutral trials, but on positive and negative trials the pattern of startle modulation was identical, with the strongest startle responses observed on *enhance* trials and the weakest startle responses observed on *decrease* trials. Similarly, an event-related potential study (Krompinger et al., 2008) found that late positive potentials (LPPs) elicited by positive pictures were modulated by reappraisal in the same way as negative pictures (Hajcak & Nieuwenhuis, 2006; Moser, Hajcak, Bukay, & Simons, 2006): Attempts to cognitively *decrease* the emotional impact of pictures reduced LPP amplitude, whether the pictures were negative or positive. The fact that the results in these studies did not differ by valence suggests that they may have reflected arousal modulation, and the lack of reappraisal effects on neutral trials in Dillon and LaBar (2005) argues against an alternative account, namely that results simply reflect cue-driven changes in arousal or attention that are independent of emotion.

However, neuroimaging research has found some evidence for valence-specific effects. Kim and Hamann (2007) directly compared reappraisal of positive and negative emotions elicited by pictures and found that reappraisal-based modulation of amygdala activity was actually more robust in the positive condition (for another example of amygdala modulation during positive emotion regulation, see Beauregard et al., 2001). Furthermore, they reported that cognitively increasing positive emotion boosted activity in the ventral striatum. A similar finding was reported in a study that explicitly combined emotion regulation and reward processing. In a functional magnetic resonance imaging (fMRI) experiment that also featured collection of skin conductance responses (SCRs), Delgado and colleagues (2008) administered an appetitive conditioning paradigm to healthy subjects. Yellow- and blue-colored squares served as conditioned stimuli (CS), and a monetary reward was presented as the unconditioned stimulus (US). At the outset of individual trials, participants saw cues instructing them to either attend to the upcoming CS or use reappraisal to reduce any emotional arousal elicited by the CS. Importantly, one CS (the CS+) was consistently paired with the US, while the other CS (the CS–) was not. As expected, in the attend condition, the CS+ elicited larger SCRs and greater ventral striatal activity than the CS–. By contrast, these differences were diminished in the reappraisal condition, such that the CS+ and CS– elicited equivalent SCRs, and the ventral striatal response to the CS+ was significantly reduced. Importantly, SCRs to the US did not differ across attend and reappraisal trials, suggesting that reappraisal specifically modulated responses to the CS rather than indiscriminately lowering arousal.

Positive Emotion Regulation and Psychopathology

With this background in place, we now consider the central question of the chapter: How do problems with positive emotion and regulation of positive emotion manifest in psychopathology? Although these types of problems may not extend to all disorders, a survey of the more recent literature indicates that they are certainly transdiagnostic, emerging in individuals with depression (e.g., Kumar et al., 2008), schizophrenia (e.g., Gard, Kring, Germans Gard, Horan, & Green, 2007; Juckel et al., 2006), posttraumatic stress disorder (e.g., Hopper et al., 2008; Sailer et al., 2008), and substance abuse (e.g., Leventhal et al., 2008). Consequently, in the closing section we argue for increased focus on dysfunction in basic processes associated with positive emotion, because these do not appear to respect nosological boundaries. Due to space limitations, in this section we restrict our discussion to MDD, substance abuse, and mania. Whereas MDD represents an illustrative case of a disorder involving deficits in positive emotions, the latter disorders provide paradigmatic examples of dysfunctions in the regulation of positive emotions.

Failures of Positive Emotion: The Role of Anhedonia in MDD

Behavior

Along with excessive negative mood, anhedonia is one of the two defining characteristics of MDD (American Psychiatric Association, 2000). Furthermore, of these two symptoms, anhedonia shows greater specificity for
depression, with excessive negative mood also characterizing anxiety disorders (e.g., de Beurs, den Hollander-Gijsman, Helmich, & Zitman, 2007).
Experimental evidence consistent with anhedonia in depressed individuals comes from a wide variety of sources. For example, behavioral studies
reveal that, when presented with appetitive or pleasant stimuli, depressed
individuals report weaker positive affect (e.g., Allen, Trinder, & Brennan,
1999; Berenbaum & Oltmanns, 1992; Kaviani et al., 2004; Rottenberg,
Kasch, Gross, & Gotlib, 2002; Sloan, Strauss, Quirk, & Sajatovic, 1997)
and blunted behavioral responsiveness (e.g., Berenbaum & Oltmanns,
1992; Sloan, Strauss, & Wisner, 2001; Tremeau et al., 2005). These findings have been complemented by psychophysiological data highlighting
reduced reactivity and elaborative processing of positive cues in depression
(e.g., Deldin, Keller, Gergen, & Miller, 2000; Nandrino, Dodin, Martin,
& Henniaux, 2004; Shestyuk, Deldin, Brand, & Deveney, 2005) as well as
diminished ability to engage in appetitively motivated behavior (Dichter &
Tomarken, 2008; Shankman, Klein, Tenke, & Bruder, 2007).

Depression has also been associated with reduced positive reinforcement (e.g., Buchwald, 1977; Hughes, Pleasants, & Pickens, 1985; Wener &
Rehm, 1975) and inability to modulate behavior as a function of reinforcement history (Pizzagalli, Iosifescu, et al., 2009). The association between
depression and failure to adjust behavior based on reinforcement history
was demonstrated using a probabilistic reward task in which participants
had to select which of two difficult-to-distinguish stimuli was briefly flashed
onscreen. Unbeknownst to the participants, correct identification of one
stimulus was rewarded three times more frequently than correct identification of the other stimulus. This manipulation consistently induces a large
response bias toward the more frequently rewarded stimulus in healthy
controls (Pizzagalli et al., 2005; Pizzagalli, Bogdan, Ratner, & Jahn, 2007;
Pizzagalli, Iosifescu, et al., 2009). By contrast, subjects with elevated depressive symptoms (Pizzagalli et al., 2005) or MDD (Pizzagalli, Iosifescu, et al.,
2009) fail to develop a response bias.

Three additional findings from this line of work deserve mention.
First, fine-grained analyses revealed that subjects with MDD were responsive to single rewards but failed to express the response bias toward the
more advantageous stimulus if it had not been rewarded in the immediately
preceding trial (Pizzagalli, Iosifescu, et al., 2009). Second, this deficit was
largest in subjects with MDD endorsing anhedonic symptoms in their daily
life and was not related to general distress or anxiety. Finally, decreased

response bias has been found to be stable (38-day test–retest reliability: $r = .57$, $p < .004$), predictive of future anhedonic symptoms (Pizzagalli et al., 2005), and heritable (Bogdan & Pizzagalli, 2009). Collectively, these findings indicate that, although responses to individual rewards appear to be intact in depression, impairments in integrating reinforcement history over time may play an important role in anhedonic symptoms characteristic of MDD.

Neuroimaging

Depression is associated with altered structure or function in many of the brain regions implicated in reward processing, including the ACC (e.g., Mayberg et al., 1999), OFC (e.g., Elliott, Sahakian, Michael, Paykel, & Dolan, 1998), and ventromedial PFC (Keedwell, Andrew, Williams, Brammer, & Phillips, 2005). However, recent work has focused on basal ganglia dysfunction in MDD. For example, Epstein and colleagues (2006) reported that, relative to healthy controls, depressed participants showed a weaker ventral striatal response to positive (but not negative or neutral) words. Furthermore, in the depressed group the magnitude of the ventral striatal response to positive words was negatively correlated with anhedonic symptoms. Similarly, in a gambling task, Steele, Kumar, and Ebmeier (2007) found that, unlike controls, subjects with MDD failed to show ventral striatal activation and faster reaction time (RT) on trials following "win" feedback. In addition, RT on trials following wins was positively correlated with anhedonic symptoms across groups. Linking basal ganglia dysfunction in MDD to its presumed neurochemical substrate, Meyer and colleagues (2006) performed an [11C]raclopride positron emission tomography study that revealed evidence (i.e., increased D_2 binding potential) of reduced DA concentration in the striatum of depressed individuals, particularly those who showed motor retardation.

To date, however, few studies involving depressed participants have attempted to disentangle various components of reward processing. One exception is a study (Knutson, Bhanji, Cooney, Atlas, & Gotlib, 2008) that used a monetary incentive delay (MID) task to investigate reward anticipation versus consummation in participants with MDD ($n = 14$) and healthy controls ($n = 11$). Surprisingly, there were no group differences in anticipatory responses to reward cues in the basal ganglia, including the nucleus accumbens. Furthermore, although individuals with MDD showed reduced bilateral putamen responses to monetary gains, there were no outcome-related differences in the nucleus accumbens or the caudate, a region that has been implicated in processing reward feedback (e.g., Tricomi et al., 2004). These null results may have reflected relatively intact reward processing in this particular MDD sample, because there were also no group differences in behavior. Indeed, using a larger sample (MDD: $n = 30$; controls: $n = 31$), we found that, relative to controls, depressed participants showed weaker nucleus accumbens and caudate responses to gains in the MID task (Pizzagalli, Holmes, et al., 2009).

Failures to Regulate Positive Emotion

Substance Abuse

Although MDD is characterized primarily by failures of positive emotion, impairments in the regulation of various aspects of positive emotion have been linked to other forms of psychopathology, most notably substance use disorders and mania. Many drugs of abuse, particularly cocaine and stimulants, act on the brain's DA system, rapidly increasing the concentration of DA in the striatum and leading to feelings of euphoria (Di Chiara & Imperato, 1988; Volkow et al., 1996; for review, see Volkow, Fowler, Wang, Baler, & Telang, 2009). Ultimately, compensatory mechanisms reduce the ability of these drugs to elicit robust changes in subjective experience (Volkow et al., 2009). However, because DA release effectively increases the salience of relevant environmental cues (Berridge & Robinson, 1998; Volkow et al., 2009), and because drugs of abuse are more powerful actors at DA receptors than natural rewards, substance abusers are motivated to compulsively pursue and consume drugs. In addition, drugs of abuse hijack encoding systems to lay down extremely durable memory traces of the context and cues associated with drug use (for a review, see Hyman & Malenka, 2001). This sets the stage for cue-induced craving and, ultimately, cue-induced relapse, which can be conceptualized as a failure to regulate positive emotion.

An early study on this topic exposed healthy controls and individuals with a history of cocaine use to audiovisual and tactile cues related to cocaine, opiates, and nondrug themes (Ehrman, Robbins, Childress, & O'Brien, 1992). In response to the cocaine cues, former users reported increases in craving and showed significant changes in heart rate, skin temperature, and skin resistance. These effects showed specificity in that (1) they were stronger in the group of users than in controls and (2) within the users they were stronger than responses to the opiate or nondrug cues. More recent reports have expanded on this work to show that, in addition to promoting craving and feelings of excitement, cues previously paired with cocaine or amphetamine can elicit DA releases in the human dorsal (e.g., Volkow et al., 2006) and ventral (e.g., Boileau et al., 2007) striatum. Thus, cue-induced changes in the subjective experience of positive emotion and DA circuitry are well established.

However, these effects are not sufficient to explain cue-induced relapse. An emerging perspective emphasizes the important contributions made by dysfunction in PFC structures (Baicy & London, 2007; Goldstein & Volkow, 2002; Jentsch & Taylor, 1999). Neurally, drug abuse is associated with dysfunction in the OFC, ACC, and dorsolateral PFC (Baicy & London, 2007; Goldstein & Volkow, 2002), regions that are important not only for reward processing but also for emotion regulation (e.g., Ochsner et al., 2002, 2004) and inhibitory functions more generally (Dillon & Pizzagalli, 2007). Although much work on this topic remains to be done, these changes are generally associated with reductions in people's ability to effortfully exert control over their emotions and actions, such that exposure to drug cues increasingly recruits rigid action tendencies associated with procuring drugs of abuse (Goldstein & Volkow, 2002). In short, with respect to cue-induced craving, the broaden-and-build functions of positive emotion are lost. The challenge for clinicians is to find ways to train substance abusers to regulate their pursuit of positive emotional experiences so as to main-tain "hedonic homeostasis" and resist the allure of a drug-induced swell in hedonic experience (Koob & Le Moal, 1997). One promising approach is to combine cognitive therapies designed to teach drug users better emo-tion regulation and coping skills with pharmacological interventions that can improve PFC function (Baicy & London, 2007).

Mania

Along with depression, mania is one of two states of emotional dysregula-tion experienced by individuals suffering from bipolar disorder (Ameri-can Psychiatric Association, 2000). Mania is characterized by extremely elevated mood and energy, often along with irritability, and is associated with deficits in a variety of executive functions related to attention, work-ing memory, problem solving, and verbal learning (for reviews, see Clark & Sahakian, 2008; Green, Cahill, & Malhi, 2007). Importantly, although many of the deficits in executive function persist across the different mood phases of the illness, including euthymia, extreme increases in positive emotion are restricted to the manic state.

In recent years, renewed interest has emerged for the hypothesis that bipolar disorder reflects dysregulation in the behavioral approach system (BAS) (Depue & Iacono, 1989; Fowles, 1993; Johnson, 2005; see Urosevic, Abramson, Harmon-Jones, & Alloy, 2008, for a recent review), which is hypothesized to regulate appetitive motivation and goal-directed behavior in response to reward-related cues in the environment (Gray, 1991). In line with this argument, increased BAS sensitivity and experiences of goal striv-ing and goal attainment events have been found to predict manic, but not depressive, symptoms (Johnson et al., 2000; Meyer, Johnson, & Winters, 2001; Nusslock, Abramson, Harmon-Jones, Alloy, & Hogan, 2007).

Moreover, Harmon-Jones and colleagues (2008) found evidence for a relationship between prefrontal EEG asymmetry and BAS dysregula-tion. Healthy controls and individuals with bipolar-spectrum disorder per-formed a task in which solving anagrams could lead to monetary wins or losses. Preparatory cues signaled whether the upcoming anagram would be easy, medium, or hard. Across all subjects, cues signaling medium trials elicited a relative leftward shift in prefrontal EEG activity. However, the two groups showed a divergent pattern during the anticipation phase of hard trials. In controls, anticipation of hard anagrams elicited a decrease in relative left PFC asymmetry across both the win and the loss conditions, a finding interpreted as reflecting an adaptive decrease in resource allocation when confronted with an especially difficult problem. By contrast, in bipolar individuals, anticipation of the hard/win condition elicited significantly stronger left PFC activity than anticipation of the hard/loss condition. In addition, in the bipolar group, self-reported approach motivation was positively correlated with left PFC activity in the hard/win condition.

Importantly, the findings were not confounded by between-group differences in performance. Instead, they appear to reflect the propensity for bipolar individuals to get "stuck" in pursuit of positive goals, even if the goals are extreme or unreasonable (e.g., Johnson & Carver, 2006). Along similar lines, another EEG study found that, relative to both controls and euthymic subjects with bipolar disorder, subjects with bipolar disorder who were currently in a mood episode (either manic or depressed) showed significantly greater left frontal activity after a positive mood induction invoking BAS-related themes (e.g., striving against difficult odds) (Hayden et al., 2008). Finally, using the same probabilistic reward task mentioned earlier (Pizzagalli et al., 2005), we recently reported that medicated euthymic subjects with bipolar disorder were characterized by reduced response bias toward the more frequently rewarded stimulus (Pizzagalli, Goetz, Ostacher, Iosifescu, & Perlis, 2008). Critically, follow-up analyses indicated that this dysfunction was largely due to patients' increased sensitivity and behavioral switching in trials immediately following positive reinforcement of the less advantageous stimulus, again consistent with an overactive BAS.

Collectively, these findings indicate that failed regulation of positive emotions, particularly those involving goal striving and goal attainment events, play an important role in triggering, maintaining, and exacerbating manic symptoms and are consistent with emerging evidence that modified cognitive therapies targeting excessive goal striving successfully reduce relapse rate in bipolar disorder (Lam et al., 2003). In spite of these promising findings and an increased recognition of the importance of emotion regulation research in bipolar disorder (Green et al., 2007; Gruber, Eidelman, & Harvey, 2008), virtually no studies have directly investigated regulation of positive emotion in bipolar disorder, and little is known about underlying neurobiological underpinnings. Based on initial reports that bipolar disorder is characterized by functional and structural abnormalities in reward-related brain regions, including the OFC and ventral striatum (e.g., Abler, Greenhouse, Ongur, Walter, & Heckers, 2008; Cotter, Hudson, & Landau, 2005; Mah et al., 2007), filling in this gap in the literature will be an important step toward understanding mania.

Future Directions for Research on Positive Emotion Regulation

As the preceding sections show, positive emotion often fails to exhibit its usual regulatory effects in depression, whereas failures to regulate one or more components of positive emotion are prominent in substance abuse and mania. It is important to note, however, that although this assignment of disorders to problems serves a heuristic purpose, it should not be taken as definitive, because depression likely involves failures to increase or up-regulate positive emotion and substance abuse is associated with anhedonia (Leventhal et al., 2008). Indeed, problems with positive emotion and regulation of positive emotion appear to be transdiagnostic. Consequently, future studies of psychopathology will likely focus less on diagnostic categories and more on deficits in basic processes related to positive (and negative) emotion.

Looking ahead, we suggest three goals for future research on positive emotion in psychopathology. First, there is a need for more theoretically driven, model-based studies of reward processing in psychopathology, so that the specific components of reward processing that are dysfunctional may be identified (for a review on the value of model-based fMRI studies of reward, see O'Doherty, Hamptom, & Kim, 2007). Recent neuroimaging studies focused on separating anticipatory versus consummatory processes in MDD are a positive step in this regard (Knutson et al., 2008; Pizzagalli, Holmes, et al., 2009) and echo similar efforts focusing on self-report assessments (e.g., Gard et al., 2006). Additional examples include an elegant study that used a temporal difference model to identify aberrant learning signals in the ventral striatum of depressed participants (Kumar et al., 2008) and a review of studies that pinpointed a deficit specifically in the representation of value in schizophrenia (Gold, Waltz, Prentice, Morris, & Heerey, 2008). Second, there is an acute need for research on the neuroscience of positive emotion regulation in psychopathology, because the small body of neuroscientific work has focused on regulation of negative emotion (Beauregard, Paquette, & Lévesque, 2006; Johnstone, van Reekum, Urry, Kalin, & Davidson, 2007). Third, and tying the two previous suggestions together, it would be useful for future studies of positive emotion regulation to take a more explicitly computational approach, so that the particular contributions made by various brain regions to emotion regulation can be specified. Simple first steps in this regard will be to (1) better specify the component psychological processes involved in conscious regulation of positive emotions (e.g., what roles are played by working memory, attention to internal states, mental imagery) and (2) dissociate brain regions implicated in these processes versus those more directly involved in modulation of emotional representations in subcortical structures such as the ventral striatum. We anticipate that a better transdiagnostic understanding of psychological and neurobiological processes underlying dysfunction in the experience and regulation of positive emotions will provide much-needed breakthroughs in the effective prevention and treatment of various forms of psychopathology.

Acknowledgments

Preparation of this chapter was supported by National Institutes of Health Grant Nos. R01 MH68376 (National Institute of Mental Health) and R21 AT002974 (National Center for Complementary and Alternative Medicine) as well as Talley Fund Awards to Diego A. Pizzagalli. Dr. Pizzagalli has received research support from GlaxoSmithKline and Merck & Co., Inc., for studies unrelated to this project.

References

Abler, B., Greenhouse, I., Ongur, D., Walter, H., & Heckers, S. (2008). Abnormal reward system activation in mania. *Neuropsychopharmacology, 33*, 2217–2227.

Allen, N. B., Trinder, J., & Brennan, C. (1999). Affective startle modulation in clinical depression: Preliminary findings. *Biological Psychiatry, 46*, 542–550.

American Psychiatric Association. (2000). *Diagnostic and statistical manual of mental disorders* (4th ed., text rev.). Washington, DC: Author.

Ashby, F. G., Isen, A. M., & Turken, A. U. (1999). A neuropsychological theory of positive affect and its influence on cognition. *Psychological Review, 106*, 529–550.

Baicy, K., & London, E. D. (2007). Corticolimbic dysregulation and chronic methamphetamine abuse. *Addiction, 102*(Suppl. 1), 5–15.

Beauregard, M., Lévesque, J., & Bourgouin, P. (2001). Neural correlates of conscious self-regulation of emotion. *Journal of Neuroscience, 21*, RC165.

Beauregard, M., Paquette, V., & Lévesque, J. (2006). Dysfunction in the neural circuitry of emotional self-regulation in major depressive disorder. *NeuroReport, 17*, 843–846.

Berenbaum, H., & Oltmanns, T. F. (1992). Emotional experience and expression in schizophrenia and depression. *Journal of Abnormal Psychology, 101*, 37–44.

Berridge, K. C., & Kringelbach, M. L. (2008). Affective neuroscience of pleasure: Reward in humans and animals. *Psychopharmacology, 199*, 457–480.

Berridge, K. C., & Robinson, T. E. (1998). What is the role of dopamine in reward: Hedonic impact, reward learning, or incentive salience? *Brain Research Reviews, 28*, 309–369.

Bogdan, R., & Pizzagalli, D. A. (2006). Acute stress reduces hedonic capacity: Implications for depression. *Biological Psychiatry, 60*, 1147–1154.

Bogdan, R., & Pizzagalli, D. A. (2009). The heritability of hedonic capacity and perceived stress: A twin study evaluation of candidate depressive phenotypes. *Psychological Medicine, 39*, 211–218.

Boileau, I., Dagher, A., Leyton, M., Welfeld, K., Booij, L., Diksic, M., et al. (2007). Conditioned dopamine release in humans: A positron emission tomography

[¹¹C]raclopride study with amphetamine. *Journal of Neuroscience, 27,* 3998–4003.

Bradley, M. M., Codispoti, M., Cuthbert, B. N., & Lang, P. J. (2001). Emotion and motivation: I. Defensive and appetitive reactions in picture processing. *Emotion, 1,* 276–298.

Brown, T. A., & Barlow, D. H. (1992). Comorbidity among anxiety disorders: Implications for treatment and *DSM-IV. Journal of Consulting and Clinical Psychology, 60,* 835–844.

Buchwald, A. M. (1977). Depressive mood and estimates of reinforcement frequency. *Journal of Abnormal Psychology, 86,* 443–446.

Clark, L., & Sahakian, B. J. (2008). Cognitive neuroscience and brain imaging in bipolar disorder. *Dialogues in Clinical Neuroscience, 10,* 153–163.

Coan, J. A., & Allen, J. J. (2004). Frontal EEG asymmetry as a moderator and mediator of emotion. *Biological Psychology, 67,* 7–49.

Cotter, D., Hudson, L., & Landau, S. (2005). Evidence for orbitofrontal pathology in bipolar disorder and major depression, but not in schizophrenia. *Bipolar Disorders, 7,* 358–369.

Davidson, R. J. (1998). Affective style and affective disorders: Perspectives from affective neuroscience. *Cognition and Emotion, 12,* 307–330.

Davidson, R. J., Ekman, P., Saron, C., Senulis, J., & Friesen, W. V. (1990). Approach-withdrawal and cerebral asymmetry: Emotion expression and brain physiology: I. *Journal of Personality and Social Psychology, 58,* 330–341.

de Beurs, E., den Hollander-Gijsman, M. E., Helmich, S., & Zitman, F. G. (2007). The tripartite model for assessing symptoms of anxiety and depression: Psychometrics of the Dutch version of the Mood and Anxiety Symptoms Questionnaire. *Behaviour Research and Therapy, 45,* 1609–1617.

Deldin, P. J., Keller, J., Gergen, J. A., & Miller, G. A. (2000). Right-posterior face processing anomaly in depression. *Journal of Abnormal Psychology, 109,* 116–121.

Delgado, M. R., Gillis, M. M., & Phelps, E. A. (2008). Regulating the expectation of reward via cognitive strategies. *Nature Neuroscience, 11,* 880–881.

Depue, R., & Iacono, W. (1989). Neurobehavioral aspects of affective disorders. *Annual Review of Psychology, 40,* 457–492.

Di Chiara, G., & Imperato, A. (1988). Drugs abused by humans preferentially increase synaptic dopamine concentrations in the mesolimbic system of freely moving rats. *Proceedings of the National Academy of Sciences USA, 85,* 5274–5278.

Dichter, G. S., & Tomarken, A. J. (2008). The chronometry of affective startle modulation in unipolar depression. *Journal of Abnormal Psychology, 117,* 1–15.

Dillon, D. G., Holmes, A. J., Jahn, A. L., Bogdan, R., Wald, L. L., & Pizzagalli, D. A. (2008). Dissociation of neural regions associated with anticipatory versus consummatory phases of incentive processing. *Psychophysiology, 45,* 36–49.

Dillon, D. G., & LaBar, K. S. (2005). Startle modulation during conscious emotion regulation is arousal-dependent. *Behavioral Neuroscience, 119,* 1118–1124.

Dillon, D. G., & Pizzagalli, D. A. (2007). Inhibition of action, thought, and emotion: A selective neurobiological review. *Applied and Preventive Psychology, 12,* 99–114.

Ehrman, R. N., Robbins, S. J., Childress, A. R., & O'Brien, C. P. (1992). Conditioned responses to cocaine-related stimuli in cocaine abuse patients. *Psychopharmacology, 107,* 523–529.

Eippert, F., Veit, R., Weiskopf, N., Erb, M., Birbaumer, N., & Anders, S. (2007). Regulation of emotional responses elicited by threat-related stimuli. *Human Brain Mapping, 28*, 409–423.

Elliott, R., Sahakian, B. J., Michael, A., Paykel, E. S., & Dolan, R. J. (1998). Abnormal neural response to feedback on planning and guessing tasks in patients with unipolar depression. *Psychological Medicine, 28*, 559–571.

Epstein, J., Pan, H., Kocsis, J. H., Yang, Y., Butler, T., Chusid, J., et al. (2006). Lack of ventral striatal response to positive stimuli in depressed versus normal subjects. *American Journal of Psychiatry, 163*, 1784–1790.

Fowles, D. C. (1993). Biological variables in psychopathology: A psychobiological perspective. In P. B. Sutker & H. E. Adams (Eds.), *Comprehensive handbook of psychopathology* (pp. 57–82). New York: Plenum Press.

Frank, M. J., & Claus, E. D. (2006). Anatomy of a decision: Striato-orbitofrontal interactions in reinforcement learning, decision making, and reversal. *Psychological Review, 113*, 300–326.

Fredrickson, B. L. (2000). Cultivating positive emotions to optimize health and well-being. *Prevention and Treatment, 3*. Retrieved September 16, 2008, from *www.unc.edu/peplab/publications/cultivating.pdf*.

Fredrickson, B. L. (2001). The role of positive emotions in positive psychology: The broaden-and-build theory of positive emotions. *American Psychologist, 56*, 218–226.

Fredrickson, B. L., Cohn, M. A., Coffey, K. A., Pek, J., & Finkel, S. M. (2008). Open hearts build lives: Positive emotions, induced through loving-kindness meditation, build consequential personal resources. *Journal of Personality and Social Psychology, 95*, 1045–1062.

Fredrickson, B. L., & Levenson, R. W. (1998). Positive emotions speed recovery from the cardiovascular sequelae of negative emotions. *Cognition and Emotion, 12*, 191–220.

Fredrickson, B. L., Mancuso, R. A., Branigan, C., & Tugade, M. M. (2000). The undoing effect of positive emotions. *Motivation and Emotion, 24*, 237–258.

Gard, D. E., Gard, M. G., Kring, A. M., & John, O. P. (2006). Anticipatory and consummatory components of the experience of pleasure: A scale development study. *Journal of Research in Personality, 40*, 1086–1102.

Gard, D. E., Kring, A. M., Germans Gard, M., Horan, W. P., & Green, M. F. (2007). Anhedonia in schizophrenia: Distinctions between anticipatory and consummatory pleasure. *Schizophrenia Research, 93*, 253–260.

Glimcher, P. W., & Rustichini, A. (2004). Neuroeconomics: The consilience of brain and decision. *Science, 306*, 447–452.

Gold, J. M., Waltz, J. A., Prentice, K. J., Morris, S. E., & Heerey, E. A. (2008). Reward processing in schizophrenia: A deficit in the representation of value. *Schizophrenia Bulletin, 34*, 835–847.

Goldstein, R. Z., & Volkow, N. D. (2002). Drug addiction and its underlying neurobiological basis: Neuroimaging evidence for the involvement of the frontal cortex. *American Journal of Psychiatry, 159*, 1642–1652.

Gray, J. A. (1991). Neural systems, emotion, and personality. In J. Madden IV (Ed.), *Neurobiology of learning, emotion, and affect* (pp. 273–306). New York: Raven Press.

Green, M. J., Cahill, C. M., & Malhi, G. S. (2007). The cognitive and neurophysiological basis of emotion dysregulation in bipolar disorder. *Journal of Affective Disorders, 103,* 29–42.

Gross, J. J. (1998). The emerging field of emotion regulation: An integrative review. *Review of General Psychology, 2,* 271–299.

Gross, J. J., & John, O. P. (2003). Individual differences in two emotion regulation processes: Implications for affect, relationships, and well-being. *Journal of Personality and Social Psychology, 85,* 348–362.

Gross, J. J., Richards, J. M., & John, O. P. (2006). Emotion regulation in everyday life. In D. K. Snyder, J. A. Simpson, & J. N. Hughes (Eds.), *Emotion regulation in couples and families: Pathways to dysfunction and health* (pp. 13–35). Washington, DC: American Psychological Association.

Gruber, J., Eidelman, P., & Harvey, A. G. (2008). Transdiagnostic emotion regulation processes in bipolar disorder and insomnia. *Behaviour Research and Therapy, 46,* 1096–1100.

Hajcak, G., & Nieuwenhuis, S. (2006). Reappraisal modulates the electrocortical response to unpleasant pictures. *Cognitive, Affective and Behavioral Neuroscience, 6,* 291–297.

Harmon-Jones, E., Abramson, L. Y., Nusslock, R., Sigelman, J. D., Urosevic, S., Turonie, L. D., et al. (2008). Effect of bipolar disorder on left frontal cortical responses to goals differing in valence and task difficulty. *Biological Psychiatry, 63,* 693–698.

Hayden, E. P., Bodkins, M., Brenner, C., Shekhar, A., Nurnberger, J. I., Jr., O'Donnell, B. F., et al. (2008). A multimethod investigation of the behavioral activation system in bipolar disorder. *Journal of Abnormal Psychology, 117,* 164–170.

Henriques, J. B., & Davidson, R. J. (1990). Regional brain electrical asymmetries discriminate between previously depressed and healthy control subjects. *Journal of Abnormal Psychology, 99,* 22–31.

Henriques, J. B., & Davidson, R. J. (1991). Left frontal hypoactivation in depression. *Journal of Abnormal Psychology, 100,* 535–545.

Hitchcock, J. M., & Davis, M. (1987). Fear-potentiated startle using an auditory conditioned stimulus: Effects of lesions of the amygdala. *Physiology and Behavior, 39,* 403–408.

Hollerman, J. R., & Schultz, W. (1998). Dopamine neurons report an error in the temporal prediction of reward during learning. *Nature Neuroscience, 1,* 304–309.

Hopper, J. W., Pitman, R. K., Su, Z., Heyman, G. M., Lasko, N. B., Macklin, M. L., et al. (2008). Probing reward function in posttraumatic stress disorder: Expectancy and satisfaction with monetary gains and losses. *Journal of Psychiatric Research, 42,* 802–807.

Hornak, J., O'Doherty, J., Bramham, J., Rolls, E. T., Morris, R. G., Bullock, P. R., et al. (2004). Reward-related reversal learning after surgical excisions in orbitofrontal or dorsolateral prefrontal cortex in humans. *Journal of Cognitive Neuroscience, 16,* 463–478.

Hughes, J. R., Pleasants, C. N., & Pickens, R. W. (1985). Measurement of reinforcement in depression: A pilot study. *Journal of Behavior Therapy and Experimental Psychiatry, 16,* 231–236.

Hyman, S. E., & Malenka, R. C. (2001). Addiction and the brain: The neurobiology of compulsion and its persistence. *Nature Reviews Neuroscience, 2,* 695–703.

Jackson, D. C, Mueller, C. J., Dolski, I., Dalton, K. M., Nitschke, J. B., Urry, H. L., et al. (2003). Now you feel it, now you don't: Frontal brain electrical asymmetry and individual differences in emotion regulation. *Psychological Science, 14,* 612–617.

Jentsch, J. D., & Taylor, J. R. (1999). Impulsivity resulting from frontostriatal dysfunction in drug abuse: Implications for the control of behavior by reward-related stimuli. *Psychopharmacology, 146,* 373–390.

Johnson, S. L. (2005). Mania and dysregulation in goal pursuit: A review. *Clinical Psychology Review, 25,* 241–262.

Johnson, S. L., & Carver, C. S. (2006). Extreme goal setting and vulnerability to mania among undiagnosed young adults. *Cognitive Therapy Research, 30,* 377–395.

Johnson, S. L., Sandrow, D., Meyer, B., Winters, R., Miller, I., Solomon, D., et al. (2000). Increases in manic symptoms after life events involving goal attainment. *Journal of Abnormal Psychology, 109,* 721–727.

Johnstone, T., van Reekum, C. M., Urry, H. L., Kalin, N. H., & Davidson, R. J. (2007). Failure to regulate: Counterproductive recruitment of top-down prefrontal-subcortical circuitry in major depression. *Journal of Neuroscience, 27,* 8877–8884.

Juckel, G., Schlagenhauf, F., Koslowski, M., Wustenberg, T., Villringer, A., Knutson, B., et al. (2006). Dysfunction of ventral striatal reward prediction in schizophrenia. *NeuroImage, 29,* 409–416.

Kalisch, R., Wiech, K., Critchley, H. D., Seymour, B., O'Doherty, J. P., Oakley, D. A., et al. (2005). Anxiety reduction through detachment: Subjective, physiological, and neural effects. *Journal of Cognitive Neuroscience, 17,* 874–883.

Kaviani, H., Gray, J. A., Checkley, S. A., Raven, P. W., Wilson, G. D., & Kumari, V. (2004). Affective modulation of the startle response in depression: Influence of the severity of depression, anhedonia, and anxiety. *Journal of Affective Disorders, 83,* 21–31.

Keedwell, P. A., Andrew, C., Williams, S. C. R., Brammer, M. J., & Phillips, M. L. (2005). The neural correlates of anhedonia in major depressive disorder. *Biological Psychiatry, 58,* 843–853.

Kennerley, S. W., Walton, M. E., Behrens, T. E. J., Buckley, M. J., & Rushworth, M. F. S. (2006). Optimal decision making and the anterior cingulate cortex. *Nature Neuroscience, 9,* 940–947.

Kim, S. H., & Hamann, S. (2007). Neural correlates of positive and negative emotion regulation. *Journal of Cognitive Neuroscience, 19,* 779–798.

Knutson, B., Adams, C. M., Fong, G. W., & Hommer, D. (2001). Anticipation of increasing monetary reward selectively recruits nucleus accumbens. *Journal of Neuroscience, 21,* RC159.

Knutson, B., Bhanji, J. P., Cooney, R. E., Atlas, L. Y., & Gotlib, I. H. (2008). Neural responses to monetary incentives in major depression. *Biological Psychiatry, 63,* 686–692.

Knutson, B., & Cooper, J. C. (2005). Functional magnetic resonance imaging of reward prediction. *Current Opinion in Neurology, 18,* 411–417.

Knutson, B., Fong, G. W., Adams, C. M., Varner, J. L., & Hommer, D. (2001). Dissociation of reward anticipation and outcome with event-related fMRI. *NeuroReport, 12,* 3683–3687.

Knutson, B., Fong, G. W., Bennett, S. M., Adams, C. M., & Hommer, D. (2003). A region of mesial prefrontal cortex tracks monetarily rewarding outcomes: Characterization with rapid event-related fMRI. *NeuroImage, 18*, 263–272.

Koch, M., Schmid, A., & Schnitzler, H. U. (1996). Pleasure-attenuation of startle is disrupted by lesions of the nucleus accumbens. *NeuroReport, 7*, 1442–1446.

Koob, G. F., & Le Moal, M. (1997). Drug abuse: Hedonic homeostatic dysregulation. *Science, 278*, 52–58.

Krompinger, J. W., Moser, J. S., & Simons, R. F. (2008). Modulations of the electrophysiological response to pleasant stimuli by cognitive reappraisal. *Emotion, 8*, 132–137.

Kumar, P., Waiter, G., Ahearn, T., Milders, M., Reid, I., & Steele, J. D. (2008). Abnormal temporal difference reward-learning signals in major depression. *Brain, 131*, 2084–2093.

Lam, D. H., Watkins, E. R., Hayward, P., Bright, J., Wright, K., Kerr, N., et al. (2003). A randomized controlled study of cognitive therapy for relapse prevention for bipolar affective disorder: Outcome of the first year. *Archives of General Psychiatry, 60*, 145–152.

Lang, P. J. (1995). The emotion probe. Studies of motivation and attention. *American Psychologist, 50*, 372–385.

Leventhal, A. M., Kahler, C. W., Ray, L. A., Stone, K., Young, D., Chelminski, I., et al. (2008). Anhedonia and amotivation in psychiatric outpatients with fully remitted stimulant use disorder. *American Journal on Addictions, 17*, 218–223.

Mah, L., Zarate, C. A., Jr., Singh, J., Duan, Y. F., Luckenbaugh, D. A., Manji, H. K., et al. (2007). Regional cerebral glucose metabolic abnormalities in bipolar II depression. *Biological Psychiatry, 61*, 765–775.

Mayberg, H. S., Liotti, M., Brannan, S. K., McGinnis, S., Mahurin, R. K., Jerabek, P. A., et al. (1999). Reciprocal limbic-cortical function and negative mood: Converging PET findings in depression and normal sadness. *American Journal of Psychiatry, 156*, 675–682.

Meyer, B., Johnson, S. L., & Winters, R. (2001). Responsiveness to threat and incentive in bipolar disorder: Relations of the BIS/BAS scales with symptoms. *Journal of Psychopathology and Behavioral Assessment, 23*, 133–143.

Meyer, J. H., McNeely, H. E., Sagrati, S., Boovariwala, A., Martin, K., Verhoeff, N. P. L. G., et al. (2006). Elevated putamen D_2 receptor binding potential in major depression with motor retardation: An [^{11}C]raclopride positron emission tomography study. *American Journal of Psychiatry, 163*, 1594–1602.

Moser, J. S., Hajcak, G., Bukay, E., & Simons, R. F. (2006). Intentional modulation of emotional responding to unpleasant pictures: An ERP study. *Psychophysiology, 43*, 292–296.

Nandrino, J.-L., Dodin, V., Martin, P., & Henniaux, M. (2004). Emotional information processing in first and recurrent major depressive episodes. *Journal of Psychiatric Research, 38*, 475–484.

Nezlek, J. B., & Kuppens, P. (2008). Regulating positive and negative emotions in daily life. *Journal of Personality, 76*, 561–580.

Nusslock, R., Abramson, L. Y., Harmon-Jones, E., Alloy, L. B., & Hogan, M. E. (2007). A goal-striving life event and the onset of hypomanic and depressive episodes and symptoms: Perspective from the behavioral approach system (BAS) dysregulation theory. *Journal of Abnormal Psychology, 116*, 105–115.

O'Doherty, J., Dayan, P., Schultz, J., Deichmann, R., Friston, K., & Dolan, R. J. (2004). Dissociable roles of ventral and dorsal striatum in instrumental conditioning. *Science, 304,* 452–454.

O'Doherty, J. P., Hampton, A., & Kim, H. (2007). Model-based fMRI and its application to reward learning and decision making. *Annals of the New York Academy of Science, 1104,* 35–53.

O'Doherty, J., Kringelbach, M. L., Rolls, E. T., Hornak, J., & Andrews, C. (2001). Abstract reward and punishment representations in the human orbitofrontal cortex. *Nature Neuroscience, 4,* 95–102.

Ochsner, K. N., Bunge, S. A., Gross, J. J., & Gabrieli, J. D. (2002). Rethinking feelings: An fMRI study of the cognitive regulation of emotion. *Journal of Cognitive Neuroscience, 14,* 1215–1229.

Ochsner, K. N., Ray, R. D., Cooper, J. C., Robertson, E. R., Chopra, S., Gabrieli, J. D. E., et al. (2004). For better or for worse: Neural systems supporting the cognitive down- and up-regulation of negative emotion. *NeuroImage, 23,* 483–499.

Olds, J., & Milner, P. (1954). Positive reinforcement produced by electrical stimulation of the septal area and other regions of rat brain. *Journal of Comparative and Physiological Psychology, 47,* 419–427.

Papa, A., & Bonanno, G. A. (2008). Smiling in the face of adversity: The interpersonal and intrapersonal functions of smiling. *Emotion, 8,* 1–12.

Pizzagalli, D. A., Bogdan, R., Ratner, K. G., & Jahn, A. L. (2007). Increased perceived stress is associated with blunted hedonic capacity: Potential implications for depression research. *Behaviour Research and Therapy, 45,* 2742–2753.

Pizzagalli, D. A., Goetz, E., Ostacher, M., Iosifescu, D. V., & Perlis, R. H. (2008). Euthymic patients with bipolar disorder show decreased reward learning in a probabilistic reward task. *Biological Psychiatry, 64,* 162–168.

Pizzagalli, D. A., Holmes, A. J., Dillon, D. G., Goetz, E. L., Birk, J. L., Bogdan, R., et al. (2009). Reduced caudate and nucleus accumbens response to rewards in unmedicated individuals with major depressive disorder. *American Journal of Psychiatry, 166,* 702–710.

Pizzagalli, D. A., Iosifescu, D., Hallett, L. A., Ratner, K. G., & Fava, M. (2009). Reduced hedonic capacity in major depressive disorder: Evidence from a probabilistic reward task. *Journal of Psychiatric Research, 43,* 76–87.

Pizzagalli, D. A., Jahn, A. L., & O'Shea, J. P. (2005). Toward an objective characterization of an anhedonic phenotype: A signal-detection approach. *Biological Psychiatry, 57,* 319–327.

Platt, M. L., & Huettel, S. A. (2008). Risky business: The neuroeconomics of decision making under uncertainty. *Nature Neuroscience, 11,* 398–403.

Rangel, A., Camerer, C., & Montague, P. R. (2008). A framework for studying the neurobiology of value-based decision making. *Nature Reviews Neuroscience, 9,* 545–556.

Rottenberg, J., Kasch, K. L., Gross, J. J., & Gotlib, I. H. (2002). Sadness and amusement reactivity differentially predict concurrent and prospective functioning in major depressive disorder. *Emotion, 2,* 135–146.

Rushworth, M. F. S., Behrens, T. E. J., Rudebeck, P. H., & Walton, M. E. (2007). Contrasting roles for cingulate and orbitofrontal cortex in decisions and social behaviour. *Trends in Cognitive Sciences, 11,* 168–176.

Russell, J. A. (1979). Affective space is bipolar. *Journal of Personality and Social Psychology, 37,* 345–356.

Sailer, U., Robinson, S., Fischmeister, F. P., Konig, D., Oppenauer, C., Lueger-Schuster, B., et al. (2008). Altered reward processing in the nucleus accumbens and mesial prefrontal cortex of patients with posttraumatic stress disorder. *Neuropsychologia, 46*, 2836–2844.

Schultz, W. (1998). Predictive reward signal of dopamine neurons. *Journal of Neurophysiology, 80*, 1–27.

Schultz, W. (2000). Multiple reward signals in the brain. *Nature Reviews Neuroscience, 1*, 199–207.

Schultz, W., Dayan, P., & Montague, P. R. (1997). A neural substrate of prediction and reward. *Science, 275*, 1593–1599.

Shankman, S. A., Klein, D. N., Tenke, C. E., & Bruder, G. E. (2007). Reward sensitivity in depression: A biobehavioral study. *Journal of Abnormal Psychology, 116*, 95–104.

Shestyuk, A. Y., Deldin, P. J., Brand, J. E., & Deveney, C. M. (2005). Reduced sustained brain activity during processing of positive emotional stimuli in major depression. *Biological Psychiatry, 57*, 1089–1096.

Sloan, D. M., Strauss, M. E., Quirk, S. W., & Sajatovic, M. (1997). Subjective and expressive emotional responses in depression. *Journal of Affective Disorders, 46*, 135–141.

Sloan, D. M., Strauss, M. E., & Wisner, K. L. (2001). Diminished response to pleasant stimuli by depressed women. *Journal of Abnormal Psychology, 110*, 488–493.

Steele, J. D., Kumar, P., & Ebmeier, K. P. (2007). Blunted response to feedback information in depressive illness. *Brain, 130*, 2367–2374.

Taylor, S. F., & Liberzon, I. (2007). Neural correlates of emotion regulation in psychopathology. *Trends in Cognitive Sciences, 11*, 413–418.

Tremeau, F., Malaspina, D., Duval, F., Corrêa, H., Hager-Budny, M., Coin-Bariou, L., et al. (2005). Facial expressiveness in patients with schizophrenia compared to depressed patients and nonpatient comparison samples. *American Journal of Psychiatry, 162*, 92–101.

Tricomi, E. M., Delgado, M. R., & Fiez, J. A. (2004). Modulation of caudate activity by action contingency. *Neuron, 41*, 281–292.

Tugade, M. M., & Fredrickson, B. L. (2004). Resilient individuals use positive emotions to bounce back from negative emotional experiences. *Journal of Personality and Social Psychology, 86*, 320–333.

Tugade, M. M., & Fredrickson, B. L. (2007). Regulation of positive emotions: Emotion regulation strategies that promote resilience. *Journal of Happiness Studies, 8*, 311–333.

Urosevic, S., Abramson, L. Y., Harmon-Jones, E., & Alloy, L. B. (2008). Dysregulation of the behavioral approach system (BAS) in bipolar spectrum disorders: Review of theory and evidence. *Clinical Psychology Review, 28*, 1188–1205.

Urry, H. L., Nitschke, J. B., Dolski, I., Jackson, D. C., Dalton, K. M., Mueller, C. J., et al. (2004). Making a life worth living: Neural correlates of well-being. *Psychological Science, 15*, 367–372.

Urry, H. L., van Reekum, C. M., Johnstone, T., Kalin, N. H., Thurow, M. E., Schaefer, H. S., et al. (2006). Amygdala and ventromedial prefrontal cortex are inversely coupled during regulation of negative affect and predict the diurnal pattern of cortisol secretion among older adults. *Journal of Neuroscience, 26*, 4415–4425.

Volkow, N. D., Fowler, J. S., Wang, G. J., Baler, R., & Telang, F. (2009). Imaging dopamine's role in drug abuse and addiction. *Neuropharmacology*, *56*(Suppl. 1), 3–8.

Volkow, N. D., Wang, G. J., Fowler, J. S., Gatley, S. J., Ding, Y. S., Logan, J., et al. (1996). Relationship between psychostimulant-induced "high" and dopamine transporter occupancy. *Proceedings of the National Academy of Sciences, USA*, *93*, 10388–10392.

Volkow, N. D., Wang, G. J., Telang, F., Fowler, J. S., Logan, J., Childress, A. S., et al. (2006). Cocaine cues and dopamine in dorsal striatum: Mechanism of craving in cocaine addiction. *Journal of Neuroscience*, *26*, 6583–6588.

Watson, D. (2005). Rethinking the mood and anxiety disorders: A quantitative hierarchical model for *DSM-V. Journal of Abnormal Psychology*, *114*, 522–536.

Wener, A. E., & Rehm, L. P. (1975). Depressive affect: A test of behavioral hypotheses. *Journal of Abnormal Psychology*, *84*, 221–227.

CHAPTER 11

The Role of Sleep
in Emotional Brain Regulation

Els van der Helm and Matthew P. Walker

The ability of the human brain to generate, regulate, and be guided by emotions represents a fundamental process governing not only our personal lives but our mental health as well as our societal structure. The recent emergence of cognitive neuroscience has ushered in a new era of research connecting affective behavior with human brain function and has provided a systems-level view of emotional processing, translationally bridging animal models of affective regulation and relevant clinical disorders.

Independent of this research area, a resurgence has also taken place within the basic sciences, focusing on the functional impact of sleep on neurocognitive processes (Walker & Stickgold, 2006). However, surprisingly less research attention has been afforded to the interaction between sleep and emotional regulation or affective brain function. We say "surprising" considering the remarkable overlap between the known physiology of sleep, especially rapid-eye-movement (REM) sleep, and the associated neurochemistry and network anatomy that modulate emotions as well as the prominent co-occurrence of abnormal sleep (including REM) in almost all affective psychiatric and mood disorders.

Despite the relative paucity of research, recent work has begun to describe a consistent and clarifying role for sleep in the selective modulation of affective information and the regulation of emotions. In this review, we survey an array of diverse findings across basic and clinical research domains, resulting in a convergent view of sleep-dependent emotional brain processing. On the basis of the unique neurobiology of sleep, we outline a model describing the overnight modulation of affective neural systems and the (re)processing of recent emotional experiences, both of which appear to redress the appropriate next-day reactivity of limbic and associated autonomic networks. Furthermore, a REM sleep hypothesis of emotional-memory processing is proposed, the implications of which may provide brain-based insights into the association between sleep abnormalities and the initiation and maintenance of mood disturbance.

It should be noted that when we use the term *emotion*, we refer to the set of physiological cascades triggered by induced feelings and whose nature can be positive or negative in context. The subsequent mental and behavioral consequences of these events we describe as emotional reactions. Furthermore, either of these (emotions or emotional reactions) can be modulated by the brain, which we describe as the process of emotional regulation.

Overview of the Neuroscience of Sleep

The sleep of mammalian species has been broadly classified into two distinct types: non-rapid-eye-movement (NREM) sleep and rapid-eye-movement (REM) sleep, with NREM sleep being further divided in primates and cats into four substages (1–4) corresponding, in that order, to increasing depth of sleep (Rechtschaffen & Kales, 1968). In humans, NREM and REM sleep alternate, or "cycle," across the night in an ultradian pattern every 90 minutes (Figure 11.1). Although this NREM–REM cycle length remains largely stable across the night, the ratio of NREM to REM within each 90-minute cycle changes, so that early in the night Stages 3 and 4 of NREM dominate, while Stage 2 NREM and REM sleep prevail in the latter half of the night. Interestingly, the functional reasons for this organizing principle (deep NREM early in the night, Stage 2 NREM and REM late in the night) remain unknown, another perplexing mystery of sleep.

As NREM sleep progresses, electroencephalographic (EEG) activity begins to slow in frequency. Throughout Stage 2 NREM, there is the presence of phasic electrical events, including K complexes (large electrical sharp waves in the EEG) and sleep spindles (short synchronized 10- to 16-Hz EEG oscillations) (Steriade & Amzica, 1998). The deepest stages of NREM, Stages 3 and 4, are often grouped together under the term *slow-wave sleep* (SWS), reflecting the occurrence of low-frequency waves (0.5–4 Hz and below <1 Hz), representing an expression of underlying mass cortical synchrony (Amzica & Steriade, 1995). During REM sleep, however, EEG waveforms once again change in their composition, associated with oscillatory activity in the theta band range (4–7 Hz), together with higher frequency synchronous activity in the 30–80 Hz range ("gamma") (Llinas & Ribary, 1993; Steriade, Amzica, & Contreras, 1996). Periodic bursts of rapid eye movement also take place, a defining characteristic of REM sleep, associated with the occurrence of phasic endogenous waveforms expressed

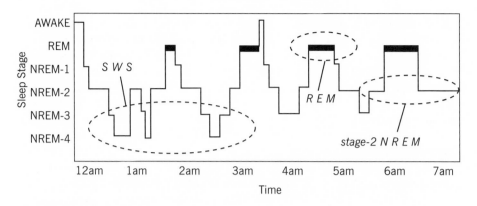

FIGURE 11.1. The human sleep cycle. Across the night, non-rapid-eye-movement (NREM) and rapid-eye-movement (REM) sleep cycle every 90 minutes in an ultradian manner, while the ratio of NREM to REM sleep shifts. During the first half of the night, NREM Stages 3 and 4 (slow-wave sleep [SWS]) dominate, while Stage 2 NREM and REM sleep prevail in the latter half of the night. Electroencephalographic patterns also differ significantly between sleep stages, with electrical oscillations such as slow delta waves developing in SWS, K complexes and sleep spindles occurring during Stage 2 NREM, and theta waves seen during REM.

in, among other brain regions, the pons (P), lateral geniculate nuclei of the thalamus (G), and the occipital cortex (O), and as such, have been termed *PGO waves* (Callaway, Lydic, Baghdoyan, & Hobson, 1987).

As the brain passes through these sleep stages, it also undergoes dramatic alterations in neurochemistry (Saper, Chou, & Scammell, 2001). In NREM sleep, subcortical cholinergic systems in the brainstem and forebrain become markedly less active (Hobson, McCarley, & Wyzinski, 1975; Lydic & Baghdoyan, 1988), while firing rates of two aminergic populations of neurons—serotonergic Raphé neurons and noradrenergic locus coeruleus neurons—are also reduced relative to waking levels (Aston-Jones & Bloom, 1981; Shima, Nakahama, & Yamamoto, 1986). During REM sleep, both the serotonergic and the noradrenergic populations are strongly inhibited while cholinergic systems become as, if not more, active compared with wake (Kametani & Kawamura, 1990; Marrosu et al., 1995), resulting in a brain state largely devoid of such aminergic modulation and dominated by acetylcholine (ACh).

At a whole-brain systems level, neuroimaging techniques have revealed complex and dramatically different patterns of functional anatomy associated with NREM and REM sleep (for a review, see Nofzinger, 2005). During NREM SWS, brainstem, thalamic, basal ganglia, prefrontal, and temporal lobe regions all appear to undergo reduced activity. However, during REM sleep, significant elevations in activity have been reported in the pontine tegmentum, thalamic nuclei, occipital cortex, mediobasal prefrontal lobes, and associated limbic groups, including the amygdala, hippocampus, and anterior cingulate cortex. In contrast, the dorsolateral prefrontal cortex, posterior cingulate, and parietal cortex appear least active in REM sleep.

Although this summary only begins to describe the range of neural processes that are affected by the brain's daily transit through sleep states, it clearly demonstrates that sleep itself cannot be treated as a homogeneous entity, offering a range of distinct neurobiological mechanisms that can support numerous brain functions. In the remaining sections, we examine the role of sleep and its specific stages in the modulation of emotional memories and the regulation of affective reactivity, culminating in a heuristic model of sleep-dependent emotional brain processing.

Sleep and Emotional Memory Processing

The impact of sleep on memory has principally been characterized at two different stages of memory: (1) before learning, in the initial formation (encoding) of new information and (2) after learning, in the long-term solidification (consolidation) of new memories (Marshall & Born, 2007; Walker & Stickgold, 2004, 2006). We now consider each of these stages and focus on reports involving affective learning.

Sleep and Affective Memory Encoding

Animal Studies

At a behavioral level, numerous studies in rodents have demonstrated the detrimental impact of prior sleep deprivation on initial memory formation, the evidence for which we only briefly summarize here. Critically, many if not all of these studies involve either appetitive or aversive learning paradigms, meaning these tasks are of an emotional nature. For example, sleep deprivation, and specifically REM deprivation, imposes detrimental effects on the encoding of one-way and two-way avoidance learning, taste aversion, and passive avoidance tasks (McGrath & Cohen, 1978; Smith, 1985). Even short (5-hour) bouts of pretraining REM sleep deprivation appear capable of disrupting the encoding of two-way avoidance learning in rats, reducing the number of avoidances, impairments that cannot be overcome by continued practice during the training session (Gruart-Masso, Nadal-Alemany, Coll-Andreu, Portell-Cortes, & Marti-Nicolovius, 1995). Therefore, sleep deprivation prior to learning in rodent models disrupts the ability to encode new affective memories.

Building on these behavioral findings, a collection of studies has explored the potential cellular mechanisms of sleep deprivation-induced encoding deficits, many of which have focused on the limbic system, specifically the hippocampus. At the cellular level, REM deprivation (ranging from 24–72 hours) not only reduces the basic excitability of hippocampal neurons but significantly impairs the formation of long-term potentiation (LTP), a foundational mechanism of memory formation, within these neurons (Davis, Harding, & Wright, 2003; McDermott et al., 2003). Furthermore, the small amount of LTP that does develop actually decays within 90 minutes, suggesting that even in the event of successful LTP induction hippocampal neurons are unable to maintain these plastic changes under conditions of REM deprivation (Davis et al., 2003). Therefore, sleep prior to learning appears to be necessary in preparing the cellular and subcellular ability of key limbic networks to acquire new memory associations.

Human Studies

Whereas early studies investigating the role of sleep in memory focused primarily on *post*training consolidation (see later sections), more recent data similarly support the need for adequate *pre*training sleep in the formation of new human episodic memories.

Some of the first studies of sleep deprivation and memory encoding focused on neutral forms of learning, indicating that "temporal memory" (memory for when events occur) was significantly disrupted by a night of pretraining sleep deprivation (Harrison & Horne, 2000; Morris, Williams, & Lubin, 1960), even when caffeine was administered to overcome nonspecific effects of lower arousal. More recent investigations have examined the importance of pretraining sleep for the formation of emotional and neutral memories (Walker & Stickgold, 2006). Subjects were either sleep deprived for 36 hours or allowed to sleep normally prior to a learning session composed of emotionally negative, positive, and neutral words and were tested following two recovery nights of sleep. Averaged across all memory categories, subjects who were sleep deprived demonstrated a 40% deficit in memory encoding relative to subjects who had slept normally prior to learning (Figure 11.2A). However, when these data were separated into the three emotional categories (negative, positive, or neutral), selective dissociations became apparent (Figure 11.2B). In subjects who had slept (control group), both positive and negative stimuli were associated with superior retention levels relative to the neutral condition, consistent with the notion that emotion facilitates memory encoding (Phelps, 2004). In the sleep-deprived group, a severe encoding impairment was evident for neutral and especially positive emotional memories, exhibiting a significant 59% retention deficit, relative to the control condition. Most interesting was the relative resistance of negative emotional memory to sleep deprivation, showing a markedly smaller and nonsignificant impairment among those who were sleep deprived.

These data first indicate that sleep loss impairs the ability to commit new experiences to memory and has recently been associated with dysfunction throughout the hippocampal complex (Yoo, Hu, Gujar, Jolesz, & Walker, 2007). Second, these findings suggest that, although the effects of

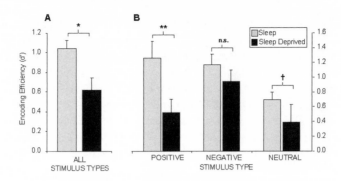

FIGURE 11.2. Sleep deprivation and encoding of emotional and nonemotional declarative memory. Effects of 38 hours of total sleep deprivation on encoding of human declarative memory (A) when combined across all emotional and non-emotional categories and (B) when separated by emotional (positive and negative valence) and nonemotional (neutral valance) categories. †p < .08; *p < .05; **p < .01; n.s., not significant; error bars represent SEM.

sleep deprivation are directionally consistent across emotional subcategories, the most profound impact is on the encoding of positive emotional stimuli and, to a lesser degree, emotionally neutral stimuli. In contrast, the encoding of negative memory appears to be more resistant to the effects of prior sleep loss. Third, these data may offer novel insights about learning and memory deficits in people with mood disorders who also express co-occurring sleep abnormalities (Buysse, 2004). Indeed, if one compares the two profiles of memory encoding in Figure 11.2B, it is clear that the sleep control group completes the encoding session with a balanced mix of both positive and negative memories. However, those in the deprivation group have a skewed distribution, finishing the encoding session with an over-riding dominance of negative memories and far fewer positive or neutral memories; an issue with clinical relevance discussed later.

As a whole, these studies indicate that prior sleep loss significantly impairs the ability for effective next-day learning of new emotion-relevant experiences across numerous species. Furthermore, sleep loss appears to differentially disrupt the learning of affective experiences, potentially creating a dominance of negative emotional memory. Most intriguing, animal models indicate that affective learning demonstrates a particular sensitivity to REM sleep deprivation, suggesting a dependency on a specific physiological stage of prior sleep for next-day emotional learning.

Sleep and Affective Memory Consolidation

Following encoding, the role of sleep after learning in subsequent memory consolidation has been demonstrated across a range of phylogeny, including human and nonhuman primates, cats, rats, mice, and birds (Walker & Stickgold, 2004, 2006), although here we again focus on affective learning paradigms.

Animal Studies

Animal studies suggest a role for sleep in the consolidation of both contextual fear and shock avoidance tasks (for a review, see Walker & Stickgold, 2004), all known to depend on intact hippocampal function. Daytime training on these tasks triggers alterations in sleep stage characteristics, predominately REM (Ambrosini et al., 1993; Ambrosini, Sadile, Gironi Carnevale, Mattiaccio, & Giuditta, 1988; Hennevin & Hars, 1987; Mandai, Guerrien, Sockeel, Dujardin, & Leconte, 1989; Sanford, Silvestri, Ross, & Morrison, 2001; Sanford, Tang, Ross, & Morrison, 2003; Smith, Young, & Young, 1980), and may reflect homeostatic demands on REM-dependent mechanisms of consolidation. Furthermore, sleep deprivation after learning such tasks has also been shown to disrupt consolidation and impair next-day memory retention (Beaulieu & Godbout, 2000; Fishbein, Kastaniotis, & Chattman, 1974; Hennevin & Hars, 1987; Marti-Nicolovius, Portell-Cortes, & Morgado-Bernal, 1988; Oniani, Lortkipanidze, & Maisuradze, 1987; Pearlman, 1969; Shiromani, Gutwein, & Fishbein, 1979; Smith & Kelly, 1988; Smith & Lapp, 1986). Interestingly, the timing of when sleep deprivation occurs appears to be critical. For example, Graves, Heller, Pack, and Abel (2003) have demonstrated that sleep deprivation 0 to 5 hours posttraining selectively impairs consolidation of contextual fear conditioning (as measured at a later 24-hour retest. However, sleep deprivation 5 to 10 hours posttraining did not block consolidation, resulting in similar memory performance at retest, relative to a non-sleep-deprived group.

These findings suggest that the consolidation of fear-associated memory occurs not only during sleep but soon after learning, during discreet sleep time windows. The implications of this temporal sensitivity are informative from a mechanistic standpoint but also from a clinical perspective, if the targeted disruption of sleep to negate overnight consolidation becomes a treatment goal, a situation perhaps most pertinent to conditions such as posttraumatic stress disorder (PTSD).

Human Studies

The role of sleep in the consolidation of fact-based memory, often referred to as declarative information, rather than being absolute, may depend on more intricate aspects of the information being learned, such as novelty, meaning to extract, and also the affective salience of the material. Independent of the field of sleep and memory, a wealth of evidence demonstrates that memory processing is modulated by emotion (Cahill, 2000; McGaugh, 2004; Phelps, 2004). Experiences that evocate emotions are not only encoded more strongly but appear to persist and even improve over time as the delay between learning and testing increases (hours/days) (Kleinsmith & Kaplan, 1963; LaBar & Phelps, 1998; Levonian, 1972; Sharot & Phelps, 2004; Walker & Tarte, 1963).

Although these findings indicate a strong influence of emotion on slow, time-dependent consolidation processes, based on the coincident neurophysiology that REM sleep provides and the neurobiological requirements of emotional memory processing (Cahill, 2000; McGaugh, 2004), work has now begun to test a selective REM-dependent hypothesis of affective human memory consolidation. For example, Hu, Stylos-Allen, and Walker (2006) have compared the consolidation of emotionally arousing and nonarousing picture stimuli following a 12-hour period across a day or after a night of sleep. A specific emotional memory benefit was observed only after sleep and not across an equivalent time awake. Wagner, Gais, and Born (2001) have also shown that sleep selectively favors the retention of previously learned emotional texts relative to neutral texts, and this affective memory benefit is present only after late-night sleep (a time period rich in Stage 2 NREM and REM sleep). Furthermore, this emotional memory enhancement has been shown to persist for several years (Wagner, Hallschmid, Rasch, & Born, 2006).

Using a nap paradigm, it has most recently been demonstrated that sleep, and specifically REM neurophysiology, may underlie this consolidation benefit (Nishida, Pearsall, Buckner, & Walker, 2009). Subjects took part in two study sessions in which they learned emotionally negative and neutral picture stimuli: one 4 hours prior and the other 15 minutes prior to a recognition memory test. In one group, participants slept (90-minute nap) after the first study session while participants in the other group remained awake. Thus, items from the first (4-hour) study sessions transitioned through different brain states in each group prior to testing, containing sleep in the nap group and no sleep in the no-nap group, yet subjects experienced identical brain state conditions following the second (15-minute) study session prior to testing.

No change in memory for emotional (or neutral) stimuli occurred across the offline delay in the no-nap group. However, a significant and selective offline enhancement of emotional memory was observed in the nap group (Figure 11.3A), the extent of which was correlated with the amount of REM sleep (Figure 11.3B) and the speed of entry into REM (latency; not shown). Most striking, spectral analysis of the EEG demonstrated that the magnitude of right-dominant prefrontal theta power during REM (activity in the frequency range of 4.0–7.0 Hz) exhibited a significant and positive relationship with the amount of emotional memory improvement (Figure 11.3C and D).

These findings go beyond simply demonstrating that affective memories are preferentially enhanced across periods of sleep and indicate that

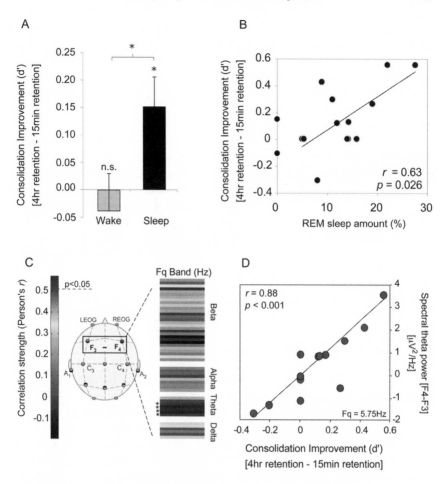

FIGURE 11.3. Rapid-eye-movement (REM) sleep enhancement of negative emotional memories. (A) Offline benefit (change in memory recall for 4-hour-old vs. 15-minute-old memories) across the day (wake, grey bar) or following a 90-minute nap (sleep, filled bar). (B) Correlation between the amount of offline emotional memory improvement in the nap group (i.e., the offline benefit expressed in filled bar of A) and the amount of REM sleep obtained within the nap. (C) Correlation strength (Pearson's *r*) between offline benefit for emotional memory in the sleep group (the benefit expressed in filled bar of A) and the relative right versus left prefrontal spectral-band power (F4–F3) within the delta, alpha, theta, and beta spectral bands, expressed in average 0.5-Hz-bin increments. Correlation strength is represented by the color range, which can be viewed in the full-color version of the figure (available at *www.guilford.com*), demonstrating significant correlations within the theta frequency band (also see * representing significance in theta range), and (D) exhibiting a maximum significance at the 5.75-Hz bin. *p < .05; error bars indicate *SEM*. From Nishida, Pearsall, Buckner, and Walker (2009). Adapted with permission from Oxford University Press.

the extent of emotional memory improvement is associated with specific REM sleep characteristics, both quantity and quality. Corroborating these correlations, it has previously been hypothesized that REM sleep represents a brain state particularly amenable to emotional memory consolidation, based on its unique biology (Hu et al., 2006; Pare, Collins, & Pelletier, 2002). Neurochemically, levels of limbic and forebrain ACh are markedly elevated during REM (Vazquez & Baghdoyan, 2001), reportedly quadruple those seen during NREM, and double those measured in quiet waking (Marrosu et al., 1995). Considering the known importance of ACh in the long-term consolidation of emotional learning (McGaugh, 2004), this procholinergic REM state may promote the selective memory facilitation of affective memories, similar to that reported using experimental manipulations of ACh (Power, 2004). Neurophysiologically, theta oscillations have been proposed as a carrier frequency, allowing disparate brain regions that initially encode information to selectively interact offline in a coupled relationship. By doing so, REM theta may afford the ability to strengthen distributed aspects of specific memory representations across related but different anatomical networks (Buzsaki, 2002; Jones & Wilson, 2005).

Sleep and Emotional Regulation

Despite substantial research focusing on the interaction between sleep and affective memory, the impact of sleep loss on basic emotional regulation and perception has received limited research attention. This absence of research is also perhaps surprising considering that nearly all psychiatric and neurological mood disorders express co-occurring abnormalities of sleep, suggesting an intimate relationship between sleep and emotion. Nevertheless, a number of studies evaluating subjective as well as objective measures of mood and affect, combined with insights from clinical domains, offer an emerging understanding for the critical role of sleep in regulating emotional brain function.

Sleep Loss, Mood Stability, and Emotional Brain (Re)activity

Together with impairments of attention and alertness, sleep deprivation is commonly associated with increased subjective reports of irritability and affective volatility (Horne, 1985). Using a sleep restriction paradigm (5 hours/night), Dinges and colleagues (1997) have reported a progressive increase in emotional disturbance across a 1-week period on the basis of questionnaire mood scales. Specifically, participants reported more fatigue, confusion, tension, and total mood disturbance as the amount of sleep deprivation increased. In addition, participants' daily journal entries also indicated increasing complaints of cognitive and emotional difficulties like concentration, lassitude, and emotional lability. Zohar, Tzischinsky, Epstein, and Lavie (2005) have also investigated the effects of sleep disruption on emotional reactivity to daytime work events among medical residents. Sleep loss was shown to amplify negative emotional consequences of disruptive daytime experiences while blunting the positive benefit associated with rewarding or goal-enhancing activities.

Although these findings help to characterize the emotional difficulties imposed by sleep loss, evidence for the role of sleep in regulating emotional brain networks is surprisingly scarce. To date, only one such study has investigated whether a lack of sleep inappropriately modulates human emotional brain reactivity (Yoo, Gujar, Hu, Jolesz, & Walker, 2007). Healthy, young participants were allowed to sleep normally prior to a functional magnetic resonance image scanning session or were sleep deprived for one night (accumulating approximately 35 hours of total sleep loss). During scanning, subjects performed an affective stimulus-viewing task involving the presentation of picture slides ranging in a gradient from emotionally neutral to increasingly negative and aversive.

Although both groups showed significant amygdala activation in response to increasingly negative picture stimuli, those in the sleep deprivation condition exhibited a remarkable +60% greater magnitude of amygdala reactivity relative to the control group (Figure 11.4A and B). In addition to this increased intensity of activation, there was also a threefold increase in the extent of amygdala volume recruited in response to the aversive stimuli in the sleep deprivation group (Figure 11.4B). Perhaps most interestingly, relative to the sleep control group, there was a significant loss of functional connectivity identified between the amygdala and the medial prefrontal cortex (mPFC) in those who were sleep deprived, a region known to have strong inhibitory projections to the amygdala (Sotres-Bayon, Bush, & LeDoux, 2004) (Figure 11.4C and D). In contrast, significantly greater connectivity was observed between the amygdala and the autonomic-activating centers of the locus coeruleus in the deprivation group.

It is interesting to note that both animal models and human imaging studies of either cognitive control or emotional responding in both healthy and psychiatric populations have implicated midline regions of the PFC in specific types of control processes and subcortical regions, such as the amygdala, in different types of emotional appraisal (Ochsner & Gross, 2005). For example, it has been proposed that the mPFC affords a degree of cognitive control over the amygdala by way of top-down inhibitory control, regulating socially appropriate limbic responses (Morgan, Romanski, & LeDoux, 1993). Furthermore, compromised interaction between the mPFC and amygdala has been implicated in the development of a number of psychiatric disorders, including depression, anxiety, and PTSD (for a review, see Sotres-Bayon et al., 2004).

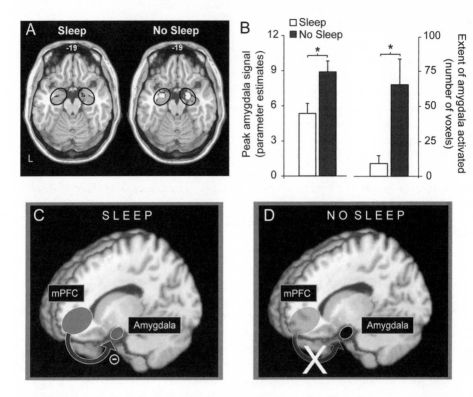

FIGURE 11.4. The impact of sleep deprivation on emotional brain reactivity and functional connectivity. (A) Amygdala response (circled areas) to increasingly negative emotional stimuli in the sleep deprivation and sleep control groups and (B) corresponding differences in intensity and volumetric extent of amygdala activation between the two groups (average ± *SEM* of left and right amygdala). (C) Depiction of associated changes in functional connectivity between the medial prefrontal cortex (mPFC) and the amygdala. With sleep, the prefrontal lobe was strongly connected to the amygdala, regulating and exerting an inhibitory top-down control (negative symbol), yet (D) without sleep the mPFC–amygdala connection was decreased, negating top-down control and resulting in an overactive amygdala. Strength of shading in C and D of mPFC, amygdala, and associated arrow represents strength of activity and connectivity, respectively. (A full-color version of this figure is available at *www.guilford.com.*) *$p < .01$; error bars indicate *SEM*. Based on Yoo, Gujar, Hu, Jolesz, and Walker (2007).

Thus, without sleep, an amplified "hyperlimbic" reaction by the human amygdala was observed in response to negative emotional stimuli. Furthermore, this altered magnitude of limbic activity was associated with a loss of functional connectivity with the mPFC in the sleep deprivation condition. It would, therefore, appear that a night of sleep may "reset" the correct affective brain reactivity to next-day emotional challenges by maintaining functional integrity of this mPFC–amygdala circuit and thus govern appropriate behavioral repertoires (e.g., optimal social judgments and rational decisions). Perhaps most intriguing, however, is that a similar pattern of anatomical dysfunction has been implicated in a number of psychiatric mood disorders that express co-occurring sleep abnormalities (Davidson, 2002; Davidson, Pizzagalli, Nitschke, & Putnam, 2002; New et al., 2007). This directly raises the issue of whether such factors (sleep loss and clinical mood disorders) are causally related.

Sleep and Mood Disorders

The implication of these findings challenges the notion that sleep disruption in mood disorders is epiphenomenal but instead a contributing (and potentially treatable) factor. Indeed, it is difficult to identify any psychiatric mood disorder where sleep disturbance not a listed formal symptom or a common feature of the condition (American Psychiatric Association, 1994). Here we focus on two psychiatric disorders of most relevance to the topic of sleep-dependent emotional processing: major depression and PTSD. However, we believe that the linkages between sleep and emotion regulation may well be useful for understanding these co-occurring difficulties across many other disorders given the pervasiveness of sleep and emotion regulation difficulties in psychopathology.

Major Depression

As the most prevalent mood disorder, major depression has consistently been linked to sleep abnormalities, found in up to 90% of patients, aspects of which are among the diagnostic criteria for this disorder (American Psychiatric Association, 1994). The inability to initiate and maintain sleep (insomnia) is a robust risk factor for the development of both the first episode of depression as well as recurrent episodes (Harvey, 2001; Perlis et al., 2006). Polysomnographic recordings of sleep in major depression are often marked by increased sleep latency, wake time after onset, and nocturnal awakenings (Berger, Doerr, Lund, Bronisch, & von Zerssen, 1982; Gillin, Duncan, Pettigrew, Frankel, & Snyder, 1979; Kupfer et al., 1985; Waller et al., 1989). Intriguingly, an additional hallmark feature appears to be reduced REM sleep latency (faster entry into REM), a prolonged first REM period, and an increase in REM density (Armitage, 2007; Gottesmann & Gottesman, 2007; Tsuno, Besset, & Ritchie, 2005). Moreover, the normalization of sleep architecture abnormalities has been associated with a reduced risk of relapse into depression, yet the persistence of abnormally short REM sleep latency is related to an increased risk of relapse (Ohayon, 2007). Short (< 65 minutes) REM latency has similarly been shown to predict both response to antidepressant treatment and risk of relapse in major depression (Giles, Jarrett, Roffwarg, & Rush, 1987; Grunhaus et al., 1994; Kupfer, Frank, McEachran, & Grochocinski, 1990; Rush et al., 1989). Furthermore, successful psychological treatments such as interpersonal therapy and cognitive-behavioral therapy have been found to decrease REM density (Buysse, Frank, Lowe, Cherry, & Kupfer, 1997; Nofzinger et al., 1994).

Interestingly, patients suffering from depression show increased activity in the midbrain reticular formation and in the anterior paralimbic activation cortex from waking to REM sleep (Nofzinger et al., 2000). Nofzinger and colleagues (2000) have suggested that the overactivation of limbic structures during REM sleep may reflect a susceptibility of depressed patients to experience (and possibly encode) stimuli in a more affectively intense, negative context, findings discussed in greater detail in the next section.

Posttraumatic Stress Disorder

Another disorder with commonly co-occurring sleep disturbance is PTSD, characterized by intrusive reexperiencing, avoidance, and hyperarousal reactions that persist after exposure to the traumatic event (American Psychiatric Association, 1994). Increasing attention has been paid to the repeated incorporation of emotionally charged waking episodes into nocturnal dreaming, a defining characteristic in the *Diagnostic and Statistical Manual of Mental Disorders* (fourth edition; American Psychiatric Association, 1994) criteria for diagnosis. Perhaps not surprisingly, PTSD has also been associated with a dysregulation of REM, together with reports of significantly increased sympathetic autonomic tone (Harvey, Jones, & Schmidt, 2003; Mellman & Hipolito, 2006). Although it is still unclear whether PTSD dream episodes reflect functional or dysfunctional processes, clearly emotional episodic memory events pervade the mental experiences of dreaming in these patients, potentially related to aberrant consolidation mechanisms and the cause of the disorder itself. In fact, the sleep disruptions that occur following trauma exposure may constitute a specific mechanism involved in the pathophysiology of chronic PTSD and poor clinical outcome. Subjective and objective sleep disturbances occurring early after trauma exposure, as well as heightened vagal tone during REM sleep, are all associated with an increased risk of meeting criteria for PTSD at subsequent assessments conducted up to 1 year later (Koren, Arnon, Lavie, & Klein, 2002; Mellman, Bustamante, Fins, Pigeon, & Nolan, 2002).

A Heuristic Model of Sleep-Dependent Emotional Processing: Explanatory Clinical Insights and Predictive Associations

On the basis of the emerging interaction between sleep and emotion at the basic experimental as well as clinical level, we next provide a synthesis of these findings, which converge on a functional role for sleep in affective brain modulation. We describe a model of sleep-dependent emotional information processing, offering provisional brain-based explanatory insights regarding the impact of sleep abnormalities in the initiation and maintenance of certain mood disorders and leading to testable predictions for future experimental investigations.

A Nexus of Experimental and Clinical Observation

The findings discussed earlier suggest a predisposition for the encoding of negative emotional memories and a hyperlimbic reactivity to negative emotional events under conditions of sleep loss, together with a strengthening of negative memories during subsequent REM, all of which have potential relevance for the understanding of major depression.

The reduction of sleep caused by insomnia (Buysse, 2004; Shaffery, Hoffmann, & Armitage, 2003) may predispose people with depression to an imbalance in memory encoding. Although based on findings from acute sleep deprivation, chronic accumulated sleep debt associated with depression may impair the ability to form and retain memories of a positive (and neutral) affective valence, yet leave preserved the formation and hence long-term dominance of negative experiences. This encoding bias would result in a perceived autobiographical history dominated by negative life events, despite being potentially filled with both positive and negative daily life experiences. Indeed, this imbalance may provide a converse mechanistic explanation for the higher incidence of depression in populations expressing impairments in sleep.

Beyond an imbalance in emotional memory formation, there may be a further sleep-dependent mnemonic dysfunction potentiating disease severity. Mounting data suggest that people with depression exhibit both a faster progression into REM (reduced REM latency) and an increase in the amount of REM, particularly early in the night (Armitage, 2007; Tsuno et al., 2005). When considered on the foundation of evidence described earlier indicating a strong positive correlation between the amplification of negative emotional memories and the amount and speed of entry into REM, this signature alteration of REM in depression may instigate the maladaptive and disproportionate consolidation of prior negative affective experiences. This would be especially pronounced when combined with the preexisting dominance of negative memories resulting from biased encoding described previously. Consistent with this hypothesis, many antidepressant medications are known to be REM sleep suppressants (Winokur et al., 2001), which, by their action, would curtail such offline emotional memory processing and in so doing reduce the strength (consolidation) of associated affective experiences. Indeed, total sleep deprivation is known to be a rapid yet short-term treatment for a subset of depressed patients. Improvement in depressive symptoms has also been shown to occur after a single night of sleep deprivation, although this is only apparent in 40 to 60% of patients (Giedke & Schwarzler, 2002; Wirz-Justice & Van den Hoofdakker, 1999) and may be related to the extent of resting baseline overactivity within the amygdala (Clark et al., 2006). Most interesting, selective deprivation of late-night sleep, rich in REM, appears to be particularly efficacious in these subgroup populations (Clark et al., 2006). It is also interesting to note the speed with which symptoms relapse following recovery sleep, which would likely contain a strong REM rebound, possibly contributing to the rapid reversal of this therapeutic effect (Wu & Bunney, 1990). It remains unclear why the efficacy of REM-suppressing antidepressants would take a number of weeks to produce clinical improvement, yet the effects of experimental sleep deprivation affords rapid symptom alterations. It may be that different mechanistic routes underlie each effect or that the magnitude of physiological REM suppression induced by antidepressant medications is significantly less than classical sleep-stage scoring actually reveals, and hence these medications require a more protracted time frame to achieve the same mechanistic impact.

Thus, at both stages of early memory processing—encoding and consolidation—the architectural sleep abnormalities expressed in major depression may facilitate an adverse prevalence and strengthening of prior negative episodic memories. Yet there may be an additional consequence of sleep-dependent memory processing beyond the strengthening of the experience itself, and one that has additional implications for mood disorders: that is, sleeping to forget.

A Hypothesis of Emotional-Memory Processing: Sleep to Forget and Sleep to Remember, Respectively

Founded on the emerging interaction between sleep and emotion, we now outline a model of affective information processing that may offer brain-based explanatory insights regarding the impact of sleep abnormalities, particularly REM, for the initiation and maintenance of mood disturbance.

Although there is abundant evidence to suggest that emotional experiences persist in our autobiographies over time, an equally remarkable but far less noted change is a reduction in the affective tone associated with their recall. Affective experiences appear to be encoded and consolidated more robustly than neutral memories because of autonomic neurochemical reactions elicited at the time of the experience (McGaugh,

2004), creating what we commonly term an *emotional memory*. However, the later recall of these experiences tends not to be associated with anywhere near the same magnitude of autonomic (re)activation as that elicited at the moment of learning/experience, suggesting that over time the affective "blanket" previously enveloped around the memory during encoding has been removed, while the information contained within that experience (the memory) remains.

For example, neuroimaging studies have shown that initial exposure and learning of emotional stimuli is associated with substantially greater activation in the amygdala and hippocampus relative to neutral stimuli (Dolcos, LaBar, & Cabeza, 2004, 2005; Kilpatrick & Cahill, 2003). In one of these studies (Dolcos et al., 2004), however, when participants were reexposed to these same stimuli during recognition testing many months later, a change in the profile of activation occurred (Dolcos et al., 2005). Although the same magnitude of differential activity between emotional and neutral items was observed in the hippocampus, this was not true in the amygdala. Instead, the difference in amygdala (re)activity compared with neutral items had dissipated over time. This would support the idea that the strength of the memory (hippocampal-associated activity) remains at later recollection, yet the associated emotional reactivity to these items (amygdala activity) is reduced over time.

Our hypothesis predicts that this decoupling preferentially takes place overnight, such that we sleep to forget the emotional tone and yet sleep to remember the tagged memory of that episode (Figure 11.5). The model further argues that if this process is not achieved, the magnitude of affective "charge" or tone remaining within autobiographical memory networks would persist, resulting in the potential condition of chronic anxiety.

Based on the consistent relationship identified between REM and emotional processing, combined with its unique neurobiology, this hypothesis proposes that REM sleep provides an optimal state for achieving such affective "therapy." Specifically, increased activity throughout the limbic network (including the hippocampus and amygdala) during REM may first offer the ability for reactivation of previously acquired affective experiences. Second, the neurophysiological signature of REM involving dominant theta oscillations within subcortical as well as cortical nodes may offer large-scale network cooperation at night, allowing the integration and, as a consequence, greater understanding of recently experienced emotional events in the context of preexisting neocortically stored semantic memory. Third, these interactions during REM (and perhaps through the conscious process of dreaming) critically and perhaps most importantly take place within a brain that is devoid of aminergic neurochemical concentration (Pace-Schott & Hobson, 2002), particularly noradrenergic input from the locus coeruleus, the influence of which has been linked to states of high stress and anxiety disorders (Sullivan, Coplan, Kent, & Gorman, 1999).

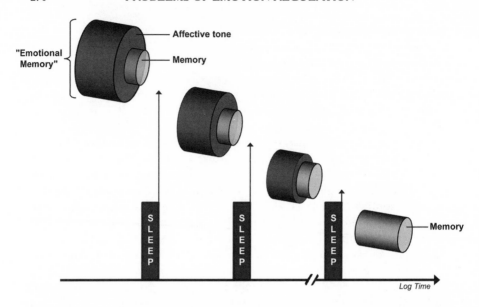

FIGURE 11.5. Model of sleep-dependent emotional-memory processing: a sleep to *forget* and sleep to *remember* hypothesis. When formed, a newly encoded "emotional-memory" is created in a milieu of high adrenergic tone, resulting in an associated affective "blanket." With multiple iterations of sleep, particularly rapid-eye-movement sleep, not only is the informational core (memory) contained within that affective experience strengthened overnight, resulting in improved memory for that event, but the autonomic tone "enveloped" around the memory becomes gradually ameliorated (emotional forgetting). Over time, the stored information of the original experience ultimately becomes decoupled and freed of its autonomic "charge," leaving just the salient memory of that emotional experience but without the affective tone previously associated with it at the time of learning.

In summary, the described neuroanatomical, neurophysiological, and neurochemical conditions of REM sleep offer a unique biological theatre in which to achieve a balanced neural potentiation of the informational core of emotional experiences (the memory), yet they may also depotentiate and ultimately ameliorate the autonomic arousing charge originally acquired at the time of learning (the emotion), negating a long-term state of anxiety (see Figure 11.5).

The model compliments previous psychological theories of dreaming by Greenberg (Greenberg, Pearlman, & Gampel, 1972; Greenberg, Pillard, & Pearlman, 1972) and also Cartwright (Cartwright, Agargun, Kirkby, & Friedman, 2006; Cartwright, Kravitz, Eastman, & Wood, 1991; Cartwright, Luten, Young, Mercer, & Bears, 1998), which suggest that the process of REM sleep mental activity aids in the resolution of previous emotional conflict, resulting in reduced next-day negative mood. Moreover, pioneering work by Cartwright and colleagues has demonstrated that not only the occurrence of dreaming but the actual content of dreams play an important role in the recovery from emotional trauma and can be predictive of clinical remission months later (Cartwright et al., 1991, 1998, 2006). Although the current model offers a neurobiological framework for the overnight modulation and alteration of emotional memories and next-day affective brain reactivity, it does not discount the potential contribution that the mental operation of dreaming itself, beyond the electrophysiological underpinnings of REM sleep, may afford to this process.

Emotional Memory Processing: Time (Wake) versus Sleep

Although many studies have described an enhancement of emotional memory across time periods containing sleep (and even when comparing sleep and wake time periods directly), several reports have demonstrated the facilitation of emotional recollection across shorter intervals (up to several hours) that are unlikely to contain sleep (Dolcos et al., 2004; Kensinger, Brierley, Medford, Growdon, & Corkin, 2002; LaBar & Phelps, 1998). This may suggest that sleep represents a preferential, although not exclusive, time when emotion memories are consolidated, and that both time and sleep modulate affective experiences by way of similar underlying mechanisms. For example, theta electrical oscillations throughout subcortical and across cortical areas appear to play an important role in promoting the strengthening and consolidation of emotional memory. Although dominant during REM sleep, such oscillatory activity could occur during the wake state, driven by prior affective learning experience.

Alternatively, however, emotional memories may be modulated by two different mechanisms—one during wake and one during sleep—which at a behavioral level (memory recollection) may appear quantitatively similar but at a mechanistic brain and autonomic-body level are qualitatively different. The contrasting neurobiology of wake and sleep states, especially REM sleep, supports this latter hypothesis. For example, across time awake, emotional memories may be processed and modulated predominately by adrenergic mechanisms, which are prolific during wakefulness (Saper et al., 2001), enabling more shorter term memory benefits without the necessity of sleep. Therefore, suppression of aminergic systems following affective learning blocks these emotional memory improvements (Cahill & McGaugh, 1998; McGaugh, 2004). The second, REM sleep-dependent process, while also facilitating the consolidation of emotional experience, may take place by way of cholinergic modulation in the absence of adrenergic influence. It is in this neurochemical distinction that the qualitative difference between wake and sleep mechanisms may emerge. Specifically, by being processed in a network that is now devoid of adrenergic neurochemistry, the visceral autonomic charge associated with the memory at the time of the emotional learning may be depotentiated during the reactivation and reprocessing of information during REM sleep. As a consequence, not only is the memory representation more robust, leading to enhanced recall, but the strength of the bound autonomic charge will be reduced.

Predictions of the Model

If this process of divorcing emotion from memory is not achieved across the first night following such an experience, the model predicts that a repeat attempt would occur on the second night, because the strength of emotional "tag" associated with the memory would remain high. If this process failed a second time, the same events would continue to repeat across ensuing nights. It is just such a cycle of REM sleep dreaming (nightmares) that represents a diagnostic key feature of PTSD (American Psychiatric Association, 1994). It may not be coincidental, therefore, that these patients continue to display hyperarousal reactions to associated trauma cues (Harvey et al., 2003; Mellman & Hipolito, 2006; Pole, 2007), indicating that the process of separating the affective tone from the emotional experience has not been accomplished. The reason why such a REM mechanism may fail in PTSD remains unknown, although the exceptional magnitude of trauma-induced emotion at the time of learning may be so great that the system is incapable of initiating or completing this process, leaving some patients unable to integrate and depotentiate the stored experience. Alternatively, it may be that the hyperarousal status of the brain during REM sleep in these patients (Harvey et al., 2003; Pole, 2007; Strawn & Geracioti, 2008), potentially suggestive of insufficient aminergic demodulation that prevents the processing and separation of emotion from memory.

This model also makes specific experimental predictions as to the fate of these two components: the memory and the emotion. As partially demonstrated, the first prediction is that, over time, the veracity of the memory itself would improve and the extent to which these [negative] emotional experiences are strengthened would be proportional to the amount of postexperience REM sleep obtained as well as the speed with which it is achieved (REM latency). Second, using autonomic physiology measures, these same predictions would hold in the inverse direction for the magnitude of emotional reactivity induced at the time of recall. Third, a pathological increase in REM (as commonly occurs in depression; Armitage, 2007; Gottesmann & Gottesman, 2007; Tsuno et al., 2005) may disproportionately amplify the strength of negative memories, so much so that, despite concomitant attempts at ameliorating the associated affective tone, it would still create a perceived autobiographical history dominated by negative memory excess (which may also facilitate disadvantageous waking rumination). In contrast, the selective decrease of REM, either experimentally or pharmacologically, would predict a decrease in negative memory consolidation and bias, although it may curtail the degree of affective decoupling that can occur. Long term, the balanced extent of accumulated REM should, therefore, not only correlate with the persistence, in memory, of the emotional experience, but also be associated with a decreased magnitude of autonomic response associated with recall, all of which are testable experimental questions.

Summary

When viewed as a whole, findings at the cellular, systems, cognitive, and clinical levels all point to a crucial role for sleep in the affective modulation of human brain function. Based on the remarkable neurobiology of sleep, and REM in particular, a unique capacity for the overnight modulation of affective networks and previously encountered emotional experiences may be possible, redressing and maintaining the appropriate connectivity and hence next-day reactivity throughout limbic and associated autonomic systems. However, if the canonical architecture and amount of sleep are disrupted, as commonly occur in mood disorders, particularly in major depression and PTSD, this symbiotic alliance of sleep-dependent emotional brain processing may fail. The predicted consequences of this failure appear to support the development and maintenance of a number of clinical symptoms expressed in mood disorders, whereas the sleep changes associated with common pharmacological treatments of these cohorts support a relief of these aberrant overnight processes, all of which lead to experimentally testable, hypothesis-driven future goals. Ultimately, the timeless maternal wisdom of mothers alike may never been more relevant—that is, when troubled, *"get a good night's sleep, and you'll feel better in the morning."*

Acknowledgments

We wish to thank Edwin Robertson, Robert Stickgold, Allison Harvey, and Ninad Gujar for thoughtful insights. This work was supported in part by grants from the National Institutes of Health (No. AG031164) and the American Academy of Sleep Medicine.

References

Ambrosini, M. V., Mariucci, G., Colarieti, L., Bruschelli, G., Carobi, C., & Giuditta, A. (1993). The structure of sleep is related to the learning ability of rats. *European Journal of Neuroscience, 5*(3), 269–275.

Ambrosini, M. V., Sadile, A. G., Gironi Carnevale, U. A., Mattiaccio, M., & Giuditta, A. (1988). The sequential hypothesis on sleep function: I. Evidence that the structure of sleep depends on the nature of the previous waking experience. *Brazilian Journal of Medical and Biological Research, 21*(1), 141–145.

American Psychiatric Association. (1994). *Diagnostic and statistical manual of mental disorders* (4th ed.). Washington, DC: Author.

Amzica, F., & Steriade, M. (1995). Short- and long-range neuronal synchronization of the slow (< 1 Hz) cortical oscillation. *Journal of Neurophysiology, 73*(1), 20–38.

Armitage, R. (2007). Sleep and circadian rhythms in mood disorders. *Acta Psychiatrica Scandinavica Supplement* (433), 104–115.

Aston-Jones, G., & Bloom, F. E. (1981). Activity of norepinephrine-containing locus coeruleus neurons in behaving rats anticipates fluctuations in the sleep–waking cycle. *Journal of Neuroscience, 1*(8), 876–886.

Beaulieu, I., & Godbout, R. (2000). Spatial learning on the Morris Water Maze Test after a short-term paradoxical sleep deprivation in the rat. *Brain and Cognition, 43*(1–3), 27–31.

Berger, M., Doerr, P., Lund, R., Bronisch, T., & von Zerssen, D. (1982). Neuroendocrinological and neurophysiological studies in major depressive disorders: Are there biological markers for the endogenous subtype? *Biological Psychiatry, 17*(11), 1217–1242.

Buysse, D. J. (2004). Insomnia, depression and aging. Assessing sleep and mood interactions in older adults. *Geriatrics, 59*(2), 47–51; quiz, 52.

Buysse, D. J., Frank, E., Lowe, K. K., Cherry, C. R., & Kupfer, D. J. (1997). Electroencephalographic sleep correlates of episode and vulnerability to recurrence in depression. *Biological Psychiatry, 41*(4), 406–418.

Buzsaki, G. (2002). Theta oscillations in the hippocampus. *Neuron, 33*(3), 325–340.

Cahill, L. (2000). Neurobiological mechanisms of emotionally influenced, long-term memory. *Progress in Brain Research, 126*, 29–37.

Cahill, L., & McGaugh, J. L. (1998). Mechanisms of emotional arousal and lasting declarative memory. *Trends in Neuroscience, 21*(7), 294–299.

Callaway, C. W., Lydic, R., Baghdoyan, H. A., & Hobson, J. A. (1987). Pontogeniculooccipital waves: Spontaneous visual system activity during rapid eye movement sleep. *Cellular and Molecular Neurobiology, 7*(2), 105–149.

Cartwright, R., Agargun, M. Y., Kirkby, J., & Friedman, J. K. (2006). Relation of dreams to waking concerns. *Psychiatry Research, 141*(3), 261–270.

Cartwright, R., Luten, A., Young, M., Mercer, P., & Bears, M. (1998). Role of REM sleep and dream affect in overnight mood regulation: A study of normal volunteers. *Psychiatry Research, 81*(1), 1–8.

Cartwright, R. D., Kravitz, H. M., Eastman, C. I., & Wood, E. (1991). REM latency and the recovery from depression: Getting over divorce. *American Journal of Psychiatry, 148*(11), 1530–1535.

Clark, C. P., Brown, G. G., Archibald, S. L., Fennema-Notestine, C., Braun, D. R., Thomas, L. S., et al. (2006). Does amygdalar perfusion correlate with antidepressant response to partial sleep deprivation in major depression? *Psychiatry Research, 146*(1), 43–51.

Davidson, R. J. (2002). Anxiety and affective style: Role of prefrontal cortex and amygdala. *Biological Psychiatry, 51*(1), 68–80.

Davidson, R. J., Pizzagalli, D., Nitschke, J. B., & Putnam, K. (2002). Depression: Perspectives from affective neuroscience. *Annual Review of Psychology, 53*, 545–574.

Davis, C. J., Harding, J. W., & Wright, J. W. (2003). REM sleep deprivation-induced deficits in the latency-to-peak induction and maintenance of long-term potentiation within the CA1 region of the hippocampus. *Brain Research, 973*(2), 293–297.

Dinges, D. F., Pack, F., Williams, K., Gillen, K. A., Powell, J. W., Ott, G. E., et al. (1997). Cumulative sleepiness, mood disturbance, and psychomotor vigilance performance decrements during a week of sleep restricted to 4–5 hours per night. *Sleep, 20*(4), 267–277.

Dolcos, F., LaBar, K. S., & Cabeza, R. (2004). Interaction between the amygdala and the medial temporal lobe memory system predicts better memory for emotional events. *Neuron, 42*, 855–863.

Dolcos, F., LaBar, K. S., & Cabeza, R. (2005). Remembering one year later: Role of the amygdala and the medial temporal lobe memory system in retrieving emotional memories. *Proceedings of the National Academy of Sciences USA, 102*(7), 2626–2631.

Fishbein, W., Kastaniotis, C., & Chattman, D. (1974). Paradoxical sleep: Prolonged augmentation following learning. *Brain Research, 79*(1), 61–75.

Giedke, H., & Schwarzler, F. (2002). Therapeutic use of sleep deprivation in depression. *Sleep Medicine Reviews, 6*(5), 361–377.

Giles, D. E., Jarrett, R. B., Roffwarg, H. P., & Rush, A. J. (1987). Reduced rapid eye movement latency: A predictor of recurrence in depression. *Neuropsychopharmacology, 1*(1), 33–39.

Gillin, J. C., Duncan, W., Pettigrew, K. D., Frankel, B. L., & Snyder, F. (1979). Successful separation of depressed, normal, and insomniac subjects by EEG sleep data. *Archives of General Psychiatry, 36*(1), 85–90.

Gottesmann, C., & Gottesman, I. (2007). The neurobiological characteristics of rapid eye movement (REM) sleep are candidate endophenotypes of depression, schizophrenia, mental retardation and dementia. *Progress in Neurobiology, 81*(4), 237–250.

Graves, L. A., Heller, E. A., Pack, A. I., & Abel, T. (2003). Sleep deprivation selectively impairs memory consolidation for contextual fear conditioning. *Learning and Memory, 10*(3), 168–176.

Greenberg, R., Pearlman, C. A., & Gampel, D. (1972). War neuroses and the adaptive function of REM sleep. *British Journal of Medical Psychology, 45*(1), 27–33.

Greenberg, R., Pillard, R., & Pearlman, C. (1972). The effect of dream (stage REM) deprivation on adaptation to stress. *Psychosomatic Medicine, 34*(3), 257–262.

Gruart-Masso, A., Nadal-Alemany, R., Coll-Andreu, M., Portell-Cortes, I., & Marti-Nicolovius, M. (1995). Effects of pretraining paradoxical sleep deprivation upon two-way active avoidance. *Behavioural Brain Research, 72*(1–2), 181–183.

Grunhaus, L., Shipley, J. E., Eiser, A., Pande, A. C., Tandon, R., Remen, A., et al. (1994). Shortened REM latency PostECT is associated with rapid recurrence of depressive symptomatology. *Biology Psychiatry, 36*(4), 214–222.

Harrison, Y., & Horne, J. A. (2000). Sleep loss and temporal memory. *Quarterly Journal of Experimental Psychology, 53*(1), 271–279.

Harvey, A. G. (2001). Insomnia: Symptom or diagnosis? *Clinical Psychology Review, 21*(7), 1037–1059.

Harvey, A. G., Jones, C., & Schmidt, D. A. (2003). Sleep and posttraumatic stress disorder: A review. *Clinical Psychology Review, 23*(3), 377–407.

Hennevin, E., & Hars, B. (1987). Is increase in post-learning paradoxical sleep modified by cueing? *Behavioural Brain Research, 24*(3), 243–249.

Hobson, J. A., McCarley, R. W., & Wyzinski, P. W. (1975). Sleep cycle oscillation: Reciprocal discharge by two brainstem neuronal groups. *Science, 189*, 55–58.

Horne, J. A. (1985). Sleep function, with particular reference to sleep deprivation. *Annals of Clinical Research, 17*(5), 199–208.

Hu, P., Stylos-Allen, M., & Walker, M. P. (2006). Sleep facilitates consolidation of emotionally arousing declarative memory. *Psychological Science, 17*(10), 891–898.

Jones, M. W., & Wilson, M. A. (2005). Theta rhythms coordinate hippocampal-prefrontal interactions in a spatial memory task. *PLoS Biology, 3*(12), e402.

Kametani, H., & Kawamura, H. (1990). Alterations in acetylcholine release in the rat hippocampus during sleep-wakefulness detected by intracerebral dialysis. *Life Sciences, 47*(5), 421–426.

Kensinger, E. A., Brierley, B., Medford, N., Growdon, J. H., & Corkin, S. (2002). Effects of normal aging and Alzheimer's disease on emotional memory. *Emotion, 2*(2), 118–134.

Kilpatrick, L., & Cahill, L. (2003). Amygdala modulation of parahippocampal and frontal regions during emotionally influenced memory storage. *NeuroImage, 20*(4), 2091–2099.

Kleinsmith, L. J., & Kaplan, S. (1963). Paired-associate learning as a function of arousal and interpolated interval. *Journal of Experimental Psychology, 65*, 190–193.

Koren, D., Arnon, I., Lavie, P., & Klein, E. (2002). Sleep complaints as early predictors of posttraumatic stress disorder: A 1-year prospective study of injured survivors of motor vehicle accidents. *American Journal of Psychiatry, 159*(5), 855–857.

Kupfer, D. J., Frank, E., McEachran, A. B., & Grochocinski, V. J. (1990). Delta sleep ratio. A biological correlate of early recurrence in unipolar affective disorder. *Archives of General Psychiatry, 47*(12), 1100–1105.

LaBar, K. S., & Phelps, E. A. (1998). Arousal-mediated memory consolidation: Role of the medial temporal lobe in humans. *Psychological Science, 9*, 490–493.

Levonian, E. (1972). Retention over time in relation to arousal during learning: an explanation of discrepant results. *Acta Psychologica, 36*(4), 290–321.

Llinas, R., & Ribary, U. (1993). Coherent 40-Hz oscillation characterizes dream state in humans. *Proceedings of the National Academy of Sciences USA, 90*(5), 2078–2081.

Lydic, R., & Baghdoyan, H. A. (1988). *Handbook of behavioral state control: Cellular and molecular mechanisms.* Boca Raton, FL: CRC Press.

Mandai, O., Guerrien, A., Sockeel, P., Dujardin, K., & Leconte, P. (1989). REM sleep modifications following a Morse code learning session in humans. *Physiology and Behavior, 46*(4), 759–762.

Marrosu, F., Portas, C., Mascia, M. S., Casu, M. A., Fa, M., Giagheddu, M., et al. (1995). Microdialysis measurement of cortical and hippocampal acetylcholine release during sleep-wake cycle in freely moving cats. *Brain Research, 671*(2), 329–332.

Marshall, L., & Born, J. (2007). The contribution of sleep to hippocampus-dependent memory consolidation. *Trends in Cognitive Science, 11*(10), 442–450.

Marti-Nicolovius, M., Portell-Cortes, I., & Morgado-Bernal, I. (1988). Improvement of shuttle-box avoidance following post-training treatment in paradoxical sleep deprivation platforms in rats. *Physiology and Behavior, 43*(1), 93–98.

McDermott, C. M., LaHoste, G. J., Chen, C., Musto, A., Bazan, N. G., & Magee, J. C.

(2003). Sleep deprivation causes behavioral, synaptic, and membrane excitability alterations in hippocampal neurons. *Journal of Neuroscience, 23*(29), 9687–9695.

McGaugh, J. L. (2004). The amygdala modulates the consolidation of memories of emotionally arousing experiences. *Annual Review of Neuroscience, 27*, 1–28.

McGrath, M. J., & Cohen, D. B. (1978). REM sleep facilitation of adaptive waking behavior: A review of the literature. *Psychological Bulletin, 85*(1), 24–57.

Mellman, T. A., Bustamante, V., Fins, A. I., Pigeon, W. R., & Nolan, B. (2002). REM sleep and the early development of posttraumatic stress disorder. *American Journal of Psychiatry, 159*(10), 1696–1701.

Mellman, T. A., & Hipolito, M. M. (2006). Sleep disturbances in the aftermath of trauma and posttraumatic stress disorder. *CNS Spectrums, 11*(8), 611–615.

Morgan, M. A., Romanski, L. M., & LeDoux, J. E. (1993). Extinction of emotional learning: Contribution of medial prefrontal cortex. *Neuroscience Letters, 163*(1), 109–113.

Morris, G. O., Williams, H. L., & Lubin, A. (1960). Misperception and disorientation during sleep. *Archives of General Psychiatry, 2*, 247–254.

New, A. S., Hazlett, E. A., Buchsbaum, M. S., Goodman, M., Mitelman, S. A., Newmark, R., et al. (2007). Amygdala-prefrontal disconnection in borderline personality disorder. *Neuropsychopharmacology, 32*(7), 1629–1640.

Nishida, M., Pearsall, J., Buckner, R. L., & Walker, M. P. (2009). REM sleep, prefrontal theta, and the consolidation of human emotional memory. *Cerebral Cortex, 19*, 1158–1166.

Nofzinger, E. A. (2005). Functional neuroimaging of sleep. *Seminars in Neurology, 25*(1), 9–18.

Nofzinger, E. A., Price, J. C., Meltzer, C. C., Buysse, D. J., Villemagne, V. L., Miewald, J. M., et al. (2000). Towards a neurobiology of dysfunctional arousal in depression: The relationship between beta EEG power and regional cerebral glucose metabolism during NREM sleep. *Psychiatry, 98*(2), 71–91.

Nofzinger, E. A., Schwartz, R. M., Reynolds, C. F., III, Thase, M. E., Jennings, J. R., Frank, E., et al. (1994). Affect intensity and phasic REM sleep in depressed men before and after treatment with cognitive-behavioral therapy. *Journal of Consulting and Clinical Psychology, 62*(1), 83–91.

Ochsner, K. N., & Gross, J. J. (2005). The cognitive control of emotion. *Trends in Cognitive Science, 9*(5), 242–249.

Ohayon, M. M. (2007). Insomnia: A ticking clock for depression? *Journal of Psychiatric Research, 41*(11), 893–894.

Oniani, T. N., Lortkipanidze, N. D., & Maisuradze, L. M. (1987). Interaction between learning and paradoxical sleep in cats. *Neuroscience and Behavioral Physiology, 17*(4), 304–310.

Pace-Schott, E. F., & Hobson, J. A. (2002). The neurobiology of sleep: Genetics, cellular physiology and subcortical networks. *Nature Reviews Neuroscience, 3*(8), 591–605.

Pare, D., Collins, D. R., & Pelletier, J. G. (2002). Amygdala oscillations and the consolidation of emotional memories. *Trends in Cognitive Science, 6*(7), 306–314.

Pearlman, C. A. (1969). Effect of rapid eye movement (dreaming) sleep deprivation on retention of avoidance learning in rats (Rep. No. 563). *Report (U.S. Naval Submarine Medical Center)*, pp. 1–4.

Perlis, M. L., Smith, L. J., Lyness, J. M., Matteson, S. R., Pigeon, W. R., Jungquist,

C. R., et al. (2006). Insomnia as a risk factor for onset of depression in the elderly. *Behavioral Sleep Medicine, 4*(2), 104–113.

Phelps, E. A. (2004). Human emotion and memory: Interactions of the amygdala and hippocampal complex. *Current Opinions in Neurobiology, 14,* 198–202.

Pole, N. (2007). The psychophysiology of posttraumatic stress disorder: A meta-analysis. *Psychological Bulletin, 133*(5), 725–746.

Power, A. E. (2004). Muscarinic cholinergic contribution to memory consolidation: With attention to involvement of the basolateral amygdala. *Current Medicinal Chemistry, 11*(8), 987–996.

Rechtschaffen, A., & Kales, A. (1968). *A manual of standardized terminology, techniques and scoring system for sleep stages of human subjects.* Bethesda, MD: Department of Health.

Rush, A. J., Giles, D. E., Jarrett, R. B., Feldman-Koffler, F., Debus, J. R., Weissenburger, J., et al. (1989). Reduced REM latency predicts response to tricyclic medication in depressed outpatients. *Biological Psychiatry, 26*(1), 61–72.

Sanford, L. D., Silvestri, A. J., Ross, R. J., & Morrison, A. R. (2001). Influence of fear conditioning on elicited ponto-geniculo-occipital waves and rapid eye movement sleep. *Archives Italiennes de Biologie, 139*(3), 169–183.

Sanford, L. D., Tang, X., Ross, R. J., & Morrison, A. R. (2003). Influence of shock training and explicit fear-conditioned cues on sleep architecture in mice: Strain comparison. *Behavior Genetics, 33*(1), 43–58.

Saper, C. B., Chou, T. C., & Scammell, T. E. (2001). The sleep switch: Hypothalamic control of sleep and wakefulness. *Trends in Neuroscience, 24*(12), 726–731.

Shaffery, J., Hoffmann, R., & Armitage, R. (2003). The neurobiology of depression: Perspectives from animal and human sleep studies. *Neuroscientist, 9*(1), 82–98.

Sharot, T., & Phelps, E. A. (2004). How arousal modulates memory: Disentangling the effects of attention and retention. *Cognitive, Affective and Behavioral Neuroscience, 4*(3), 294–306.

Shima, K., Nakahama, H., & Yamamoto, M. (1986). Firing properties of two types of nucleus raphe dorsalis neurons during the sleep–waking cycle and their responses to sensory stimuli. *Brain Research, 399*(2), 317–326.

Shiromani, P., Gutwein, B. M., & Fishbein, W. (1979). Development of learning and memory in mice after brief paradoxical sleep deprivation. *Physiology and Behavior, 22*(5), 971–978.

Smith, C. (1985). Sleep states and learning: A review of the animal literature. *Neuroscience and Biobehavioral Reviews, 9*(2), 157–168.

Smith, C., & Kelly, G. (1988). Paradoxical sleep deprivation applied two days after end of training retards learning. *Physiology and Behavior, 43*(2), 213–216.

Smith, C., & Lapp, L. (1986). Prolonged increases in both PS and number of REMS following a shuttle avoidance task. *Physiology and Behavior, 36*(6), 1053–1057.

Smith, C., Young, J., & Young, W. (1980). Prolonged increases in paradoxical sleep during and after avoidance-task acquisition. *Sleep, 3*(1), 67–81.

Sotres-Bayon, F., Bush, D. E., & LeDoux, J. E. (2004). Emotional perseveration: An update on prefrontal-amygdala interactions in fear extinction. *Learning and Memory, 11*(5), 525–535.

Steriade, M., & Amzica, F. (1998). Coalescence of sleep rhythms and their chronology in corticothalamic networks. *Sleep Research Online, 1*(1), 1–10.

Steriade, M., Amzica, F., & Contreras, D. (1996). Synchronization of fast (30–40

Hz) spontaneous cortical rhythms during brain activation. *Journal of Neuroscience, 16*(1), 392–417.

Strawn, J. R., & Geracioti, T. D., Jr. (2008). Noradrenergic dysfunction and the psychopharmacology of posttraumatic stress disorder. *Depression and Anxiety, 25*(3), 260–271.

Sullivan, G. M., Coplan, J. D., Kent, J. M., & Gorman, J. M. (1999). The noradrenergic system in pathological anxiety: A focus on panic with relevance to generalized anxiety and phobias. *Biological Psychiatry, 46*(9), 1205–1218.

Tsuno, N., Besset, A., & Ritchie, K. (2005). Sleep and depression. *Journal of Clinical Psychiatry, 66*(10), 1254–1269.

Vazquez, J., & Baghdoyan, H. A. (2001). Basal forebrain acetylcholine release during REM sleep is significantly greater than during waking. *American Journal of Physiology: Regulatory, Integrative and Comparative Physiology, 280*(2), R598–601.

Wagner, U., Gais, S., & Born, J. (2001). Emotional memory formation is enhanced across sleep intervals with high amounts of rapid eye movement sleep. *Learning and Memory, 8*(2), 112–119.

Wagner, U., Hallschmid, M., Rasch, B., & Born, J. (2006). Brief sleep after learning keeps emotional memories alive for years. *Biological Psychiatry, 60*(7), 788–790.

Walker, E. L., & Tarte, R. D. (1963). Memory storage as a function of arousal and time with homogeneous and heterogeneous lists. *Journal of Verbal Learning and Verbal Behavior, 2*, 113–119.

Walker, M. P., & Stickgold, R. (2004). Sleep-dependent learning and memory consolidation. *Neuron, 44*, 121–133.

Walker, M. P., & Stickgold, R. (2006). Sleep, memory and plasticity. *Annual Review of Psychology, 10*(57), 139–166.

Waller, D. A., Hardy, B. W., Pole, R., Giles, D., Gullion, C. M., Rush, A. J., et al. (1989). Sleep EEG in bulimic, depressed, and normal subjects. *Biological Psychiatry, 25*(5), 661–664.

Winokur, A., Gary, K. A., Rodner, S., Rae-Red, C., Fernando, A. T., & Szuba, M. P. (2001). Depression, sleep physiology, and antidepressant drugs. *Depression and Anxiety, 14*(1), 19–28.

Wirz-Justice, A., & Van den Hoofdakker, R. H. (1999). Sleep deprivation in depression: What do we know, where do we go? *Biological Psychiatry, 46*(4), 445–453.

Wu, J. C., & Bunney, W. E. (1990). The biological basis of an antidepressant response to sleep deprivation and relapse: Review and hypothesis. *American Journal of Psychiatry, 147*(1), 14–21.

Yoo, S. S., Gujar, N., Hu, P., Jolesz, F. A., & Walker, M. P. (2007). The human emotional brain without sleep—A prefrontal amygdala disconnect. *Current Biology, 17*(20), R877–R878.

Yoo, S. S., Hu, P. T., Gujar, N., Jolesz, F. A., & Walker, M. P. (2007). A deficit in the ability to form new human memories without sleep. *Nature Neuroscience, 10*(3), 385–392.

Zohar, D., Tzischinsky, O., Epstein, R., & Lavie, P. (2005). The effects of sleep loss on medical residents' emotional reactions to work events: A cognitive-energy model. *Sleep, 28*(1), 47–54.

PART III

Treatment of Problems
in Emotion Regulation

CHAPTER 12

Emotions, Emotion Regulation, and Psychological Treatment

A UNIFIED PERSPECTIVE

Christopher P. Fairholme, Christina L. Boisseau,
Kristen K. Ellard, Jill T. Ehrenreich, and David H. Barlow

We begin this chapter by presenting how emotion is conceptualized within the unified protocol for the treatment of emotional disorders (Barlow et al., 2008), a transdiagnostic approach to psychological intervention, briefly reviewing emotion theory and research most relevant to this treatment. Following this, we outline the process model of emotion regulation (Gross, 1998, 2002; Gross & Thompson, 2007) and how this model is conceptualized in regard to the unified protocol, highlighting (1) how emotion regulation processes become maladaptive across the emotional disorders and (2) the extant research supporting this model. We then outline the intervention components specified in the unified protocol that map directly onto the theoretical model of emotion regulation and discuss how we operationalize and track progress during treatment. We present a case example to illustrate how these intervention components are practically implemented during treatment. Finally, we briefly discuss future directions for our work, specifically in continuing our investigations on emotional processes, as we work toward evaluation and eventual dissemination of the unified protocol.

A Unified Treatment Protocol

The unified protocol was developed to be applicable to all anxiety and unipolar mood disorders and possibly other disorders with strong emotional components such as many somatoform and dissociative disorders. Since its introduction in 2004 (Barlow, Allen, & Choate, 2004), this treatment has undergone several revisions consistent with developments in the field of emotion science and experiences of our own research group. Here we present and illustrate the main components of the current, modular version of our protocol (Barlow et al., 2008).

Grounded in traditional cognitive-behavioral principles, the protocol is unique in the particular emphasis placed on the way individuals with emotional disorders experience and respond to their emotions. The unified protocol is based upon the premise that the ways in which individuals with anxiety and mood disorders experience and respond to their emotions represents an underlying, unifying factor across these disorders. Specifically, individuals with these disorders tend to experience negative affect more frequently and more intensely than healthy individuals (e.g., Campbell-Sills & Barlow, 2007) and tend to view these experiences as more aversive (e.g., Roemer, Salters, Raffa, & Orsillo, 2005), a point we return to in further detail later in this chapter. Clinical experience suggests that aversive reactions to emotional experiences in these disorders may not be limited to negative emotions but may also include positive emotions. For example, positive emotions have been observed to paradoxically trigger negative experiences in some individuals, such as eliciting anxious reactions as one "waits for the other shoe to drop." As such, inappropriate processing of a full range of emotional experiences plays a role in the development and maintenance of symptoms in anxiety and mood disorders. Treatment is designed to help patients learn how to confront and experience uncomfortable emotions and develop ways to respond to those emotions in more adaptive ways. By adjusting patients' emotional regulation habits, this treatment aims to reduce the intensity and incidence of disordered emotions, reduce impairment, and improve functioning.

Emotions in the Unified Protocol

In the unified protocol, emotions are viewed as essential phenomena that help organize behavior in service of people's goals, allowing individuals to navigate their environment and meet situational demands (Barlow, 2002; Campbell-Sills & Barlow, 2007; Gross & Thompson, 2007). At any given time, these goals may be immediate (survival), ongoing (well-being), or long term (security, reproduction). As such, emotions are viewed in their primary state as functional and adaptive (e.g., Barlow, 1988; Levenson, 1994). Emotions function to interrupt ongoing cognitive processes or behavior, redirect attention to stimuli relevant to the preservation of goal-directed states, and trigger action tendencies in service of these goals (Fridja, 1986). Whereas delineating the functional role of emotions can be relatively straightforward, defining emotion is somewhat more complex. As

Gross and Thompson (2007) describe, emotions are "famously difficult to pin down" (p. 4). A concise, all-inclusive definition of emotion is often elusive because discrete emotions themselves represent a wide and incredibly variable array of experiences (Barlow, 1988; Gross & Thompson, 2007).

In the unified treatment, emotions are not limited to discrete categories of experience; rather, they are conceptualized as emergent phenomena resulting from the dynamic interaction of three modes of responding: cognitions, behaviors (or action tendencies), and physiological sensations (Izard, 1993; Lang, 1979, 1985; Mauss, Levenson, McCarter, Wilhelm, & Gross, 2005). As such, the unified treatment follows a "modal" model of emotion (Barrett, Ochsner, & Gross, 2007; Gross & Thompson, 2007). Emotion generation and regulation may be initiated from any one of these three modes (Berkowitz & Harmon-Jones, 2004; Duclos et al., 1989; Ochsner et al., 2004; Riskind & Gotay, 1982; Schacter & Singer, 1962; Siemer, Mauss, & Gross, 2007; Stepper & Strack, 1993) and emerge as a result of ongoing implicit and explicit appraisals as to the relevance and significance of both external stimuli and internal experiences to the attainment of individual goals (Arnold, 1960; Ellsworth & Scherer, 2003; Fridja, 1986; Scherer, 2001; Siemer & Reisenzein, 2007).

The dynamic nature of the relationship among the modes of cognition, physiological responses, and action tendencies conceptualized in the unified treatment departs somewhat from traditional dual-processing approaches to emotion and is more in line with recent extensions of the modal model (e.g., Barrett et al., 2007). Traditional dual-processing models suggest that two distinct forms of processing are involved in the generation of emotional experiences: automatic and controlled. Emotions are the result of the interaction between the two such that automatic, subconscious, reflexive processing is modulated by more conscious, systematic, controlled processing. This suggests that more conscious processes, such as thoughts, serve to control more automatically generated feelings and behaviors. In the unified treatment, however, thoughts, behaviors, and feelings are viewed as dynamic and interacting, each contributing to and influencing emotional experiences. In support of this view, newer models, emerging from both behavioral studies and accumulating evidence from cognitive neuroscience, suggest the absence of a controlled–automatic distinction and indicate instead that emotions emerge out of parallel processing along an automatic–controlled continuum (Barrett et al., 2007; Siemer et al., 2007).

Parallel processing models also support the idea that emotion generation can proceed from any one of the three domains of thoughts, feelings, or behaviors (Barlow, 2002; Lang, 1985), a concept that is, in turn, supported by behavioral evidence of the influence of cognitive appraisals (e.g., Siemer et al., 2007), behaviors (Duclos et al., 1989; Riskind & Gotay, 1982; Stepper & Strack, 1993), and physiological sensations (Levitt, Brown, Orsillo, & Barlow, 2004; Schacter & Singer, 1962; Veleber &

Templer, 1984) on emotion generation. Importantly, these models also allow for the possibility of both bottom-up and top-down generation of emotional experiences. They depart from the idea that emotions emerge primarily out of automatic, stimulus-driven responses and permit a greater role for controlled, cognitive processes and behaviors in the production of emotion, lending support to a more dynamic model of emotion generation. In support of this idea, recent neuroimaging studies by Ochsner and colleagues (Ochsner, Bunge, Gross, & Gabrieli, 2002; Ochsner et al., 2004) demonstrated that conscious, controlled, cognitive appraisals can directly influence activation of limbic structures implicated in the generation of emotional responses.

Recent extensions of the modal model of emotion, based on the premise of parallel processing, are particularly illustrative of the ways in which emotional experiences may emerge from dynamic interactions among thoughts, feelings, and behaviors. Barrett and colleagues' (2007) *constraint–satisfaction* model of emotion suggests that automatic and controlled processes combine in a componential fashion, whereby bottom-up, stimulus driven and top-down, goal-driven processes comprise a heterogeneous network that together form coherent interpretations of events and determine plans of action. In this model, emotions represent the final "solution" arrived at through parallel processing networks. Possible interpretations of stimuli are *constrained* at each level of processing that proceeds, for example, from evaluating the emotional and motivational significance of stimuli (amygdala, ventral striatum), to interpreting the meaning of stimuli by comparing and determining a match between current and past situational contexts (hippocampus), to determining situationally appropriate behavior based on learned experience and instrumental action (orbitofrontal cortex), to reflecting on and drawing inferences from one's affective state and behavioral intentions or interpreting the affective state or intentions of others (medial prefrontal cortex), to monitoring conflicts between competing response tendencies (dorsal anterior cingulate), to coordinating responses by implementing control processes such as narrowing attention and coordinating motor responses (dorsolateral prefrontal cortex), and ultimately bringing behavior in line with goals (Barrett et al., 2007). Parallel connections between structures throughout these distributed networks suggest that emotional processing proceeds in a dynamic, feedback, and feed-forward fashion.

Understanding the dynamic interaction of both top-down and bottom-up generation of emotional experiences has particular clinical relevance. Many patients describe their emotional experiences as overwhelming or out of control. However, the emotions described may be generated from both bottom-up and top-down processes. As Barrett and colleagues' (2007) indicate, emotions generated from bottom-up processes tend to be experienced as happening *to* individuals, causing them to act or feel in certain ways. However, emotions may also emerge from, or be compounded by, top-down processes. Many of the emotional experiences individuals with anxiety and mood disorders describe are intensified by the top-down generation of emotional responses through processes such as judgmental or self-critical thinking, rejection of emotional experiences, worry, rumination, or the engagement of cognitive "thinking traps." Increasing patients' awareness of the ways in which these processes serve to intensify their emotional experiences may help to reduce the compounding effect of top-down generated emotional experiences and bring factors contributing toward bottom-up generated experiences into greater awareness. In addition, increasing awareness of the ways in which thoughts, feelings, and behaviors interact in the emergence of emotional experiences allows individuals to make adjustments in each of these domains in more adaptive ways, a topic discussed in greater detail in the next section.

Emotion Regulation in the Unified Protocol

Defining and differentiating emotions and emotion regulation are central issues for the study of emotion regulation and psychopathology, and the theoretical separation and empirical delineation of these ostensibly interdependent constructs remain important tasks for researchers (Gross & Thompson, 2007; Kring & Werner, 2004). We consider emotion and emotion regulation to be theoretically separable constructs. However, from a practical perspective within the unified protocol, we consider them to be interdependent constructs. This is because individuals with emotional disorders presenting for treatment are experiencing emotions that have become disordered, largely because of the ways in which they have gone about trying to regulate their emotions. In this case, we view emotion regulation as referring to the modification of any aspect of an emotional response, including the valence, intensity, duration, and expression of the emotion. Such processes occur at multiple degrees of conscious awareness, with varying levels of control processes involved. Both positive and negative emotions serve as targets for such processes, while the amplification, attenuation, and maintenance of such emotions are the goals.

Despite such an all-encompassing definition, much of the research on the role of emotion regulation in psychopathology has focused on attenuating or down-regulating negative emotions. Increasing evidence suggests that certain forms of psychopathology are marked not just by an excess of negative emotions but also by a paucity of positive emotions, particularly depression and social phobia (Brown, 2007; Brown, Chorpita, & Barlow, 1998; Kashdan, 2007). Additional research on the role of positive emotions and their regulation will undoubtedly further our understanding of psychopathology and enrich existing interventions for several disorders, including bipolar disorder (Ehrenreich, Fairholme, Buzzella, Ellard, & Barlow, 2007). With this in mind, for the purposes of this chapter, we primarily focus on the down-regulation of negative emotions in our discussion, because this has received the majority of attention in the research on emotion regulation and psychopathology.

Emotion regulation is a dynamic process that unfolds over time and often involves multiple or iterative attempts to regulate emotions as they unfold. The process model of emotion regulation (Gross, 1998, 2002; Gross & Thompson, 2007) identifies five separate components of the emotion regulation process or points at which regulation strategies can be used: (1) situation selection, (2) situation modification, (3) attentional deployment, (4) cognitive change, and (5) response modulation. These five intervention points provide a useful heuristic in defining how emotion regulation processes are targeted across the range of emotional disorders with the unified protocol.

Treatment and Assessment of Emotion Regulation Components in the Unified Protocol

Treatment from the perspective of the unified protocol maps onto the process model of emotion regulation. Moreover, each of the five emotion regulation components identified within Gross's process model are directly targeted with a total of seven different modules in the unified protocol. A modularized approach to treatment is relatively new to the unified protocol and represents a recent modification from previous presentations (Allen, McHugh, & Barlow, 2008; Barlow et al., 2004; Ehrenreich, Buzzella, & Barlow, 2007). As currently conceived, the modular approach consists of seven modules that progressively build on one another. Functional assessment, coupled with a focus on emotions and emotion regulation, serves as a common thread across the different modules, tying together concepts and providing coherence across the flexible structure. For the purposes of initial treatment validation, all seven modules are administered in a set order to ensure that the same treatment components are being evaluated across patients. However, each treatment module has a suggested range for number of sessions required to complete the module, allowing the unified protocol to be flexibly administered based on the specific needs of the patient. Ultimately, the modular approach provides for the intriguing possibility of fully tailoring treatment to the specific pattern of emotion regulation deficits for a particular patient. Although further research is needed before such an approach is feasible or prudent, initial attempts at developing assessment procedures are currently underway.

We now discuss each of the components of the process model in turn, highlighting how each process can become maladaptive across the emotional disorders (Figure 12.1), how the process is targeted in treatment within the unified protocol (Figure 12.2), and how progress is monitored during the course of treatment (Table 12.1). Following this presentation,

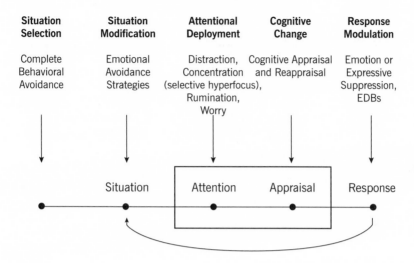

FIGURE 12.1. Emotion regulation in the unified protocol (EDBs, emotion-driven behaviors).

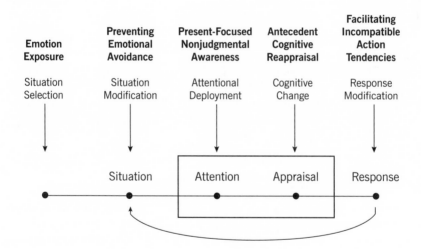

FIGURE 12.2. Interventions targeting emotion regulation in the unified protocol.

TABLE 12.1. Assessment of Emotion Regulation Components in the Unified Protocol

Emotion regulation component	Assessment measure
Situation selection	Emotional Avoidance Hierarchy (EAH)
Situation modification	Emotional Avoidance Strategy Inventory (EASI)
	Checklist for Emotional Avoidance Strategy Engagement (CEASE)
	Idiographic patient self-monitoring form
Attentional deployment	Penn State Worry Questionnaire (PSWQ)
	Ruminative Response Scale (RRS)
	Trait Meta-Mood Scale (TMMS)—Attention to Feelings subscale
	TMMS—Clarity in Discrimination of Feelings subscale
Cognitive change	Emotion Regulation Questionnaire (ERQ)— Reappraisal subscale
Response modulation	ERQ—Suppression subscale

we illustrate how these principles are applied based on a case treated in our setting using the unified protocol. For the purposes of this chapter, the modules are presented in an order consistent with the process model of emotion regulation (Gross & Thompson, 2007), although this is not the order that treatment typically progresses (see Case Illustration and Future Directions sections, as well as Barlow et al., 2008, for further discussion).

Situation Selection and Emotion Exposure

Maladaptive Situation Selection

Situational avoidance is an emotion regulation strategy commonly used among individuals with emotional disorders. For instance, an individual who experiences anxiety in social situations might decline a party invitation in an attempt to avoid the embarrassment she believes entering such a situation will elicit. Similarly, in panic disorder, individuals will avoid situations where the perceived likelihood of experiencing fear or fear-related physical reactions is high, such as enclosed spaces, drinking caffeine, or exercising. Individuals with generalized anxiety disorder (GAD) might put off opening and paying bills in order to avoid the anxiety triggered by worries of not having enough money to pay the bills. In the short term, situational avoidance provides an immediate sense of relief or an immediate reduction in negative affect. Thus, the avoidance behavior is negatively reinforced for the immediate, temporary reduction in negative affect it provides the individual in a given situation. However, the long-term consequences become problematic, because avoidance prevents the normative process of habituation from occurring, leading to impairment and interference in daily living and an overall reduction in quality of life (Barlow et al., 2004).

Treatment

Maladaptive situation selection is a hallmark of the emotional disorders and often results in significant impairment in people's lives. This emotion regulation component is directly targeted in the unified protocol using situationally based emotion exposure. Substantial evidence supports the efficacy of situational exposure in treating anxiety and mood disorders (Barlow, Gorman, Shear, & Woods, 2000; Borkovec & Ruscio, 2001; Dimidjian et al., 2006; Foa et al., 1999, 2005; Heimberg et al., 1998). As traditionally carried out, exposure therapy has focused on exposing individuals to feared situations as a way of facilitating fear extinction, viewing the external situation as the primary context under which the original fear learning took place. Thus, exposures would proceed in a hierarchical fashion, exposing individuals to different situations to buttress the new learning that was taking place in previously avoided situations. Emotion exposures differ in that the focus of the exposure is the emotional experience itself that arises in these situations. The emotional experience is conceptualized as the context under which new learning must occur and situations are highlighted only to the extent that they trigger emotions. Within the unified protocol, emotion exposures proceed in a hierarchical fashion, beginning in early sessions with exposure to nonspecific (or clinically irrelevant) emotion cues (Allen et al., 2008) and progressing toward exposure to situations that evoke stronger or more uncomfortable emotions. Key considerations when conducting such emotion exposures include eliminating concurrent emotional avoidance strategies (including maladaptive situation modification and attentional deployment emotion regulation attempts) and eliciting authentic emotions.

Assessment

In the unified protocol, the emotional avoidance hierarchy (EAH; Ehrenreich et al., 2008) is used to track progress over the course of treatment and to help guide and structure situational emotion exposures over the latter stages of treatment. The EAH was adapted based on the traditional fear and avoidance hierarchy that is commonly used to identify situations that the individual is apprehensive of and avoiding in anxiety disorders (e.g., Barlow & Craske, 2007). The EAH asks patients to list situations or events that might produce strong or uncomfortable emotions for them. They then rate the intensity of the emotion that these situations produce and the extent to which they are avoiding them currently. Although some nomothetic measures of situational avoidance do exist (e.g., Albany Panic and Phobia Questionnaire; Rapee, Craske, & Barlow, 1995), they tend to be disorder specific and do not lend themselves well to assessing outcome across the range of emotional disorders. Thus, the EAH was adopted as an idiographic measure of situational avoidance in order to monitor progress over the course of treatment.

Situation Modification and Preventing Emotional Avoidance

Maladaptive Situation Modification

Once the situation has been entered or if a situation/encounter is unavoidable, individuals with emotional disorders will sometimes attempt to modify the situation in order to make their emotions more manageable. Safety behaviors, a form of situation modification, are ubiquitous across the emotional disorders. For instance, individuals who experience panic disorder will often carry items (e.g., cell phone, medication) with them into a feared situation in order to reduce the anxiety and fear they experience in the situation and to make the situation itself more manageable (Barlow & Craske, 2007). Persons with social anxiety often rehearse precisely what they will say prior to having a conversation or giving a speech. An individual with GAD might set a wristwatch alarm to help manage anxiety associated with worry about being late for an appointment.

The use of situation modification or safety signals as an emotion regulation strategy has been found to be associated with poorer outcomes, including increased negative affect, reduced habituation, and poorer treatment response (Kim, 2005; Salkovskis, 1991; Salkovskis, Clark, Hackmann, Wells, & Gelder, 1999; Sloan & Telch, 2002; Wells et al., 1995). In a randomized controlled trial (RCT), Powers, Smits, and Telch (2004) randomized individuals meeting diagnostic criteria for specific fear of enclosed spaces to one of three conditions: (1) exposure with no safety behavior available, (2) exposure with safety behavior utilization, and (3) exposure with safety behavior availability. Response rates at posttreatment were 94% for the no safety behavior condition versus 45% and 44% for the safety behavior availability and utilization conditions, respectively. This suggests that maladaptive situation modification can be both behavioral (e.g., opening an air vent while locked in a box) and cognitive (e.g., knowing that one *could* open an air vent if the emotions become "too intense" or overwhelming), in that an "unmanageable situation" becomes manageable with the knowledge that help is available, not simply with the actual use of such strategies.

It is interesting to note that there is some preliminary evidence that the "judicious use" of safety behaviors can have facilitative effects on treatment retention and perhaps even treatment outcome (Rachman, Radomsky, & Shafran, 2008). Rachman and colleagues (2008) describe a study by Milosevic and Radomsky evaluating the use of safety behaviors in the context of exposure treatment of snake phobia. Participants were randomly assigned to either select the safety behaviors they wished to use (e.g., helmet, gloves, goggles) or to a no safety behavior condition. Safety behavior use did not affect either reports of anxiety or overall approach distance in a behavioral approach test following a 45-minute in vivo exposure session. Although the results of this study await replication and evaluation across different emotional disorders, it raises questions about the contexts under which safety behaviors might be adaptive.

More research is needed to further elucidate the circumstances under which safety behaviors might be beneficial and, if so, what the limits to such facilitative effects might be. For instance, the Milosevic and Radomsky study only reported outcome immediately following a single in vivo exposure session. As discussed earlier, the detrimental effects of safety behaviors are hypothesized to manifest in the long-term maintenance of negative affect via negative reinforcement. It is possible that short-term "forgetting" occurs or "exceptions" are made, which might show up if assessment occurs shortly following exposure (e.g., immediate fear reduction). However, the durability of such changes might be less than exposure without the use or availability of safety behaviors (e.g., fear reinstatement or long-term maintenance). Ostensibly conflicting findings such as these might indicate that the rigid application of such techniques is what becomes truly problematic and suggests that encouraging the flexible application of multiple emotion regulation strategies might be an important treatment target (Bonanno, 2001; Bonanno, Papa, Lalande, Westphal, & Coifman, 2004; Ehrenreich et al., 2007).

Treatment

The prevention of emotional avoidance is essential for successful emotion exposure. As discussed previously, individuals with emotion disorders frequently use maladaptive situation modification as an attempt to regulate strong or uncomfortable emotions. The unified protocol directly targets maladaptive situation modification with a module focused on preventing emotional avoidance. The module begins with identification of emotional avoidance strategies the individual uses both with nomothetic (individual difference measures discussed earlier) and idiographic (having patients monitor and list avoidance strategies they notice over the course of treatment) measures. Individuals are presented with the rationale for how emotional avoidance can maintain maladaptive cycles of emotional responding, including a discussion about how such behaviors are negatively reinforced by the immediate temporary sense of relief they often provide. However, the long-term consequences of such strategies are demonstrated using in-session exercises demonstrating the ironic effects of suppression (Wegner, Schneider, Carter, & White, 1987; Wegner & Zanakos, 1994). Patients are asked to recall an emotionally relevant memory that happened over the previous week, having them recall specific details so as to increase the salience of the associated emotions, and then they are instructed to do whatever they can to not think about any details of the memory. Typically, after a brief suppression period, patients state that they were not very successful at suppressing any thoughts about the event. This exercise can help the therapist introduce, and allows patients to experience firsthand, the counterproductive effects of emotion suppression. This exercise provides experiential evidence supporting the rationale for preventing emotional suppression and avoidance and their importance to treatment outcome. Once the rationale has been provided and some strategies relevant to the presenting complaint have been identified, the therapist and patient work together to systematically eliminate them from the patient's emotion regulation repertoire.

Assessment

A number of assessment instruments are used to gather data during this module, including nomothetic self-report scales and idiographic self-monitoring forms. Despite the increased recognition and widespread discussion of emotional avoidance as a central concept across the emotional disorders, currently there is a dearth of instruments specifically designed to assess this construct. Three primary measures are used to assess and track emotional avoidance in the unified protocol: the Emotional Avoidance Strategy Inventory (EASI), the Checklist for Emotional Avoidance Strategy Engagement (CEASE), and an idiographic patient self-monitoring form. Validation of these measures is currently underway, and their utility in research and practice remains to be demonstrated. However, the measures are briefly introduced here because we believe they fill an important gap in our current assessment arsenal.

The EASI is a 33-item self-report questionnaire designed to assess individual differences in the dispositional tendency to avoid strong or uncomfortable emotional experiences (Fairholme et al., 2008). Example items include "I do all I can to avoid feeling depression and anxiety" and "I avoid watching 'heavy' or 'intense' movies." Higher scores are presumed to indicate a greater dispositional tendency to avoid strong or uncomfortable emotional experiences. As mentioned previously, scale development and validation are currently underway; however, the scale appears promising for both research and practice.

The CEASE was developed by the authors of the unified protocol as a nomothetic measure of the frequency with which individuals engage in common emotional avoidance strategies (Barlow et al., 2008). The CEASE was created based on, and modified from, the Texas Safety Maneuvers Scale

(TSMS; Kamphuis & Telch, 1998), which was designed to assess the use of safety behaviors in individuals with panic disorder. The scale is administered at the beginning of the emotional avoidance module. It is useful in identifying emotional avoidance strategies that are commonly used among individuals with emotional disorders and is often successful in helping patients begin to think about ways in which they might be avoiding strong or uncomfortable emotions. Although the TSMS has demonstrated strong internal consistency and construct validity (Kamphuis & Telch, 1998), validation for the modified CEASE is currently ongoing.

In addition to the EASI and the CEASE, therapists administer an idiographic self-monitoring form so patients can begin to identify the unique strategies they use on a day-to-day basis. Patients simply record any strategies they noticed themselves using in order to reduce or avoid strong, uncomfortable emotions. Patients generally find this extremely useful, after having been provided with the rationale, completing the CEASE, and discussing with the therapist ways in which they might be avoiding emotional experiences. Idiographic and nomothetic assessment instruments both have their own unique strengths, and using both methods offers a more complete assessment.

Attentional Deployment and Present-Focused Nonjudgmental Awareness

Maladaptive Attentional Deployment

Perhaps one of the more prevalent emotion regulation strategies among individuals with emotional disorders is the use of attentional deployment, either by intentionally focusing on or away from, for example, the trigger, emotion, or thought. Worry, rumination, and distraction are all examples of maladaptive attentional deployment strategies characteristic across the range of emotional disorders. For instance, GAD is characterized by excessive, uncontrollable worry. Individuals with generalized anxiety have positive expectancies and beliefs regarding their worry and report that they are engaging in worry to prevent a negative consequence (Borkovec & Roemer, 1995; Davey, Thallis, & Capuzzo, 1996; Freeston, Rheaume, Letarte, Dugas, & Ladouceur, 1994), indicating worry is a form of emotion regulation, one that likely serves an avoidance function (Borkovec, Alcaine, & Behar, 2004). Such positive expectancies and beliefs do not bear out in research, however, because worry has not been shown to decrease the likelihood of negative consequences or to increase effective coping efforts (Borkovec, Hazlett-Stevens, & Diaz, 1999). Similar to worry, rumination is largely a verbal-linguistic strategy that involves cognitively focusing on past negative events or perceived failures (Nolen-Hoeksema, Wisco, & Lyubomirsky, 2008). Rumination is a common emotion regulation strategy among individuals with mood disorders. Maladaptive attentional deployment strategies are presumed to be maintained or reinforced by (1) offering an active, as opposed to passive, way for individuals to address situations or issues that are out of their control and (2) serving as a way of distracting oneself from the emotions associated with the situation or issue.

Treatment

Individuals with emotional disorders commonly attempt to regulate emotions by either focusing attention on or away from emotional experiences or potential triggers. Common examples of maladaptive attentional deployment include distraction, thought suppression, worry, and rumination. Each of these strategies diverts attentional resources from the "here and now" in an attempt to modify the emotions perceived to be tied to such events. Such attempts are believed to be prefaced on perceptions of such emotional experiences as threatening coupled with low expectancies for successful regulation of such emotions. Increasing evidence suggests that mindfulness or acceptance-based emotion regulation strategies are a worthy foil for maladaptive strategies such as suppression (Campbell-Sills, Barlow, Brown, & Hofmann, 2006; Levitt et al., 2004). In a sample of patients with panic disorder, Levitt and colleagues (2004) found that individuals provided with an acceptance-based rationale (i.e., "If you are willing to feel happy, sad, anxious, unsure, joyful and any other emotions that come up for you, you can choose your directions in life, instead of letting your fear of anxious thoughts and feelings make those choices for you"; p. 754) experienced less negative affect during a carbon dioxide challenge and were more likely to participate in a subsequent challenge than the suppression comparison condition. In a more diverse clinical sample of patients with mixed anxiety and depressive disorders, Campbell-Sills and colleagues (2006) found that patients provided with an acceptance rationale experienced similar distress to a suppression comparison condition during a negative mood induction but exhibited less negative affect during a postinduction recovery period. Together, these findings suggest that acceptance-based strategies might serve as an adaptive alternative to emotional and expressive suppression.

Building on the literature indicating that acceptance-based emotion regulation strategies confer benefits beyond other emotion regulation strategies such as suppression, the unified protocol targets maladaptive attentional deployment strategies with a module designed to promote present-focused nonjudgmental awareness. The emotional awareness training module begins with general didactic presentation of the concept of present-focused emotional awareness, judgments individuals place on their experiences, and a brief discussion of emotional avoidance. The therapist and patient then conduct an in-session exercise to demonstrate the concept of present-focused nonjudgmental awareness, based on the Mindfulness of the Breath exercise from Williams, Teasdale, Segal, and Kabat-Zinn (2007). Once the patient has had chance to walk through the exercise once, the therapist conducts a nonspecific emotion exposure using an idiographic music mood induction, allowing the patient to practice present-focused nonjudgmental awareness in the context of personally relevant emotions. The remainder of the module focuses on practicing present-focused nonjudgmental awareness and helping patients practice anchoring themselves in the present moment.

Assessment

A number of assessment measures are used to operationalize and assess outcome for the attentional deployment component. Measures of maladaptive attentional deployment strategies, such as the Penn State Worry Questionnaire (Meyer, Miller, Metzger, & Borkovec, 1990) and the Ruminative Response Scale (Nolen-Hoeksema & Morrow, 1991; Treynor, Gonzalez, & Nolen-Hoeksema, 2003) are used to track progress in reducing maladaptive strategies such as worry and rumination. Progress in the emotional awareness training module is tracked using the Attention to Feelings and Clarity in Discrimination of Feelings subscales of the Trait Meta-Mood Scale (Salovey, Mayer, Goldman, Turvey, & Palfai, 1995). The Attention subscale has been found to be inversely associated with depressed mood, while the Clarity subscale was found to be negatively associated with depressed mood and neuroticism and successfully predicted decline in ruminative thought following a negative mood induction (Salovey et al., 1995). Although to date no studies have directly evaluated the relationship between the Attention and Clarity subscales and maladaptive attention deployment, there is a strong theoretical and conceptual basis for predicting an inverse relationship (John & Gross, 2007).

Cognitive Change and Antecedent Cognitive Reappraisal

Maladaptive Cognitive Change

Another form of emotion regulation that individuals can engage in is cognitive change, or altering the way they appraise or ascribe meaning to the situation or emotional triggering event. This component of the emotion regulation process has primarily been studied with respect to cognitive reappraisal, or changing the meaning individuals assign to a given situation so as to change the emotional meaning it holds for them (Gross & Thompson, 2007). Campbell-Sills and Barlow (2007) distinguished between *reappraisal*, in which individuals provide realistic evidence-based interpretations of a situation, and *rationalization*, in which individuals rationalize away the problem or tell themselves something about the situation to alter its emotional impact without regard to its validity. For example, a man with social phobia might reappraise concern about an upcoming work presentation by telling himself that he "doesn't care about the presentation" and that it "isn't a big deal." This reappraisal is adaptive to the extent that it accurately represents the person's actual value system. However, if a raise were riding on the outcome of the presentation or if the person was significantly invested in his job and cared about his performance, then this reappraisal would be maladaptive. Interestingly, this distinction is one that often manifests clinically; however, it has received little to no empirical attention. Upon reviewing the literature, it seems there are at least two dimensions along which cognitive change can occur: (1) *temporal*, or whether the reappraisal occurs before, during, or after the emotional-triggering event and (2) *veracity*, or the degree to which the reappraisal is realistic and evidence based. Inevitably, future research will further refine these dimensions or perhaps identify additional dimensions. However, it seems that this might be a useful heuristic for guiding and clarifying subsequent emotion regulation research to better understand when and under what circumstances cognitive change might be harmful and most beneficial.

Treatment

The unified protocol has a module designed to promote cognitive reappraisal, because this has been shown to be an effective emotion regulation strategy in a number of different studies using a variety of methods (Gross & John, 2003; John & Gross, 2007; Ray, Wilhelm, & Gross, 2008). The cognitive reappraisal module begins with a discussion of the reciprocal relationship between cognitive appraisals and emotions. This relationship is then illustrated with an in-session exercise in which the patient is asked to interpret an ambiguous picture. The therapist discusses common traps people with emotional disorders can fall into when appraising situations and introduces cognitive reappraisal as a way of altering this process. The remainder of the module focuses on practicing cognitive reappraisal, ultimately moving toward doing so in the context of emotion provocation exercises.

Assessment

Consistent with previous components, the cognitive change component in the unified protocol is assessed with a combination of idiographic and nomothetic measures. Cognitive reappraisal is assessed using the Reappraisal subscale of the Emotion Regulation Questionnaire (ERQ; Gross & John, 2003), a nomothetic individual difference measure indexing habitual tendencies to use reappraisal as an emotion regulation strategy. Idiographic self-monitoring forms are also used during treatment to track progress in identifying appraisals and generating alternate appraisals of the situation or the emotion-triggering event.

Response Modulation and Facilitating Incompatible Action Tendencies

Maladaptive Response Modulation

Individuals with emotional disorders often regulate their emotions by attempting to directly alter the subjective, physiological, or behavioral components of their emotional responses. Modulating how one responds to an emotion that has already been triggered and attempting to alter the manifestation of an emotional response is referred to as *response modulation*. Suppression is one of the most researched forms of response modulation and is most often operationalized as attempts to hide what one is feeling, or *expressive suppression* (Gross & Thompson, 2007). Some investigations have defined suppression as attempts to inhibit the emotional experience itself, or *emotion suppression* (Campbell-Sills et al., 2006). A number of laboratory studies have found that, although suppression successfully mutes emotionally expressive behavior, it also reduces subjective experience of positive emotions (Gross, 1998; Gross & Levenson, 1993, 1997). Ironically, the subjective experience of the negative emotion remains unchanged (e.g., efforts to regulate the emotion itself fail) and sympathetic arousal actually increases with suppression. In addition to laboratory studies, individual differences in trait levels of suppression have been found to be associated with lower levels of positive affect and higher levels of negative affect, poorer interpersonal functioning, and decreased psychological well-being (Gross & John, 2003).

Theorists have long recognized the link between emotions and behavior, and action tendencies, or motivated behavioral responses associated with emotions, have a long history in the emotion science literature (Barlow, 1988, 2000, 2002). Based on these long-standing tenets of emotion science, one of us suggested in 1988 that changing action tendencies (which we now refer to as *emotion-driven behavior* [EDB]) would become an essential step in the treatment of emotional disorders (Barlow, 1988). Within the unified protocol, EDB refers to any of a number of specific behaviors that are driven by the height of the emotional experience itself. Consistent with the functionalist perspective, EDBs are presumed to be adaptive under certain circumstances (e.g., immediate danger triggers fear, which elicits an escape response). However, they can contribute to the maintenance of emotional disorders when they lose congruence with the context, occurring in inappropriate situations (e.g., fear triggered by perceived danger associated with potential embarrassment in a social situation elicits the same escape response). From an emotion regulation perceptive, EDBs can be considered a form of response modulation because the behavior is aimed at altering the ongoing emotional response. Such responses are negatively reinforced and contribute to the maintenance of emotional disorders by preventing habituation from occurring (Campbell-Sills & Barlow, 2007).

Treatment

Maladaptive response modulation is directly targeted in the unified protocol with the EDB module. The module begins with a discussion of the nature of EDBs, including how they can be natural and adaptive, how they can become maladaptive, and the emotional avoidance or suppressive function that such behaviors can serve. During this module, the therapist draws heavily on the ongoing functional assessment initiated when the intake assessment was conducted or the patient began treatment. Over the course of treatment, patients are helped to internalize the process of conducting a functional assessment of their own emotional experiences, because the context in which the disordered emotion or behavior occurs is central in the maintenance of emotional disorders. Once patients and their therapists have identified maladaptive EDBs, they work together to generate incompatible behaviors that patients can implement in the situation to allow both natural habituation and more adaptive regulation of their emotional experience. Patients are taught this general approach of acting opposite to their emotions (by implementing incompatible behaviors) in order to alter their emotional experiences. Linehan (1993) also adopted the strategy to great effect in dialectical behavior therapy. The therapist emphasizes how *acting consistent* with an emotion reinforces the stimulus properties of that emotional experience and the emotion-triggering event (e.g., public speaking is to be feared or anxiety is to be avoided) and offers *acting opposite* as a key skill for changing such maladaptive patterns.

Assessment

Habitual use of expressive suppression as an emotion regulation strategy is assessed with the Suppression subscale of the ERQ (Gross & John, 2003). EDBs are difficult to operationalize and assess given their highly idiosyncratic, context-sensitive nature. We have not yet found or created a measure that can adequately capture this aspect of emotion regulation. Currently, idiographic self-monitoring forms are used throughout treatment to help identify and monitor EDBs, practice countering EDBs, and track progress in applying this skill. However, a measure that assessed the frequency with which an individual engaged in common action tendencies associated with specific emotions would be useful in tracking progress through this module. For instance, "How often do you escape a situation when you feel fearful or afraid?" or "How often do you yell or become aggressive when you feel angry?"

Case Illustration

The current version of the unified protocol uses a modular approach to target five components of emotion regulation. Treatment progresses through the modules culminating in exposure not only to anxiety-provoking situations but also intense emotional experiences that may be associated with these situations in order to facilitate recognition and acceptance of emotional responding and create new behavioral habits that promote better psychosocial functioning and eventual symptom alleviation. In this section, we focus on the application of the protocol to a specific case, noting how the different components of emotion regulation may be applied sequentially in a way that fosters therapeutic change.

One main advantage of a transdiagnostic treatment approach is that it allows for treatment of patients presenting with comorbid conditions or multiple emotional disorders. To illustrate this point, we present the case of "Steve," a 40-year-old businessman who presented to our clinic with clinical diagnoses of obsessive–compulsive disorder (OCD) and social phobia. His primary concern at the time of the assessment surrounded aggressive impulses that were interfering in his marital relationship. Steve was avoiding being alone with his wife out of fear that he might hurt her, and the couple often argued over his persistent need for reassurance, as he would often ask questions such as "I won't actually hurt someone, right?" Additionally, he reported difficulty engaging in social situations, including speaking in front of groups, being assertive, and speaking with unfamiliar people out of the concern that he would be negatively evaluated. His social anxiety was negatively impacting his career because it decreased his ability to pursue jobs consistent with his level of expertise.

Attentional Deployment:
Promoting Present-Focused Nonjudgmental Awareness

After a psychoeducation component common to all cognitive-behavior treatments, we focus on helping patients become more aware of their emotions and their reactions to those emotions. When introducing emotional awareness, we stress the importance of nonjudgment and accepting emotions even when they are uncomfortable, because attempts to suppress emotions or push them away prolongs them and typically increases their intensity. For Steve this was demonstrated by having him avoid thinking about the sadness a gruesome image evoked. He noticed (as do most patients) that in trying to avoid thinking about his emotions, he thought about them more.

We assist patients in developing a more present-focused emotional awareness via in-session mindfulness exercises and inducing different emotions, including positive ones, because all emotions (not just anxiety and depression) may contribute to the development of emotional disorders. Steve was asked to listen to a CD of music designed to provoke different emotions and practice being aware of them without labeling or judging his experience using the mindfulness exercise conducted earlier in-session.

Cognitive Change: Antecedent Cognitive Reappraisal

We focus on two appraisals that seem central to anxious and depressive thinking: (1) overestimating the probably of negative events happening and (2) overestimating the consequences of that negative event if it did happen. Patients are taught to recognize these appraisals and to use cognitive restructuring to reappraise these situations in a more adaptive manner, with the ultimate goal of increased flexibility in thinking. For example, Steve identified numerous fearful cognitions before attending business meetings relating to both his social phobia (e.g., "I have nothing to contribute;" "My voice will shake so bad that I won't be able to answer the questions asked") and his OCD (e.g., "I'll see a knife and be incapacitated by intrusive thoughts about killing my boss").

Steve recognized that he was overgeneralizing based on the rare experience of being unable to answer a question or having an intrusive thought and magnifying the importance of anxiety symptoms like a shaky voice. Through cognitive reappraisal, he was able to consider a more adaptive and realistic interpretation of the situation (e.g., "Even if my voice shakes, I can still answer a question;" "Just because I see a knife does not mean I'll have an intrusive thought, and even if I have an intrusive thought it will not leave me incapacitated or mean I will act on that thought"). These skills are practiced prior to emotion-provoking situations, because the goal is to alter the cognitive conditions under which patients encounter emotion-provoking stimuli, not to dampen the emotional salience of a situation they are currently in. From our perspective, patients' attempts to dampen the intensity of emotions (or to avoid emotions) are maladaptive and only serve to maintain their emotional disorder. Thus, we discuss cognitive reappraisal as antecedent-based strategy that leads directly into the next target of treatment: preventing emotional avoidance.

Situation Modification: Preventing Emotional Avoidance

Continual use of behavioral and cognitive avoidance strategies prevents patients from benefiting from the positive functions of emotions and reinforces disordered emotion. Steve, for example, would arrive to business meetings early in order reserve a seat where he could remain hidden. Most patients report that such strategies are successful (e.g., hiding behind others decreased Steve's anxiety over being called on) and are reluctant to relinquish them; however, increased awareness of the long-term consequences of avoiding emotion coupled with slow withdrawal of those strategies helps patients recognize them as maladaptive. Steve learned how hiding behind others perpetuated his anxiety, both reinforcing the notion that being called on was something to be feared and preventing him from learning that he could cope with the situation despite his anxiety.

When Steve was asked to view images of knives and films clips of people being physically assaulted, he noticed that he averted his gaze, focused his attention on trivial details (e.g., the wristwatch of the person holding a knife), or rationalized his emotion (e.g., "I know this is a movie and not real") to subtly control his affect. Instead of hiding, Steve was encouraged to sit at the conference table; instead of turning away from gruesome images, he was asked to look at them and describe them in detail.

Response Modulation: Facilitating Incompatible Action Tendencies

Before treatment, Steve had stopped entering the kitchen when his wife was present because he was too fearful to be around knives in his wife's presence. He also avoided taking jobs where he might have to present in front of groups. Thus, our protocol helps patients recognize EDBs that occur in response to both emotionally provoking situations and to internal triggers such as physical sensations, cognitions, and emotions. Patients are then taught to act contrary to their EDBs in treatment, which ultimately decreases the disordered emotion. Thus, instead of leaving the kitchen when his wife was present, Steve was instructed to remain in the situation despite his anxiety; instead of seeking reassurance (e.g., "I won't actually hurt someone, right?"), he was asked to sit with his emotions without doing anything to reduce the intensity of them.

Situation Selection: Emotion Exposure

For patients to learn to implement new responses to emotionally intense situations and not avoid those situations, we deliberately provoke these types of experiences both in and out of session through hierarchical emotion exposure. Confronting emotionally provoking situations allows several things to occur, including (1) interpretations and appraisals about the dangerousness of the situation begin to change without direct therapeutic attention; (2) newer, more adaptive interpretations and appraisals begin to emerge; (3) avoidance and subsequent impairment begin to be reversed; and (4) EDBs are recognized and modified. For Steve, exposures meant seeing picture of knives, standing in the kitchen with his wife, holding a knife in session, writing about how it would feel to kill a loved one, holding a knife with his wife nearby, and so on. It also meant running in place to mimic the physiological symptoms of social anxiety (e.g., rapid heart rate, flushing), giving a speech to colleagues, and presenting at work. Important to this process is confronting all the associated emotions, not just anxiety. For instance, Steve also confronted shame, sadness, guilt, and frustration as well as anxiety.

Throughout the course of treatment, Steve was able to learn to respond to his emotions in more adaptive ways. At the end of treatment, he no longer met diagnostic criteria for any emotional disorder. Functionally, Steve significantly improved and was able to hold his wife, cook and dice vegetables with her, and attend and even ask questions at business meetings.

Future Directions

Following from models of treatment dissemination such as the one proposed by Weisz, Southam-Gerow, Gordis, and Connor-Smith (2003), it is critical to first establish the efficacy of a novel intervention in a controlled research setting. An RCT of the unified protocol is currently nearing completion. This trial and the open trial preceding it have already significantly informed the protocol's development and aim to provide preliminary evidence of the protocol's acceptability, feasibility, and clinical utility across patients presenting with an array of emotional disorders. The current RCT necessitated a more structured application of the modular design, with a set ordering of treatment components (e.g., proceeding sequentially from Module 1 through 7), although flexibility in the number of sessions was retained (e.g., session ranges, allowing treatment to extend from nine to 18 sessions). The current modular design of the protocol has set the stage for better identifying treatment response relative to both individual modules and guiding emotion regulation theory. Assessing the nature of treatment response as a function of specific modules and emotion regulation skills entails a number of more future-oriented empirical questions. Preliminary steps toward this agenda have already been taken by generating assessment measures (e.g., EAH, EASI, CEASE) relevant to specific modules in the protocol.

Clearly, the ultimate realization of this protocol would entail a fully modular format (e.g., with order of module presentation and decisions about module use defined by idiographic algorithms or other guides to clinical decision making) and to test it in real-world clinical settings (Weisz, Donenberg, Han, & Weiss, 1995). Much of the pioneering work on such modular approaches has been in the domain of child and adolescent intervention. Chorpita and colleagues (Chorpita, 2007; Chorpita, Daleiden, & Weisz, 2005), for example, have described a modular treatment approach to anxiety disorders in youth that follows a default order of treatment (determined by primary diagnosis) but allows clinicians to add modules relevant to interfering comorbid problems (e.g., parent training interventions). Southam-Gerow and colleagues have applied this modular approach and added a functional analytic module (cf. Henggeler, Schoenwald, Rowland, & Cunningham, 2002) as a selection method that permits a very flexible ordering of treatment (Southam-Gerow, 2005).

It follows that a natural extension of such work would be to apply a theoretically driven, transdiagnostic approach, such as the unified protocol (Barlow et al., 2008) and its developmentally informed companion protocol for adolescents (Ehrenreich et al., 2008) within community clinics using a fully modular format. Such work is clearly on the horizon for our research lab. By setting the stage for both emotion-oriented and dissemination-focused research questions, we hope to inform the link between theory and practice with emotional disorders over time.

References

Allen, L. B., McHugh, R. K., & Barlow, D. H. (2008). Emotional disorders: A unified protocol. In D. H. Barlow (Ed.), *Clinical handbook of psychological disorders: A step-by-step treatment manual* (4th ed., pp. 216–249). New York: Guilford Press.

Arnold, M. B. (1960). *Emotions and personality.* New York: Columbia University Press.

Barlow, D. H. (1988). *Anxiety and its disorders: The nature and treatment of anxiety and panic.* New York: Guilford Press.

Barlow, D. H. (2000). Unraveling the mysteries of anxiety and its disorders from the perspective of emotion theory. *American Psychologist, 55,* 1247–1263.

Barlow, D. H. (2002). *Anxiety and its disorders: The nature and treatment of anxiety and panic* (2nd ed.). New York: Guilford Press.

Barlow, D. H., Allen, L. B., Boisseau, C. L., Ehrenreich, J. T., Ellard, K. K., Farchione, T., et al. (2008). *Unified protocol for treatment of emotional disorders: Modular version 2.0.* Unpublished manuscript, Boston University.

Barlow, D. H., Allen, L. B., & Choate, M. (2004). Toward a unified treatment for emotional disorders. *Behavior Therapy, 35,* 205–230.

Barlow, D. H., & Craske, M. G. (2007). *Mastery of your anxiety and panic: Client workbook for anxiety and panic* (4th ed.). New York: Oxford University Press.

Barlow, D. H., Gorman, J. M., Shear, M. K., & Woods, S. W. (2000). Cognitive-behavioral therapy, imipramine, or their combination for panic disorder: A randomized controlled trial. *Journal of the American Medical Association, 283,* 2529–2536.

Barrett, L. F., Ochsner, K. N., & Gross, J. J. (2007). On the automaticity of emotion. In J. A. Bargh (Ed.), *Social psychology and the unconscious: The automaticity of higher mental processes* (pp. 173–217). New York: Psychology Press.

Berkowitz, L., & Harmon-Jones, E. (2004). Toward an understanding of the determinants of anger. *Emotion, 4,* 107–130.

Bonanno, G. A. (2001). Emotion self-regulation. In T. J. Mayne & G. A. Bonanno (Eds.), *Emotions: Current issues and future directions* (pp. 251–285). New York: Guilford Press.

Bonanno, G. A., Papa, A., Lalande, K., Westphal, M., & Coifman, K. (2004). The importance of being flexible: The ability to both enhance and suppress emotional expression predicts long-term adjustment. *Psychological Science, 15,* 482–487.

Borkovec, T. D., Alcaine, O., & Behar, E. (2004). Avoidance theory of worry and generalized anxiety disorder. In R. G. Heimberg, C. L. Turk, & D. S. Mennin (Eds.), *Generalized anxiety disorder: Advances in research and practice* (pp. 77–108). New York: Guilford Press.

Borkovec, T. D., Hazlett-Stevens, H., & Diaz, M. L. (1999). The role of positive beliefs about worry in generalized anxiety disorder and its treatment. *Clinical Psychology and Psychotherapy, 6,* 126–138.

Borkovec, T. D., & Roemer, L. (1995). Perceived functions of worry among generalized anxiety disorder subjects: Distraction from more emotionally distressing topics? *Journal of Behavior Therapy and Experimental Psychiatry, 26,* 25–30.

Borkovec, T. D., & Ruscio, A. M. (2001). Psychotherapy for generalized anxiety disorder. *Journal of Clinical Psychiatry, 62,* 37–45.

Brown, T. A. (2007). Temporal course and structural relationships among dimensions of temperament and DSM-IV anxiety and mood disorder constructs. *Journal of Abnormal Psychology, 116,* 313–328.

Brown, T. A., Chorpita, B. F., & Barlow, D. H. (1998). Structural relationships among dimensions of the DSM-IV anxiety and mood disorders and dimensions of negative affect, positive affect, and autonomic arousal. *Journal of Abnormal Psychology, 107,* 179–192.

Campbell-Sills, L., & Barlow, D. H. (2007). Incorporating emotion regulation into conceptualizations and treatments of anxiety and mood disorders. In J. J. Gross (Ed.), *Handbook of emotion regulation* (pp. 542–559). New York: Guilford Press.

Campbell-Sills, L., Barlow, D. H., Brown, T. A., & Hofmann, S. G. (2006). Effects of suppression and acceptance on emotional responses of individuals with anxiety and mood disorders. *Behaviour and Research Therapy, 44,* 1251–1263.

Chorpita, B. F. (2007). *Modular cognitive-behavioral therapy for childhood anxiety disorders.* New York: Guilford Press.

Chorpita, B. F., Daleiden, E. L., & Weisz, J. R. (2005). Indentifying and selecting the common elements of evidence based interventions: A distillation and matching model. *Mental Health Services Research, 7,* 5–20.

Davey, G. C. L., Thallis, F., & Capuzzo, N. (1996). Beliefs about the consequences of worrying. *Cognitive Therapy and Research, 20,* 499–520.

Dimidjian, S., Hollon, S. D., Dobson, K. S., Schmaling, K. B., Kohlenberg, R. J., Addis, M., et al. (2006). Randomized trial of behavioral activation, cognitive therapy, and antidepressant medication in the acute treatment of adults with major depression. *Journal of Consulting and Clinical Psychology, 74,* 658–670.

Duclos, S. E., Laird, J. D., Schneider, E., Sexter, M., Sterm, L., & Van Lighten, O. (1989). Emotion-specific effects of facial expressions and postures on emotional experience. *Journal of Personality and Social Psychology, 57,* 100–108.

Ehrenreich, J. T., Buzzella, B. A., & Barlow, D. H. (2007). General principles for the treatment of emotional disorders across the lifespan. In S. Hofmann & J. Weinberger (Eds.), *The art and science of psychotherapy* (pp. 191–210). New York: Brunner-Routledge.

Ehrenreich, J. T., Buzzella, B. A., Trosper, S., Bennett, S. M., Wright, L. R., & Barlow, D. H. (2008). *Unified treatment for adolescents with emotional disorders.* Unpublished manuscript, Boston University.

Ehrenreich, J. T., Fairholme, C. P., Buzzella, B. A., Ellard, K. K., & Barlow, D. H. (2007). The role of emotion in psychological therapy. *Clinical Psychology: Science and Practice, 14,* 422–428.

Ellsworth, P. C., & Scherer, K. R. (2003). Appraisal processes in emotion. In R. J. Davidson, K. R. Scherer, & H. H. Goldsmith (Eds.), *Handbook of affective sciences* (pp. 572–595). New York: Oxford University Press.

Fairholme, C. P., Ellard, K. K., Boisseau, C. L., Farchione, T., & Barlow, D. H. (2008). *The Emotional Avoidance Strategy Inventory (EASI).* Unpublished manuscript, Boston University.

Foa, E. B., Dancu, C. V., Hembree, E. A., Jaycox, L. H., Meadows, E. A., & Street, G. P. (1999). A comparison of exposure therapy, stress inoculation training, and their combination for reducing posttraumatic stress disorder in female assault victims. *Journal of Consulting and Clinical Psychology, 67,* 194–200.

Foa, E. B., Liebowitz, M. R., Kozak, M. J., Davies, S., Campeas, R., Franklin, M. E., et al. (2005). Randomized, placebo-controlled trial of exposure and ritual prevention in the treatment of obsessive–compulsive disorder. *American Journal of Psychiatry, 162,* 151–161.

Freeston, M. H., Rheaume, J., Letarte, H., Dugas, M. J., & Ladouceur, R. (1994). Why do people worry? *Personality and Individual Differences, 17,* 791–802.

Fridja, N. H. (1986). *The emotions.* Cambridge, UK: Cambridge University Press.

Gross, J. J. (1998). The emerging field of emotion regulation: An integrative review. *Review of General Psychology, 2,* 271–299.

Gross, J. J. (2002). Emotion regulation: Affective, cognitive, and social consequences. *Psychophysiology, 39,* 281–291.

Gross, J. J., & John, O. P. (2003). Individual differences in two emotion regulation processes: Implications for affect, relationships, and well-being. *Journal of Personality and Social Psychology, 85,* 348–362.

Gross, J. J., & Levenson, R. W. (1993). Emotional suppression: Physiology, self-report, and expressive behavior. *Journal of Personality and Social Psychology, 64,* 970–986.

Gross, J. J., & Levenson, R. W. (1997). Hiding feelings: The acute effects of inhibiting negative and positive emotion. *Journal of Abnormal Psychology, 106,* 95–103.

Gross, J. J., & Thompson, R. A. (2007). Emotion regulation: Conceptual foundations. In J. J. Gross (Ed.), *Handbook of emotion regulation* (pp. 3–24). New York: Guilford Press.

Heimberg, R. G., Liebowitz, M. R., Hope, D. A., Schneier, F. R., Holt, C. S., Welkowitz, L. A., et al. (1998). Cognitive behavioral group therapy vs. phenelzine therapy for social phobia. *Archives of General Psychiatry, 55,* 1133–1141.

Henggeler, S. W., Schoenwald, S. K., Rowland, M. D., & Cunningham, P. B. (2002). *Serious emotional disturbance in children and adolescents: Multisystemic therapy.* New York: Guilford Press.

Izard, C. E. (1993). Four systems for emotion activation: Cognitive and noncognitive processes. *Psychological Bulletin, 100,* 68–90.

John, O. P., & Gross, J. J. (2007). Individual differences in emotion regulation. In J. J. Gross (Ed.), *Handbook of emotion regulation* (pp. 351–372). New York: Guilford Press.

Kamphuis, J. H., & Telch, M. J. (1998). Assessment of strategies to manage or avoid perceived threats among panic disorder patients: The Texas Safety Maneuvers Scale (TSMS). *Clinical Psychology and Psychotherapy, 5,* 177–186.

Kashdan, T. B. (2007). Social anxiety spectrum and diminished positive experiences: Theoretical synthesis and meta-analysis. *Clinical Psychology Review, 27,* 348–365.

Kim, E. J. (2005). The effect of decreased safety behavior on anxiety and negative thoughts in social phobics. *Journal of Anxiety Disorders, 19,* 69–86.

Kring, A. M., & Werner, K. H. (2004). Emotion regulation and psychopathology. In P. Philippot & R. S. Feldman (Eds.), *The regulation of emotion* (pp. 359–385). Mahwah, NJ: Erlbaum.

Lang, P. J. (1979). A bio-informational theory of emotional imagery. *Psychophysiology, 16,* 495–512.

Lang, P. J. (1985). The cognitive psychophysiology of emotion: Fear and anxiety. In A. H. Tuma & J. D. Maser (Eds.), *Anxiety and the anxiety disorders* (pp. 131–170). Hillsdale, NJ: Erlbaum.

Levenson, R. W. (1994). Human emotions: A functional view. In P. Ekman & R. J. Davidson (Eds.), *The nature of emotion: Fundamental questions* (pp. 123–126). New York: Oxford University Press.

Levitt, J. T., Brown, T. A., Orsillo, S. M., & Barlow, D. H. (2004). The effects of acceptance versus suppression of emotion on subjective and psychophysiological response to carbon dioxide challenge in patients with panic disorder. *Behavior Therapy, 35,* 747–766.

Linehan, M. M. (1993). *Cognitive-behavioral treatment of borderline personality disorder.* New York: Guilford Press.

Mauss, I. B., Levenson, R. W., McCarter, L., Wilhelm, F. H., & Gross, J. J. (2005). The tie that binds?: Coherence among emotion experience, behavior, and physiology. *Emotion, 2,* 175–190.

Meyer, T. J., Miller, M. L., Metzger, R. L., & Borkovec, T. D. (1990). Development and validation of the Penn State Worry Questionnaire. *Behaviour Research and Therapy, 28,* 487–495.

Nolen-Hoeksema, S., & Morrow, J. (1991). A prospective study of depression and distress following a natural disaster: The 1989 Loma Prieta earthquake. *Journal of Personality and Social Psychology, 61,* 105–121.

Nolen-Hoeksema, S., Wisco, B. E., & Lyubomirsky, S. (2008). Rethinking rumination. *Perspectives on Psychological Science, 3,* 400–424.

Ochsner, K. N., Bunge, S. A., Gross, J. J., & Gabrieli, J. D. E. (2002). Rethinking feelings: An fMRI study of the cognitive regulation of emotion. *Journal of Cognitive Neuroscience, 14,* 1215–1229.

Ochsner, K. N., Ray, R. D., Cooper, J. C., Robertson, E. R., Chopra, S., Gabrieli, J. D. E., et al. (2004). For better or for worse: Neural systems supporting the cognitive down- and up-regulation of negative emotion. *NeuroImage, 23,* 483–499.

Powers, M. B., Smits, J. A. J., & Telch, M. J. (2004). Disentangling the effects of safety-behavior and safety-behavior availability during exposure-based treatment: A placebo-controlled trial. *Journal of Consulting and Clinical Psychology, 72,* 448–454.

Rachman, S., Radomsky, A. S., & Shafran, R. (2008). Safety behaviour: A reconsideration. *Behaviour Research and Therapy, 46,* 163–173.

Rapee, R. M., Craske, M. G., & Barlow, D. H. (1995). Assessment instrument for panic disorder that includes fear of sensation-producing activities: The Albany Panic and Phobia Questionnaire. *Anxiety, 1,* 114–122.

Ray, R. D., Wilhelm, F. H., & Gross, J. J. (2008). All in the mind's eye?: Anger, rumination and reappraisal. *Journal of Personality and Social Psychology, 94,* 133–145.

Riskind, J. H., & Gotay, C. C. (1982). Physical posture: Could it have regulatory or feedback effects on motivation and emotion? *Motivation and Emotion, 6,* 273–298.

Roemer, L., Salters, K., Raffa, S. D., & Orsillo, S. M. (2005). Fear and avoidance of internal experiences in GAD: Preliminary tests of a conceptual model. *Cognitive Therapy and Research, 29,* 71–88.

Salkovskis, P. M. (1991). The importance of behavior in the maintenance of anxiety and panic: A cognitive account. *Behavioural Psychotherapy, 19,* 6–19.

Salkovskis, P. M., Clark, D. M., Hackmann, A., Wells, A., & Gelder, M. G. (1999). An experimental investigation of agoraphobia. *Behavior Research and Therapy, 37,* 559–574.

Salovey, P., Mayer, J. D., Goldman, S. L., Turvey, C., & Palfai, T. P. (1995). Emotional attention, clarity, and repair: Exploring emotional intelligence using the Trait Meta-Mood Scale. In J. W. Pennebaker (Ed.), *Emotion, disclosure, and health* (pp. 125–154). Washington, DC: American Psychological Association.

Schacter, S., & Singer, J. E. (1962). Cognitive, social, and physiological determinants of emotional state. *Psychological Review, 69,* 379–399.

Scherer, K. R. (2001). Appraisal considered as a process of multi-level sequential checking. In K. R. Scherer, A. Schorr, & T. Johnstone (Eds.), *Appraisal processes in emotion: Theory, methods, research* (pp. 92–120). New York: Oxford University Press.

Siemer, M., Mauss, I., & Gross, J. J. (2007). Same situation—different emotions: How appraisals shape our emotions. *Emotion, 7,* 592–600.

Siemer, M., & Reisenzein, R. (2007). The process of emotion inference. *Emotion, 7,* 1–20.

Stepper, S., & Strack, F. (1993). Proprioceptive determinants of emotional and nonemotional feelings. *Journal of Personality and Social Psychology, 64,* 211–220.

Sloan, T., & Telch, M. J. (2002). The effects of safety-seeking behavior and guided threat reappraisal on fear reduction during exposure: An experimental investigation. *Behaviour Research and Therapy, 40,* 235–251.

Southam-Gerow, M. A. (2005, Summer). Using partnerships to adapt evidence-based mental health treatments for use outside labs. *Report on Emotional and Behavioral Disorders in Youth, 5,* 58–60, 77–79.

Treynor, W., Gonzalez, R., & Nolen-Hoeksema, S. (2003). Rumination reconsidered: A psychometric analysis. *Cognitive Therapy and Research, 27,* 247–259.

Veleber, D. M., & Templer, D. I. (1984). Effects of caffeine on anxiety and depression. *Journal of Abnormal Psychology, 93,* 120–122.

Wegner, D. M., Schneider, D. J., Carter, S. R., & White, T. L. (1987). Paradoxical effects of thought suppression. *Journal of Personality and Social Psychology, 52,* 5–13.

Wegner, D. M., & Zanakos, S. (1994). Chronic thought suppression. *Journal of Personality, 62,* 615–640.

Weisz, J. R., Donenberg, G. R., Han, S. S., & Weiss, B. (1995). Bridging the gap between laboratory and clinic in child and adolescent psychotherapy. *Journal of Consulting and Clinical Psychology, 63,* 688–701.

Weisz, J. R., Southam-Gerow, M. A., Gordis, E. B., & Connor-Smith, J. (2003). Primary and secondary control enhancement training for youth depression: Applying the deployment-focused model of treatment development and testing. In A. E. Kazdin & J. R. Weisz (Eds.), *Evidenced-based psychotherapies for children and adolescents* (pp. 165–182). New York: Guilford Press.

Wells, A., Clark, D. M., Salkovskis, P., Ludgate, J., Hackmann, A., & Gelder, M. (1995). Social phobia: The role of in-situation safety behaviors in maintaining anxiety and negative beliefs. *Behavior Therapy, 26,* 153–161.

Williams, J. M. G., Teasdale, J. D., Segal, Z. V., & Kabat-Zinn, J. (2007). *The mindful way through depression: Freeing yourself from chronic unhappiness.* New York: Guilford Press.

CHAPTER 13

Acceptance and Commitment Therapy in an Emotion Regulation Context

Sonsoles Valdivia-Salas, Sean C. Sheppard, and John P. Forsyth

The topic of emotion regulation is gaining currency in psychopathology research (e.g., Barlow, Allen, & Choate, 2004; Eifert & Forsyth, 2005) and mental health care more generally (Gross & Muñoz, 1995). Historically, the field of emotion regulation research and theory has remained agnostic with regard to the positive and negative consequences of various emotion regulation strategies and their implications for psychological health and wellness. Increasingly, however, we are learning that certain forms of emotion regulation may be healthier than others and that some strategies tend to yield human suffering (Garnefski, Teerds, Kraaij, Legerstee, & Van den Kommer, 2004; Hayes, Wilson, Gifford, Follette, & Strosahl, 1996; Moore, Zoellner, & Mollenholt, 2008). In the present chapter, we examine the implications of emotion regulatory processes in the cause, maintenance, and treatment of psychopathology from a contemporary behavior-analytic perspective on the nature of human suffering and vitality. This approach, in turn, is the foundation for newer third-generation behavior therapies such as acceptance and commitment therapy (ACT) (Hayes & Strosahl, 2004; Hayes, Strosahl, & Wilson, 1999).

ACT explicitly seeks to undermine rigidly applied emotion regulatory processes via experiential, metaphorical, and somewhat paradoxical (even counterintuitive) strategies and links those strategies with explicit behavior change strategies in the service of valued ends. This approach is predicated on relational frame theory (RFT) (Hayes, Barnes-Holmes, & Roche, 2001), a modern behavior-analytic account of language and cognition. Thus, to understand how ACT conceptualizes and targets emotion regulation, it is important to outline how language and cognition operate from an RFT perspective. In this chapter, we begin with a basic overview of emotion regulation itself and then emotion regulation from an RFT point of view. We then follow this discussion with an introduction to ACT within an emotion regulation context.

Emotion Regulation: Concept, Strategies, and Evidence

Emotion regulation is a topic that means different things to different people. For instance, developmental psychopathologists tend to emphasize the regulatory effects of emotion itself on behavior (e.g., extreme anxiety). Adult psychopathologists tend to focus on emotion regulation as behavior, or what people do with and about their emotional experience. In this chapter, we focus on emotion regulation as a behavior, while recognizing that emotional responding itself can, at times, limit or narrow behavioral options. In this direction, emotion regulation refers to a heterogeneous set of actions that are designed to influence "which emotions we have, when we have them, and how we experience and express them" (Gross, 2002, p. 282). This move is, in part, strategic because humans have limited control over the onset, frequency, duration, and intensity of emotional responses but do have control over what they do with it and how they respond to it (i.e., their behavior; Hayes et al., 1999). This distinction, as we show, is central to ACT.

Emotion regulatory behavior can manifest in many obvious and subtle ways, including reappraisal, distraction, avoidance, escape, suppression, emotion and problem-focused coping, and use of substances to enhance or blunt emotional experience. Each of these strategies subsumes numerous actions that can be applied to both positive and negative emotional states (Parrott, 1993). Most of them, however, can be characterized by actions that aim to alter the form, frequency, duration, or situational occurrence of events that may precede an emotional response as well as the events that may follow an emotional response (Gross, 1998). The former has been described as antecedent-focused emotion regulation (e.g., reappraisal, cognitive avoidance), whereas the latter refers to response-focused emotion regulation (e.g., suppression, distraction, escape). Additionally, regulatory strategies may sometimes serve to alter the emotional response itself. Some regulatory processes may be relatively autonomic or habitual, occurring in or outside of awareness (e.g., selective attention), whereas others may be more purposeful or deliberate (e.g., blame, rumination, suppression, avoidance).

Some research has indicated that reappraisal can be a flexible and effective means of minimizing the negative impact of an aversive event (Gross, 1998, 2002; Ochsner, Bunge, Gross, & Gabrieli, 2002). However, a significant body of evidence has demonstrated that suppression of aversive emotions, including suppression of expressive outward emotion, does not provide relief from the psychological experience of that emotion. In fact, just the opposite tends to occur. Typically, the emotion becomes stronger and more salient, resulting in increased sympathetic nervous system activity as well as a range of undesired psychological content (see Butler & Gross, 2004, for a review).

For instance, it has been shown that attempts to suppress and control unwanted thoughts and feelings can result in more (not less) unwanted thoughts and emotions (for reviews, see Purdon, 1999; Wegner, 1994). Moreover, emotion suppression has been shown to impair memory and problem solving (e.g., Richards & Gross, 2000), tends to contribute to suffering and pain (e.g., Cioffi & Holloway, 1993; McCracken, Spertus, Janeck, Sinclair, & Wetzel, 1999), increases distress and restricts life functioning (e.g., Marx & Sloan, 2002), diminishes contact with meaningful and valued life activities, and reduces overall quality of life (see Hayes, Luoma, Bond, Masuda, & Lillis, 2006, for a summary of outcome studies). The emerging consensus here is that response-focused emotion regulation requires considerable effort, only works to a point, is counterproductive when the emotions are intense and highly aversive, and may get in the way of meaningful life activities (i.e., regulation itself competes with powerful approach contingencies) (see Forsyth, Eifert, & Barrios, 2006; Hayes, 1976).

From a functional view, the utility of emotion regulation depends on whether it achieves desired outcomes and can be flexibly applied depending on context (Forsyth et al., 2006). Flexibility, or the ability to discriminate when emotion regulation is a workable option, is crucial to the functional utility of emotion regulation strategies (Bonanno, Papa, Lalande, Westphal, & Coifman, 2004). In fact, discrimination failure has recently emerged as a core feature that distinguishes problematic from functional forms of emotion regulation (John & Gross, 2004). In line with this, the RFT/ACT perspective maintains that it is not the presence of unwanted thoughts and emotions but rather the inflexible efforts to control or eliminate them that constitute the problem. In short, excessive emotion regulation itself is what exacerbates psychological pain and limits the life of the individual. These notions may initially seem counterintuitive given the effectiveness of control-based strategies in our physical environment, but as we outline, the uncontrollability of our own thoughts and emotions is entirely expected from what we know about the way language and cognition function in verbal organisms.

In the next sections, we address how the properties of language and cognition, as described within RFT, lead to inflexible and unhealthy forms of emotion regulation given certain circumstances and how ACT undermines the regulation agenda itself as a prerequisite for (or in the service of) effective action. As we proceed through the chapter, we frame our discussion around the processes illustrated in Figure 13.1, or what are referred to in the ACT research and clinical community as hexaflex mod-

ACT Model of Psychopathology

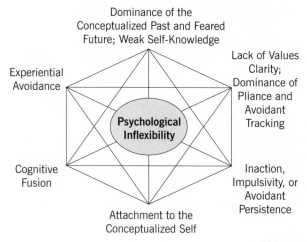

ACT Targets of Intervention

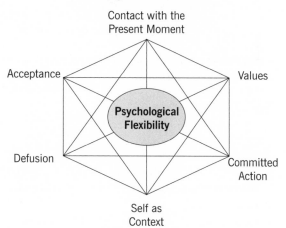

These illustrations are referred to as the hexaflex model (adapted from Hayes et al., 2006). Notice that points on top correspond to those at the bottom. The intersecting lines show how different process elements tend to be linked with one another both in feeding human suffering and in its successful alleviation. Next, a brief description of each of the ACT targets for intervention, as opposed to the processes contributing to psychopathology, is presented.

Defusion versus Cognitive Fusion: Clients are taught to notice words (emotions, thoughts) for what they are (sounds with particular meanings and emotional functions as a result of the way the client interacts with them) and not for what they advertise themselves to be (threatening events linked with action or inaction).

(cont.)

FIGURE 13.1. Acceptance and commitment therapy (ACT) model of psychopathology linked with ACT targets of intervention.

Self and Context versus Attachment to the Conceptualized Self: Clients learn the difference between the self as a space or place for psychological activity versus the self as linked with thoughts, feelings, memories, and unavoidable products of a personal history.

Contact with the Present Moment versus Dominance of the Conceptualized Past and Future: Clients learn a difference between thoughts about the past or a future that has yet to be and the now. Traumatic memories, for instance, happen now; futures are constructed, but that construction is happening now. Now, or the present, is the place where life is engaged and where actions can be taken. Contact with the present moment, along with defusion and self-as-context work, increases sensitivity to "here and now" contingencies that may be helpful in guiding behavior.

Acceptance versus Experiential Avoidance: Avoidance and acceptance are two ways of relating with a wide range of private events. Acceptance entails changing what can be changed (i.e., what clients do with their mouth, hands, and feet), while making room for what cannot be changed (i.e., presence, frequency, and intensity of thoughts, emotions, evaluations of private and public experiences, relating, sense making).

Values versus Lack of Values Clarity: The acceptance of private contents that have been avoided for so long makes sense only in the context of personally held values or done in the service of meaningful life directions. These will be established very early in treatment, revisited throughout therapy, and serve as the referent to determine the effectiveness of treatment.

Committed Action versus Avoidant Persistence: Clients learn to distinguish choices in the service of compliance with others or those to avoid or attenuate forms of discomfort versus making commitments and choices in the service of what they value, even when those choices are accompanied by discomfort that they do not like or wish not to have.

FIGURE 13.1. *(cont.)*

els. In the first half of the chapter, we address emotion regulation within the context of the ACT model of psychopathology and follow in the second half of the chapter with a discussion of its role in ACT interventions (see Figure 13.1).

The Language Trap: Why Emotion Regulation Does Not Always Work

Language serves an important symbolic function by providing humans with (emotional) experiences without the necessary exposure to the actual physical stimuli or events that ordinarily elicit those responses (Forsyth & Eifert, 1996; Staats & Eiffert, 1990). For instance, humans are able to reexperience, countless times and with great intensity, emotions associated with a first romantic relationship or the birth of their first child. They can also enjoy pleasant emotions while planning a first vacation to the Caribbean, even before setting foot on a plane or experiencing the warmth of the tropical sun directly. With this same intensity, humans can reexperience a traumatic event that may have happened years ago simply by thinking about or visualizing the event. They can also get anxious about a future that has not occurred yet simply by thinking or talking about it as if it was actually happening in the "here and now."

The principles that explain why this happens within a modern approach to language and cognition are described in RFT. It is beyond the scope of the present chapter to present RFT in detail, but we illustrate the principles that explain why humans suffer with their histories, futures, emotions, and thoughts and why deliberate efforts to end suffering often fail. We also examine why humans persist in using unworkable emotion regulation strategies rather than exploring new and presumably more effective ways of dealing with their psychological pain. Addressing issues such as these seems crucial to understanding and alleviating a wide range of human suffering. A central aim of RFT and ACT is to tackle these central issues head on.

Psychological Inflexibility as a Model of Psychopathology

To better capture the relevance of RFT principles and findings as they relate to the development of psychological suffering and unhealthy forms of emotion regulation, we describe RFT principles in the context of the six processes that make up the ACT model of psychopathology (see Figure 13.1, top). For the sake of clarity and fluency, we organize the six processes into two groups: cognitive fusion and experiential avoidance. Cognitive fusion and experiential avoidance have both been regarded as core processes that give rise to psychological inflexibility and maladaptive emotion regulation strategies (Hayes & Strosahl, 2004).

Cognitive Fusion

Cognitive fusion entails buying into the content of our thoughts and feelings (e.g., "Life is overwhelming") as if they were true statements (e.g., "Life cannot be handled, I would rather give up"). Certain properties of language, as regarded from the RFT perspective, explain not only why cognitive fusion occurs but also the role it plays in maladaptive emotion regulation strategies and psychological suffering (Blackledge, 2003; Hayes et al., 2001).

Consider the following example. A verbally able individual is told that a particular pain reliever (that we refer to as *aspi*, or A in general terms) is "better than" pain reliever *melgi* (B). Without further specification and in the absence of necessary direct experience with either of them, the individual will automatically *derive* that melgi (B) is worse than aspi (A). If the individual is now told that pain reliever melgi (B) is "better than" pain reliever *nolo* (C), he will derive that nolo (C) is worse than melgi (B) and, more interestingly, that nolo (C) is worse than aspi (A) and that aspi (A) is better than nolo (C)—and all of this can occur without actually having to experience any of the stimuli in question! Even more interesting, if the individual usually takes nolo for his regular headaches, it is most likely that in the case of a particularly painful headache he will take aspi, which has been arbitrarily established as the best of the three brands available.

This example comprises several key aspects that characterize the way humans respond to events (in contrast with nonhumans). First, aspi and nolo do not need to share any formal stimulus properties (e.g., color, size, weight, shape) in order to be related. Instead, humans can and do relate events in accordance with *relational cues* whose function is established by social whim or convention (e.g., same as, different to, opposite of, if . . . then, better than). Once relational learning is established early on during normal development (Luciano, Gómez-Becerra, & Rodríguez-Valverde, 2007), relational cues can by applied to any stimuli in the appropriate context.[1] For instance, a verbally able human can readily establish that, in the context of monetary value, a half-inch piece of gold is "more than" a one-gallon bottle of milk, despite the fact that the latter is bigger than the former. The arbitrary application of relational cues is at the basis of the emergence or *derivation* of private contents or events such as thoughts, feelings, memories, expectations, fears, and the like. Also, it is at the basis of the formation of evaluations of those private contents. Much as in the example of the pain relievers, a person exposed to messages like "Being anxious is contrary to feeling at ease" and "Feeling at ease helps you in social situations" may derive "Being anxious will not help me in social situations" or "Anxiety is bad, anxiety is a barrier to a full life, and I have to find a way to control my anxiety before I can have a full life." The derivation of thoughts and emotions is automatic and unavoidable, or, in other words, is not under the voluntary control of the individual.

Second, and intimately related to the former, as a result of the arbitrary application of relational cues, humans can and do respond to novel events in "appropriate" ways, that is, in ways that are concordant with relations already established in the behavioral repertoire. Imagine a child is told that the word *fire* is *the same as* (or stands for) the actual fire. If the actual flames of a fire had acquired avoidant functions (e.g., the child runs

---

[1]RFT uses the generic term *relational frame* to describe several patterns of responding under the control of verbal relational cues. Examples of these include relational frames of coordination (or relational responding under the control of the arbitrary cue "same as" or its functional equivalent), distinction ("different to"), opposition ("opposite of"), comparison ("more/less than"), temporal ("before . . . after"), and conditional ("if . . . then"), among others. See Hayes and colleagues (2001) for a book-length approach to relational frames; and Luciano and colleagues (2009) for a detailed description of the emergence of relational cues.

away from them), then hearing somebody scream "Fire!" would probably evoke similar avoidant functions (e.g., the child would look around for fire and prepare to run if necessary). It is through the arbitrary application of relational cues that words stand for persons, places, and things (e.g., "anxiety" stands for, or is the *same as*, the experience of certain bodily reactions, thoughts, and feelings) and that words acquire psychological functions when presented in the appropriate context. For instance, in the context of feeling good (understood as the absence of discomfort), the thought "I'm an anxious person" may be as aversive as feeling anxious.

There is now a considerable amount of research showing that novel or arbitrary stimuli may acquire functions through the arbitrary application of relational cues (i.e., by verbal means and social convention). For instance, several lines of research suggest that humans can behave under the control of consequences that they have never directly contacted with but whose reinforcing properties have been established via language (e.g., Valdivia-Salas, Dougher, & Luciano, 2009; Whelan & Barnes-Holmes, 2004; Whelan, Barnes-Holmes, & Dymond, 2006). These findings may be at the basis of or may partially explain why humans sometimes reach for "perfection," fear "failure," or avoid a panic attack they have never had. It has also been shown that novel events can elicit strong emotional functions because they are arbitrarily related to actual punishers or reinforcers (e.g., Dougher, Augustson, Markham, Greenway, & Wulfert, 1994; Dougher, Hamilton, Fink, & Harrington, 2007; Roche & Barnes, 1997; Rodríguez-Valverde, Luciano, & Barnes-Holmes, 2009). This may partially explain why someone with agoraphobia panics when her job requires her to go to a mall she has been told is *bigger than*, or *more crowded than*, the one in her city she consistently avoids because of fears of having a panic attack.

Cognitive fusion entails reacting to derived functions (the ones that result from the arbitrary application of relational cues) as if they are direct (the formal or nonarbitrary properties of the stimuli), based on the failure to distinguish the products of thinking (e.g., "What a jerk") from the process of thinking (e.g., "I am having a thought that a person is a jerk") and context where both occur (e.g., a situation where I was expecting something in return for my generous efforts). Cognitive fusion may occur with a variety of thoughts and feelings, like those that relate to the self, the past, and the future. For instance, someone exposed to a message like "Anxiety is terrible" may easily derive "I am terrible" when anxious. Cognitive fusion with a conceptualized self, past, or future considerably narrows behavioral options. That is, people can quite literally live in their heads, their pasts, or futures that have yet to be and engage in actions to support or defend the stories they tell about themselves and their world and about what they must do to be happy, successful, and so on (for further details, see Hayes et al., 1996; Törneke, Luciano, & Valdivia-Salas, 2008; Wilson, Hayes, Gregg, & Zettle, 2001).

Experiential Avoidance

Experiential avoidance is the inflexible and indiscriminate pattern of deliberate efforts to avoid or escape from aversively experienced private events such as emotions, thoughts, memories, and bodily sensations (Hayes et al., 1996, see Boulanger, Hayes, & Pistorello, Chapter 5, this volume). Experiential avoidance is heavily supported by cognitive fusion with the content of thoughts and feelings. That is, it is because the person buys into the content "Feeling worthless is a barrier to a full life" that *feeling worthless* becomes something to fight against.

As has been illustrated, thoughts and other private events, including the evaluations of such thoughts, are derived products of the individual's personal history that occur automatically given certain circumstances. From an ACT/RFT point of view, the content of private events is not directly problematic unless contextual features establish relations between emotional content and unhelpful regulation strategies. These contextual features (literality, evaluation, reason giving, and control of causes, discussed next) are largely sustained by our "feel good" culture, which promotes the idea that psychological health means the absence of certain emotions (e.g., sadness, fear, insecurity, anxiety, worries, guilt, and unpleasant thoughts or images). For instance, painful reminders of a traumatic past can be relived many times, and some people have difficulty distinguishing the painful memory occurring now from the experience of the trauma then and engage in efforts to avoid, minimize, or escape from the painful past showing up in the present, some of which may be self-destructive and self-defeating (e.g., drinking alcohol, acting out, or withdrawing from the world).

The contexts of *literality, evaluation,* and *reason giving* involve cognitive fusion with naturally derived products of our history. Literality is the tendency to treat words as the events they stand for. An example of this might be a person reacting to the thought "I'm stupid" by abandoning work on a project he was perfectly capable of completing. Evaluation is the tendency to evaluate the world around us, and by extension our own private experiences, as good, bad, helpful, or toxic and the failure to see that the evaluation is not a property of the event but rather mere thoughts (e.g., "beautiful" or "lousy" could be applied to a fresh rose, and yet these evaluations are not physical properties of roses). Reason giving is the tendency to give a causal role to our thoughts and feelings regardless of their emotional valence, as when we attribute our success to our self-confidence and our misery to our low mood (for a detailed description, see Luciano, Rodríguez, & Gutiérrez, 2004).

The context *control of causes* involves the extension of our control strategies in the outside world (e.g., replacing a broken cell phone with a new one) to the world within our skin (e.g., "If I could just stop worrying, I would finally be happy"). Control efforts are strongly potentiated by the immediate and momentary removal of the source of discomfort.

For instance, only by staying away from social interactions do many anxious clients find momentary relief from the discomfort of meeting new people (e.g., thoughts like "I will not know what to talk about," "They may not like me," and "I will look stupid," temporarily disappear). In the long term, however, the effects are paradoxical. The feared private events may increase in frequency, variety, and strength while life satisfaction becomes reduced.[2] The paradoxical effect of control efforts is related to both the additive nature of language and the insensitivity of rule-governed behavior (Luciano et al., 2004). We now turn to a brief discussion of these two phenomena.

The additive nature of language means that once a particular set of relations, or relational network, has been established, it will be brought to bear given the proper circumstances and despite any efforts to change or suppress it. These efforts to change, suppress, or otherwise modulate private events will, contrary to the intention of the individual, tend to expand and elaborate the network by adding new elements and relations (Wegner, 1994; Wilson & Hayes, 1996; Wilson et al., 2001). For instance, each time an anxious individual tries unsuccessfully to get rid of anxiety, he or she may derive the following: "I am doing something wrong," "This should work," "I must be stupid," "I cannot control myself," "I am weak person," "Others will notice how weak I am," "Thinking this about myself will turn things worse," "I am good; I can handle this," "No, I guess I cannot," "Stop thinking that! . . . Try harder," and so on. This results in a vicious self-perpetuating cycle that will expand to new contexts and private events as more effort is devoted to control thoughts, feelings, and bodily reactions.

In general terms, the additive nature of language is well illustrated by some clients who describe how their discomfort changes over time, from being relatively discrete and circumscribed to overwhelming, omnipresent, and associated with a variety of unpleasant emotional content and important life activities, some of which were not previously linked with the original problem. Control efforts also exacerbate aversive emotional responding (its frequency, intensity, and variety), even in individuals with no known history of psychopathology (Forsyth et al., 2006).

Fusion with thoughts and feelings may yield formalized rules about how to think, feel, and behave (e.g., "Having fears means I am a weak person; I have to get rid of them"). It has been repeatedly demonstrated in the laboratory that rule-governed behavior tends to dominate other sources of behavioral regulation such as contingency-shaped learning (see Catania, Matthews, & Shimoff, 1990, for a review of the empirical evidence in

---

[2] In the work with our clients, it is crucial to detect the contingencies that maintain the control agenda because it will guide how the intervention should proceed. The three types of contingencies are known as pliance, tracking, and augmenting. For further details, see Hayes, Gifford, and Hayes (1998). For a detailed description of the relation between the three types of problematic rule following and psychopathology, see Törneke and colleagues (2008).

laboratory settings). Moreover, it does not take much for this to set into motion, in part, because rules are enormously helpful in many areas of life. In fact, problem solving is partly based on rules. For instance, suppose you've learned this simple problem-solving set: "If something is not working, do something to fix it, and you will get a good outcome." So, when your flashlight stops working, you can replace the batteries and once again have light, which is good. From this simple rule set, you can also get "I will be anxious and embarrass myself if I go to the party, so I will avoid it altogether, and then I won't feel anxious, which is good." In the extreme, this simple relational set can be applied in irreversible ways, such as "If I kill myself, then I will end my suffering, which is good."

In the laboratory, we see that rigidly and inflexibly followed rules (self-generated or provided by others) can interfere with normal adjustment to ever-changing life conditions and contribute to individuals becoming less sensitive to real-life outcomes. A good deal of superstitious and safety behavior (e.g., carrying a charm or empty pill bottle) would seem to fit this category. Experiential avoidance characterizes a set of actions that tend to be more rule governed than contingency shaped and thus yield behavior that appears more rigid and inflexible than circumstances warrant (Forsyth et al., 2006; Törneke et al., 2008). So we see that fusion with rules about how and when it is acceptable to experience private content that has been established as toxic can result in more struggle, even when the experience shows that control-based strategies do not work and are actually expanding and exacerbating the psychological discomfort and hence suffering.

Rigid and inflexible patterns of avoidant behavior maintained over a long period of time will result in a life limited to doing anything and everything necessary to down-regulate thoughts, emotions, bodily sensations, and other private events that are experienced as barriers to important action. That is, life is spent trying to eliminate content that cannot be eliminated (because of the way language works) instead of pursuing meaningful activities that really matter to the individual (Hayes et al., 1996). In short, all of the elements depicted within the hexaflex model in Figure 13.1 (top)—fusion, experiential avoidance, dominance of a conceptualized past of future, avoidant persistence, and lack of values clarity—interact to yield psychological inflexibility, or a narrowing of behavioral options. These are the processes that drive excessive forms of emotion regulation, and those very processes are thus central targets within ACT.

Experiential Acceptance as a Healthy Form of Emotion Regulation within ACT

"If I cannot change how I think or feel, then what is left?" This question often arises as clients confront the unworkability of the control agenda itself. This process creates room for clients to consider acceptance as an alternative.

Acceptance means to "take what is offered" or to have an experience without engaging in efforts to somehow change that experience. More broadly, acceptance involves changing what can be changed (behavior) without attempting to change the private contents (thoughts and emotions) that often show up as people take steps in directions they wish to go. Acceptance has been regarded as a deregulation strategy because its purpose is not to regulate emotional experiences (in the sense of changing or eliminating them) but to make contact with what one experiences on the inside as a conscious human being while persisting in purposeful behavior given what the situation affords (Forsyth et al., 2006).

Acceptance also entails taking an active and courageous stance that undermines the notion that one must change what one thinks and feels in order to live better. Instead, acceptance allows room to live better with whatever one thinks or feels. This is a choice to lay down arms in a war with facets of our emotional life. While recognizing that humans cannot control how they think or feel (because the nature of the mind or language is fundamentally about relating, sense making, and deriving new relations), they can control what it is they do while thinking or feeling a particular way. To get a sense of this, take a moment to sit in your chair and say aloud, "I cannot get up and touch the wall." Repeat this for a few moments and then stand up, move forward, and touch the wall all the while repeating the phrase aloud. This very simple exercise illustrates a central idea within ACT that thoughts need not be barriers to effective action and can be had just as they are while doing what we care about.

The research on the benefits of acceptance over control rationales, particularly with psychological suffering that is maintained over long periods of time and of high intensity, is becoming increasingly more extensive. These benefits, measured by prolonged persistence in aversive tasks and with less subjective distress, have been demonstrated in coping with laboratory-induced panic-like symptoms (Eifert & Heffner, 2003; Levitt, Brown, Orsillo, & Barlow, 2004; Spira, Zvolensky, Eifert, & Feldner, 2004) and pain (e.g., Gutiérrez, Luciano, Rodríguez, & Fink, 2004; Masedo & Esteve, 2007; McMullen et al., 2008; Páez-Blarrina, Luciano, Gutiérrez, Valdivia, Ortega, & Rodríguez, 2008; Páez-Blarrina, Luciano, Gutiérrez, Valdivia, Rodríguez, & Ortega, 2008). Research has also moved from analogue laboratory studies to clinical settings. The efficacy of acceptance-based protocols has been demonstrated in the treatment of such diverse problems as chronic pain (e.g., McCracken, Vowles, & Eccleston, 2005; Vowles & McCracken, 2008), decreasing self-harm in women with borderline personality disorder (Gratz & Gunderson, 2006), smoking cessation (Gifford et al., 2004; Hernández-López, Luciano, Bricker, Roales-Nieto, & Montesinos, 2008), improving quality of life for individuals with epilepsy (Lundgren, Dahl, & Hayes, 2008) and breast cancer (Páez-Blarrina,

Luciano, & Gutiérrez, 2007), and undermining the believability of delusions and decreasing the frequency of rehospitalization in individuals with schizophrenia (Bach & Hayes, 2002; Gaudiano & Herbert, 2006).

Taken together, mounting evidence points to the utility of using acceptance-based strategies to undermine toxic processes linked with experiential avoidance in the alleviation of human suffering. The remainder of this chapter integrates this evidence within a discussion of the core principles, processes, and clinical applications of ACT.

ACT: Basic Principles and Core Processes

ACT is one of several newer third-generation, or "third-wave," behavior therapies, with roots in a wing of behavior therapy known as applied behavior analysis. The emergence of the third wave stemmed from empirical and theoretical issues with traditional cognitive-behavioral therapy as well as the larger movement to develop and disseminate empirically based clinical interventions (see Hayes, 2004).

By moving beyond the therapeutic goals of symptom alleviation and control, ACT offers an expanded view of human suffering and what it means to foster psychological health and wellness. Integrated with RFT at the level of basic science, the basic premise of ACT is that people cannot choose the emotions they have, whether they be happiness, excitement, fear, anxiety, or anger to name a few. They can, however, choose how they respond to their thoughts, feelings, and physical sensations, particularly the ones experienced as aversive, when they arise. From this premise, the ultimate goal of ACT is to alter rigid and inflexible patterns of reacting to private events (e.g., suppression, avoidance, distraction) in favor of more flexible responding. The choice about how to relate with and respond to private events (either avoidance or acceptance) becomes a matter of workability toward valued life goals and directions. Psychological flexibility is established through intense work in six core processes (see Figure 13.1, bottom).

The core processes of acceptance, defusion, self as context, contact with the present moment, values, and committed action are not unique to ACT, but they are organized and integrated in a consistent theory of the functional properties of human language and cognition and provide a useful way to organize treatment targets (Hayes, Strosahl, Bunting, Twohig, & Wilson, 2004). The ACT Targets for Intervention in Figure 13.1 contain six processes that can be divided into two larger and overlapping groups. The four processes to the left refer to acceptance and mindfulness processes. The four processes to the right represent commitment and behavior change processes. Combining the two larger groups, ACT may be defined as a "therapy approach that uses acceptance and mindfulness processes, as well as commitment and behavior change processes, to produce greater psychological flexibility" (Hayes, Strosahl, et al., 2004, p.13). A detailed description of the six processes is provided in the next section, along with the clinical methods usually used to promote them.

ACT: Application and Methods

Rather than a technology, ACT is an approach to understanding and treating the diverse forms of experiential avoidance. It is built on metaphors, exercises, and paradoxes but is not *just* a set of those technologies. For this reason, the therapist is encouraged to use the exercises and metaphors in a flexible and creative fashion as opposed to a memorized or formulaic approach. In a way, the application of ACT in clinical practice is like a dance, where therapist and client move among and between elements of the hexaflex (see Targets of Intervention in Figure 13.1) to foster greater psychological flexibility in the service of valued ends. Likewise, the therapist is encouraged to tailor and match the techniques to the functional characteristics of the conceptualized case. That is, ACT is a functional approach that demands attention to relevant processes as they emerge in and outside the therapeutic context (Eifert & Forsyth, 2005). Because all ACT components and clinical methods have the same goal (i.e., fostering psychological flexibility in the service of valued ends), their ordering can be varied to meet the needs of individual clients. We now turn to a description of ACT processes presented in the order that is generally utilized in the work with a broad range of clients and problems (see Hayes & Strosahl, 2004, for a book-length review).

Establishing Valued Action as a Healthy Alternative to Struggle and Control

Acceptance and Willingness

The therapist initially begins by addressing the cost of control and avoidance-based agendas as measured against what the client really values in his or her life. As part of this process, the therapist and client explore several issues described next (for more details, see Wilson & Byrd, 2004; Wilson & Luciano, 2002). First, avoidant repertoires and avoided events need to be assessed. In the case of a client suffering from alcohol abuse, for instance, it is important to identify what occasions the drinking behavior (contexts, thoughts, and other private contents that increase the likelihood of drinking). Additionally, the therapist will seek to clarify what the client has tried in order to alleviate suffering, such as social withdraw, procrastination, or staying in bed, with an eye on the short- and long-term costs and benefits of such avoidance strategies.

Beyond symptoms of depression, phobias, insecurity, anxiety, and the like, the therapist explores what aspects of life the problem (as perceived by the client) is limiting or interfering with. A typical way of accomplishing this is to inquire of the client, "What would you be doing if [insert problem or complaint] wasn't such a problem for you?" "How would you spend your time?" "What is anxiety in the way of?" This also constitutes a first approach to identifying the client's values, something that is covered in more detail later. Finally, therapist and client assess the workability of staying in bed, drinking, and other avoidant behaviors in the sense of moving the client closer to valued life goals. Here, the aim is to help the client make experiential contact with the obvious: that increased effort to gain control of or regulate unpleasant facets of emotional experiences (by doing whatever it takes to be away from discomfort) has not worked all that well and, in fact, paradoxically leads to feeling less in control over life.

This process we just outlined is commonly referred to as *creative hopelessness*. This term emphasizes the sense of creativeness and empowerment that comes from the realization that the control agenda itself (i.e., various forms of control, struggle, emotion regulation) is unworkable or hopeless, not the person. This, in turn, helps to create space for doing something new that may be more workable. The therapist emphasizes shifting the client's attention from the logic and literal content of solutions ("I cannot work while I am so depressed," "The urges are so strong that I cannot help myself") to their workability.

When acceptance is presented as the alternative to the control agenda, it is addressed neither as tolerance nor as resignation but rather as taking responsibility for the choices we make in life. Being responsible, in turn, means assuming that every choice we make will bring along thoughts and other private events because of the way language and cognition work. More metaphorically, suppose a coin represented a full, rich life, with heads representing all that we desire and cherish and tails being symbolic of all that is unpleasant and uncomfortable. In order to have that coin and the possibility of heads, one must also be willing to have the tails. If you throw out the coin because of the dark and scary events associated with tails, you also throw out all that is cherished on the heads side. A similar process is at work when people devote enormous time, energy, and effort to quelling their psychological and emotional pain, for in this process the resources necessary to engage important life areas are simply not available.

This is a critical moment in treatment because in cases where there is not strong cognitive fusion with the contents of feared private events, this intervention may be enough by itself to have the client engage in valued life directions (for laboratory evidence, see, for instance, Gutiérrez et al., 2004). In cases where cognitive fusion is stronger, work on cognitive defusion should then begin. It is advisable, however, to start establishing valued life directions early, in part, because it will dignify the cognitive defusion practice, including exposure-like exercises.

Values

The assessment and clarification of values are key components of ACT insofar as suffering and the subsequent experience of creative hopelessness would be impossible if values had not been abandoned somewhere along the way (Hayes et al., 1999). Within ACT, values are conceptualized as individual dynamic ongoing patterns of behavior in different life domains that organize behavior and provide a sense of direction (Wilson & Byrd, 2004). Values are not about beliefs, morality, and so on.

Let's consider for a moment a value most of us can identify with: that of being "caring and loving in intimate relationships and friendships." In contrast to specific actions (discrete in nature) and goals (achievable outcomes), values have no endpoint or sense of finality. There is no way to cross values off a "to-do" list. In other words, no matter how much love and care you provide to a significant other or close friend, you always can do more. Values identification also supports the overarching aim of ACT of redirecting attention from unworkable goals (i.e., getting unpleasant thoughts and feelings under control) to actions that truly define what clients wish their lives to stand for (Eifert & Forsyth, 2005). Valued action, therefore, becomes an important benchmark for therapeutic success.

At times during therapy, clients are encouraged to face, openly and without struggle, the most feared and avoided thoughts, feelings, memories, and physical sensations that they have been otherwise struggling with. The therapist will introduce this practice *only if* the strategy of not looking at such private contents for what they really are (automatic derived products of clients' histories that have acquired their aversive functions primarily because of the way the clients react to them) has functioned as a barrier to a fulfilling life. Clients with a long history of avoidant behavior will rarely be fully receptive to making contact with aversive private content they have been battling for so long. Yet clients are more likely to contact unwanted private events when they are linked to living out their values. In this sense, values clarification can be an important motivating factor.

There are many ways of assessing values, including empirically supported standardized measures (see, for instance, Wilson, Sandoz, Kitchens, & Roberts, in press), but the general intent is for clients to discover or define what matters most in their lives. Answers to questions such as the following are frequently helpful in the process to identify values: "What do you want your life to stand for?" "What do you want to be about?" "If you only had today to live, then how would you spend it?" This process can be time consuming and hard, and it is common to find clients who say they do not have any values, consistently report that their value is to stop feeling miserable, are confused about what they want, or report someone else's values as their own, such as those held by a parent, friend, lover, or employer. All these different patterns usually share the same underlying phenomenon: inflexible fusion with their most feared private content and a heavy degree of pliance, as when clients do something to please others, gain approval, make others feel better, avoid conflict, and so on (Törneke et al., 2008). In these situations, therapists will often devote more time and effort than usual to building a solid therapeutic relationship so that the various unhelpful sources of influence over client choices diminish, while also supporting client choices in the service of what they value.

Once clarified, values are revisited throughout therapy and serve as the referent for the clients and their therapists to ascertain whether the intervention is working in terms of helping clients use their hands and feet to move in valued life directions, regardless of the private content that may show up on the way. This is also a key place where acceptance and mindfulness processes become linked with commitment and values processes. In short, clients learn to let go of the struggle to regulate their private world in order to engage their lives more fully.

Committed Action

The major goal of this process is to help the client develop a pattern of value-driven committed action that is progressively broader, deeper, and more elaborate. Broad-based achievement of committed action rests on the establishment of successively larger commitments over time as well as practice in defusing from unpleasant private events (through the variety of methods presented in the next section). In a client with multiple problems, for instance, these little commitments may be "simple" in-session acts like keeping eye contact with the therapist while speaking, especially when this action supports, for example, improving communication with loved ones outside the session (Wilson & Luciano, 2002). This focus lets the client know from the very beginning that therapy is not about blaming others or oneself, nor is it about making sense of the misery already endured.

ACT is about finding a way to live well while noticing the aspects of one's history that may be painful. Valued action will naturally trigger psychological barriers, which, after being identified, serve as opportunities to practice acceptance strategies. Consider someone who avoids intimate relationships because he is afraid of being hurt. On one level, this person clearly values intimacy and yet views fear as a barrier to such intimacy. At another level, real intimacy requires risking being hurt. ACT helps draw this out so that clients can hold the thought of being hurt while also engaging in the value of intimacy and connection with another human being.

Here, it is important to point out that committing to one's values does not mean committing to never experiencing failure. Instead, slips are treated as opportunities to notice what the client's mind brings along ("I must be stupid," "This will not work either," "Mine is a very special case," "I'm always wrong," "The depression is coming back"). The client is further encouraged to respond with "response-ability," or the recognition that we are the products of our own history (thus, certain thoughts will show up upon slipping) and are nonetheless able to respond by standing up to rejoin the commitment to doing what matters most. The progress in ACT is measured not by the absence of slips but by increased ability to discriminate when one is slipping and to do something that is more functional or workable.

Developing patterns of broader and deeper committed actions involves, to a greater or lesser extent, undermining the fusion with language processes. We turn now to a description of the three ACT processes that move the client toward this goal.

Using Mindful Acceptance and Defusion to Move with Emotional Barriers

Letting go, or detaching from contents and processes of literal language and thought, is a skill that can be acquired over time and only with practice. Thus, therapy sessions should be a context to *go for* feared thoughts and feelings while practicing defusion and mindfulness in the service of living fully in the present moment. Through the work toward undermining psychological barriers, the client recognizes that these assorted private contents (sensations, labels, evaluations) are automatic products of their personal history that occur from the self-as-context, or the safe place from where one can observe how this all happens. For instance, "I am depressed" may become "I am having the thought that I am depressed. Thanks, Mind!" Seeing all this, instead of seeing *from* this, increases the client's flexibility or ability to responsibly choose what to do in the presence of the unwanted private events. Over time, the client comes to understand that therapy, and life more generally, is not about accepting pain, anxiety, urges, and obsessions (discomfort in general) but rather is about learning to notice discomfort for what it really is (a label referring to certain sensations) and sensing that the experience of discomfort is part of moving in life directions that are freely and responsibly chosen.

Cognitive Defusion

Cognitive defusion strategies are aimed at undermining cognitive fusion (see Figure 13.1). Here, it is important to note that cognitive fusion is neither good nor bad; it just is. As outlined, fusion can be problematic when the products of thinking are linked with actions and emotions that, when bought into, tend to lead to other actions that pull the client out of their lives. Consider the thought "I am banana." Thinking or saying those words does not turn you into a yellow-skinned piece of fruit. It is just a thought, right? However, for someone suffering from a psychosis, the thought "I am a banana" may be treated as literally true, and this may be linked with wearing yellow-colored clothing and distress and fear of being picked, bought, sold, pealed, or eaten by others. In short, delusional thought is an extreme example of the problematic nature of fusion, and yet fusion operates at many levels and is far more pervasive than seen in psychotic disorders.

The general goal of cognitive defusion is to teach the client to experience private contents for what they really are (e.g., thoughts as thoughts, sensations as sensations, memories as memories), not what they advertise themselves to be (Strosahl, Hayes, Wilson, & Gifford, 2004). Various ACT exercises may be used to teach defusion (e.g., see Hayes et al., 1999; McKay & Sutker, 2007) and all have multiple purposes.

One goal is to teach the client about the automatic and programmable nature of language that leads to certain contents as well as evaluations. To get a sense of that, imagine that you must not think the thought that fills in the blank appearing at the end of the following phrase: "Twinkle, twinkle, little, _____." You didn't ask for that thought, and yet "star" is present and notoriously difficult to avoid or dismiss.

Another purpose is to show how thoughts, feelings, evaluations, and other private events do not cause behavior, even though they may appear to do so. Recall the exercise involving touching the wall while thinking "I cannot get up and touch the wall." A third goal is to teach clients how words have different effects depending on how they are used (see Valdivia-Salas, Luciano, & Molina, 2006, for laboratory evidence). Last, they help the client change verbal conventions that may be potentiating fusion (i.e., those that establish private events as causes of behavior, as in "When I think and feel better, then I will live better"). As an example, take the sentence "I want to go to the party, *but* I am feeling depressed," which establishes the verbal relation opposite of, between partying and feeling depressed. In fact, the literal function of *but* is to undo what comes before; in the prior example, *but* undoes wanting to go to a party. As a consequence, the person may not go to the party. As an alternative, an ACT therapist may encourage use of statements like "I want to go to the party *and* I am feeling depressed." Unlike *but*, which literally keeps people on their butts, *and* allows both elements to coexist and is a more open and honest reflection of what is going on: The client wants to go to the party, is feeling depressed, and can experience both without needing to resolve one or the other first. The *and* also helps the client notice that the content experienced as unpleasant can arise when people engage in valued directions, and that's okay. Another example is the statement "I am worthless—I can't handle this any longer." Instead, the client would be encouraged to say "I am having the thought of being worthless and the thought of not being able to handle this." Such statements may seem awkward, and yet they nonetheless help clients to create space between the products of thinking and the person doing that thinking.

Getting in Contact with the Present Moment: Self as Process

A client showing up to therapy is typically stuck living in a past that once was or a future that has yet to be. Fusion with either the contents of the past or future precludes living in the present moment, or the place where living is enacted. An important piece of the work involves helping the client experience life not as something that will be lived once certain private content is eliminated but as it is actually occurring in the present moment (Strosahl et al., 2004). Through acceptance and mindfulness exercises, thoughts and emotions are brought to the same level where content is experienced in the "here and now" and from the same "I" perspective.

Mindfulness exercises are useful for clients because they encourage paying attention, on purpose, in the present, and without evaluation, judgment, or suppression of content that is being experienced (see Kabat-Zinn, 2003). They teach clients to allow private events to come and go, simply sitting with and noticing them as they are in the moment (Eifert & Forsyth, 2005). In other words, the goal of mindfulness and other exposure exercises is to *feel and think* better (i.e., become better at thinking and feeling), not to feel *better* (i.e., feeling less discomfort; Forsyth et al., 2006). Acceptance and mindfulness exercises are meant to broaden the client's behavioral repertoire and increase flexibility. Such exercises teach new skills and ways of relating with the world within and outside the skin by creating "space" between the person doing the experiencing and the content being experienced (Eifert & Forsyth, 2005). As previous authors have noted (Strosahl et al., 2004) and as is further discussed later, there is overlap between self-as-context and self-as-process insofar as exercises directed toward noticing what is being experienced in the present moment (process) also serve as opportunities to point to the "you" who is noticing (context).

Self as Context

Normally, language processes (e.g., RFT processes reviewed early on) obscure distinctions between events and thoughts about events, including distinctions between the person as a place of emotional experiences versus being part of or identifying with those emotional experiences (e.g., "I am a loser," "I am depressed," or "I am empty and unlovable," etc.). In short, humans tend to see the world through language and thought and fail to see that they are not their thoughts or feelings (what we have called *cognitive fusion*).

Self-as-context exercises within ACT—and there are many—are designed to create space between the observer and what is observed, the thinking and what is thought, the feeler and what is felt, and the like. For instance, clients may be encouraged to see themselves as a movie screen upon which thousands of experiences are played out. The screen, or you "the person," will host millions of thoughts, memories, and feelings in a lifetime, whereas you "the screen" are not those experiences but rather provide the place and space for those experiences. The screen does not care what is projected on it; it merely allows those projections to be. Much as a house provides the context for people to live within and remains the same regardless of changing inhabitants, furniture, and wall colors, the self provides the context for our changing experiences to occur over time.

If the client cannot make contact with this psychological space and is instead fused with the content of some particular feared private event, the content is threatening and invites struggle. On the other hand, the client can learn to experience the ongoing stream of thoughts, memories, images, and bodily sensations as merely the products of a personal history along with his or her emotional valences from an "I" that has always been there welcoming all such experiences. Without something to fight against or resist, there is no struggle and no need to regulate the experience to make it something other than it is. Fighting against a particular set of thoughts is akin to fighting against a part of ourselves, and the emerging literature on emotion regulation suggests that such efforts do not work particularly well (Gross & Munoz, 1995; John & Gross, 2004).

When clients learn to discriminate between private events and the context in which they occur, a major step in building long-term psychological flexibility is reached. That is, the very definition of psychological flexibility hinges on an affirmative "yes" to the following question (see Figure 13.1, bottom): "Given a distinction between you and the stuff you are struggling with and trying to change (self-as-context), are you willing to have that stuff, fully and without defense (acceptance), as it is and not as what it says it is (defusion), *and* do what takes you in the direction (committed action), of your chosen values (values), at this time, in this situation (contact with the present)?" Here, "yes" means that clients choose, with the necessary perspective, what they want their lives to stand for, noticing when thoughts and old histories serve them well on that path and when they don't and then committing themselves to doing what matters to them right where they are, even when their old history screams "Don't do it."

An Evaluation of ACT as a Transdiagnostic Approach

As the material in this chapter suggests, the ACT model of psychopathology explicitly assumes that underlying problems (e.g., cognitive fusion, experiential avoidance) are common to many forms of human suffering, and thus may span traditional boundaries between psychological disorders. From this perspective, it follows that the transdiagnostic approach of ACT should be effective across many types of problems and settings, and the current state of evidence supports this view in showing ACT to be effective for a broad range of problems (for a meta-analysis, see Hayes et al., 2006).

This work includes both effectiveness and efficacy studies in diverse areas such as generalized anxiety disorder (Dalrymple & Herbert, 2007), obsessive–compulsive disorder (Twohig, Hayes, & Masuda, 2006), comorbid anxiety and depressive disorders (Forman, Herbert, Moitra, Yeomans, & Geller, 2007), work site stress (Bond & Bunce, 2000), depression (Dougher & Hackbert, 1994; Zettle & Rains, 1989), substance use disorders (Gifford et al., 2004; Hayes, Wilson, et al., 2004; Hernández-López et al., 2008; Twohig, Shoenberger, & Hayes, 2007), chronic pain (Dahl, Wilson, & Nilsson, 2004; McCracken et al., 2005), diabetes (Gregg, Callaghan, Hayes, & Glenn-Lawson, 2007), sexual dysfunction (Montesinos, 2003), epilepsy (Lundgren et al., 2008; Lundgren, Dahl, Melin, & Kies, 2006), breast cancer (Páez-Blarrina et al., 2007), eating disorders (Baer, Fischer, & Huss, 2005; Heffner, Sperry, & Eifert, 2002), stigma toward clients (Hayes, Bissett, et al., 2004), and psychosis (Bach & Hayes, 2002; Gaudiano & Herbert, 2006). To date, there have been approximately 20 randomized controlled trials evaluating ACT outcomes, and despite relatively small sample sizes, the outcomes have been generally supportive.

This kind of breadth is unusual in the current mental health care climate, where the tendency has been to develop and test treatments matched to specific disorders. ACT, by contrast, is a model of processes that feed many forms of human suffering (Hayes et al., 1996). If the model is correct, then areas where those processes show up ought to be amenable to ACT interventions. Thus, it is not surprising that ACT is working for such a broad range of problems that are linked to the model.

It is important to note that ACT is beginning to be subjected to criticisms from within the behavior therapy community (Arch & Craske, 2008; Hofmann & Asmundson, 2008; Öst, 2008). Although a review of these criticisms is beyond the scope of this chapter, the theme of the discussion generally involves the differences and similarities between ACT and more traditional cognitive-behavioral therapies. Beyond this, ACT has yet to reach the level of an empirically supported psychosocial intervention by conventional standards (Task Force on Promotion and Dissemination of Psychological Procedures, 1995). Yet it is well on its way to doing that.

Summary and Conclusions

Emotion regulation is not necessarily a maladaptive phenomenon, but its potential to be problematic is connected to human language and cognition. Avoidance, for instance, has greatly contributed to the survival of human and other species. Problems arise when the avoidance efforts are inflexibly directed toward targets such as emotions, thoughts, bodily sensations, and other private events that cannot, in fact, be avoided. These problems are compounded when these efforts progressively keep the individual away from personally meaningful life directions and goals. There is no other nonverbal species that struggles with the contents of unpleasant private events in the way humans do. In a way, humans turn strategies that have enabled survival and enormous accomplishments in the world outside the skin on its host and fight a war with themselves that need not be fought in order to live well. This is a trap that can transform pain into suffering and highlights where and why emotion regulation is problematic.

According to the characteristics of human language and cognition as described in RFT, thoughts and other private contents are derived products of our personal history whose occurrence is, by definition, not under the voluntary control of the individual. Humans, however, are immersed in a culture in which the contents that relate to fear, anxiety, loneliness, regret, painful memories, and so on are demonized as the reasons of our suffering and misery, are barriers to a fulfilling live, and thus become objects to resist and overcome. Research has shown that this war tends not to work well and, in fact, amplifies and expands the very pain that people so desperately wish to avoid. When taken to the extreme, emotion regulation can quite literally become what life is about, and this is no way to live.

For a time, behavior therapy was about helping people to think and feel better in order to live better. With the evolution of the third generation of behavior therapies, however, the goal has been to help people to live well with whatever they may feel or think. ACT does this by incorporating contextual and experiential methods within direct-change strategies, with the final purpose of increasing psychological flexibility in the service of personally meaningful life directions and goals. Research on ACT is growing and the results so far are quite promising (see Hayes et al., 2006, for a recent review). ACT-based interventions are being adapted and subjected to empirical scrutiny with a wide variety of psychological problems in diverse setting, from clinical to work contexts. Basic research on processes of change, as well as on RFT and experimental psychopathology, is also growing at a fast pace. We have come a long way but still have a long way to go.

Acknowledgments

The preparation of this material was partially supported by grants from the Spanish Fulbright Alumni Association and the Department of Education and Science, Government of Spain, to Sonsoles Valdivia-Salas.

References

Arch, J. J., & Craske, M. G. (2008). Acceptance and commitment therapy and cognitive behavioral therapy for anxiety disorders: Different treatments, similar mechanisms? *Clinical Psychology: Science and Practice, 15,* 263–279.
Bach, P., & Hayes, S. C. (2002). The use of acceptance and commitment therapy to

prevent the rehospitalization of psychotic patients: A randomized controlled trial. *Journal of Consulting and Clinical Psychology, 70,* 1129–1139.

Baer, R. A., Fischer, S., & Huss, D. B. (2005). Mindfulness and acceptance in the treatment of disordered eating. *Journal of Rational-Emotive and Cognitive-Behavior Therapy, 23,* 281–299.

Barlow, D. H., Allen, L. B., & Choate, M. L. (2004). Toward a unified treatment for emotional disorders. *Behavior Therapy, 35,* 205–230.

Blackledge, J. T. (2003). An introduction to relational frame theory: Basics and applications. *The Behavior Analyst Today, 3,* 421–433.

Bonanno, G. A., Papa, A., Lalande, K., Westphal, M., & Coifman, K. (2004). The importance of being flexible: The ability to both enhance and suppress emotional expression predicts long-term adjustment. *Psychological Science, 15,* 482–487.

Bond, F. W., & Bunce, D. (2000). Mediators of change in emotion-focused and problem-focused worksite stress management interventions. *Journal of Occupational Health Psychology, 5,* 156–163.

Butler, E. A., & Gross, J. J. (2004). Hiding feelings in social contexts: Out of sight is not out of mind. In P. Philippot & R. S. Feldman (Eds.), *The regulation of emotion* (pp. 101–126). Mahwah, NJ: Erlbaum.

Catania, A. C., Matthews, A., & Shimoff, E. (1990). Properties of rule-governed behavior and their implications. In D. E. Blackman & H. Lejeune (Eds.), *Behavior analysis in theory and practice* (pp. 215–230). Hillsdale, NJ: Erlbaum.

Cioffi, D., & Holloway, J. (1993). Delayed costs of suppressed pain. *Journal of Personality and Social Psychology, 64,* 274–282.

Dahl, J., Wilson, K. G., & Nilsson, A. (2004). Acceptance and commitment therapy and the treatment of persons at risk for long-term disability resulting from stress and pain symptoms: A preliminary randomized trial. *Behavior Therapy, 35,* 785–802.

Dalrymple, K. L., & Herbert, J. D. (2007). Acceptance and commitment therapy for generalized social anxiety disorder: A pilot study. *Behavior Modification, 31,* 543–568.

Dougher, M. J., Augustson, E. M., Markham, M. R., Greenway, D. E., & Wulfert, E. (1994). The transfer of respondent eliciting and extinction functions through stimulus equivalence classes. *Journal of the Experimental Analysis of Behavior, 62,* 331–351.

Dougher, M. J., & Hackbert, L. (1994). A behavior-analytic account of depression and a case report using acceptance-based procedures. *The Behavior Analyst, 17,* 321–334.

Dougher, M. J., Hamilton, D. A., Fink, B. C., & Harrington, J. (2007). Transformation of the discriminative and eliciting functions of generalized relational stimuli. *Journal of the Experimental Analysis of Behavior, 88,* 179–197.

Eifert, G. H., & Forsyth, J. P. (2005). *Acceptance and commitment therapy for anxiety disorders: A practitioner's treatment guide to using mindfulness, acceptance, and value-based behavior change strategies.* Oakland, CA: New Harbinger.

Eifert, G. H., & Heffner, M. (2003). The effects of acceptance versus control contexts on avoidance of panic-related symptoms. *Journal of Behavior Therapy and Experimental Psychiatry, 34,* 293–312.

Forman, E. M., Herbert, J. D., Moitra, E., Yeomans, P. D., & Geller, P. A. (2007). A randomized controlled effectiveness trial of acceptance and commitment therapy and cognitive therapy for anxiety and depression. *Behavior Modification, 31,* 772–799.

Forsyth, J. P., & Eifert, G. H. (1996). The language of feeling and the feeling of anxiety: Contributions of the behaviorisms toward understanding the function-altering effects of language. *Psychological Record, 46,* 607–649.

Forsyth, J. P., Eifert, G. H., & Barrios, V. (2006). Fear conditioning research as a clinical analog: What makes fear learning disordered? In M. G. Craske, D. Hermans, & D. Vansteenwegen (Eds.), *Fear and learning: From basic processes to clinical implications* (pp. 133–156). Washington, DC: American Psychological Association.

Garnefski, N., Teerds, J., Kraaij, V., Legerstee, J., & Van den Kommer, T. (2004). Cognitive emotion regulation strategies and depressive symptoms: Differences between males and females. *Personality and Individual Differences, 36,* 267–276.

Gaudiano, B. A., & Herbert, J. D. (2006). Acute treatment of inpatients with psychotic symptoms using acceptance and commitment therapy: Pilot results. *Behaviour Research and Therapy, 44,* 415–437.

Gifford, E. V., Kohlenberg, B. S., Hayes, S. C., Antonuccio, D. O., Piasecki, M. M., Rasmussen-Hall, M. L., et al. (2004). Applying a functional acceptance based model to smoking cessation: An initial trial of acceptance and commitment therapy. *Behavior Therapy, 35,* 689–705.

Gratz, K. L., & Gunderson, J. G. (2006). Preliminary data on an acceptance-based emotion regulation group intervention for deliberate self-harm among women with borderline personality disorder. *Behavior Therapy, 37,* 25–35.

Gregg, J. A., Callaghan, G. M., Hayes, S. C., & Glenn-Lawson, J. L. (2007). Improving diabetes self-management through acceptance, mindfulness, and values: A randomized controlled trial. *Journal of Consulting and Clinical Psychology, 75,* 336–343.

Gross, J. J. (1998). Antecedent- and response-focused emotion regulation: Divergent consequences for experience, expression, and physiology. *Journal of Personality and Social Psychology, 74,* 224–237.

Gross, J. J. (2002). Emotion regulation: Affective, cognitive, and social consequences. *Psychophysiology, 39,* 281–291.

Gross, J. J., & Muñoz, R. F. (1995). Emotion regulation and mental health. *Clinical Psychology: Science and Practice, 2,* 151–164.

Gutiérrez, O., Luciano, C., Rodríguez, M., & Fink, B. C. (2004). Comparison between an acceptance-based and a cognitive-control-based protocol for coping with pain. *Behavior Therapy, 35,* 767–783.

Hayes, S. C. (1976). The role of approach contingencies in phobic behavior. *Behavior Therapy, 7,* 28–36.

Hayes, S. C. (2004). Acceptance and commitment therapy, relational frame theory, and the third wave of behavioral and cognitive therapies. *Behavior Therapy, 35,* 639–666.

Hayes, S. C., Barnes-Holmes, D., & Roche, B. (2001). *Relational frame theory: A post-Skinnerian account of human language and cognition.* New York: Kluwer.

Hayes, S. C., Bissett, R., Roget, N., Padilla, M., Kohlenberg, B. S., Fisher, G., et al. (2004). The impact of acceptance and commitment training and multicultural training on the stigmatizing attitudes and professional burnout of substance abuse counselors. *Behavior Therapy, 35,* 821–835.

Hayes, S. C., Gifford, E. V., & Hayes, G. J. (1998). Moral behavior and the development of verbal regulation. *The Behavior Analyst, 21,* 253–279.

Hayes, S. C., Luoma, J. B., Bond, F. W., Masuda, A., & Lillis, J. (2006). Acceptance and commitment therapy: Model, processes, and outcomes. *Behaviour Research and Therapy, 44,* 1–25.

Hayes, S. C., & Strosahl, K. D. (2004). *A practical guide to acceptance and commitment therapy.* New York: Springer-Verlag.

Hayes, S. C., Strosahl, K. D., Bunting, K., Twohig, M., & Wilson, K. G. (2004). What is acceptance and commitment therapy? In S. C. Hayes & K. D. Strosahl (Eds.), *A practical guide to acceptance and commitment therapy* (pp. 1–29). New York: Springer-Verlag.

Hayes, S. C., Strosahl, K. D., & Wilson. K. G. (1999). *Acceptance and commitment therapy: An experiential approach to behavior change.* New York: Guilford Press.

Hayes, S. C., Wilson, K. G., Gifford, E. V., Bissett, R., Piasecki, M., Batten, S. V., et al. (2004). A preliminary trial of twelve-step facilitation and acceptance and commitment therapy with polysubstance-abusing methadone-maintained opiate addicts. *Behavior Therapy, 35,* 667–688.

Hayes, S. C., Wilson, K. G., Gifford, E. V., Follette, V. M., & Strosahl, K. (1996). Experiential avoidance and behavioral disorders: A functional dimensional approach to diagnosis and treatment. *Journal of Consulting and Clinical Psychology, 64,* 1152–1168.

Heffner, M., Sperry, J., & Eifert, G. H. (2002). Acceptance and commitment therapy in the treatment of an adolescent female with anorexia nervosa: A case example. *Cognitive and Behavioral Practice, 9,* 232–236.

Hernández-López, M., Luciano, M. C., Bricker, J. B., Roales-Nieto, J. G., & Montesinos, F. (2008). *Acceptance and commitment therapy for smoking cessation: A study of its effectiveness in comparison with a multicomponent cognitive-behavioral treatment.* Manuscript submitted for publication.

Hofmann, S. G., & Asmundson, G. J. (2008). Acceptance and mindfulness-based therapy: New wave or old hat? *Clinical Psychology Review, 28,* 1–16.

John, O. P., & Gross, J. J. (2004). Healthy and unhealthy emotion regulation: Personality processes, individual differences, and life span development. *Journal of Personality, 72,* 1301–1333.

Kabat-Zinn, J. (2003). Mindfulness-based interventions in context: Past, present, and future. *Clinical Psychology Science and Practice, 10,* 144–156.

Levitt, J. T., Brown, T. A., Orsillo, S. M., & Barlow, D. H. (2004). The effects of acceptance versus suppression of emotion on subjective and psychophysiological response to carbon dioxide challenge in patients with panic disorder. *Behavior Therapy, 35,* 747–766.

Luciano, M. C., Gómez-Becerra, I., & Rodríguez-Valverde, M. (2007). The role of multiple-exemplar training and naming in establishing derived equivalence in an infant. *Journal of the Experimental Analysis of Behavior, 87,* 349–365.

Luciano, M. C., Rodríguez-Valverde, M., & Gutiérrez, O. (2004). A proposal for synthesizing verbal contexts in experiential avoidance disorder and acceptance and commitment therapy. *International Journal of Psychology and Psychological Therapy, 4,* 377–394.

Luciano, M. C., Valdivia-Salas, S., Berens, N., Rodríguez-Valverde, M., Ruiz, F., & Mañas, I. (2009). Acquiring the earliest relational operants: Coordination, difference, opposition, comparison, and hierarchy. In R. A. Rehfeldt &

Y. Barnes-Holmes (Eds.), *Derived relational responding: Applications for learners with autism and other developmental disabilities* (pp. 149–170). Oakland, CA: New Harbinger.

Lundgren, T., Dahl, J., & Hayes, S. C. (2008). Evaluation of mediators of change in the treatment of epilepsy with acceptance and commitment therapy. *Journal of Behavior Medicine, 31*, 225–235.

Lundgren, T., Dahl, J., Melin, L., & Kies, B. (2006). Evaluation of acceptance and commitment therapy for drug refractory epilepsy: A randomized controlled trial in South Africa—A pilot study. *Epilepsia, 47*, 2173–2179.

Marx, B. P., & Sloan, D. M. (2002). The role of emotion in the psychological functioning of adult survivors of childhood sexual abuse. *Behavior Therapy, 33*, 563–577.

Masedo, A. I., & Esteve, R. (2007). Effects of suppression, acceptance and spontaneous coping on pain tolerance, pain intensity and distress. *Behaviour Research and Therapy, 45*, 199–209.

McCracken, L. M., Spertus, I. L., Janeck, A. S., Sinclair, D., & Wetzel, F. T. (1999). Behavioral dimensions of adjustment in persons with chronic pain: Pain-related anxiety and acceptance. *Pain, 80*, 283–289.

McCracken, L. M., Vowles, K. E., & Eccleston, C. (2005). Acceptance-based treatment for persons with complex, long standing chronic pain: A preliminary analysis of treatment outcome in comparison to a waiting phase. *Behaviour Research and Therapy, 43*, 1335–1346.

McKay, M., & Sutker, C. (2007). *Leave your mind behind: The everyday practice of finding stillness amid the rushing thoughts.* Oakland, CA: New Harbinger.

McMullen, J., Barnes-Holmes, D., Barnes-Holmes, Y., Stewart, I., Luciano, M. C., & Cochrane, A. (2008). Acceptance versus distraction: Brief instructions, metaphors, and exercises in increasing tolerance for self-delivered electric shocks. *Behaviour Research and Therapy, 46*, 122–129.

Montesinos, F. (2003). ACT, sexual desire orientation, and erectile dysfunction: A case study. *Análisis y Modificación de Conducta, 29*, 291–320.

Moore, S. A., Zoellner, L. A., & Mollenholt, N. (2008). Are expressive suppression and cognitive reappraisal associated with stress-related symptoms? *Behaviour Research and Therapy, 46*, 993–1000.

Ochsner, K. N., Bunge, S. A., Gross, J. J., & Gabrieli, J. D. (2002). Rethinking feelings: An fMRI study of the cognitive regulation of emotion. *Journal of Cognitive Neuroscience, 14*, 1215–1229.

Öst, L. G. (2008). Efficacy of the third wave of behavior therapies: A systematic review and meta-analysis. *Behaviour Research and Therapy, 46*, 296–321.

Páez-Blarrina, M., Luciano, M. C., & Gutiérrez, O. (2007). Tratamiento psicológico para el tratamiento del cáncer de mama: Estudio comparativo entre estrategias de aceptación y de control cognitivo [Psychological treatment for breast cancer: Comparison between acceptance-based and cognitive control-based strategies]. *Psicooncología, 4*, 75–95.

Páez-Blarrina, M., Luciano, M. C., Gutiérrez, O., Valdivia, S., Ortega, J., & Rodríguez, M. (2008). The role of values with personal examples in altering the functions of pain: Comparisons between acceptance-based and cognitive-control-based protocols. *Behavior Research and Therapy, 46*, 84–97.

Páez-Blarrina, M., Luciano, M. C., Gutiérrez, O., Valdivia, S., Rodríguez, M., & Ortega, J. (2008). Coping with pain in the motivational context of values:

A comparison between an acceptance-based and a cognitive-control-based protocol. *Behavior Modification, 32*, 403–422.

Parrott, W. G. (1993). Beyond hedonism: Motives for inhibiting good moods and for maximizing bad moods. In D. M. Wegner & J. W. Pennebaker (Eds.), *Handbook of mental control* (pp. 278–308). Englewood Cliffs, NJ: Prentice Hall.

Purdon, C. (1999). Thought suppression and psychopathology. *Behaviour Research and Therapy, 37*, 1029–1054.

Richards, J. M., & Gross, J. J. (2000). Emotion regulation and memory: The cognitive costs of keeping one's cool. *Journal of Personality and Social Psychology, 79*, 410–424.

Roche, B., & Barnes, D. (1997). A transformation of respondently conditioned stimulus functions in accordance with arbitrarily applicable relations. *Journal of the Experimental Analysis of Behavior, 67*, 275–301.

Rodríguez-Valverde, M., Luciano, M. C., & Barnes-Holmes, D. (2009). Transfer of aversive respondent elicitation in accordance with equivalence relations. *Journal of the Experimental Analysis of Behavior, 92*, 85–111.

Spira, A. P., Zvolensky, M. J., Eifert, G. H., & Feldner, M. T. (2004). Avoidance-oriented coping as a predictor of anxiety-based physical stress: A test using biological challenge. *Journal of Anxiety Disorders, 18*, 309–323.

Staats, A. W., & Eifert, G. H. (1990). The paradigmatic behaviorism theory of emotions: Basis for unification. *Clinical Psychology Review, 10*, 539–566.

Strosahl, K. D., Hayes, S. C., Wilson, K. G., & Gifford, E. (2004). An ACT primer: Core therapy processes, intervention strategies, and therapist competencies. In S. C. Hayes & K. D. Strosahl (Eds.), *A practical guide to acceptance and commitment therapy* (pp. 31–58). New York: Springer-Verlag.

Task Force on Promotion and Dissemination of Psychological Procedures. (1995). Training in and dissemination of empirically-validated psychological treatments. *The Clinical Psychologist, 48*, 3–23.

Törneke, N., Luciano, M. C., & Valdivia-Salas, S. (2008). Rule-governed behavior and psychological problems. *International Journal of Psychology and Psychological Therapy, 8*, 141–156.

Twohig, M. P., Hayes, S. C., & Masuda, A. (2006). Increasing willingness to experience obsessions: Acceptance and commitment therapy as a treatment for obsessive-compulsive disorder. *Behavior Therapy, 37*, 3–13.

Twohig, M. P., Shoenberger, D., & Hayes, S. C. (2007). A preliminary investigation of acceptance and commitment therapy as a treatment for marijuana dependence in adults. *Journal of Applied Behavior Analysis, 40*, 619–632.

Valdivia-Salas, S., Dougher, M. J., & Luciano, M. C. (2009). *Transfer of the function-altering functions of the events.* Manuscript submitted for publication.

Valdivia-Salas, S., Luciano, M. C., & Molina, F. J. (2006). Verbal regulation of motivational states. *Psychological Record, 56*, 577–595.

Vowles, K. E., & McCracken, L. M. (2008). Acceptance and values-based action in chronic pain: A study of treatment effectiveness and process. *Journal of Consulting and Clinical Psychology, 76*, 397–407.

Wegner, D. M. (1994). Ironic processes of mental control. *Psychological Review, 101*, 34–52.

Whelan, R., & Barnes-Holmes, D. (2004). The transformation of consequential function in accordance with the relational frames of same and opposite. *Journal of the Experimental Analysis of Behavior, 82*, 177–195.

Whelan, R., Barnes-Holmes, D., & Dymond, S. (2006). Transformation of consequential functions in accordance with the relational frames of more-than and
less-than. *Journal of the Experimental Analysis of Behavior, 86*, 317–335.

Wilson, K. G., & Byrd, M. R. (2004). ACT for substance abuse and dependence. In
S. C. Hayes & K. D. Strosahl (Eds.), *A practical guide to acceptance and commitment therapy* (pp. 153–184). New York: Springer-Verlag.

Wilson, K. G., & Hayes, S. C. (1996). Resurgence of derived stimulus relations.
Journal of the Experimental Analysis of Behavior, 66, 267–281.

Wilson, K. G., Hayes, S. C., Gregg, J., & Zettle, R. (2001). Psychopathology and
psychotherapy. In S. C. Hayes, D. Barnes-Holmes, & B. Roche (Eds.), *Relational frame theory: A post-Skinnerian account of human language and cognition*
(pp. 211–238). New York: Kluwer Academic.

Wilson, K., & Luciano, M. C. (2002). *Terapia de Aceptación y Compromiso: Un
Tratamiento conductual orientado a los valores* [Acceptance and commitment
therapy: A behavioral therapeutic approach focused in values]. Madrid:
Pirámide.

Wilson, K. G., Sandoz, E. K., Kitchens, J., & Roberts, M. E. (in press). The Valued
Living Questionnaire: Defining and measuring valued action within a behavioral framework. *Psychological Record*.

Zettle, R. D., & Rains, J. C. (1989). Group cognitive and contextual therapies in
treatment of depression. *Journal of Clinical Psychology, 45*, 438–445.

CHAPTER 14

• — — • — — • — — •

Mindfulness and Emotion Regulation

OUTCOMES AND POSSIBLE MEDIATING MECHANISMS

**Kathleen M. Corcoran, Norman Farb, Adam Anderson,
and Zindel V. Segal**

Over the past 10 years, the topic of mindfulness has figured increasingly prominently in accounts of physical and emotional illness and health maintenance. Often described in terms of its attentional and affective parameters, mindfulness encourages a nonelaborative, nonjudgmental, present-centered awareness in which thoughts, feelings, or bodily sensations that arise in the attentional field are acknowledged and accepted as they are (Kabat-Zinn, 1990; Segal, Williams, & Teasdale, 2002; Shapiro & Schwartz, 2000). Mindfulness is developed through the practice of various meditation techniques that have their origin in Buddhist spiritual practices (Hanh, 1976) but can easily be taught within a secular framework. Evidence has accumulated that both the practice of mindfulness meditation and trait levels of mindfulness are associated with increased well-being, reduced stress, negative affectivity, and robust physical health outcomes (Baer, 2003) across a variety of patient groups, including those with anxiety, depression, pain, stress, and chronic illnesses. Indeed, the integration of mindfulness practice into a number of established clinical treatments has aided the wider dissemination of these practices in both clinical and research realms.

Although the benefits of mindfulness practice are generally accepted, the specific mechanisms and processes that operate in their attainment are largely unknown. This is true in terms of the work needed to rule out competing explanations, such as active relaxation or cognitive distraction, as accounting for the observed gains. Similarly, the psychological and neural processes triggered by the practice of mindfulness have yet to be identified. A reasonable starting point might be the nature of the connection between mindfulness and emotion. For example, these practices have traditionally been taught as a method for compassionately calming the mind in the face of negative affect. It has been suggested that the repetitive labeling of thoughts, feelings, and sensations as events in the mind reduces identification with their literal content and creates an attentional buffer between stimulus and response. In this chapter, we describe mindfulness training, discuss the empirical findings on mindfulness, and review possible psychological and neural mechanisms through which these practices aid in the processing of disturbed affect and cognition.

Emotions and Emotion Regulation

The study of emotion has a long history in psychology, with a good deal of attention paid to describing individual differences in the regulation of emotional states. Our view of emotion is drawn largely from Ekman and Davidson (1994), who conceived of emotions as a complex set of cognitive, behavioral, and physiological responses to internal and external stimuli (Gross & Thompson, 2007). We believe that emotions are adaptive and provide vital information regarding internal or external events. They help motivate action (often triggering behavioral responses such as approach or avoidance) and communicate information to others. Although the experience of negative emotion is found in many forms of psychopathology, we do not view negative emotion itself as unhealthy. Instead, we believe that problems with emotion regulation often underlie psychopathology. Our view of emotion regulation corresponds in many ways to the definition put forward by Gross (1998), who describes emotion regulation as "the processes by which individuals influence which emotions they have, when they have them, and how they experience and express these emotions" (p. 275). Gross also suggests that the process of regulating emotions can lie along a continuum, from "conscious, effortful, and controlled regulation to unconscious, effortless, and automatic regulation" (p. 275). In psychopathology, this often involves regulation of negative emotional experiences, such as anxiety or low mood, but it also can involve the regulation of the experience and expression of positive mood.

Problems with emotion regulation are central to many forms of psychopathology (e.g., Cicchetti, Ackerman, & Izard, 1995; Gross, 1998). One way to classify psychiatric disorders is to consider the degree to which emotions, reported within their syndromal presentation, are over- or underregulated. For example, emotion underregulation is common to disorders such as borderline personality disorder, posttraumatic stress disorder, and many of the anxiety disorders, in which individuals experience intense emotions that they find difficult to regulate. On the other end of the spectrum lie disorders in which overregulation of emotion becomes problematic, such as in obsessive–compulsive personality disorder. In still other disorders, such as bipolar disorder, problems exist with emotion dysregulation. Indeed, problems with emotion regulation have been implicated as a key factor in mood and anxiety disorders (Campbell-Sills & Barlow, 2007; Mennin, Heimberg, Turk, & Fresco, 2005).

Several maladaptive emotion regulation strategies are commonly found in psychiatric disorders. One such strategy is avoidance, which can take on many forms, including distraction, suppression of thoughts or emotions, or actual avoidance of people, places, or situations. Emotional avoidance can also be achieved through the use of substances or other methods to numb emotional experience, such as dissociation, self-harm, or risky behaviors (Linehan, 1993). A related concept, experiential avoidance, has been characterized as an unwillingness to remain in contact with internal experiences such as thoughts, emotions, and physical sensations (Hayes, Strosahl, & Wilson, 1999; see also Boulanger, Hayes, & Pistorello, Chapter 5, this volume). Standing in contrast to avoidance, overengagement with emotions is another commonly used emotion regulation strategy that involves, for example, rumination, obsessions, worry, and compulsions (Hayes & Feldman, 2004; see also Joorman, Yoon, & Siemer, Chapter 8, this volume).

Strategies to help enhance adaptive emotion regulation lie at the heart of many forms of treatment. Most commonly, treatments for the mood and anxiety disorders involve strategies to down-regulate negative emotional experiences. Cognitive-behavioral treatments, for example, focus on reducing negative emotion by identifying and challenging negative thinking through the use of thought records and core belief work and by encouraging behavior change to promote enhanced emotion regulation (i.e., through exposure to feared stimuli in the anxiety disorders or behavioral activation in depression). In doing so, cognitive-behavioral therapies appear to be working at the levels of reappraisal and response modulation, as described by Gross (1998).

Mindfulness Interventions

Mindfulness-based therapies mark an important departure from the more traditional cognitive-behavioral treatments in that they promote changing one's relationship to thoughts and feelings rather than directly changing the content of thoughts per se. Moreover, mindfulness training emphasizes developing greater awareness and acceptance of emotions rather than teaching methods to change emotional experience. As discussed by Linehan (1993), adaptive emotional regulation involves both change strategies, such as those emphasized in cognitive-behavioral treatments, and acceptance strategies, such as those taught in mindfulness-based treatments.

Mindfulness-based interventions have been developed to treat a wide variety of populations and disorders. Mindfulness-based stress reduction (MBSR; Kabat-Zinn, 1990) and mindfulness-based cognitive therapy (MBCT; Segal et al., 2002) include a predominant focus on mindfulness practices, with the former used to treat anxiety and chronic pain difficulties and the latter used to help prevent the relapse of depression. Acceptance and commitment therapy (Hayes et al., 1999) and dialectical behavior therapy (Linehan, 1993) also incorporate elements of mindfulness into their treatments, although mindfulness strategies form but one of many strategies utilized in these treatments.

Both MBCT and MBSR are offered in an 8-week group format that combines sustained attentional training (drawn from Vipassana meditation) with psychoeducation about physical and emotional disorders. Each session is approximately 2 to 2.5 hours in length and provides a series of experiential exercises, guided discussion of participants' reactions to the exercises, and training in cognitive techniques. Experiential exercises, which make up the largest component of the programs, facilitate greater awareness of present-moment experience, including thoughts, emotions, and bodily sensations such as tension and pain. Formal mindfulness practices include the body scan, an exercise in which each body region is briefly attended to, mindfulness of the breath, mindfulness of the body, mindful stretching, and short mindfulness exercises such as the 3-minute breathing space. Participants are also taught informal mindfulness practices, in which they are encouraged to be attentive to seemingly "routine" activities in their day-to-day lives, such as eating and walking and to monitor their thoughts, emotions, and bodily sensations during pleasant and unpleasant activities.

MBCT differs from MBSR in its inclusion of cognitive techniques borrowed from traditional cognitive-behavioral therapy strategies. These techniques were included in the program to address the residual mood-linked reactivity that has been shown to place remitted patients at risk for relapse (Segal et al., 2006). These cognitive techniques include psychoeducation about depressive symptoms and the connection between thoughts, moods, and behavior; exercises such as monitoring the relationship between activities and mood; questioning and challenging negative automatic thoughts; and developing a relapse prevention plan. MBCT also includes a specific technique called the "3-minute breathing space," which was designed to help individuals develop nonjudgmental awareness of upsetting thoughts and emotional experiences. In this exercise, participants are taught to actively shift the focus of attention across three different foci over the course of 3 minutes. The first focus is an open monitoring of thoughts, sensations, and emotions as they occur on a moment-by-moment basis. This is done without any demand that the quality of these elements be altered. Rather, the intention is to stay attentive and notice any changes that may occur. The second focus is introduced by asking participants to let go of watching thoughts, sensations, and feelings and to shift their attention to a more narrow attending to the breath at the belly. In the third stage of this exercise, attention is broadened once again, as participants are asked to expand their awareness and become aware of the body as a whole. One hypothesis about the 3-minute breathing space is that the purposeful shifting of attention can disrupt ruminative processing of negative emotion by reallocating scarce cognitive resources to competing demands (Teasdale, Segal, & Williams, 1995).

Woven throughout the training, MBSR and MBCT facilitate greater emotional awareness and the development of a different relationship to troubling emotions. In MBCT, for example, participants complete negative and pleasant events calendars, in which they take note of situations that are associated with negative and positive mood. Through these exercises, individuals learn to recognize how affectively charged situations have correlates in the body and how these signals are often overlooked. For many participants, this turns out to be a novel way of understanding their emotional triggers. Emotion regulation skills are also learned during sustained mindfulness practice. Mindfulness training promotes observing the qualities of an emotional experience, noticing how these qualities change from moment to moment, and attending to accompanying somatic and cognitive cues. With time, individuals become more adept at recognizing subtle changes in their bodies that may signal the presence of an emotional state. They also learn new ways to deal with emotions, becoming better able to observe, notice, and approach emotions rather than to engage in potentially maladaptive strategies such as suppression or rumination.

Scientific investigation on the use of mindfulness training as a treatment for pain, illness, anxiety, and mood disorders has increased markedly over the past two decades (Baer, 2003). MBCT has been shown to reduce relapse rates in individuals who have experienced episodic depression (Ma & Teasdale, 2004; Teasdale et al., 2000), and MBSR has been found to improve psychological and physical well-being (Kabat-Zinn, 1982). Reviews suggest that the practice of mindfulness is associated with significant improvements across broad domains of functioning, including reductions in anxiety and depression and increases in physical and psychological well-being (Baer, 2003; Shapiro, Carlson, Astin, & Freedman, 2006), and meta-analyses confirm these findings, demonstrating a moderate effect size for mindfulness-based interventions (Baer, 2003; Grossman, Niemann, Schmidt, & Walach, 2004).

Mindfulness and Emotion Regulation

The act of watching one's experience with equanimity rather than attempting to alter or control one's experience is central to mindfulness training (Brown & Ryan, 2006; Creswell, Way, Eisenberger, & Lieberman, 2007), yet mindfulness as a form of emotion regulation is in many ways foreign to the framing of emotion regulation in conventional scientific literature. Traditionally, emotion regulation has been cast in terms of two major strategies: suppression and reappraisal (Gross, 1998). Suppression attempts to limit or exaggerate the representation of emotion itself (Kim & Hamann, 2007), whereas reappraisal strategies seek to alter the context in which an emotion-inducing stimulus is viewed, thereby altering the emotion provoked (Ochsner, Bunge, Gross, & Gabrieli, 2002). Unlike effortful suppression or reappraisal strategies, however, mindfulness does not seek to achieve an idealized, nonaversive goal state, but rather attempts to create psychological distance between the emotion and the individual, thereby limiting its behavioral consequences (Kabat-Zinn, Lipworth, & Burney, 1985). Establishing psychological distance from aversive emotions may be part of the reappraisal process (Ochsner & Gross, 2008), but mindfulness differs importantly from such processes in that it treats the labeling or monitoring of experience as an end unto itself rather than a means by which to then control the emotion.

A central component of mindfulness practice is the repetitive and deliberate training of attention. As described by Lutz, Slagter, Dunne, and Davidson (2008), mindfulness encompasses competence in both "concentrative" and "open" attentional foci. Unlike traditional reappraisal methods, mindfulness training teaches patients to develop moment-to-moment awareness of available stimuli, decoupling the sensory and affective/evaluative aspects of emotion. Through repeated observation of affective states as "objects" of attention (Creswell et al., 2007), patients learn that emotions have their own somatic signatures, whose fluctuations in intensity and duration provide a continuous cue for refocusing attention (Brefczynski-Lewis, Lutz, & Schaefer, 2007), especially when allocation of scarce mental resources to ruminative processing has been the default (Slagter et al., 2007). Indeed, research on even short-term mindfulness practitioners has provided evidence for improved attentional control (Chambers, Lo, & Allen, 2008; Jha, Krompinger, & Baime, 2007), specifically in areas of overcoming distraction and conflicting information (Wenk-Sormaz, 2005).

There is also evidence that mindfulness training is associated with increases in metacognitive awareness, which is the ability to experience thoughts and feelings from a decentered perspective, one in which thoughts and emotions are seen as "mental events" rather than as accurate reflections of reality (Teasdale et al., 1995, 2002). Mindfulness training promotes the development of a decentered perspective by encouraging participants to better attend to thoughts, emotions, and physical sensations and to view these experiences as passing events. For example, during guided mindfulness exercises, participants are provided with metaphors to help foster this decentered perspective, such as the suggestion to view their thoughts as clouds, floating through the sky. Metacognitive awareness was examined in a study by Teasdale and colleagues (2002), in which 100 patients, who were in either remission or recovery from major depression, were randomized to receive treatment as usual or treatment as usual augmented with MBCT. The patients who participated in MBCT showed greater metacognitive awareness, as assessed by an interview that measured the degree to which individuals adopted a "decentered set" with respect to their thoughts and feelings, at the end of treatment than did patients who received treatment as usual. Moreover, those who completed the MBCT training were less likely to suffer a depressive relapse following treatment. The authors suggest that the ability to approach one's thoughts and feelings from a decentered perspective may be an important mediator in the effectiveness of this treatment. Metacognitive awareness was also examined in a series of two studies by Frewen, Evans, Maraj, Dozois, and Partridge (2008), who found that individuals high in dispositional mindfulness reported greater ease in disengaging from negative thoughts. These correlations were replicated in a second study that involved a help-seeking student sample who underwent an 8-week mindfulness training course. Participation in this mindfulness program resulted in increases in mindfulness and decreases in both the frequency and the difficulty of letting go of negative thoughts.

The development of greater attentional training and metacognitive awareness should result in concomitant changes in the strategies used to deal with negative internal experiences, with increased openness to, and acceptance of, thoughts and feelings. Indeed, there is evidence that mindfulness training is associated with decreases in maladaptive emotion regulation strategies such as rumination and avoidance. Rumination, a passive mode of responding to negative emotions through a focus on the causes, consequences, and meaning of one's problems (Nolen-Hoeksema, 1991), is associated with increased levels of anxiety and depression (Nolen-Hoeksema, 2000). Ramel, Goldin, Carmona, and McQuaid (2004) examined changes in rumination following an 8-week mindfulness training course and found that mindfulness was associated with significant reductions in ruminative tendencies, with decreases in rumination predicted by the amount of meditation practiced by study participants. Similarly, reflexive rumination was found to decrease significantly following an intensive 10-day mindfulness course (Chambers et al., 2008). Mindfulness-based strategies have also proven more effective in reducing dysphoric mood than rumination or distraction strategies in a laboratory study (Broderick, 2005). Thus, there is mounting evidence that one of the beneficial effects of mindfulness training is that it promotes the use of alternate strategies such as acceptance and, in so doing, reduces the reliance of ruminative strategies. Indeed, in at least one study, decreases in rumination were found to mediate the relationship between mindfulness training and decreased dysphoria following a mindfulness course (McKim, 2008).

There is also evidence that mindfulness training is associated with greater ability to tolerate negative emotions and reduced emotional reactivity. Arch and Craske (2006) conducted an analogue study of mindfulness in which they examined the effects of a 15-minute focused-breathing induction on emotional intensity and willingness to tolerate emotion during a slide-viewing task. Participants with no previous experience in mindfulness practice were trained to focus their attention on the breath. Compared with participants in worry induction and unfocused attention conditions, participants who followed mindfulness instructions were more willing to remain in contact with highly aversive slides, and they reported less emotional volatility and negative reactivity across the task. Similarly, in a correlational study, Ortner, Kilner, and Zelazo (2007) found that individuals with greater meditation experience reported lower levels of emotional reactivity in response to negative picture slides. In a second experimental study by the same authors, individuals who participated in a mindfulness training course demonstrated increases in mindfulness over the course of treatment, and at posttreatment they were found to demonstrate lower emotional reactivity than individuals who had participated in a relaxation course or those in a wait-list control. These results suggest that another benefit of mindfulness training is that it promotes the ability to disengage from emotionally provocative material, freeing individuals to refocus their attention on other aspects of experience.

Mindfulness and Emotion Regulation Viewed from the Perspective of Cognitive Neuroscience

In addition to the significant interest in behavioral correlates of mindfulness training, significant advances have taken place with respect to understanding the neural correlates of mindfulness. When attempting to discover how mindfulness operates on a neural level, it is useful to discuss the literature on neural response to emotional stressors. The generally accepted view is that the limbic system represents an evolutionarily more primitive part of the mammalian brain, integrating physiological information to provide immediate behavioral cues to the organism; in human beings this information can eventually reach conscious awareness and reflection, forming the basis for mood and more complicated and nuanced emotional responses (Lane, 2008). The frontal cortices likely act as an attentional control system, which responds to such emotion (Corrigan, 2004). The rostral anterior cingulate cortex has been implicated in maintained attention to self (Kelley et al., 2002) and emotion (Lane, Fink, Chau, & Dolan, 1997), dorsolateral prefrontal cortices with maintaining information in awareness (Courtney, Ungerleider, Keil, & Haxby, 1997; Goldman-Rakic, 1995; Smith & Jonides, 1999), and ventrolateral prefrontal cortices with inhibitory processes critical to resisting distraction (Aron, Robbins, & Poldrack, 2004; D'Esposito, Postle, Jonides, & Smith, 1999; Jonides, Smith, Marshuetz, Koeppe, & Reuter-Lorenz, 1998). The medial prefrontal cortices can, therefore, be thought of as attentional control centers helping to regulate the flow of information from memory and the senses to one's internally represented goals and self-knowledge (Beauregard, Lévesque, & Bourgouin, 2001; Fossati et al., 2003; Kelley et al., 2002; Ochsner et al., 2002), while the dorsolateral and ventrolateral prefrontal cortices seem related to keeping things in and out of mind, respectively (Bunge, Ochsner, Desmond, Glover, & Gabrieli, 2001; Dolcos, Miller, Kragel, Jha, & McCarthy, 2007).

While suppression and reappraisal processes may serve as effective, normative regulatory strategies (e.g., Goldin, McRae, Ramel, & Gross, 2008), a number of studies now point to compromised frontal cortical modulation of limbic circuitry as underlying ineffective regulation of negative emotion (Johnstone, van Reekum, Urry, Kalin, & Davidson, 2007; Ressler & Mayberg, 2007). The ventromedial prefrontal cortex (vmPFC) serves to link the limbic cortices with the medial prefrontal cortices (mPFC), areas implicated in higher order executive functions such as self-referential thought, voluntary memory recall, and effortful emotion regulation (Amodio & Frith, 2006; Craik et al., 1999; Fossati et al., 2003; Johnson et al., 2002; Kelley et al., 2002; Macrae, Moran, Heatherton, Banfield, & Kelley, 2004; Northoff & Heinzel, 2006; Ochsner et al., 2005). Physically situated directly between the limbic cortices and the mPFC, the vmPFC presents a likely candidate for regulating the interplay between executive function and the representation of emotion. The vmPFC receives connections from all exteroceptive (Barbas, 2000) and interoceptive (Carmichael & Price, 1996) modalities and has been viewed as a polymodal convergence zone (Rolls, 2000), supporting the integration of external and internal stimuli with judgments about their affective relevance to the self (Ochsner & Gross, 2005).

The action of mindfulness training on ventral frontal cortical networks, the systems bridging emotional and self-referential processing, is of special interest when one considers evidence of neural activation disparities between dysphoric patients and healthy controls. In studies of sad mood provocation, for example, patients currently diagnosed with or at risk for an affective disorder show altered activation in these same regions, notably the medial prefrontal, orbital frontal, and subgenual cingulate cortices (e.g., Keightley et al., 2003). Dysphoria-linked changes in the configurations of prefrontal engagement may signal compromised cognitive or attentional control over emotion, leading to maladaptive behavioral efforts at regulation by vulnerable patients (e.g., Ramel et al., 2007). In Johnstone and colleagues (2007), depressed patients showed reduced connectivity between limbic and frontal cortices though the vmPFC relative to controls, and this lack of connectivity was used to explain why the depressed group was less able to decrease limbic activation to a dysphoric stimulus. The cause of these patients' inability to use the vmPFC as a "limbic filter" is unknown and likely has a range of influences, from genetics to personal history.

Until it becomes clear exactly how one can repair vmPFC regulation of emotional information, strategies reducing the aversive reactivity to emotion could be vital in building resilience and reducing illness risk. Mindfulness presents itself as one such approach to combating dysphoric reactivity by seeking to develop metacognitive skills for tolerating and approaching negative affect from a wider attentional frame (Teasdale, 1999). The ability to suppress distracting influences and engage in sensation without necessarily restricting the flow of information may represent an important first step in combating affective disorders, in which the aversive reaction to one's feelings may ironically serve to perpetuate the depressed state in what has been termed a *depressogenic cycle* (Teasdale et al., 1995).

Suppression versus Equanimity in the Brain

If vmPFC hyperactivity is commonly correlated with depressive states, its specific functions may be to perpetuate habits in cognitive control on emotion representation. In the Farb and colleagues (2007) study, participants engaging in verbal self-elaboration showed strong vmPFC activity, and of the MBSR treatment and wait-list control groups, only the MBSR group were able to disengage vmPFC when performing self-reflection tasks. It is important to note that the mindfulness training did not eliminate activation in areas of emotion representation themselves; in fact, the MBSR group showed heightened activation in limbic cortices. Thus, the neural correlates of mindfulness lie less in the ability to eliminate emotional processing and more in narrowing the neural link between such processing with higher cognitive function like self reference, memory retrieval, and verbal elaboration. Heightened neural representation of emotion has also been found in a study with experienced meditators (> 4 years of regular practice): Lazar and colleagues (2000) found widespread cortical deactivation during meditation but widespread activation in the limbic cortices and hippocampus. Indeed, a further study by Lazar and colleagues (2005) found that hours of meditation practice ranging from novice to expert positively predicted grey matter volume in the right anterior insula and prefrontal cortex, areas involved in interoceptive awareness and viscerosomatic representation (Craig, 2004). These functional differences in neural connectivity between those who do and do not meditate represent a key distinction between mindfulness training and maladaptive emotion regulation. Rather than labeling the emotion as something negative to be controlled and ruminated upon or suppressed, the momentary assessment of emotion is performed with greater precision and attention to nuanced changes. In this way, higher resolution processing of emotion can occur, and with it the possibility for variability in an otherwise categorically negative emotional experience. By freeing the individual from conceiving negative emotion as a uniform category to be controlled, the possibility of emotional change, of an ebb and flow to positive and negative emotions, can potentially be realized.

The results summarized previously suggest that, while the mindfulness practice might be impairing the narrative and analytic processing of self-related information, the bodily representations themselves are actually heightened by the mindfulness training. An account for the mechanisms underlying mindfulness training efficacy must, therefore, take into consideration this central concept: that the emotion itself is not a problem to be dealt with, but rather that the pervasiveness and strength of the cognitive reactions to the emotion are the issues at stake. From such results, it seems likely that in healthy people the regulatory response to dysphoric affective challenge is one primarily of successful inhibition: Strong vmPFC gating of limbic activation weakens the somatic marker's ability to influence cognition and present itself to conscious awareness. On the other hand, the Johnstone and colleagues (2007) study demonstrates the inadequacy of such an approach in depression and perhaps other affective disorders as well. In the case of patients with mood disorder, attempts to down-regulate or suppress the affective content serve only to maintain that pattern of neural activity. In such a population, an alternative approach such as mindfulness may hold the greatest promise. Rather than seeking to suppress the dysphoric neural representations, the training removes the conflict by removing the suppressive tendency. It remains to be demonstrated whether the time course of representing dysphoric information paradoxically shortens when efforts to suppress it are abated.

Conclusion

With the growing evidence that mindfulness training can help people moderate distressing emotions and enhance positive affect, there is a concomitant need to clarify the mechanisms through which these effects occur. As reviewed in this chapter, we hypothesize that mindfulness training enhances emotion regulation through the development of increased attentional capacity and greater metacognitive awareness (Figure 14.1), which, in turn, are associated with reduced avoidance of thoughts and feelings, increased ability to tolerate negative emotions, and decreased reliance on strategies such as rumination and overengagement with thoughts. These changes, we believe, enhance emotion regulation. However, clinically based mindfulness interventions, especially those offered in a group format, contain elements that, apart from specific mental training, may contribute to effective emotion regulation, making it difficult to conclusively link the practice of mindfulness to observed outcomes. A step in this direction was reported by Carmody and Baer (2008), who conducted mediation analyses of symptom change following an 8-week MBSR program. They found that reductions in symptom severity and increases in

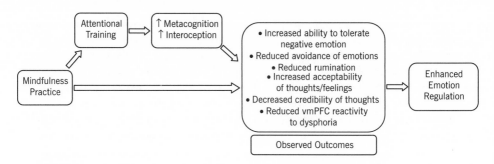

FIGURE 14.1. Hypothesized relation between mindfulness and emotion regulation.

personal well-being were associated with increased mindfulness in course participants and that this relationship was mediated by the duration of actual mindfulness practice. Going forward, it will be helpful to examine the relative contribution of mindfulness training, over and above the other nonspecific factors, to enhanced psychological health. Moreover, many studies of mindfulness have used relatively weak control groups. The field would benefit from studies that directly compare the effectiveness of mindfulness-based emotion regulation strategies, such as acceptance, metacognitive awareness, and interoceptive awareness, with cognitive reappraisal and perspective-taking strategies, to better elucidate whether mindfulness interventions make a unique contribution to emotion regulation.

In addition, it will be important to examine whether the strategies learned through mindfulness practice are simply variants of the traditional emotion regulation strategies such as cognitive reappraisal or whether they are qualitatively different. Mindfulness training and cognitive reappraisal strategies share a focus on cognitive processes, attention, and concentration. However, mindfulness differs from more traditional reappraisal strategies in its emphasis on acceptance of, rather than control over, difficult thoughts and feelings. Moreover, mindfulness practice promotes attending to all aspects of internal experience, including somatic and interoceptive information, rather than focusing exclusively on the content of thoughts and emotions. It will be important to determine whether these differences are associated with concomitant differences in emotion regulation.

Finally, although there is a growing literature on the neural correlates of mindfulness practice, very little of this work has linked these changes with behavioral outcomes. To date, the evidence for neural changes shows associations with molar clinical variables, such as psychological well-being and reduced symptomatology. However, it will be important to explore whether specific behavioral correlates associated with the amount of time spent practicing mindfulness also track the magnitude of the neural changes that are observed. In this way, we would be able to move from simply saying that "mindfulness practice changes the brain" to perhaps being more specific about those regions that are activated when adaptive or maladaptive emotion regulation occurs.

References

Amodio, D. M., & Frith, C. D. (2006). Meeting of minds: The medial frontal cortex and social cognition. *Nature Reviews Neuroscience, 7*, 268–277.

Arch, J. J., & Craske, M. G. (2006). Mechanisms of mindfulness: Emotion regulation following a focused breathing induction. *Behaviour Research and Therapy, 44*, 1849–1858.

Aron, A. R., Robbins, T. W., & Poldrack, R. A. (2004). Inhibition and the right inferior frontal cortex. *Trends in Cognitive Sciences, 8*, 170–177.

Baer, R. A. (2003). Mindfulness training as a clinical intervention: A conceptual and empirical review. *Clinical Psychology: Science and Practice, 10*, 125–143.

Barbas, H. (2000). Proceedings of the human cerebral cortex: From gene to structure and function. *Brain Research Bulletin, 52*, 319–330.

Beauregard, M., Lévesque, J., & Bourgouin, P. (2001). Neural correlates of conscious self-regulation of emotion. *Journal of Neuroscience, 21*, 1–6.

Brefczynski-Lewis, J., Lutz, A., & Schaefer, H. (2007). Neural correlates of attentional expertise in long-term mediation practitioners. *Proceeding of the National Academy of Sciences USA, 104*, 11483–11488.

Broderick, P. C. (2005). Mindfulness and coping with dysphoric mood: Contrasts with rumination and distraction. *Cognitive Therapy and Research, 29*, 501–510.

Brown, K. W., & Ryan, R. M. (2006). Perils and promise in defining and measuring mindfulness: Observations from experience. *Clinical Psychology: Science and Practice, 11*, 242–248.

Bunge, S. A., Ochsner, K. N., Desmond, J. E., Glover, G. H., & Gabrieli, J. D. (2001). Prefrontal regions involved in keeping information in and out of mind. *Brain, 124*, 2074–2086.

Campbell-Sills, L., & Barlow, D. H. (2007). Incorporating emotion regulation into conceptualizations and treatments of anxiety and mood disorders. In J. J. Gross (Ed.), *Handbook of emotion regulation* (pp. 542–559). New York: Guilford Press.

Carmichael, S. T., & Price, J. L. (1996). Connectional networks within the orbital and the medial prefrontal cortex of macaque monkeys. *Journal of Comparative Neurology, 371*, 179–207.

Carmody, J., & Baer, R. A. (2008). Relationships between mindfulness practice and levels of mindfulness, medical and psychological symptoms and well-being in a mindfulness based stress reduction program. *Journal of Behavioral Medicine, 31*, 23–33.

Chambers, R., Lo, B. C., & Allen, N. B. (2008).The impact of intensive mindfulness training on attentional control, cognitive style and affect. *Cognitive Therapy and Research, 32*, 303–322.

Cicchetti, D., Ackerman, B. P., & Izard, C. E. (1995). Emotions and emotion regulation in developmental psychopathology. *Development and Psychopathology, 7*, 1–10.

Corrigan, F. M. (2004). Psychotherapy as assisted homeostasis: Activation of emotion processing mediated by the anterior cingulate cortex. *Medical Hypotheses, 63,* 968–973.

Courtney, S. M., Ungerleider, L. G., Keil, K., & Haxby, J. V. (1997). Transient and sustained activity in a distributed neural system for human working memory. *Nature, 386,* 608–611.

Craig, A. D. (2004). Human feelings: Why are some more aware than others? *Trends in Cognitive Science, 8,* 239–241.

Craik, F. I. M., Moroz, T. M., Moscovitch, M., Stuss, D. T., Winocur, G., Tulving, E., et al. (1999). In search of the self: A positron emission tomography study. *Psychological Science, 10,* 26–34.

Creswell, J. D., Way, B. M., Eisenberger, N. I., & Lieberman, M. D. (2007). Neural correlates of dispositional mindfulness during affect labelling. *Psychosomatic Medicine, 69,* 560–565.

D'Esposito, M., Postle, B. R., Jonides, J., & Smith, E. E. (1999). The neural substrate and temporal dynamics of interference effects in working memory as revealed by event-related functional MRI. *Proceedings of the National Academy of Sciences USA, 96,* 7514–7519.

Dolcos, F., Miller, B., Kragel, P., Jha, A., & McCarthy, G. (2007). Regional brain differences in the effect of distraction during the delay interval of a working memory task. *Brain Research, 1152,* 171–181.

Ekman, P., & Davidson, R. J. (Eds.). (1994). *The nature of emotion: Fundamental questions.* New York: Oxford University Press.

Farb, N., Segal, Z. V., Mayberg, H., Bean, J., McKeon, D., Fatima, Z., et al. (2007). Attending to the present: Mindfulness meditation reveals distinct neural modes of self-reference. *Social Cognitive and Affective Neuroscience, 2,* 313–322.

Fossati, P., Hevenor, S. J., Graham, S. J., Grady, C., Keightley, M. L., Craik, F., et al. (2003). In search of the emotional self: An fMRI study using positive and negative emotional words. *American Journal of Psychiatry, 160,* 1938–1945.

Frewen, P. A., Evans, E. M., Maraj, N., Dozois, D. J. A., & Partridge, K. (2008). Letting go: Mindfulness and negative automatic thinking. *Cognitive Therapy and Research, 32,* 758–774.

Goldin, P., McRae, K., Ramel, W., & Gross, J. J. (2008). The neural bases of emotion regulation: Reappraisal and suppression of negative emotion. *Biological Psychiatry, 63,* 577–586.

Goldman-Rakic, P. S. (1995). Cellular basis of working memory. *Neuron, 14,* 477–485.

Gross, J. J. (1998). The emerging field of emotion regulation: An integrative review. *Review of General Psychology, 2,* 271–299.

Gross, J. J., & Thompson, R. A. (2007). Emotion regulation: Conceptual foundations. In J. J. Gross (Ed.), *Handbook of emotion regulation* (pp. 3–24). New York: Guilford Press.

Grossman, P., Niemann, L., Schmidt, S., & Walach, H. (2004). Mindfulness-based stress reduction and health benefits: A meta-analysis. *Journal of Psychosomatic Research, 57,* 35–43.

Hanh, T. N. (1976). *The miracle of mindfulness* (M. Ho, Trans.). Boston: Beacon Press.

Hayes, A. M., & Feldman, G. (2004). Clarifying the construct of mindfulness in the context of emotion regulation and the process of change in therapy. *Clinical Psychology: Science and Practice, 11,* 255–262.

Hayes, S. C., Strosahl, K. D., & Wilson, K. G. (1999). *Acceptance and commitment therapy: An experiential approach to behavior change.* New York: Guilford Press.

Jha, A., Krompinger, J., & Baime, M. (2007). Mindfulness training modifies subsystems of attention. *Cognitive, Affective and Behavioral Neuroscience, 7,* 109–119.

Johnson, S. C., Baxter, L. C., Wilder, L. S., Pipe, J. G., Heiserman, J. E., & Prigatano, G. P. (2002). Neural correlates of self-reflection. *Brain, 125,* 1808–1814.

Johnstone, T., van Reekum, C., Urry, H., Kalin, N., & Davidson R. (2007). Failure to regulate: Counterproductive recruitment of top-down prefrontal subcortical circuitry in major depression. *Journal of Neuroscience, 27,* 577–586.

Jonides, J., Smith, E. E., Marshuetz, C., Koeppe, R. A., & Reuter-Lorenz, P. A. (1998). Inhibition in verbal working memory revealed by brain activation. *Proceedings of the National Academy of Sciences USA, 95,* 8410–8413.

Kabat-Zinn, J. (1982). An outpatient program in behavioral medicine for chronic pain patients based on the practice of mindfulness meditation: Theoretical considerations and preliminary results. *General Hospital Psychiatry, 4,* 33–47.

Kabat-Zinn, J. (1990). *Full catastrophe living.* New York: Delacorte Press.

Kabat-Zinn, J., Lipworth, L., & Burney, R. (1985). The clinical use of mindfulness meditation for the self-regulation of chronic pain. *Journal of Behavioral Medicine, 8,* 163–190.

Keightley, M., Seminowicz, D., Bagby, R., Costa, P., Fossati, P., & Mayberg, H. (2003). Personality influences limbic-cortical interactions during sad mood induction. *NeuroImage, 20,* 2031–2039.

Kelley, W., Macrae, C., Wyland, C., Caglar, S., Inati, S., & Heatherton, T. (2002). Finding the self?: An event-related fMRI study. *Journal of Cognitive Neuroscience, 14,* 785–794.

Kim, S. H., & Hamann, S. (2007). Neural correlates of positive and negative emotion regulation. *Journal of Cognitive Neuroscience, 19,* 776–798.

Lane, R. D. (2008). Neural substrates of implicit and explicit emotional processes: A unifying framework for psychosomatic medicine. *Psychosomatic Medicine, 70,* 214–221.

Lane, R. D., Fink, G. R., Chau, P. M.-L., & Dolan, R. J. (1997). Neural activation during selective attention to subjective emotional responses. *Cognitive Neuroscience and Neuropsychology, 8,* 3969–3972.

Lazar, S. W., Bush, G., Gollub, R. L., Fricchione, G., Khalsa, G., & Benson, H. (2000). Functional brain mapping of the relaxation response and meditation. *NeuroReport, 11,* 1581–1585.

Lazar, S. W., Kerr, C. E., Wasserman, R. H., Gray, J. R., Greve, D. N., Treadway, M. T., et al. (2005). Meditation experience is associated with increased cortical thickness. *NeuroReport, 16,* 1893–1897.

Linehan, M. M. (1993). *Cognitive-behavioral treatment of borderline personality disorder.* New York: Guilford Press.

Lutz, A., Slagter, H. A., Dunne, J. D., & Davidson, R. J. (2008). Cognitive-emotional interactions—Attention regulation and monitoring in meditation. *Trends in Cognitive Sciences, 12,* 163–169.

Ma, S. H., & Teasdale, J. (2004). Mindfulness-based cognitive therapy for depression: Replication and exploration of differential relapse prevention effects. *Journal of Consulting and Clinical Psychology, 72,* 31–40.

Macrae, C. N., Moran, J. M., Heatherton, T. F., Banfield, J. F., & Kelley, W. M.

(2004). Medial prefrontal activity predicts memory for self. *Cerebral Cortex, 14,* 647–654.

McKim, R. D. (2008). Rumination as a mediator of the effects of mindfulness: Mindfulness-based stress reduction (MBSR) with a heterogeneous community sample experiencing anxiety, depression, and/or chronic pain. *Dissertation Abstracts International: Section B. The Sciences and Engineering, 68*(11-B).

Mennin, D. S., Heimberg, R. G., Turk, C. L., & Fresco, D. M. (2005). Preliminary evidence for an emotion dysregulation model of generalized anxiety disorder. *Behaviour Research and Therapy, 43,* 1281–1310.

Nolen-Hoeksema, S. (1991). Responses to depression and their effects on the duration of depressive episodes. *Journal of Abnormal Psychology, 100,* 569–582.

Nolen-Hoeksema, S. (2000). The role of rumination in depressive disorders and mixed anxiety/depressive symptoms. *Journal of Abnormal Psychology, 109,* 504–511.

Northoff, G., & Heinzel, A. (2006, March). First-person neuroscience: A new methodological approach for linking mental and neuronal states. *Philosophy, Ethics, and Humanities in Medicine, 1*(1), E3.

Ochsner, K. N., Beer, J. S., Robertson, E. R., Cooper, J. C., Gabrieli, J. D., Kihlstrom, J. F., et al. (2005). The neural correlates of direct and reflected self-knowledge. *NeuroImage, 28,* 797–814.

Ochsner, K. N., Bunge, S., Gross, J., & Gabrieli, J. (2002). Rethinking feelings: An fMRI study of the cognitive regulation of emotion. *Journal of Cognitive Neuroscience, 14,* 1215–1229.

Ochsner, K. N., & Gross, J. J. (2005). The cognitive control of emotion. *Trends in Cognitive Sciences, 9,* 242–249.

Ochsner, K. N., & Gross, J. J. (2008). Cognitive emotion regulation: Insights from social cognitive and affective neuroscience. *Current Directions in Psychological Science, 17,* 153–158.

Ortner, C. N. M., Kilner, S. J., & Zelazo, P. D. (2007). Mindfulness meditation and reduced emotional interference on a cognitive task. *Motivation and Emotion, 31,* 271–283.

Ramel, W., Goldin, P. R., Carmona, P. E., & McQuaid, J. R. (2004). The effects of mindfulness meditation on cognitive processes and affect in patients with past depression. *Cognitive Therapy and Research, 28,* 433–455.

Ramel, W., Goldin, P. R., Eykel, L., Brown, G., Gotlib, I., & McQuaid, J. (2007). Amygdala reactivity and mood-congruent memory in individuals at risk for depressive relapse. *Biological Psychiatry, 61,* 231–239.

Ressler, K., & Mayberg, H. (2007). Targeting abnormal neural circuits in mood and anxiety disorders: From the laboratory to the clinic. *Nature Neuroscience, 10,* 1116–1124.

Rolls, E. T. (2000). Précis of the brain and emotion. *Behavioral and Brain Sciences, 23,* 177–234.

Segal, Z. V., Kennedy, S., Gemar, M., Hood, K., Pedersen, R., & Buis, T. (2006). Cognitive reactivity to sad mood provocation and the prediction of depressive relapse. *Archives of General Psychiatry, 63,* 749–755.

Segal, Z. V., Williams, J. M. G., & Teasdale, J. D. (2002). *Mindfulness-based cognitive therapy for depression: A new approach to preventing relapse.* New York: Guilford Press.

Shapiro, S. L., Carlson, L. E., Astin, J. A., & Freedman, B. (2006). Mechanisms of mindfulness. *Journal of Clinical Psychology, 62,* 373–386.

Shapiro, S. L., & Schwartz, G. E. R. (2000). Intentional systemic mindfulness: An integrative model for self-regulation and health. *Advances in Mind–Body Medicine, 16,* 128–134.

Slagter, H., Lutz, A., Greischar, L., Francis, A., Nieuwenhuis, S., Davis, J., et al. (2007). Mental training affects distribution of limited brain resources. *PLoS Biology, 5,* 1228–1235.

Smith, E. E., & Jonides, J. (1999). Storage and executive processes in the frontal lobes. *Science, 283,* 1657–1661.

Teasdale, J. D. (1999). Emotional processing, three modes of mind and prevention of relapse in depression. *Behaviour Research and Therapy, 37,* S53–S77.

Teasdale, J. D., Moore, R. G., Hayhurst, H., Pope, M., Williams, S., & Segal, Z. V. (2002). Metacognitive awareness and prevention of relapse in depression: Empirical evidence. *Journal of Consulting and Clinical Psychology, 70,* 275–287.

Teasdale, J. D., Segal, Z. V., & Williams, J. M. G. (1995). How does cognitive therapy prevent depressive relapse and why should attentional control (mindfulness) training help? *Behaviour Research and Therapy, 33,* 25–39.

Teasdale, J. D., Segal, Z. V., Williams, J. M. G., Ridgeway, V. A., Soulsby, J. M., & Lau, M. A. (2000). Prevention of relapse/recurrence in major depression by mindfulness-based cognitive therapy. *Journal of Consulting and Clinical Psychology, 68,* 615–623.

Wenk-Sormaz, H. (2005). Meditation can reduce habitual responding. *Alternative Therapy in Health and Medicine, 11,* 42–58.

CHAPTER 15

Emotion Regulation as an Integrative
Framework for Understanding
and Treating Psychopathology

Douglas S. Mennin and David M. Fresco

Investigations of emotional processes such as sadness, elation, fear, and anxiety have historically been viewed as core components of numerous psychopathological conditions (Barlow, 2002; Kring & Werner, 2004). Despite their centrality in psychopathology, emotions have historically been a source of confusion and disagreement in clinical psychology, in part because of a lack of conceptual clarity in the definition of emotion, awareness of the purpose it serves, and an understanding of how psychopathology can be generated from absence, deficits, or excesses in efforts to regulate emotions (Greenberg, 2002; Samoilov & Goldfried, 2000). The affective science field (e.g., Davidson, Jackson, & Kalin, 2000) provides an opportunity to expand our paradigms regarding the role of emotion-related processes in conceptualizing and treating psychopathology. In this chapter, we review (1) a conceptualization of emotion regulation that stresses distinctions in generative and regulatory characteristics; (2) the application of an emotion dysregulation perspective to various forms of psychopathology; and (3) the utilization of an emotion regulation framework for integrating various emotion-related approaches to treatment.

Emotions and Emotion Regulation

Emotions can be discussed in terms of their (1) *generative* characteristics, including their purpose (i.e., function, motivational properties) and structure (i.e., multiple response domains), as well as (2) *regulatory* characteristics, including the altering of response trajectories to be more congruent with contextual demands and constraints as well as one's personal values or goals (cf. Cole, Martin, & Dennis, 2004).

Emotion Generation

Generative Function

Emotions arise purposefully to promote action toward survival as well as personal and societal functions by signaling the relevance of our basic motivations or higher order values and goals to given external or internal contexts (Keltner & Haidt, 1999). Because of this informational role, emotions can be integral in making decisions regarding particular actions or plans. Negative emotions focus us toward a particular direction to solve a problem or clarify our goals (Parrott, 2001). For instance, fear can narrow our attention to a possible threat, sadness can orient us toward a possible loss, and disgust can spur us to elude an indigestible object or idea. Similarly, positive emotions (e.g., joy or interest) help widen the array of thoughts and actions and build new approaches through the generation of enduring personal resources (Fredrickson, 2001).

Emotional responding arises from our innate motivational systems, which are activated in response to punishment and reward as well as a need for momentary action (i.e., fight–flight system) (Carver & Scheier, 1998; Gray & McNaughton, 2000; Higgins, 1997). One motivational function of emotions is protection, which is reflective of a behavioral inhibition (BIS), or prevention, system that instigates avoidance of novel or potentially threatening or painful stimuli or end states. For instance, anxiety signals an impetus to avoid people, objects, or events perceived as harmful. Conversely, the behavioral activation, or promotion, system relates to approach in the face of rewarding or appetitive stimuli or end states. Promotion and prevention systems are independent and can be activated alone or in unison in response to a stimulus or event such as when an individual becomes both excited and anxious about an anticipated career change, increasing both motivations to approach rewards and avoid risks associated with this life change (Dollard & Miller, 1950). Motivational conflicts can be resolved through higher order values-based decision making (Wilson & Murrell, 2004).

Generative Structure

In addition to function, emotion generation can be characterized by activation in one or more response components (e.g., Lang, Bradley, & Cuthbert, 1998). Although no single brain area or body part is dedicated solely to emotions, a series of components may be engaged during emotional

responding, including (1) *physiological responses* (e.g., heart rate, musculature responses, body temperature, blood pressure) and their coordination in subcortical and brainstem areas; (2) *behavioral responses*, including
expressive elements (e.g., facial displays) and motor actions (e.g., physical
escape or avoidance); and (3) *subjective responses*, including verbally mediated thought as well as "feelings," which have been hypothesized to involve
a directing of attention to changes in the other components, such as feeling
"scared" when experiencing an increase in heart rate (LeDoux, 1996).

   This multisystemic structure serves an important purpose for survival because it allows for the rapid, simultaneous coordination of many
response systems in preparation for action. For instance, in fear, physiological changes are enacted to prepare the body for mobilization, subjective awareness directs attention toward threatening stimuli for appraisal
of danger value, and behavioral patterns are enacted to thwart or escape
possible harm. In such instances, these multiple systems increase the odds
for survival through their coordinated responses (Cosmides & Tooby,
2000). However, most emotionally eliciting events in our modern age do
not require this level of mobilization. Indeed, findings indicate loose coordination of these response components in various instances of induced
emotional experience (cf. Lang et al., 1998; Mauss, Levenson, McCarter,
Wilhelm, & Gross, 2005). Neurobiological evidence supports the notion
that there are multiple pathways to emotion generation, including automated, "hard-wired," or lower order systems (largely involving physiological responses and their subcortical control) and more controlled, higher
order systems (largely involving subjective, cortical responses), separate
but interactive and mutually essential for differing aspects of emotional
experience (LeDoux, 1996).

Emotion Regulation

Dynamic Systems

Higher order and lower order neural systems related to emotions actively
regulate each other (Davidson et al., 2000; LeDoux, 1996). As such, theorists have begun to view regulatory functions of emotion through the
lens of homeostatic mechanisms, in which the overarching goal of self-
regulation is maintenance of organismic equilibrium (e.g., Bonnano,
2001). The challenge of an emotional landscape, however, is that conditions are ever changing. For an emotional system to be effective, it needs to
be flexible and responsive to changing environmental needs. Indeed, the
ability to adaptively regulate emotions for a given context is associated with
well-being (cf. Mayer, Salovey, & Caruso, 2004) and the promotion of mental health (cf. Kring & Werner, 2004). Functioning may be a product of
the ability to balance the need for behavioral stability and behavioral flexibility (i.e., maintaining *allostasis*; McEwen, 2003). Emotional response sys-

tems regulate each other through mutual communication that is dynamic, consistent, and, when most effective, flexible (Bonnano, 2001; Cole et al., 2004). Thus, emotions can be seen as responding to the need to balance contextual demands and personal goals or values with regulatory efforts by acting as (1) regulators of other processes such as cognition and behavior and (2) recipients of regulatory efforts by these other processes to modulate strength or weakness of responses (cf. Cole et al., 2004).

Emotions Regulate

Despite considerable evidence that emotions negatively bias cognitive processes (cf. Mineka, Rafaeli, & Yovel, 2003), few studies have examined the conditions under which individuals benefit from emotional information. Although intense or inappropriate activation of emotional responses may indeed characterize maladaptive cognitive functioning, emotions activated at low or moderate levels can also be regulatory by facilitating cognitive activities in situations beyond survival needs. Through motivation, emotions can direct attention toward goal-relevant features in the environment and can facilitate their perceptual processing to increase the probability of goal attainment (e.g., Anderson & Phelps, 2001). Also, promotional motivations elicited by positive emotions have been shown to enhance verbal working memory while preventive motivations elicited by negative emotions have been found to enhance spatial working memory (Gray, 2004). Finally, neuroimaging, psychophysiological, and behavioral evidence suggests that initial affective responses can guide advantageous decision making (cf. Bargh & Williams, 2007).

Emotions are Regulated

A significant aspect of emotions is the manner by which we attempt to influence their experience and expression. Although emotions serve adaptive functions, their presence is not always functional. Conversely, in some contexts, emotion absence might be seen as dysfunctional. Regulation of emotion by cognitive and behavioral processes can take the form of up-regulation (i.e., enhance) or down-regulation (i.e., dampen) of emotion (Gross, 2002). Emotional processes unfold over time; thus, emotion regulation is best conceptualized and measured temporally congruent with the unfolding of emotional responses (cf. Davidson et al., 2000). Gross's (2002) process model of emotion regulatory strategies distinguishes between strategies that modulate emotion before (i.e., *antecedent-focused strategies*) versus after (i.e., *response-focused strategies*) an emotional response (see Werner & Gross, Chapter 1, this volume). Antecedent-focused strategies include selecting a situation, modifying an ongoing situation, directing one's attention toward or away from emotional stimuli, and changing the conditions of the situation itself (e.g., reappraising one's beliefs regarding a situation).

Adaptive forms of response-focused strategies might include self-soothing (e.g., relaxation; Borkovec & Sharpless, 2004), emotional expression (Bonnano, 2001), and engagement of positive stimuli (Fredrickson, 2001). However, empirical research demonstrates that some response-focused strategies such as suppression, the active inhibition of ongoing emotion expressive behavior, tax cognitive resources and, paradoxically, increase physiological arousal, making suppression a potentially costly form of regulation (cf. Gross, 2002).

Emotion Dysregulation and Psychopathology

Although emotions serve important functions, they can take detrimental forms when characterized by contextually invariant excesses, deficits, or lability or when regulatory efforts are not utilized, are deficient, are used excessively, or are enacted in rigid and inflexible ways (Kring & Werner, 2004). Given advances in the affective sciences, understanding how fear, anxiety, sadness, and elation—which are, in fact, common, often humanity-defining experiences—can become associated with psychopathology may be an important avenue for inquiry (Samoilov & Goldfried, 2000). An understanding of functional and dysfunctional emotion processes may elucidate our conceptualization of these disorders and provide a broader framework for understanding how other factors (e.g., cognitive, behavioral, interpersonal, and biological) interrelate in the pathogenesis and maintenance of anxiety pathology (Barlow, 2002).

Important to applying affective science to psychopathology is the development of overarching frameworks to organize the roles of emotion-related factors. Rottenberg and Gross (2003) have stressed that when examining the relationship between emotion dysregulation and psychopathology, investigators need to parse emotion-generative processes from regulation deficits and to recognize that, similar to conceptualizations of healthy regulation, dysregulatory efforts occur dynamically throughout different points in the emotion-generative process. This distinction is quite congruent with classical conceptualizations of pathological learning. For instance, Mowrer (1947) distinguished characteristics of fear acquisition (i.e., associative conditioning) from resultant avoidance behaviors, which reinforce fear and anxiety (i.e., operant conditioning). Recent evidence further supports the distinction of emotion-generative and dysregulatory factors in psychopathology. For example, we found that characteristics of one's emotional experience and components of dysregulation were distinct and had differential relationships with anxiety and mood pathology (Mennin, Holaway, Fresco, Moore, & Heimberg, 2007). With this distinction in mind, we present an updated emotion dysregulation model that distinguishes dysfunction in emotion-generative processes (e.g., heightened intensity of emotions) from regulatory efforts (e.g., poor understanding of emotional experience, negative cognitive reactions to emotions, or maladaptive management of emotions).

Elevated Emotion Generation

Generative characteristics of emotion experience include its intensity, valence, duration, and lability (Thompson, 1994). Dysfunction may occur in one or more of these characteristics (cf. Berenbaum, Raghavan, Le, Vernon, & Gomez, 2003). The subjective intensity of emotional experience refers to frequently experiencing emotions more strongly and having reactions that occur more intensely, easily, and quickly than others. Intensity of emotions has been linked to borderline personality disorder (cf. Linehan, 1993) as well as both anxiety and mood disorders (e.g., Mennin et al., 2007). Furthermore, recent evidence has demonstrated that heightened subjective intensity of emotions is particularly relevant for individuals with generalized anxiety disorder (GAD) compared with those with social anxiety disorder (SAD) (Mennin et al., 2007; Mennin, McLaughlin, & Flanagan, in press) or depression (Mennin et al., 2007). Also important to understanding the relationship between emotion-generative characteristics and psychopathology is delineating the role of motivational components (cf. Gray & McNaughton, 2000). Indeed, prevention motivations (i.e., BIS) are strongly related to both neuroticism and the anxiety and mood disorders (Campbell-Sills, Liverant, & Brown, 2004). Despite the relevance of emotion-generative processes to dysfunction, Kring and Werner (2004) point out that intensity alone may not be pathological (e.g., someone who reacts strongly at weddings with tears of joy or screams loudly at a horror movie). It may take the presence of emotion regulation deficits for intense emotions to be problematic (Linehan, 1993; Lynch, Robins, Morse, & MorKrause, 2001). The presence of intensity may become detrimental by heightening a need for regulation such that emotionally intense individuals are confronted with a greater need for regulation and, without these skills, emotional processes become dysfunctional.

Emotion Dysregulation

Our emotion dysregulation model (Mennin, Heimberg, Turk, & Fresco, 2005; Mennin et al., 2007) defines dysregulation broadly as represented by maladaptive emotional responsiveness reflected in dysfunctional understanding, reactivity, and management. This formulation is congruent with others who define regulation both in terms of processes related to managing emotions and processes involved in evaluating and responding to emotions (e.g., Cole et al., 2004; Gratz & Roemer, 2004). *Poor understanding of emotional experience* refers to difficulties in clarifying, labeling, and differentiating emotions and their underlying motivational messages in order to draw meanings from these experiences, elucidate choices for action, and respond more effectively to changing contexts. A lack of understanding of emotional information has been shown to be characteristic of those with depression (e.g., Mennin et al., 2007; Rude & McCarthy, 2003), anxiety disorders (e.g., Mennin et al., 2005, 2007; Parker, Taylor, Bagby, & Acklin, 1993), and substance use disorders (e.g., Haviland, Hendryx, Shaw, & Henry, 1994).

Rather than processing emotion information and utilizing its motivational value, individuals with various forms of psychopathology may negatively react to emotions as reflected in the activation of negative beliefs about emotions and avoidance of emotional awareness (i.e., *negative cognitive reactions to emotions*). For instance, anxiety sensitivity, which refers to beliefs regarding the harmfulness of fear- or anxiety-related sensations, is associated with a number of anxiety disorders, particularly panic disorder (Taylor, Koch, & McNally, 1992). More generally, individuals with anxiety and mood disorders have demonstrated both negative judgments and cognitive avoidance of a number of emotional experiences, including anxiety, sadness, anger, and elating emotions (e.g., Kashdan, Morina, & Priebe, 2009; Leahy, 2002; Mennin et al., 2005, 2007; Salters-Pedneault, Roemer, Tull, Rucker, & Mennin, 2006; Tull & Roemer, 2007).

Emotion dysregulation is also indicated by difficulty knowing when or how to enhance or diminish emotional experiences in a manner that is appropriate to a particular environmental context (i.e., *maladaptive management of emotions*). Maladaptive emotion management skills have been observed in individuals with anxiety disorders (Baker, Holloway, Thomas, Thomas, & Owens, 2004; Mennin et al., 2005, 2007, in press; Salters-Pedneault et al., 2006), child abuse–related posttraumatic stress disorder (PTSD) (Cloitre, Koenen, Cohen, & Han, 2002), depression (Flett, Blankstein, & Obertynski, 1996; Mennin et al., 2007), and borderline personality disorder (Yen, Zlotnick, & Costello, 2002; Zittel Conklin, Bradley, & Westen, 2006). Furthermore, studies have found poor emotion management to be associated with functional impairment beyond the effects of symptoms (Cloitre, Miranda, Stovall-McClough, & Han, 2005). Identified management problems have included difficulty self-soothing, repairing negative moods, engaging in goal-directed behaviors when distressed, displaying impulse control, and ability to access effective regulation strategies.

Clinical Application of an Emotion Regulation Perspective

In addition to expanding our understanding of psychopathology, a focus on emotion dysfunction may also have treatment implications. Although psychotherapeutic interventions for numerous disorders demonstrate considerable efficacy (cf. Roth & Fonagy, 2004), some conditions remain characterized by relapse (e.g., depression) (Segal, Williams, & Teasdale, 2002), poor ability to function adaptively (e.g., chronic PTSD) (Cloitre et al., 2002), or persistent symptomatic recurrence (e.g., GAD) (Borkovec & Ruscio, 2001). For these disorders, further intervention may be required to instill a consistent level of symptom amelioration, functionality, and life satisfaction (Newman, 2000). Understanding the role of emotions in functioning may aid in generating new targets for intervening in refractory forms of psychopathology (cf. Mennin & Farach, 2007). Although several investigators have utilized an emotion regulation framework for depression (e.g., Hayes & Feldman, 2004), PTSD (e.g., Cloitre et al., 2002), and transdiagnostic (e.g., Barlow, Allen, & Choate, 2004) treatments, we focus on our own efforts to develop an integrative, emotion-based, treatment: emotion regulation therapy (ERT). Thus far, ERT is being applied to GAD, a disorder for which treatments have shown only moderate long-term efficacy (cf. Borkovec & Ruscio, 2001). Given the findings supporting emotion dysregulatory factors in GAD reviewed previously, treatments for this disorder may further benefit from incorporation of an emotion regulatory framework. However, given the broader framework the treatment draws from, other related forms of psychopathology such as depression, SAD, and PTSD may also be viable targets for ERT.

ERT utilizes an emotion regulatory framework (i.e., focus on functional emotions, motivation, and emotion regulation) to integrate components of (1) cognitive-behavioral therapy (CBT) treatments (e.g., psychoeducation, self-monitoring, cognitive perspective taking, problem solving, relaxation and diaphragmatic breathing exercises) (Borkovec & Sharpless, 2004; Dugas & Robichaud, 2007); (2) acceptance-, dialectic-, and mindfulness-based behavioral treatments (e.g., mindfulness exercises to broaden awareness of sensations, bodily responses, and emotions in the present moment; exercises to increase willingness to accept emotions, commitment to action related to personal values) (Hayes, Strosahl, & Wilson, 1999; Linehan, 1993; Roemer & Orsillo, 2008; Segal et al., 2002); and (3) experiential therapy (e.g., focus on empathic attunement, importance of agency, delineation of emotion function, engagement of experiential tasks) (e.g., Elliott, Watson, Goldman, & Greenberg, 2004; Gendlin, 1996; Greenberg, 2002). We expect clients successfully treated with ERT to show significant decreases in reactive efforts to control emotions (e.g., worry, suppression) and commensurate increases in the ability to accept emotional experience, flexibly balance responses to emotions according to contextual demands, and utilize emotional information to adaptively problem solve, make decisions, and take action according to their personal values, which, we argue, will lead to improvements in quality of life and adaptive functioning. Successfully treated clients should also have a greater ability to be self-reliant in the face of distress and uncertainty.

Acceptance-and mindfulness-based approaches increasingly have been developed as stand-alone, supplemental, or integrated interventions with CBT for anxiety and mood disorders (e.g., Eifert & Forsyth, 2005; Roemer & Orsillo, 2008; see also Valdivia-Salas, Sheppard, & Forsyth, Chapter 13, this volume). These interventions view the allowance of emotional experiences as essential to breaking maladaptive intrapersonal and interpersonal patterns. Linehan's (1993) dialectical behavior therapy (DBT), which consists of mindfulness-based and emotion regulatory skills-based intervention for individuals with borderline personality disorder, has served as a resource for individuals developing mindfulness-based approaches to the treatment of anxiety disorders (Gratz, Tull, & Wagner, 2005). In acceptance and commitment therapy (ACT), clients are given extensive training in attending to and examining their internal experiences without avoiding them (Hayes et al., 1999). Elements of this intervention have been combined with mindfulness techniques and integrated with CBT for GAD to help clients increase awareness of their emotional state and to allow them to utilize this information to set, prioritize, and achieve adaptive personal goals (cf. Roemer & Orsillo, 2008).

ERT continues to be actively developed, but preliminary data from our open trial appear promising (Mennin, Fresco, Ritter, Heimberg, & Moore, 2008). Presently, ERT consists of 20 weekly sessions. The first four weekly sessions (Phase I) focus on psychoeducation about the emotion regulation model (i.e., role of emotions, motivations, and reactive and control-oriented responses to emotions such as suppression, worry, reassurance seeking, and behavioral avoidance and skills training in mindful sensation, somatic, and emotion awareness). The next six weekly sessions (Phase II) focus on the development of skills aimed at balancing responses to emotions through decentering, acceptance, and management. The following six sessions (Phase III) focus on making a proactive commitment to taking actions reflective of personal values (involving balancing actions related to promotion and prevention motivations). Obstacles to taking these actions are explored, in session, through experiential exposure to emotionally evocative motivational themes through the use of emotion-focused techniques from the experiential tradition (Elliott et al., 2004; Greenberg, 2002) and, out of session, through active skills application during planned valued-action exercises. The final four sessions (Phase IV) focus on skills consolidation, taking larger steps toward valued action, handling lapses and relapses, and termination.

Consistent with DBT (Linehan, 1993) and other treatments (e.g., Cloitre et al., 2005), ERT utilizes a phasic structure that helps clients build skills in the first half of treatment that are utilized in the second half of therapy during exposure exercises. In ERT, this progression also draws largely from Gross's (2002) emotion regulation model, which distinguishes between efforts to regulate emotions later (i.e., response-focused strategies) and earlier (i.e., antecedent-focused strategies) in the emotion-generative process. ERT follows a progression wherein emotion dysregulation is addressed in Phase I through the exploration of unhealthy response-focused strategies (discussed as "reactive responding" to the client), such as worrying, suppression, rumination, self-critical thinking, reassurance seeking toward others, and behavioral avoidance. In Phase II, healthier response-focused strategies are taught (discussed as "counteractive responding" to the client) that are enacted when clients notice themselves being overtaken by intense emotions such as anxiety, anger, or sadness. These strategies encourage a healthier cognitive distance from emotions while not depleting resources by trying to control emotions and, rather, attending to all possible information that emotions might be conveying. Finally, congruent with Gross, the most healthy form of emotion regulation, antecedent-focused strategies (discussed as "proactive responding"), is explored in Phase III through committing to actions that are guided by one's values rather than solely "putting out the fires" that strong emotions signal. In Phase IV, counteractive and proactive skills utilization help clients respond most effectively to challenges and opportunities that may arise after therapy. This progression is also congruent with ACT, in which therapists help clients move from an emotionally avoidant mode of responding to one that is values based (Hayes et al., 1999).

Phase I: Psychoeducational Model and Skills Training in Mindful Awareness

In Phase I, clients learn a psychoeducation model of ERT, begin to self-monitor components of their experience related to this conceptualization (i.e., motivations, emotions, responses to emotions), and begin skills training in mindful awareness of emotions and their perceptual and somatic elements.

Psychoeducational Model

In the initial sessions of ERT, clients are introduced to a psychoeducation module that currently highlights GAD and centers on (1) motivations that, as in all humans, naturally pull us to prevent harm and promote rewards and how, at times, these "pulls" are in conflict (Dollard & Miller, 1950; Higgins, 1997); (2) intense emotional reactions (e.g., Mennin et al., 2007) that, coupled with a history that challenged a sense of security (cf. Borkovec & Sharpless, 2004), have led to an increased focus on prevention motivations (Dugas & Robichaud, 2007; Woody & Rachman, 1994); (3) rapid and rigid reactive responses such as worrying, suppression, and reassurance seeking that are enacted in service of controlling these strong emotions (Borkovec & Sharpless, 2004; Hayes et al., 1999), which, subsequently, lead to losses in emotional clarity; and (4) a decreased likelihood to balance promotion and prevention motivations according to either contextual demands (Rodebaugh & Heimberg, 2008) or one's personal value system (Hayes et al., 1999; Wilson & Murrell, 2004). Throughout ERT, clients solidify their awareness of these model components through out-of-session self-monitoring and unstructured writing exercises (e.g., Sloan, Marx, & Epstein, 2005), which are meant to increase awareness of anxiety-related themes through developing a narrative of these experiences.

Skills Training in Mindful Awareness of Sensations, Soma, and Emotion

Phase I sessions also focus on developing skills that encourage greater awareness of components of the emotion process, including bodily responses, sensations, and subjective experience. In ERT, *mindfulness* is utilized to increase a healthy awareness of the emotional process. By practicing mindfulness exercises, individuals flexibly but purposefully (i.e., engaging one thing at a time) encourage attention to immediate experience with curiosity, openness, and nonjudgment, thereby allowing for increased recognition of experience in the present moment (Bishop et al., 2004; Kabat-Zinn, 1990). Drawing from both mindfulness-based stress reduction (Kabat-Zinn, 1990) and mindfulness-based cognitive therapy (MBCT; Segal et al., 2002), ERT includes both in-session and between-session mindfulness skill-building exercises. Out of session, clients are encouraged to practice mindful awareness skills related to bodily responses, sensations, and emotions in a daily practice that stresses a new exercise each session as well as the continued practice of previously learned exercises. In session, practitioners utilize numerous exercises to help client's increase present-moment awareness. For example, in the *body scan*, one slowly examines each part of their body from head to toe, including imagining internal organ functioning, to gain a better awareness of bodily responses (Kabat-Zinn, 1990). In ERT, established behavioral techniques (cf. Bernstein, Borkovec, & Hazlett-Stevens, 2000) are adapted to be congruent with a mindfulness perspective. Clients are taught *diaphragmatic breathing* and a modified *progressive muscle relaxation* training, which includes an abbreviated body scan to increase flexibility in somatovisceral and muscular responses rather than solely to regulate high levels of arousal (cf. Roemer & Orsillo, 2008). In addition, broadened awareness to appetitive and aversive stimuli alike are encouraged through practices that increase mindful ingestion of senses, including the *raisin exercise*, in which clients are asked to slowly ingest a raisin while taking notice of its tactile, olfactory, and visual features (Kabat-Zinn, 1990).

Gendlin (1996), in his focusing-oriented psychotherapy, has stressed the importance of awareness of the immediate emotional experience, especially as it relates to bodily sensations. In his treatment, individuals learn to identify emotions through a process of *focusing* to gain a "felt sense," which refers to a better understanding of implicit meanings associated with often-experienced bodily responses. Both focusing and increasing mindfulness toward positive and negative emotions (Kabat-Zinn, 1990; Segal et al., 2002) are utilized in ERT to broaden awareness of the emotional process. Although not every emotion experienced should be considered adaptive, broadening awareness to the full spectrum of emotional experience can help clients move through "cloudy" (i.e., secondary emotional reactions) toward "clear" (i.e., primary emotions that convey initial action tendencies and their associated meanings for behavior) emotions, including the presence of all motivational cues that may be present (Greenberg, 2002; Linehan, 1993; Roemer & Orsillo, 2008).

Phase II: Skills Training in Balancing Responses to Emotions

In Phase II, clients work to build skills to flexibly balance their responses to emotions by (1) decentering from immediate emotional experience (rather than distracting or perseverating); (2) allowing and accepting emotions; and (3) mindfully managing difficult emotional responses. Clients engage in a daily practice of these skills and utilize briefer forms of these skills during moments when they become aware that they are responding reactively (e.g., worrying) to external and internal emotional events.

Decentering from Immediate Emotional Experience

The first response-balancing skill set that clients learn promotes cultivating a response to emotions and emotional thoughts with a *slightly* distanced observational perspective. Termed *decentering* (similar constructs include metacognitive awareness [Segal et al., 2002], cognitive defusion [Hayes et al., 1999], reflective functioning [Fonagy, Gergely, Jurist, & Target, 2002]), this is the ability to define one's thoughts and feelings as temporary, objective events in the mind as opposed to reflections of the self that are necessarily true. In a decentered perspective, "the reality of the moment is not absolute, immutable, or unalterable" (Safran & Segal, 1990, p. 117). Fresco and colleagues (2007) found a measure of decentering to be negatively related to emotional avoidance and suppression strategies but positively related to reappraisal strategies. Teasdale and colleagues (2002) found that MBCT resulted in larger increases in decentering than treatment as usual, highlighting its potential as a possible mediator. Similarly, Masuda, Hayes, Sackett, and Twohig (2004) found that a cognitive defusion task reduced discomfort in and believability of negative, self-relevant thoughts more so than distraction or cognitive control.

Decentering is not synonymous with mindfulness, but practices of the latter can promote the ability of the former. Consequently, ERT includes the mountain meditation (Kabat-Zinn, 1990), a mindfulness practice to help clients gain perspective on a difficult emotional state by imagining themselves as a sturdy mountain that is continually awash in the effects of changing climates and seasons, yet essentially still, consistent, and grounded. A central principle in this practice is the encouragement of equanimity, which refers to approaching the diversity of human experiences and emotions with an evenhandedness and equilibrium (Kabat-

Zinn, 1990; Segal et al., 2002). Thus, clients are able to decenter when they recognize that emotional storms, like real ones, are experiences rather than defining entities. In the observer exercise (Hayes et al., 1999), clients learn to notice internal emotional processes (i.e., emotional sensations, thoughts, memories) as transient experiences rather than defining characteristics. Also consistent with ACT, which stresses the importance of language as a conduit for mental events (i.e., cognitive fusion) (Hayes et al., 1999), ERT clients are encouraged to practice defusion (i.e., decentering) from the impact of language-reinforcing associations. For example, clients might be encouraged to say "I am *having* anxiety right now" instead of "I *am* anxious." In experiential therapies, the ability to find this decentered or slightly distanced stance is called *working distance* (Gendlin, 1996), a term that highlights the importance of not only generating cognitive distance but also encouraging observation or exploration of the emotional state from this distance. Drawing on Linehan (1993), ERT clients learn the concept of "wise mind" to promote a decentered stance. *Wise mind* refers to a flexible integration of both rational and emotional states of mind. Engaging a wise mind is to respond to emotional events with the ability to pull back from immediate emotional experience and motivations and flexibly attend to both rational and emotive aspects of experience as is necessary to attain desired outcomes, tolerate distress, and properly adapt to life's inevitable challenges (cf. Teasdale, 1999).

Allowing and Accepting Emotions

Efforts to suppress or constrain emotional experience paradoxically increase physiological arousal (cf. Gross, 2002). Conversely, studies indicate that experimentally induced regulation strategies to accept, allow, or mindfully broaden attention to emotions have demonstrated a greater ameliorative effect on symptoms compared with efforts to suppress (e.g., Campbell-Sills, Barlow, Brown, & Hofmann, 2006; Levitt, Brown, Orsillo, & Barlow, 2004). The skills utilized in ERT to encourage allowance of emotions are drawn primarily from acceptance- and mindfulness-based behavioral practices (e.g., Hayes et al., 1999; Roemer & Orsillo, 2008; Segal et al., 2002). Mindfulness facilitates the reduction of reactive urges to avoid or control difficult experiences by promoting the allowance of the rise and passage of emotions (Segal et al., 2002). Accepting emotional experiences is central to the goals of ACT (Hayes et al., 1999). Although not an explicit skill, metaphors, commonly used in ACT, are utilized as a conduit to internalize a *willingness* to allow emotions to be present. Exercises from ACT, such as "carrying your keys," are used in ERT to promote willingness and build upon clients' developing ability to decenter. In this task, clients physically place their keys in front of them and then mentally assign characteristics of one's emotional experience (i.e., motivations, worries, critical thoughts) to different keys and then carry these keys (and their representational meanings) with them rather than trying to rid themselves of these experiences despite how distressing they may feel.

Encouraging the allowance of emotional responses reduces reactive emotional responses and increases receptiveness to information conveyed by emotion (Roemer & Orsillo, 2008). If emotion responses impart motivational information, then increasing allowance of experience through an expanded, present-moment focus may enhance one's ability to detect and use early emotional cues to guide actions, solve conflicts, and make important decisions. Drawing from emotion-focused therapy (see Greenberg, 2002), ERT allowance skills target the functional role of emotions in the acceptance process. Clients learn through allowing and engaging emotional experiences, distressing or otherwise, that emotions are not truths but, rather, are a means to provide information regarding one's values, judgments, and well-being (Greenberg, 2002). By accepting and exploring emotions, clients gain an ability to be present with emotions and learn how to determine their functional utility in guiding actions. Becoming more comfortable with emotions and the motivational information they impart may also be automated, through repeated exposure, into a greater ability to utilize their felt sense more rapidly in facilitating cognitive processes such as decision making (Damasio, 1994).

Mindfully Managing Difficult Emotional Responses

A debate remains over whether efforts to manage emotions are therapeutic or even possible. Traditional cognitive therapy emphasizes the control of emotional responses, particularly through conscious thought (e.g., Beck, Rush, Shaw, & Emery, 1979). In contrast, acceptance-based behavioral therapies do not involve the direct manipulation of emotional states because control efforts are seen as countertherapeutic and ultimately futile (Hayes et al., 1999; Valdivia-Salas et al., Chapter 13, this volume), especially when used habitually because they become contextually nonfunctional as flexibility in emotional responses gets reduced (Wilson & Murrell, 2004). ERT adopts a dynamic systems approach to emotion function and regulation, recognizing the merits of both the allowance and management of emotional responses used in a functional manner. Some environmental contingencies (either external or internal) may be engaged best through allowance and acceptance of emotions (e.g., nervous anticipation of biopsy results), whereas others may call for more immediate efforts to effect change in the emotional process (e.g., focusing away from sad feelings after a breakup while in a board meeting).

In ERT, we introduce skills to help soothe intense and distressful emotional thoughts, bodily sensations, and action tendencies in service of maintaining mindful contact and clarification with the emotional experience rather than in service of disengaging from or quelling the emotional state. Specifically, clients utilize the "breathing space" (Segal et al., 2002), a brief mindfulness practice, to assist in locating their wise mind (Linehan, 1993) in a moment of distress so that management skills are not enacted in a manner to escape or remove emotional experience. Mindfulness, by broadening attentional processes, can counter the action tendencies associated with the narrowed focus inherent in threat-based emotions such as fear and anxiety. The nonjudgmental stance encouraged by mindfulness exercises may also help individuals gain perspective on a situation that might have inherent negative emotion-reducing properties (Roemer & Orsillo, 2008). Management skills are discussed in terms of their ability to lessen emotional intensity to not only reduce distress but also to gain a clearer signal of the range of emotional messages in an important life situation.

ERT uses several strategies to promote mindful management of emotions. An important strategy, given the central role of divergent motivations in the treatment, is engaging in *opposite action* (Linehan, 1993), *changing emotions with emotion* (Greenberg, 2002), or *modifying emotional action tendencies* (Barlow et al., 2004). These approaches involve assessing whether an emotion is functional in a given situation, examining cues that may exacerbate emotional responses, deliberately not engaging behavioral responses associated with context-specific maladaptive emotions, and replacing the responses with behavior that is counter to the actions tendency compelled by the emotion. For instance, positive emotional experiences may be used to widen one's attentional frame after prolonged exposure to negative emotions. In addition, ERT clients can utilize recall relaxation (cf. Borkovec & Sharpless, 2004), which follows from the mindfulness-enriched progressive muscle relaxation practice discussed previously, to promote more flexibility in musculature response during periods of physical tension. Finally, reappraisal (Gross, 2002) processes are utilized in conjunction with the promotion of mindful self-compassion in response to self-critical thoughts (Segal et al., 2002). A "softening" of critical self-statements during intense emotional episodes is encouraged through the invoking of alternative, compassionate statements.

Phase III: Values-Based, Experiential Exposure

Exposure therapies typically focus on fear-evoking cues (cf. Foa & Kozak, 1986). However, advances in affective sciences support a broader focus on various emotions and disorders beyond fear as well as an expansion of the goal of emotional processing from reducing emotions to the creation of new personal meanings through facilitated attention to the motivational information conveyed through emotion (cf. Greenberg, 2002; Teasdale, 1999). In this regard, new meanings occur from the utilization of emotional information rather than its mere reduction. Indeed, modern learning theory suggests that exposure is effective not because previously associated emotional meanings are unlearned or erased but because new emotional meanings are strengthened (Bouton, 2002). Also, the promotion of new, rewarding behaviors is a central treatment goal for behavioral activation therapy (Martell, Addis, & Jacobson, 2001; see also Syzdek, Addis, & Martell, Chapter 17, this volume), which has demonstrated efficacy for depression.

After having worked in Phase II to develop effective, "counteractive" (i.e., response-focused) strategies in response to emotional states, Phase III centers on helping clients to engage a "proactive" (i.e., antecedent-focused) stance toward change by making choices about how they may want to be balancing protecting and promoting endeavors in service of what matters most to them. Consistent with ACT, this objective is accomplished by focusing clients on their personal values, which represent their highest priorities and most cherished principles (Hayes et al., 1999; Wilson & Murrell, 2004). In Phase III, clients experientially explore acting in accordance with their values and confronting any accompanying perceived obstacles that arise both within and between sessions. Specifically, Phase III sessions consist of three main exposure components to promote valued living: (1) imaginal action related to values-informed goals; (2) experiential tasks to explore perceived internal conflicts that impede engaging valued actions (Greenberg, 2002); and (3) planned homework exercises wherein clients engage valued actions outside of session. Clients also utilize the awareness and response-balancing skills to help facilitate engagement during the in-session experiential tasks and to facilitate valued action outside of session.

Proactive Valued Action

ERT draws from ACT (Hayes et al., 1999) in stressing the importance of *commitment*, involving a willingness to act in accordance with one's values despite whether strong security motivations and accompanying anxiety, worry, and distress are present. This willingness may also involve an allowance of enhancement (i.e., promotion) motivations to become more salient and to follow these motivations in service of valued action. In ERT, commitment is considered to be proactive because it involves intentional actions toward goals that are reflective of stated values. However, outcome and goal achievement are not the purpose of engaging values (Hayes et al., 1999; Wilson & Murrell, 2004). Rather, values are engaged to be more congruent with what matters most to the client and to open up to the opportunities that come with that flexibility. In the outset of Phase III, therapists and clients collaborate to identify cherished values in the domains (e.g., family, friends, relationships, work, personal care) where clients report discrepancies between the importance they place on this value and how consistently they have been living accordingly (Wilson & Murrell, 2004). Therapists then encourage clients to think about a salient value with a large discrepancy and how they want their actions to reflect this value *today*, even if it involves only a small action step.

Wilson and Murrell (2004) note that clients often have difficulty engaging in values work. Given that clients may still be committed to not experiencing their emotions and could utilize the skills in an avoidant manner, valued action is explored through systematic experiential exploration. By encouraging active exploration of valued actions, clients can form a better blueprint for how to live by their values and create new meaningful change. Specifically, imaginal exposure tasks that focus on engaging in *specific* valued actions are conducted (1) to provide clients with an experientially rich rehearsal of the steps that might be necessary to live by their values and (2) to confront the emotional challenges that are likely to arise as clients imagine engagement of valued action. In this imagery exposure task, therapists help clients imagine each step involved in engaging this action while noting changes in motivational levels and encouraging utilization of skills to address difficulties in awareness and balancing of emotional responses. Utilizing imagery to consolidate skills and promote functional action is also congruent with interventions such as *cognitive rehearsal* (Beck et al., 1979).

Exploring Conflict Themes in Obstacles to Valued Living

The second component of exposure work in ERT involves addressing perceived obstacles to taking valued action. Obstacles reflect clients' own internal struggle that holds them back from engaging in this valued action. In ERT, obstacles are addressed through the lens of "conflict themes," including (1) a *motivational conflict* (e.g., security motivations are blocking or interrupting enhancement efforts); (2) *self-critical reactive responses to emotions* (i.e., judgmental negative beliefs about one's emotional responses and associated motivations); and (3) *unfinished business with a security-challenging or critical figure* (i.e., lingering painful feelings related to the perception that an important other has been profoundly judgmental and dismissive or disrupted a sense of safety and, possibly, the emergence of enhancement motivations). These conflict themes are addressed within session using experiential techniques from emotion-focused therapy (i.e., chair dialogues) (Elliott et al., 2004; Greenberg, 2002; for an alternative approach to chair dialogues in treatment for GAD, see Newman, Castonguay, Borkovec, Fisher, & Nordberg, 2008). Respective thematic experiential exposure tasks address each of these conflict themes. In ERT, the *motivational conflict* is most central to interrupting valued action and is addressed by encouraging clients to engage a dialogue between the part of themselves that is strongly motivated to obtain security and the part that is motivated toward self-reliance to arrive at a more unified motivational stance that is conducive to valued action. The purpose of these tasks is to reduce negative emotional responses that are activated when obstacles reflecting these conflicts are perceived (i.e., exposure), generate a new perspective (i.e., new meaning) on these obstacles, and engage more adaptive emotions that are facilitative of valued-action engagement.

Engaging Proactive Valued Action Outside of Session

Finally, valued action is promoted through between-session exercises that build on the work conducted during the valued-action exploration and obstacles-confrontation exposure tasks. Clients are reminded that protection and avoidance will always preclude the ability to live in their most cherished ways. Thus, commitment involves clients agreeing to bring some of this struggle with them in the week following therapy by making choices to engage valued actions. Therapists encourage clients to engage both planned (i.e., specific valued actions related to salient values explored in session and committed to in the presence of therapists) and spontaneous (i.e., any other valued actions clients notice themselves engaging in) valued actions outside of session (Hayes et al., 1999). Furthermore, clients are encouraged to utilize skills both proactively (in an antecedent-focused manner) when they are planning to engage valued actions and counteractively (in a response-focused manner) when they notice themselves getting unexpectedly anxious and beginning to respond reactively with worry, reassurance seeking, self-criticism, or behavioral avoidance. Finally, external barriers (i.e., obstacles in the environment that are outside clients' control), which might have been deferred during exposure tasks, can also be addressed more actively in between session exercises. Therapists can help clients problem solve these obstacles or utilize skills such as acceptance to further facilitate valued action.

Phase IV: Consolidating Gains, Anticipating Lapses and Relapses, and Termination Processing

In this final phase of ERT, sessions focus on consolidating gains and preparing for termination. Initial goals are reviewed to determine whether changes have occurred as well as determining what goals still need to be addressed. Clients and therapists discuss how to apply skills following therapy termination in service of (1) taking larger steps toward valued action and (2) addressing lapses so that they do not become full-blown relapses during difficult life periods that may arise (Dugas & Robichaud, 2007). Specifically, discussion focuses on ways to help prevent clients from becoming once again reliant on obtaining security and responding reactively (e.g., excessive worry and behavioral avoidance) once therapy is terminated. Clients and therapists discuss how emotion awareness and response-balancing skills can continue to be utilized in service of taking new valued actions and responding to difficult events. Ability to tolerate possible future stressful and painful life circumstances is also further explored by reviewing skills and applying them to experiential exposure exercises that center on hypothetical situations related to core themes that may arise in the future. An open discussion of termination and "life after therapy" helps to fully address feelings associated with termination and the loss of the therapeutic relationship.

Conclusions

Utilizing an integrative, emotion-based framework may provide a promising, novel direction for conceptualization of psychopathology and its treatment. Nonetheless, it is important to acknowledge the limitations and challenges that should be addressed as this field of inquiry moves forward. First, thus far, ERT has been utilized only for GAD. Its applicability to other conditions remains unknown. However, given the broad framework that the treatment draws from and the relevance of emotion dysregulation to a number of conditions, including major depression, bipolar disorders, SAD, PTSD, and eating disorders, a common treatment approach such as ERT may be viable for seemingly disparate, yet highly co-occurring, disorders (Barlow et al., 2004). Second, the construct validity of many of these ideas has not been established, although efforts are already underway (e.g., Bishop et al., 2004). Future research in this area must continue to operationalize these constructs as well as examine their validity in relation to more established constructs. Third, it will be important to determine whether these new treatments have incremental efficacy for refractory disorders compared with existing treatments and whether emotion regulatory factors are central mechanisms in this change. Finally, given the complexity inherent in integrating approaches, striving for parsimony will be an important challenge to address in future research. With these caveats in mind, future endeavors will no doubt expand inquiry into the nexus of affective and clinical psychological approaches and, it is hoped, in so doing, expand our knowledge base of psychopathological conceptualization and treatment.

References

Anderson, A., & Phelps, E. (2001). Lesions of the human amygdala impair enhanced perception of emotionally salient events. *Nature, 411*, 305–309.

Baker, R., Holloway, J., Thomas, P., Thomas, S., & Owens, M. (2004). Emotional processing and panic. *Behaviour Research and Therapy, 42*, 1271–1287.

Bargh, J. A., & Williams, L. E. (2007). On the nonconscious of emotion regulation. In J. J. Gross (Ed.), *Handbook of emotion regulation* (pp. 429–445). New York: Guilford Press.

Barlow, D. H. (2002). *Anxiety and its disorders: The nature and treatment of anxiety and panic* (2nd ed.). New York: Guilford Press.

Barlow, D. H., Allen, L., & Choate, M. (2004). Toward a unified treatment for emotional disorders. *Behavior Therapy, 35,* 205–230.

Beck, A. T., Rush, A. J., Shaw, B. F., & Emery, G. (1979). *Cognitive therapy for depression.* New York: Guilford Press.

Berenbaum, H., Raghavan, C., Le, H. N., Vernon, L., & Gomez, J. (2003). A taxonomy of emotional disturbances. *Clinical Psychology: Science and Practice, 10,* 206–226.

Bernstein, D. A., Borkovec, T. D., & Hazlett-Stevens, H. (2000). *New directions in progressive relaxation training.* Westport, CT: Praeger.

Bishop, S. R., Laue, M., Shapiro, S., Carlson, L., Anderson, N. D., Carmody, J., et al. (2004). Mindfulness: A proposed operational definition. *Clinical Psychology: Science and Practice, 11,* 230–241.

Bonnano, G. (2001). Emotion self-regulation. In T. J. Mayne & G. A. Bonnano (Eds.), *Emotions: Current issues and future directions* (pp. 251–285). New York: Guilford Press.

Borkovec, T. D., & Ruscio, A. M. (2001). Psychotherapy for generalized anxiety disorder. *Journal of Clinical Psychiatry, 62*(Suppl. 11), 37–42.

Borkovec, T. D., & Sharpless, B. (2004). Generalized anxiety disorder: Bringing cognitive-behavioral therapy into the valued present. In S. C. Hayes, V. M. Follette, & M. M. Linehan (Eds.), *Mindfulness and acceptance: Expanding the cognitive-behavioral tradition* (pp. 209–242). New York: Guilford Press.

Bouton, M. E. (2002). Context, ambiguity, and unlearning: Sources of relapse after behavioral extinction. *Biological Psychiatry, 52,* 976–986.

Campbell-Sills, L., Barlow, D. H., Brown, T. A., & Hofmann, S. G. (2006). Effects of emotional suppression and acceptance in anxiety and mood disorders. *Behaviour Research and Therapy, 44,* 1251–1263.

Campbell-Sills, L., Liverant, G. I., & Brown, T. A. (2004). Psychometric evaluation of the Behavioral Inhibition/Behavioral Activation Scales in a large sample of outpatients with anxiety and mood disorders. *Psychological Assessment, 16,* 244–254.

Carver, C. S., & Scheier, M. F. (1998). *On the self-regulation of behavior.* New York: Cambridge University Press.

Cloitre, M., Koenen, K. C., Cohen, L. R., & Han, H. (2002). Skills training in affective and interpersonal regulation followed by exposure: A phase-based treatment for PTSD related to childhood abuse. *Journal of Consulting and Clinical Psychology, 70,* 1067–1074.

Cloitre, M., Miranda, R., Stovall-McClough, K. C., & Han, H. (2005). Beyond PTSD: Emotion regulation and interpersonal problems as predictors of functional impairment in survivors of childhood abuse. *Behavior Therapy, 36,* 119–124.

Cole, P. M., Martin, S. E., & Dennis, T. A. (2004). Emotion regulation as a scientific construct: Methodological challenges and directions for child development research. *Child Development, 75,* 317–333.

Cosmides, L., & Tooby, J. (2000). Evolutionary psychology and the emotions. In M. Lewis & J. M. Haviland-Jones (Eds.), *Handbook of emotions* (2nd ed., pp. 91–115). New York: Guilford Press.

Damasio, A. R. (1994). *Descartes' error.* New York: Putnam.

Davidson, R. J., Jackson, D. C., & Kalin, N. H. (2000). Emotion, plasticity, context, and regulation: Perspectives from affective neuroscience. *Psychological Bulletin, 126,* 890–909.

Dollard, J., & Miller, N. E. (1950). *Personality and psychotherapy.* New York: McGraw-Hill.

Dugas, M. J., & Robichaud, M. (2007). *Cognitive-behavioral treatment for generalized anxiety disorder.* New York: Routledge.

Eifert, G. H., & Forsyth, J. P. (2005). *Acceptance and commitment therapy for anxiety disorders: A practitioner's treatment guide to using mindfulness, acceptance, and values-based behavior change strategies.* Oakland, CA: New Harbinger.

Elliott, R., Watson, J., Goldman, R. N., & Greenberg, L. S. (2004). *Learning emotion-focused therapy: The process-experiential approach to change.* Washington, DC: American Psychological Association.

Flett, G. L., Blankstein, K. R., & Obertynski, M. (1996). Affect intensity, coping styles, mood regulation expectancies and depressive symptoms. *Personality and Individual Differences, 20,* 221–228.

Foa, E. B., & Kozak, M. J. (1986). Emotional processing of fear: Exposure to corrective information. *Psychological Bulletin, 99,* 20–35.

Fonagy, P., Gergely, G., Jurist, E. L., & Target, M. (2002). *Affect regulation, mentalization and the development of the self.* New York: Other Press.

Fredrickson, B. L. (2001). The role of positive emotions in positive psychology: The broaden-and-build theory of positive emotions. *American Psychologist, 56,* 218–226.

Fresco, D. M., Moore, M. T., van Dulman, M. H. M., Segal, Z. V., Ma, S. H., Teasdale, J. D., et al. (2007). Initial psychometric properties of the Experiences Questionnaire: Validation of a self-report measure of decentering. *Behavior Therapy, 38,* 234–246.

Gendlin, E. T. (1996). *Focusing-oriented psychotherapy: A manual of the experiential method.* New York: Guilford Press.

Gratz, K. L., & Roemer, L. (2004). Multidimensional assessment of emotion regulation and dysregulation: Development, factor structure, and validation of the Difficulties with Emotion Regulation Scale. *Journal of Psychopathology and Behavioral Assessment, 26,* 41–54.

Gratz, K. L., Tull, M. T., & Wagner, A. W. (2005). Applying DBT mindfulness skills to the treatment of clients with anxiety disorders In S. M. Orsillo & L. Roemer (Eds.), *Acceptance and mindfulness-based approaches to anxiety: Conceptualization and treatment* (pp. 147–164). New York: Springer.

Gray, J. A., & McNaughton, N. (2000). *The neuropsychology of anxiety: An enquiry into the functions of the septo-hippocampal system* (2nd ed.). New York: Oxford University Press.

Gray, J. R. (2004). Integration of emotion and cognitive control. *Current Directions in Psychological Science, 13,* 46–48.

Greenberg, L. S. (2002). *Emotion-focused therapy: Coaching clients to work through their feelings.* Washington, DC: American Psychological Association.

Gross, J. J. (2002). Emotion regulation: Affective, cognitive, and social consequences. *Psychophysiology, 39,* 281–291.

Haviland, M. G., Hendryx, M. S., Shaw, D. G., & Henry, J. P. (1994). Alexithymia in women and men hospitalized for psychoactive substance dependence. *Comprehensive Psychiatry, 35,* 124–128.

Hayes, A. M., & Feldman, G. (2004). Clarifying the construct of mindfulness in the context of emotion regulation and the process of change in therapy. *Clinical Psychology: Science and Practice, 11,* 255–262.

Hayes, S. C., Strosahl, K. D., & Wilson, K. G. (1999). *Acceptance and commitment therapy: An experiential approach to behavior change.* New York: Guilford Press.

Higgins, E. T. (1997). Beyond pleasure and pain. *American Psychologist, 52,* 1280–1300.

Kabat-Zinn, J. (1990). *Full catastrophe living: Using the wisdom of your body and mind to face stress, pain, and illness.* New York: Delta.

Kashdan, T. B., Morina, N., & Priebe, S. (2009). Post-traumatic stress disorder, social anxiety disorder, and depression in survivors of the Kosovo War: Experiential avoidance as a contributor to distress and quality of life. *Journal of Anxiety Disorders, 23*(2), 185–196.

Keltner, D., & Haidt, J. (1999). Social functions of emotions at four levels of analysis. *Cognition and Emotion, 13,* 505–521.

Kring, A. M., & Werner, K. H. (2004). Emotion regulation and psychopathology. In P. Philippot & R. S. Feldman (Eds.), *The regulation of emotion* (pp. 359–385). Mahwah, NJ: Erlbaum.

Lang, P. J., Bradley, M. M., & Cuthbert, B. N. (1998). Emotion, motivation, and anxiety: Brain mechanisms and psychophysiology. *Biological Psychiatry, 44,* 1248–1263.

Leahy, R. L. (2002). A model of emotional schemas. *Cognitive and Behavioral Practice, 9,* 177–190.

LeDoux, J. E. (1996). *The emotional brain: The mysterious underpinnings of emotional life.* New York: Simon & Schuster.

Levitt, J. T., Brown, T. A., Orsillo, S. M., & Barlow, D. H. (2004). The effects of acceptance versus suppression of emotion on subjective and psychophysiological response to carbon dioxide challenge in patients with panic disorder. *Behavior Therapy, 35,* 747–766.

Linehan, M. M. (1993). *Cognitive-behavioral treatment for borderline personality disorder.* New York: Guilford Press.

Lynch, T. R., Robins, C. J., Morse, J. Q., & MorKrause, E. D. (2001). A mediational model relating affect intensity, emotion inhibition, and psychological distress. *Behavior Therapy, 32,* 519–536.

Martell, C. R., Addis, M. E., & Jacobson, N. S. (2001). *Depression in context: Strategies for guided action.* New York: Norton.

Masuda, A., Hayes, S. C., Sackett, C. F., & Twohig, M. P. (2004). Cognitive defusion and self-relevant negative thoughts: Examining the impact of a ninety year old technique. *Behaviour Research and Therapy, 42,* 477–485.

Mauss, I. B., Levenson, R. W., McCarter, L., Wilhelm, F., & Gross, J. J. (2005). The tie that binds?: Coherence among emotion experience, behavior, and physiology. *Emotion, 5,* 175–190.

Mayer, J. D., Salovey, P., & Caruso, D. (2004). Emotional intelligence: Theory, findings, and implications. *Psychological Inquiry, 15,* 197–215.

McEwen, B. S. (2003). Mood disorders and allostatic load. *Biological Psychiatry, 54,* 200–207.

Mennin, D. S., & Farach, F. J. (2007). Emotion and evolving treatments for adult psychopathology. *Clinical Psychology: Science and Practice, 14,* 329–352.

Mennin, D. S., Fresco, D. M., Ritter, M., Heimberg, R. G., & Moore, M. T. (2008, November). Emotion regulation therapy for generalized anxiety disorder: Integrating emotion-related approaches using an affect science framework.

In C. T. Taylor & N. Amir (Chairs), *Novel approaches to the treatment of generalized anxiety disorder*. Paper presented at the annual meeting of the Association for Behavioral and Cognitive Therapies, Orlando, FL.

Mennin, D. S., Heimberg, R. G., Turk, C. L., & Fresco, D. M. (2005). Preliminary evidence for an emotion dysregulation model of generalized anxiety disorder. *Behaviour Research and Therapy, 43*, 1281–1310.

Mennin, D. S., Holaway, R., Fresco, D. M., Moore, M. T., & Heimberg, R. G. (2007). Delineating components of emotion and its dysregulation in anxiety and mood psychopathology. *Behavior Therapy, 38*, 284–302.

Mennin, D. S., McLaughlin, K. A., & Flanagan, T. (in press). Emotion regulation deficits in generalized anxiety disorder, social anxiety disorder, and their co-occurrence. *Journal of Anxiety Disorders*.

Mineka, S., Rafaeli, E., & Yovel, I. (2003). Cognitive biases in emotional disorders: Information processing and social-cognitive perspectives. In R. J. Davidson, K. R. Scherer, & H. H. Goldsmith (Eds.), *Handbook of affective sciences* (pp. 976–1009). New York: Oxford University Press.

Mowrer, O. H. (1947). On the dual nature of learning: A re-interpretation of "conditioning" and "problem-solving." *Harvard Educational Review, 17*, 102–148.

Newman, M. G. (2000). Recommendations for a cost offset model of psychotherapy allocation using generalized anxiety disorder as an example. *Journal of Consulting and Clinical Psychology, 68*, 549–555.

Newman, M. G., Castonguay, L. G., Borkovec, T. D., Fisher, A. J., & Nordberg, S. S. (2008). An open trial of integrative therapy for generalized anxiety disorder. *Psychotherapy Theory, Research, Practice, Training, 45*, 135–147.

Parker, J. D., Taylor, G. J., Bagby, R. M., & Acklin, M. W. (1993). Alexithymia in panic disorder and simple phobia: A comparative study. *American Journal of Psychiatry, 150*, 1105–1107.

Parrott, W. G. (2001). Implications of dysfunctional emotions for understanding how emotions function. *Review of General Psychology, 5*, 180–186.

Rodebaugh, T. L., & Heimberg, R. G. (2008). Emotion regulation and the anxiety disorders: Adopting a self-regulation perspective. In A. Vingerhoets, I. Nyklícek, & J. Denollet (Eds.), *Emotion regulation: Conceptual and clinical issues* (pp. 140–149). New York: Springer.

Roemer, L., & Orsillo, S. M. (2008). *Mindfulness- and acceptance-based behavioral therapies in practice*. New York: Guilford Press.

Roth, A., & Fonagy, P. (2004). *What works for whom?: A critical review of psychotherapy research* (2nd ed.). New York: Guilford Press.

Rottenberg, J., & Gross, J. (2003). When emotion goes wrong: Realizing the promise of affective science. *Clinical Psychology: Science and Practice, 10*, 227–232.

Rude, S. S., & McCarthy, C. T. (2003). Emotional functioning in depressed and depression-vulnerable college students. *Cognition and Emotion, 17*, 799–806.

Safran, J. D., & Segal, Z. V. (1990). *Interpersonal process in cognitive therapy*. New York: Basic Books.

Salters-Pedneault, K., Roemer, L., Tull, M. T., Rucker, L., & Mennin, D. S. (2006). Evidence of broad deficits in emotion regulation associated with chronic worry and generalized anxiety disorder. *Cognitive Therapy and Research, 30*, 469–480.

Samoilov, A., & Goldfried, M. R. (2000). Role of emotion in cognitive-behavior therapy. *Clinical Psychology: Science and Practice, 7*, 373–385.

Segal, Z., Williams, J. M. G., & Teasdale, J. D. (2002). *Mindfulness-based cognitive therapy for depression: A new approach to preventing relapse.* New York: Guilford Press.

Sloan, D. M., Marx, B. P., & Epstein, E. M. (2005). Further examination of the exposure model underlying the efficacy of written emotional disclosure. *Journal of Counseling and Clinical Psychology, 73,* 549–554.

Taylor, S., Koch, W. J., & McNally, R. J. (1992). How does anxiety sensitivity vary across the anxiety disorders? *Journal of Anxiety Disorders, 6,* 249–259.

Teasdale, J. D. (1999). Emotional processing, three modes of mind, and the prevention of relapse in depression. *Behaviour Research and Therapy, 37,* S53–S78.

Teasdale, J. D., Moore, R. G., Hayhurst, H., Pope, M., Williams, S., & Segal, Z. V. (2002). Metacognitive awareness and prevention of relapse in depression: Empirical evidence. *Journal of Consulting and Clinical Psychology, 70,* 275–287.

Thompson, R. A. (1994). Emotion regulation: A theme in search of a definition. In N. Fox (Ed.), *Monographs of the Society for Research in Child Development, 59*(2/3), 25–52.

Tull, M. T., & Roemer, L. (2007). Emotion regulation deficits among a non-treatment seeking sample of individuals with uncued panic attacks: Evidence of emotional avoidance, non-acceptance, and decreased emotional clarity. *Behavior Therapy, 38,* 378–391.

Wilson, K. G., & Murrell, A. R. (2004). Values work in acceptance and commitment therapy: Setting a course for behavioral treatment. In S. C. Hayes, V. M. Follette, & M. M. Linehan (Eds.), *Mindfulness and acceptance: Expanding the cognitive-behavioral tradition* (pp. 120–151). New York: Guilford Press.

Woody, S., & Rachman, S. (1994). Generalized anxiety disorder (GAD) as an unsuccessful search for safety. *Clinical Psychology Review, 14,* 743–753.

Yen, S., Zlotnick, C., & Costello, E. (2002). Affect regulation in women with borderline personality disorder traits. *Journal of Nervous and Mental Disease, 190,* 693–696.

Zittel Conklin, C., Bradley, R., & Westen, D. (2006). Affect regulation in borderline personality disorder. *Journal of Nervous and Mental Disease, 194,* 69–77.

●————————●————————●————————●

CHAPTER 16

Attention and Emotion Regulation

Charles T. Taylor and Nader Amir

Dysregulation of attention has long been implicated in the pathogenesis and maintenance of emotional disorders (e.g., Mathews & MacLeod, 2005; Williams, Watts, MacLeod, & Mathews, 1997). As reviewed earlier in this volume (see Denny, Silvers, & Ochsner, Chapter 3), basic processes involving attention and emotion regulatory systems are fundamentally related at the genetic, neural, physiological, cognitive, and behavioral levels (see also Ochsner & Gross, 2007, 2008; Pessoa, 2008). Therefore, as our understanding of the role of basic attention processes in the generation and regulation of emotions continues to grow, so does our understanding of the way normal attention processes go awry and ultimately contribute to various forms of psychopathology (see Joorman, Yoon, & Seimer, Chapter 8, this volume). In this chapter, we focus on clinical interventions designed to explicitly modify pathological attention processes in disorders of emotion, reviewing the extant literature on attention-based treatments and emotional disorders broadly defined. However, because aberrant functioning in attention and emotion regulation are implicated in the pathophysiology of a wide range of psychiatric conditions (Harvey, Watkins, Mansell, & Shafran, 2004), we also consider transdiagnostic applications of attention modification interventions in the treatment of psychopathology in general.

We begin with operational definitions of attention and emotion regulation. Here, we underscore the importance of distinguishing key subcomponents of each system. Given the diversity of techniques purportedly designed to modify attention, we argue that understanding the complexity of basic attention processes is essential when considering the implications of this literature. We then review basic research demonstrating that attentional manipulations influence subjective emotional experiences both within laboratory settings and naturalistically, which establishes that aberrant attention processes are etiologically significant in the development and maintenance of emotional disorders. Next, we turn to empirical findings regarding the efficacy of attention-based treatments across emotional disorders as well as research that examines change in the attention processes purported to underlie treatment effects. We conclude with a consideration of unresolved issues and future directions in the clinical domain of attention and emotion regulation.

Definitions

Attention

Broadly defined, attention refers to any cognitive process that results in the selection of some information over other information (Posner, 1988, Weierich, Treat, & Hollingworth, 2008). Attention is arguably the most fundamental cognitive operation, serving as a universal gatekeeper that grants access to some stimuli for further processing while limiting access to other types of information. However, attention is *not* a unitary construct. This is particularly important because basic attention research implicates the role of attention subsystems in the spatial allocation of attention (e.g., Fan, McCandliss, Sommer, Raz, & Posner, 2002; Pashler, 1998). For example, Posner (1988) suggested that visual–spatial attention involves facilitation and inhibition of various spatial locations. The presentation of a cue increases alertness and directs attention to that spatial location, enhancing the processing of targets in this location. As attention is directed to that specific location, a second mechanism is initiated, resulting in less efficient (i.e., inhibited) processing of all other locations. Posner referred to this second mechanism as the "cost" of attending. More specifically, Posner decomposed spatial attention into a series of basic processes: (1) interruption of ongoing activity, (2) disengaging attention from the present stimulus, (3) moving attention to the new location, and (4) reengaging attention to the new stimulus. Given this complexity of basic attention processes, it is important to design effective and efficient attention-based treatments as well as assessment tools that appropriately tap the underlying processes purported to change as a result of treatment.

To further complicate matters, some cognitive psychologists posit that information processing occurs at different stages (e.g., Bargh, 1989; Shiffrin & Schneider, 1977). One parsimonious conceptualization divides information processing into automatic and strategic processes (Shiffrin & Schneider, 1977). *Automatic* processes are thought to be (1) relatively capacity free with respect to resources, effort, and energy, (2) unconscious, not requiring awareness, and (3) involuntary, nonvolitional or obligatory. *Strategic* processes, on the other hand, are thought to be (1) resource limited, (2) effortful, involving conscious attention, and (3) under voluntary control. McNally (1995) suggested that examination of the role of automatic versus strategic processing of information in anxious individuals is motivated by the observation that threat-relevant thoughts are often ego-dystonic. Therefore, they seem to be involuntary and may imply that they operate automatically. Others (e.g., Foa & Kozak, 1986; Mathews & MacLeod, 1994) have suggested that at least some individuals with emotional dysregulation (e.g., anxiety disorders) are characterized by voluntary cognitive avoidance, which seems to involve strategic processes. Accordingly, one aim of basic research on attention is to examine abnormalities in both stages of processing. This research underscores the importance of considering the specific subcomponents or stages of attention processing that may be important in the persistence of emotional disorders as well as their treatment outcome.

Emotion Regulation

Consistent with earlier descriptions in this volume (see Chapters 1–4), we use the term *emotion regulation* to refer to any process an individual uses to influence the *type* of emotion experienced, *when* it is experienced, and *how* it is experienced (see also Gross, 1998, 2001). Contemporary models of emotion regulation argue that specific emotion regulatory acts can be differentiated according to the point along the time line of the unfolding emotion-generative process where they have their primary impact (e.g., Gross, 1998, 2001). At the broadest level, Gross's model distinguishes between *antecedent*-focused and *response*-focused strategies. Antecedent-focused strategies refer to what one does *before* the generation of emotion occurs, while response-focused strategies are implemented once an emotion and its associated response tendencies (i.e., behavioral and physiological responses) have already been activated. Although this model highlights at least two points along the emotion-generative process where emotions can be regulated, most relevant to the present chapter is the notion that *attentional deployment* is one method of modulating emotions (see Gross, 2001). More specifically, emotions can be regulated by *bottom-up* (i.e., stimulus-driven; Yantis, 1998) or *top-down* (i.e., goal-directed; Corbetta & Shulman, 2002) processes (see also Ochsner & Gross, 2007), and attention deployment is one example of a top-down regulatory process that can be used to place particular stimuli in the focus of attention. Thus, attention has the ability to both generate *and* regulate emotions by determining which stimuli have access to bottom-up processes that generate emotions (Ochsner & Gross, 2007).

Attention and Emotion Regulation:
Applications to the Treatment of Emotional Disorders

Adaptive self-regulation involves the ability to exert control over attentional processes that allow us to choose *which* stimuli we attend to and *when* to attend to them. In this way, the flexible use of *attention control* can be used to facilitate top-down emotion regulation by determining which stimuli are granted access for further emotional processing (e.g., Ochsner & Gross, 2007). In contrast, emotional disorders are characterized by rigid, inflexible attentional processing, most notably in the presence of emotionally evocative stimuli (e.g., Mathews & MacLeod, 2005; see also Derryberry & Reed, 2002). In particular, selective processing biases that automatically favor negatively valenced emotional information are thought to be a hallmark of emotional disorders (see Bar-Haim, Lamy, Pergamin, Bakermans-Kranenburg, & van IJzendoorn, 2007; Mathews & MacLeod, 2005). More specifically, deficits in attention control thought to arise from an undue influence of the stimulus-driven (bottom-up) attention system at the expense of the goal-directed (top-down) attention system in the context of salient emotional cues may be one cause of excessive emotional arousal (e.g., Eysenck, Derakshan, Santos, & Calvo, 2007). According to this perspective, an overactive stimulus-driven attention system biased in favor of emotionally salient cues, combined with a diminished capacity to use top-down attention control to regulate affective responses, may place individuals at heightened risk for experiencing emotional dysregulation.

In light of the evidence documenting the relationship between basic attention and emotion regulatory processes (see Ochsner & Gross, 2007, 2008; Pessoa, 2008), the current chapter focuses on the link between basic research and the treatment of emotional disorders. Although manipulating attention has long been a part of treatments for anxiety and depression, earlier studies conceptualized and treated attention in a uniform way, and the results have been inconsistent (see Wells & Matthews, 1994). One reason for some of these inconsistencies may be a lack of precision in defining processes that underlie the attention–emotion relationship (see Weierich et al., 2008). Such precision may also help develop novel treatments and enhance the efficacy and efficiency of existing treatments. Treatment development efforts may benefit from findings in basic research that have identified mechanisms thought to be involved in the maintenance of pathological emotions. Ideally, such mechanisms would possess the following characteristics. First, they should originate from reliable findings in the experimental psychopathology literature. Second, the purported mechanism should predict emotional symptoms in longitudinal studies. Finally, modification of the mechanism should lead to changes in emotional symptoms. We now review the evidence that speaks to each of these points.

Attention and Vulnerability to Negative Emotion

Cognitive theories of emotional disorders suggest that vulnerability to negative emotion arises in part from the operation of selective processing biases that automatically favor negative emotional information (e.g., Mathews & MacLeod, 2005; Williams et al., 1997). Consistent with the diathesis-stress model of psychopathology, attention bias is thought to become activated under conditions of heightened stress and subsequently contributes to the persistence of negative mood states by facilitating preferential processing of negative information at the expense of benign or positive cues. In turn, this attention bias may negatively skew interpretations and memories of contemporary and past events and promote the use of maladaptive behaviors designed to modulate affective experiences. Although there are differences across emotional disorders regarding (1) the types of emotional stimuli that elicit selective attention (e.g., social vs. physical threat), (2) the time course of activation, in the temporal stream of emotional stimuli (500 ms vs. 1,000 ms), and (3) the attention subsystems responsible for processing biases (e.g., facilitation vs. disengagement), the extant literature supports a general association between attention biases toward negative emotional information and emotional disorders (see Mathews & MacLeod, 2005, for a review).

Although cognitive models assume that selective attention to emotionally evocative stimuli is *causally* involved in the maintenance of emotional disorders, this causal hypothesis remains largely untested because previous research has relied on correlational designs (e.g., Bar-Haim et al., 2007; Mathews & MacLeod, 2005). More direct evidence for the causal role of aberrant attention processes in anxiety and depression comes from either prospective studies or direct experimental manipulations of attention (see Joorman et al., Chapter 8, this volume, for a review). Several studies have demonstrated that baseline measures of attention bias toward threat (MacLeod & Hagan, 1992) as well as the degree to which attentional allocation toward negative information shifts following experimental attention manipulations (Clarke, MacLeod, & Shirazee, 2008) or negative mood induction procedures (Beevers & Carver, 2003) predict the subsequent development of negative emotions (anxiety and depression) following exposure to naturally occurring stressors. Importantly, the relationship between attention bias to threat and subsequent affective response remains significant, even after controlling for baseline levels of negative affect.

Researchers have also examined the causal role of attention bias to negative information in increasing affective vulnerability by experimentally manipulating attentional deployment prior to exposing participants to a laboratory-based stressor. Several studies have used experimental instruction sets designed to manipulate strategic attentional focus. For example, instructing participants with social anxiety disorder (SAD) to increase self-focused attention heightens anticipated anxiety and anxious appearance in the context of a laboratory speech task (e.g., Woody, 1996), while instructing individuals with SAD to focus externally decreases anxiety during exposure to idiosyncratic fear-provoking situations (Wells & Papageorgiou, 1998).

More recently, researchers have modified computerized experimental tests of attention in order to selectively induce *automatic* processing of negative or benign cues and subsequently examined effects of the manipulation on emotional reactivity in the context of a laboratory-based stressor. In a seminal study, MacLeod, Rutherford, Campbell, Ebsworthy, and Holker (2002), used a variation of the probe-detection task to modify attention in the presence of threat-relevant stimuli in undergraduate participants scoring in the middle third of the distribution on a self-report measure of trait anxiety. In the original dot-probe task (MacLeod, Mathews, & Tata, 1986), participants see two words, one above the other, on a computer screen. One word is neutral, and the other word is threatening. On critical trials, either the upper or the lower word is replaced with a probe, and participants are asked to press a button to identify the probe. Faster response latencies in detecting probes replacing words that represent threatening content versus probes replacing neutral words reflect an attention bias toward threatening information. MacLeod and colleagues trained participants to orient their attention either toward or away from threatening cues by requiring them to respond to a visual probe that appeared consistently following words of negative valence or neutral valence, respectively. Results revealed that, although participants did not differ in self-reported negative affect before and after the training procedure, participants trained to attend to the threatening stimuli reported higher levels of depression and anxiety in response to the experimental stressor (i.e., attempting to solve insoluble anagrams) than those trained to orient toward neutral cues.

Amir, Weber, Beard, Bomyea, and Taylor (2008) extended those findings by examining whether attention-training procedures were capable of modifying attention bias and emotional reactivity in individuals with high levels of social anxiety. Participants completed a modified probe-detection task with pictures of faces with either a threatening (i.e., disgust) or neutral emotional expression cuing different locations on the computer screen (500-ms stimulus presentation). Using an adaptation of the attention modification procedure reported by MacLeod and colleagues (2002), attentional allocation was trained by including a contingency between the location of the nonthreatening stimuli (i.e., neutral face) and the probe in one group (attention modification program [AMP]) and not in the other (attention control condition [ACC]). Participants also completed an independent measure of attention bias using a task and stimuli not encountered during training in order to examine the generalizability of the AMP. Following training, participants completed a videotaped speech task and provided ratings of state anxiety throughout the procedures. Consistent with the findings of MacLeod and colleagues, participants in the AMP condition reported lower levels of anxiety in response to the public speaking task and were judged as having superior speech performance relative to control participants. Importantly, reductions in attention bias from pre- to posttraining mediated the relationship between attention training and negative emotional and behavioral reactivity to the social stressor. Recent research also suggests that the beneficial stress-buffering effects of computerized attention manipulations observed in the laboratory may also extend to naturalistic stressors (Dandeneau, Baldwin, Baccus, Sakellaropoulo, & Pruessner, 2007). Considered together, these experimental studies provide the strongest support to date for the hypothesis that individual differences in the allocation of attention to threat-relevant and negative information are causally important in mediating vulnerability to negative affectivity.

Modifying Attention in the Treatment of Emotional Disorders

Although the studies just mentioned have established a causal relationship between change in attention and change in negative emotions, questions remain regarding the use of attention manipulations as a treatment for emotional disorders. The first and most basic question concerns whether attention-based treatments are efficacious in reducing symptoms of emotional disorders. The second question pertains to elucidating the processes that underlie observed treatment effects. That is, do attention-based interventions modify the specific attention processes they were designed to change? If so, do changes in attention correspond to changes in treatment outcome?

Given that attention comprises multiple subsystems that may guide emotional processing in distinctive ways (e.g., Fan et al., 2002; Pashler, 1998; Weierich et al., 2008), various attention manipulations could ostensibly facilitate change in pathological emotion processes in different ways. For the purposes of this review, we group existing attention-based treatments into three categories: (1) attention control training (e.g., Bögels, Mulkens, & De Jong, 1997; Siegle, Ghinassi, & Thase, 2007; Wells, 2000), (2) mindfulness-based treatments (e.g., Kabat-Zinn, 2003; Roemer & Orsillo, 2007; Segal, Williams, & Teasdale, 2002), and (3) computerized attention bias modification procedures (e.g., Amir, Beard, Burns, & Bomyea, 2009; Schmidt, Richey, Buckner, & Timpano, 2009).

Attention Control Training

Within the broad category of attention control training, we consider interventions designed to facilitate strategic control over attention, including Wells's (2000) attention-training technique (ATT), Bögels and colleagues' task-concentration training (TCT—Bögels, 2006; Bögels et al., 1997), and Siegle and colleagues' cognitive control training (CCT—Siegle et al., 2007). These interventions share the common goal of facilitating voluntary control over basic attention processes designed to short-circuit dysfunctional habitual information-processing routines characteristic of anxiety and depression.

ATT (Wells, 2000) originated from Wells and colleagues' cognitive-attentional model of psychopathology, which argues that the persistence of emotional disorders lies in dysfunctional appraisals and beliefs that are the product of habitual cognitive processing configurations characterized by excessive and inflexible self-focused attention (see Wells, 2000; Wells & Matthews, 1994, 1996, for details). Accordingly, the goal of ATT is to strengthen attentional control in order to reduce self-focus, broaden attentional scope, and increase cognitive processing flexibility. ATT consists of monitoring competing external auditory signals in a manner that requires progressively greater attentional capacity as the procedure unfolds. Participants are asked to remain focused on a visual fixation point while a series of competing sounds are introduced (or identified if naturally occurring sounds already exist) in the immediate vicinity of the participant, outside of the room but within the near distance, and in the far distance. During the selective-attention phase, individuals are required to focus on one sound while excluding all others for 30 seconds before shifting to another sound. In the attention-switching phase, individuals focus on one sound to the exclusion of all others, but this time they are required to shift their attention to a new sound approximately every 5 seconds. Finally, the divided-attention phase requires individuals to simultaneously focus on as many sounds as possible. Task difficulty is increased by requiring individuals to identify progressively less distinct sounds, increasing the speed of attention switching, and ending the procedure with a sustained divided-attention instruction.

Given that ATT was not intended to be used as a distraction strategy during heightened states of negative affect, the technique is practiced when patients are not exposed to emotionally evocative cues. Moreover, ATT was designed to modify basic attention regulation and, therefore, does not require tailoring to specific disorders. As a result, ATT has been applied to the treatment of numerous psychiatric conditions. To date, several studies using single-case designs have demonstrated that ATT is associated with clinical improvements in self-report measures of affect, behavior, and cognition in panic disorder and social phobia (Wells, White, & Carter, 1997), health anxiety (Papageorgiou & Wells, 1998), and major depression (Papageorgiou & Wells, 2000). In these latter two studies, measures of self-reported focus of attention indicated that ATT produced reductions in self-focus as intended. Although these preliminary studies suggest that ATT is associated with consistent effects across a range of psychiatric conditions, these studies await replication in larger randomized controlled trials. Furthermore, although consistent with the cognitive-attentional model of Wells and Mathews (1994, 1996), it remains unclear whether changes in self-focused attention and rumination from pre- to posttreatment are a direct effect of the ATT or merely a consequence of symptomatic improvement. An important question for future research will be to examine whether the ATT modifies other basic attention control processes (i.e., attention switching, divided attention) as hypothesized by the model and whether those changes mediate treatment outcome. Finally, one recent study found that supplementing group cognitive-behavioral therapy (CBT) for SAD with ATT did not potentiate treatment effects for symptoms of social anxiety, depression, or attention control (McEvoy & Perini, 2009). It is notable, however, that across both treatment conditions greater improvements in self-reported attention control were associated with greater symptom reduction, suggesting that the beneficial effects of CBT may lie in part in changes in basic attention processes.

Siegle and colleagues (2007) developed CCT to complement existing treatments for unipolar depression. The conceptual and empirical basis for CCT comes from basic neurobehavioral research suggesting that diminished prefrontal control may contribute to the increased and sustained emotional reactivity characteristic of depression. Accordingly, it was hypothesized that attentional tasks that enhance prefrontal inhibitory control (e.g., sustained attention and working memory exercises) may be beneficial in modifying information-processing biases characteristic of depression (see Siegle et al., 2007). The treatment itself consists of Wells's (2000) ATT, intended to improve strategic control of attention, and a variant of the Paced Auditory Serial Attention Task (PASAT; Gronwall, 1977), intended to activate the prefrontal cortex in the context of a mildly stressful task associated with heightened emotional reactivity. The modified PASAT involves continuously adding serially presented digits in working memory, while task difficulty is manipulated by varying the speed at which the items are presented according to individuals' performance. In a preliminary investigation, a small group of inpatients diagnosed with unipolar major depression were randomly assigned to receive six sessions of CCT over a 2-week period as part of their ongoing participation in an intensive outpatient program, or treatment as usual (TAU), which included medication management, supportive group psychotherapy based on dialectical behavior therapy principles, and milieu therapy. Results revealed that the addition of CCT was superior to TAU, as evidenced by significantly larger decreases in depression and self-reported rumination from pre- to post-assessment. Furthermore, in a subsample of six patients receiving CCT, neuroimaging data collected from pre- to posttreatment revealed that CCT-treated patients demonstrated decreased disruptions in amygdala reactivity and prefrontal cortex activity on cognitive-affective tasks. The authors interpreted these findings to suggest that CCT was associated with a normalization in the functioning of brain regions implicated in the basic control of attention and emotion regulation.

Another version of strategic attention control training, TCT (Bögels et al., 1997), was designed as a treatment for SAD and extreme blushing to reduce excessive self-focused attention hypothesized to play a central role in the maintenance of those conditions. Using a series of progressively more challenging concentration exercises, first in nonthreatening situations and then gradually applied to anxiety-provoking situations, TCT teaches patients to redirect their attention away from aspects of the self (e.g., bodily symptoms, negative cognitions) and toward the specific tasks required in the situation. A number of studies have supported the beneficial effects of TCT in reducing symptoms of social anxiety and anxiety-related beliefs (e.g., fear of bodily symptoms and dysfunctional beliefs about blushing) (Bögels, 2006; Bögels et al., 1997; Mulkens, Bögels, de Jong, & Louwers, 2001). Additionally, Bögels (2006) found that TCT produced greater reductions in self-consciousness and self-focused attention relative to active comparison treatments (i.e., applied relaxation and cognitive therapy), which was responsible for the superior effect of TCT on fear of showing bodily symptoms at 1-year follow-up. Although these initial studies support the efficacy of TCT in reducing symptoms of social anxiety, research is needed to establish whether TCT extends to clinical conditions beyond SAD that are characterized by excessive self-focused attention (e.g., depression).

In summary, the extant literature provides preliminary support for the use of strategic attention control training interventions in the treatment of emotional disorders. Although promising, existing studies are limited by modest sample sizes, the lack of randomized controlled trials, and a paucity of evidence regarding the mechanisms purported to underlie treatment effects.

Mindfulness-Based Treatments

In recent years there has been growing interest in the use of mindfulness meditation practices in the treatment of emotional dysfunction. Despite operational challenges, generally, *mindfulness* refers to a particular quality of awareness that emerges through intentional paying attention, in the present moment and nonjudgmentally, to the unfolding of experience moment by moment (e.g., Baer, 2003; Kabat-Zinn, 2003). Because mindfulness aims to facilitate control over attention and awareness of current-moment internal and external experience *irrespective* of the nature or valence of that experience, it has potential for transdiagnostic applications in the treatment of psychopathology (see Corcoran, Farb, Anderson, & Segal, Chapter 14, this volume). Applied to the treatment of emotional disorders, mindfulness-based therapies share the common goal of teaching patients to recognize and disengage from dysfunctional modes of thinking (i.e., rumination) (see Teasdale, 1999) and self-regulation (e.g., cognitive and emotional avoidance) (see Linehan, 1993; Roemer & Orsillo, 2007). Accumulating evidence suggests that mindfulness-based treatments are effective in treating a range of emotional disorders, including relapse in recurrent major depression (i.e., mindfulness-based cognitive therapy) (Ma & Teasdale, 2004; Teasdale et al., 2000), medical patients with generalized anxiety disorder (GAD) or panic disorder (mindfulness-based stress reduction [MBSR]; Kabat-Zinn et al., 1992), and individuals presenting with a primary diagnosis of GAD (Roemer & Orsillo, 2007; see Corcoran et al., Chapter 14, this volume, for a review). Despite these promising findings, some have argued that because few studies have compared mindfulness interventions to credible control conditions, it becomes difficult to disentangle mindfulness-specific outcomes from common treatment effects (e.g., psychoeducation) and nonspecific therapy effects such as group contact and therapist support (e.g., Coelho, Canter, & Ernst, 2007; see, however, Williams, Russell, & Russell, 2008, for a discussion of ongoing research in this regard). Moreover, interpretation of treatment effects attributable to mindfulness practices is not clear given that those procedures are rarely used in isolation but instead are often incorporated as part of a more comprehensive treatment regimen. Therefore, treatment effects uniquely attributable to mindfulness procedures remain to be established.

Recent debates regarding the unique clinical utility of mindfulness-based treatments (e.g., Coelho et al., 2007; Hofmann & Asmundson, 2008) notwithstanding, little is known about the processes purported to be responsible for clinical change in these regimens. According to operational definitions of mindfulness (e.g., Bishop et al., 2004), the self-regulation of attention (i.e., attention control) is argued to be central to the cultivation of a mindful state. It has been proposed that a number of distinct attentional processes are affected by mindfulness meditation practice, for example, sustained attention (required to maintain awareness of present-moment experience) and attention switching (required to bring attention back to the present moment when it wanders; Bishop et al., 2004).

To elucidate the role of basic attention processes during mindfulness mediation, a number of studies have examined changes in attentional processing occurring in the context of mindfulness practices in nonclinical samples of novice meditators. In one study, Jha, Krompinger, and Baime (2007) compared changes on the Attention Network Test (ANT; Fan et al., 2002) in a group of naïve meditators who completed an 8-week MBSR course with changes in a no-intervention control group. The ANT was designed to assess attention systems involved in alerting (thought to reflect operations of the bottom-up/stimulus-driven attention system) and orienting and conflict monitoring (argued to involve top-down or voluntary attention systems). Results revealed that participants in the MBSR course improved on the measure of orienting relative to controls (but not conflict monitoring or alerting), suggesting that mindfulness training improved specific aspects of voluntary top-down attention control. In a similar vein, Chambers, Lo, and Allen (2008) found that novice meditators who participated in a 10-day intensive mindfulness meditation retreat demonstrated significant improvements in self-reported mindfulness and rumination and on performance measures of working memory and sustained attention (but not internal attention switching) relative to a comparison group who did not undergo any meditation training. Furthermore, the mindfulness-trained group reported reductions on some indices of negative affect (i.e., depression but not anxiety). Notably, change in self-reported mindfulness was associated with improvements in working memory. However, the mediating role of changes in attention processes in explaining the relationship between mindfulness training and reduction in negative emotions was not formally assessed.

Not all studies, however, have found changes in attention processes following mindfulness-based interventions. For example, although individuals completing an 8-week MBSR course displayed greater improvements in self-reported mindfulness and emotional well-being (e.g., anxiety, depression, anger, positive affect) relative to a wait-list control group, they did not differ on behavioral indices of attention control (e.g., sustained attention, attention switching, Stroop interference, and nondirected attention) (Anderson, Lau, Segal, & Bishop, 2007). Moreover, although self-reported improvements in mindfulness were associated with greater emotional well-being, changes in mindfulness were only associated with one of four measures of attention control. These latter findings point to an incongruity between self-report assessments of mindfulness and behavioral measures of the basic attention processes purported to be affected by mindfulness practices. Research is needed to clarify these discrepancies.

In summary, although the unique treatment effects of mindfulness-based practices require further empirical scrutiny (e.g., Coelho et al., 2007), emerging research provides preliminary support suggesting that mindfulness-based interventions may influence a number of basic attention processes thought to be important in the persistence of emotional disorders. However, empirical findings to date have been mixed. Moreover, existing studies have examined change in attentional processing using nonclinical samples, and it remains to be established whether those results would generalize to individuals presenting with clinically significant levels of emotional dysfunction. Nonetheless, these initial studies represent an encouraging first step in examining the basic attention processes purported to underlie mindfulness-based treatments. Further work is needed to replicate and extend these findings in the context of mindfulness-based treatments for emotional disorders (e.g., Roemer & Orsillo, 2007; Segal et al., 2002) and to examine whether changes in attentional functioning resulting from mindfulness practices lead to symptom reduction.

Computerized Attention Bias Modification Procedures

Thus far, we have focused on the extant empirical literature regarding treatments designed to facilitate strategic control over attention. However, there is compelling evidence to suggest that biased attention processes characteristic of some emotional disorders (e.g., anxiety) originate *automatically*, that is, without voluntary or conscious control (see Mathews & MacLeod, 2005). Accordingly, researchers have become increasingly interested in examining procedures designed to modify *automatic* attention processes in order to reduce clinical symptoms of emotional disorders. Although a number of the previously reviewed studies examined the effects of training selective processing biases on subsequent emotional reactivity to laboratory stressors (e.g., Amir et al., 2008; MacLeod et al., 2002), the following series of studies were interested in evaluating the efficacy of administering similar computerized attention bias modification programs over *multiple* sessions in reducing symptoms of specific emotional disorders.

To our knowledge, three published studies have examined the efficacy of computerized attention modification procedures in reducing symptoms in individuals meeting diagnostic criteria for a psychiatric condition. In one, Amir and colleagues (2009) examined the effect of an eight-session attention modification program (administered twice weekly over 4 weeks) on participants' attentional allocation toward threat-relevant information as well as symptoms of anxiety in a sample of 29 individuals seeking treatment for GAD. Attention training comprised a probe-detection task where pairs of words that were either emotionally evocative (i.e., represented threatening information, e.g., illness) or emotionally neutral (e.g., couch) cued different locations on the computer screen, and participants were simply required to respond to a probe, immediately replacing one of the words as quickly and as accurately as possible. To selectively train attention in the active condition, the contingency between the probe and threat-relevant cues was manipulated, such that the probe always replaced a word depicting neutral content during neutral-threat trials, thereby directing attention away from negative emotional information (AMP). A sham condition was created such that the probe appeared with equal frequency in the position of the threatening and neutral words (ACC). Participants were randomly allocated to the AMP or ACC conditions, and participants, experimental assistants, and diagnostic interviewers remained blind to condition. Results of this study revealed that patients who were trained to repeatedly direct their attention away from threatening cues displayed a significant reduction in attention bias toward threat and a decrease in anxiety, as indicated by both self-report and interviewer measures relative to the control group. Change in attention bias from pre- to postassessment mediated the relationship between attention training and interviewer-rated change in anxiety. Furthermore, 50% of participants who received the attention training program no longer met diagnostic criteria for GAD at postassessment compared with only 13% of control participants. The magnitude of treatment of effects in this study (i.e., between-group controlled Cohen's $d = 0.72–0.88$) were comparable to those reported in recent meta-analyses for both psychosocial (0.71–0.90; Borkovec & Ruscio, 2001) and pharmacological (0.42–0.90; Lydiard & Monnier, 2004) treatments for GAD.

Using the attention-training program described in Amir and colleagues (2008), Schmidt and colleagues (2009) randomly assigned 36 individuals meeting criteria for generalized SAD (GSAD) to either an attention-training condition designed to facilitate attentional disengagement from threatening (i.e., disgust) faces or to a control condition. Consistent with the GAD study, GSAD patients in the attention-training condition exhibited significantly greater reductions in social anxiety and trait anxiety compared with patients in the control condition. Remarkably, at postassessment, 72% of patients in the active treatment condition no longer met diagnostic criteria for SAD, relative to 11% of patients in the control condition. Clinical improvement was maintained at 4-month follow-up. It is also noteworthy that all but one participant in the attention-training condition did not believe they were receiving an active intervention, suggesting that experimental demand was unlikely to account for the results.

Using an identical attention-training program, we have provided independent replication of these results in a sample of 44 individuals diagnosed with GSAD (Amir et al., in press). The convergence of findings across sites using identical procedures bolsters confidence that the effects of the AMP were not due to idiosyncratic characteristics of the treatment setting (see also Li, Tan, Qian, & Liu, 2008, for similar findings in a sample of socially anxious undergraduates receiving daily attention training over a 1-week period). In light of research suggesting that different subcomponents of attention may be involved in the maintenance of anxiety (e.g., hypervigilance toward threat; difficulties disengaging from threat; see Weierich et al., 2008), we sought to examine the effect of the AMP on a measure of attention disengagement that used a task and stimuli different from those used during training. The results suggested that the AMP facilitated participants' ability to disengage their attention from social threat cues and that change in attention bias from pre- to postassessment mediated change in clinician-reported social anxiety symptoms. Taken together, emerging evidence suggests that altering attention mechanisms using computerized bias modification procedures may effectively reduce pathological anxiety symptoms in clinical samples. Those findings are notable given the relatively short duration of the treatments and limited therapist contact. Research is needed to replicate and extend those findings to other psychological disorders characterized by pathological attention and emotional processes.

Summary

Existing empirical evidence provides support for the use of attentional manipulations in the treatment of emotional disorders. Clinical improvement has been observed across a range of anxiety disorders and major depression using strategic attention control techniques, mindfulness practices, and computerized bias modification procedures. Despite these encouraging findings, a number of methodological issues have made interpretation of the treatment effects challenging. Numerous studies have used case-controlled designs and suffer from small sample sizes. Other studies have failed to use credible control conditions, which obscures detection of treatment effects uniquely attributable to the attention-based intervention under study. A particularly notable omission from numerous studies is the use of assessment instruments that specifically tap into the attention processes purported to underlie clinical improvement. Even fewer studies have examined relationships between change in attention processes and treatment outcome. We recognize that many attentional manipulations are routinely incorporated into larger treatment regimens, which presents challenges in clarifying the degree to which the attention-based component of treatment is responsible for the observed treatment effect. Nonetheless, elucidating the unique contribution of attention-based interventions to clinical change, as well as the processes that underlie these changes, is essential if we are to maximize the potential of these treatments in ameliorating symptoms of emotional disorders.

It is encouraging, however, that a number of studies have begun to address some of these issues. For example, recent studies have examined the attentional mechanisms hypothesized to underlie treatment effects in mindfulness-based interventions (e.g., Anderson et al., 2007; Chambers et al., 2008; Jha et al., 2007). Replication and extension of these studies to clinical populations are important avenues for future research. Siegle and colleagues' (2007) emerging work using attention control training in depressed populations is an example of a research agenda designed to test changes in the underlying neurobiological mechanisms argued to be important in the effective regulation of emotion. Studies examining the effectiveness of ATT point to research efforts directed at distilling attention-based treatments into their pure form (e.g., Wells et al., 1997). Finally, recent research examining the application of computer-based attention modification procedures to the treatment of clinical disorders has underscored the importance of developing credible control conditions against which treatment effects can be compared as well as testing the purported mechanisms responsible for clinical change (e.g., Amir et al., 2009). These types of studies are crucial for us to clarify the source of treatment effects, which will facilitate improvements in existing treatments as well as refinements in the conceptual model upon which these treatments are based.

Future Directions

Attention Modification and Transdiagnostic Clinical Applications

The rapidly accumulating empirical evidence documenting that attention is fundamentally involved in the regulation of emotion (see Ochsner & Gross, 2007, 2008; Pessoa, 2008) has implications for the transdiagnostic application of clinical interventions designed to modify attention. Recent years have seen a growing interest in treatment approaches that cut across disorder-based categorizations and address common underlying pathologies (e.g., Barlow, Allen, & Choate, 2004; Harvey et al., 2004). Justification for transdiagnostic treatment approaches is grounded in research pointing to commonalities in the cause and pathophysiology of emotional disorders (see Allen, McHugh, & Barlow, 2008, for a review). A robust empirical literature points to common heritable factors across disorders characterized by emotion dysregulation (e.g., Kendler, Neale, Kessler, & Heath, 1993). Moreover, emerging evidence suggests that dysfunctional attention processes may be proximal to the basic genetic predisposition for emotional disorders. For example, polymorphisms in genes involved in the expression of specific neurotransmitters that are important in the regulation of emotion (e.g., serotonin) have been linked to biased attention toward negative emotional information (Beevers, Gibb, McGeary, & Miller, 2007) as well as heightened reactivity of limbic circuitries (i.e., amygdala and perigenual cingulate) during the processing of emotional stimuli (see Hariri & Holmes, 2006, for a review). Considered together, this literature points to individual differences in genetic susceptibility to dysregulation of basic attention systems involved in the processing of emotion cues, which may confer heightened vulnerability to the development of emotion-related pathology.

Because aberrant functioning in basic attention and emotion regulation processes are implicated in the pathophysiology of a wide range of psychological disorders (see Harvey et al., 2004), interventions that specifically target these deficits offer great promise for transdiagnostic approaches to treatment of psychopathology. The attention-based treatments reviewed previously aim to modify pathological cognitive *operations* characteristic of emotional dysregulation rather than targeting the *content* of those cognitive processes that may be more unique to particular psychological disorders. For example, whereas cognitive restructuring techniques typically target disorder-specific cognitive misappraisals (e.g., fear of bodily sensations in panic disorder; fear of negative evaluation in SAD; inflated appraisals of responsibility in obsessive–compulsive disorder), attention interventions are intended to target basic underlying cognitive functions (e.g., attention control) hypothesized to play a role in the persistence of psychopathology. Thus, attention-based interventions may more directly target fundamental psychopathological vulnerabilities (e.g.,

Beevers et al., 2007), while the maladaptive cognitions and behaviors characteristic of emotional disorders may be viewed as more distal expressions of those basic vulnerabilities. One implication of this distinction is that a two-pronged approach that uses attention modification procedures to complement existing empirically supported treatments (e.g., CBT) may produce more effective or efficient interventions. Research is needed to address that issue.

Given the transdiagnostic appeal of attention modification procedures, it is not surprising that these interventions have made their way into contemporary treatment regimens for an array of psychiatric conditions. Although much of this research is still in its infancy, initial studies suggest that, in addition to anxiety and depression, attention modification interventions may offer benefits in the treatment of attention-deficit/hyperactivity disorder (Posner, Rothbart, & Sheese, 2007), substance use disorders (Witkiewitz, Marlatt, & Walker, 2005), schizophrenia and psychotic-spectrum disorders (e.g., Suslow, Schonauer, & Arolt, 2001; Valmaggia, Bouman, & Schuurman, 2007), and personality disorders (e.g., Linehan, 1993). The transdiagnostic application of attention-based treatments also suggests that these procedures, through modifying common psychopathological mechanisms, may be effective in treating the comorbid conditions that often present in emotional disorders. Finally, the transdiagnostic perspective suggests that attention-based treatments have the potential for increasing the accessibility and dissemination of empirically supported and cost-effective interventions. Such treatments would likely be more efficient in the training of health professionals in the community (cf. disorder-focused treatments) as well as more cost-effective by reducing the amount of therapist contact.

Attention Control versus Distraction

An important consideration raised during our review concerns the optimal *target* toward which one's attention should be trained. According to emotional processing theory (e.g., Foa, Huppert, & Cahill, 2006; Foa & Kozak, 1986), treatments for emotional disorders are effective to the extent that they encourage active engagement with emotional stimuli in order to facilitate complete processing of that material. Consistent with this proposition, mindfulness-based interventions encourage full attentional awareness of present-moment experience, including thoughts, feelings, and cues of arousal regardless of their valence (i.e., negative, positive, or neutral). This treatment approach is consistent with existing empirically supported cognitive and behavioral regimens that promote active engagement with emotional stimuli through exposure. In contrast, computerized attention bias modification exercises repeatedly redirect attention *away* from emotionally evocative cues. One might argue that this approach, through encouraging attentional avoidance of emotional stimuli, would prevent elaborative processing of emotional material necessary for symptom reduction. How do we reconcile these seemingly opposing positions?

Accumulating empirical evidence regarding the link between basic attention and emotional processing may provide some insights into this puzzle. Recent models of the cognitive control of emotion (Oschner & Gross, 2007, 2008) differentiate between two related but distinct types of attentional deployment, namely selective attention and attention distraction. *Selective attention* is defined as the process wherein an individual selects some environmental cues for further processing while screening out or minimizing the processing of other cues. In contrast, *attention distraction* occurs when an individual engages in a secondary task that diverts attention from processing a primary target stimulus. Attention distraction is differentiated from selective attention in that the former type of attention deployment does not involve screening out unwanted distractions per se, but instead involves managing the competing demands of doing two things at once (Oschner & Gross, 2007). For example, a number of studies have demonstrated that exposure to emotionally evocative cues (e.g., threatening faces) resulted in heightened amygdala reactivity, but only when sufficient attention resources were available to process the emotional stimuli (e.g., Pessoa, McKenna, Gutierrez, & Ungerleider, 2002). In contrast, when participants were required to complete a competing attention-demanding task during exposure to the emotional stimuli (e.g., judging whether two lines were or were not of similar orientations), differential activation of emotion-generative brain regions was not observed. This accumulating body of evidence suggests that top-down attention processes regulate the processing of emotional cues *before* emotion generation has occurred. Thus, computerized attention-training programs may recruit attentional processes before emotion-generative operations are activated by requiring individuals to perform a primary task (i.e., make a judgment about the probe type) in the context of emotionally evocative stimuli (e.g., threatening faces), and consequently may regulate emotions before they are generated. In contrast, encouraging avoidance of emotional stimuli may be less effective or even detrimental once the behavioral response tendencies associated with a particular emotion are already activated (e.g., Gross, 1998).

Considered in the context of process models of emotion regulation (e.g., Gross, 2001), computerized attention bias modification programs and mindfulness-based interventions target different stages of the emotion-generative process. Mindfulness techniques target maladaptive response-focused strategies (e.g., suppression), while computerized bias modification programs facilitate adaptive antecedent-focused emotion regulation. It is notable that cognitive and behavioral treatments (CBT) also target antecedent strategies through cognitive reappraisal (e.g., Hofmann & Asmundson, 2008). One key difference, however, is that whereas CBT requires controlled, conscious modification of dysfunctional cognitions, computerized attention-training programs modify automatic cognitive processes and, therefore, require fewer cognitive resources. This distinction is noteworthy because existing treatments often require people to use cognitive resources to reevaluate cognitions in the context of emotionally arousing situations, a time when cognitive resources are most taxed. An important direction for future research will be to examine the potential to enhance the impact of treatments by directly targeting automatic attention biases in conjunction with traditional CBT approaches.

Attention, Positive Stimuli, and Positive Emotions

There is growing recognition that positive emotions are important in facilitating therapeutic change in the treatment of emotional disorders (e.g., Ehrenreich, Fairholme, Buzzella, Ellard, & Barlow, 2007). For example, positive affect has been shown to facilitate recovery from the physiological and behavioral effects of negative emotions, promote social approach behaviors, broaden attentional focus, and induce selective attentional processing toward positive stimuli and away from negative stimuli (e.g., Fredrickson, 2001; Gable, Reis, & Elliot, 2000; Isaacowitz, 2005; Tugade & Fredrickson, 2004). In contrast, a number of emotional disorders (e.g., depression, SAD) are characterized by low positive affect (e.g., Brown, Chorpita, & Barlow, 1998). Moreover, diminished emotional responsiveness to positive stimuli in currently depressed individuals was found to predict a more severe subsequent course of depression (Rottenberg, Kasch, Gross, & Gotlib, 2002).

One explanation for these hedonic deficiencies is that some individuals may process positive information in a biased manner, which places them at greater risk for emotional dysfunction. Consistent with this proposition, several studies have demonstrated that a variety of emotional disorders are characterized by diminished processing of positive stimuli (e.g., Joorman & Gotlib, 2007). For example, following a negative mood induction, girls identified as at risk for depression displayed an attentional shift toward negative emotional information, while their low-risk control counterparts tended to shift their attention toward positive emotional cues (e.g., Joorman, Talbot, & Gotlib, 2007). These researchers interpreted those findings to suggest that allocating attention toward positive stimuli may promote adaptive emotion regulation under conditions of heightened stress, thereby protecting individuals from resultant increases in negative mood states. Those findings raise the possibility that training attention toward positive stimuli may serve to buffer people against adverse consequences associated with negative life experiences. Consistent with that possibility, Wadlinger and Isaacowitz (2008) found that individuals repeatedly trained to allocate their attention toward positive stimuli using a similar computerized attention task to those described earlier (e.g., Amir et al., 2008 ; MacLeod et al., 2002) directed their attention significantly less toward novel negative images during a visual stress task. Those findings suggest that positive attention training may promote effective emotion regulation by facilitating a broader and more flexible attentional set, thereby preventing the attentional narrowing toward negative stimuli characteristic of emotional disorders. Future research is needed to examine whether changes in the processing of positive stimuli are important in facilitating enduring recovery from emotional disorders and whether attention training toward positive information can augment existing treatments.

Conclusion

Our goals in this chapter were to examine the current empirical status of attention-based interventions in the treatment of emotional disorders and to elucidate unresolved issues and directions for future research. While the extant literature suggests that attention-based treatments are effective in reducing symptoms of emotional disorders, much less is known about the unique contribution of attention manipulations to the amelioration of pathological emotion processes as well as the specific mechanisms purported to underlie observed treatment effects. However, given the steadily accumulating evidence documenting the relationship between basic processes involving attention and emotion regulatory systems, translation of this basic research to the treatment of emotional dysfunction can only enhance the efficacy and efficiency of existing treatments as well as promote the development of novel treatments and their transdiagnostic application.

References

Allen, L. B., McHugh, R. K., & Barlow, D. H. (2008). Emotional disorders: A unified protocol. In D. H. Barlow (Ed.), *Clinical handbook of psychological disorders: A step-by-step treatment manual* (4th ed., pp. 216–249). New York: Guilford Press.

Amir, N., Beard, C., Burns, M., & Bomyea, J. (2009). Attention modification program in individuals with generalized anxiety disorder. *Journal of Abnormal Psychology, 118*(1), 28–33.

Amir, N., Beard, C., Taylor, C. T., Klumpp, H., Elias, J., Burns, M., et al. (in press). Attention training in individuals with generalized social phobia: A randomized controlled trial. *Journal of Consulting and Clinical Psychology.*

Amir, N., Weber, G., Beard, C., Bomyea, J., & Taylor, C. T. (2008). The effect of a single-session attention modification program on response to a public speaking challenge in socially anxious individuals. *Journal of Abnormal Psychology, 117*(4), 860–868.

Anderson, N. D., Lau, M. A., Segal, Z. V., & Bishop, S. R. (2007). Mindfulness-based stress reduction and attentional control. *Clinical Psychology and Psychotherapy, 14*, 449–463.

Baer, R. A. (2003). Mindfulness training as a clinical intervention: A conceptual and empirical review. *Clinical Psychology: Science and Practice, 10*, 125–143.

Bargh, J. A. (1989). Conditional automaticity: Varieties of automatic influence in social perception and cognition. In J. S. Uleman & J. A. Bargh (Eds.), *Unintended thought* (pp. 3–51). New York: Guilford Press.

Bar-Haim, Y., Lamy, D., Pergamin, L., Bakermans-Kranenburg, M. J., & van IJzendoorn, M. H. (2007). Threat-related attentional bias in anxious and nonanxious individuals: A meta-analytic study. *Psychological Bulletin, 133*, 1–12.

Barlow, D. H., Allen, L. B., & Choate, M. L. (2004). Toward a unified treatment for emotional disorders. *Behavior Therapy, 35*, 205–230.

Beevers, C. G., & Carver, C. S. (2003). Attentional bias and mood persistence as prospective predictors of dysphoria. *Cognitive Therapy and Research, 27*, 619–637.

Beevers, C. G., Gibb, B. E., McGeary, J. E., & Miller, I. W. (2007). Serotonin transporter genetic variation and biased attention for emotional word stimuli among psychiatric inpatients. *Journal of Abnormal Psychology, 116*, 208–212.

Bishop, S. R., Lau, M., Shapiro, S., Carlson, L., Anderson, N. D., Carmody, J., et al. (2004). Mindfulness: A proposed operational definition. *Clinical Psychology: Science and Practice, 11*, 230–241.

Bögels, S. M. (2006). Task concentration training versus applied relaxation, in combination with cognitive therapy, for social phobia patients with fear of blushing, trembling, and sweating. *Behaviour Research and Therapy, 44*, 1199–1210.

Bögels, S. M., Mulkens, S., & De Jong, P. J. (1997). Task concentration training and fear of blushing. *Clinical Psychology and Psychotherapy, 4*, 251–258.

Borkovec, T. D., & Ruscio, A. (2001). Psychotherapy for generalized anxiety disorder. *Journal of Clinical Psychiatry, 62*, 37–45.

Brown, T. A., Chorpita, B. F., & Barlow, D. H. (1998). Structural relationships among dimensions of DSM-IV anxiety and mood disorders and dimensions of negative affect, positive affect, and autonomic arousal. *Journal of Abnormal Psychology, 107*, 179–192.

Chambers, R., Lo, B. C. Y., & Allen, N. B. (2008). The impact of intensive mindfulness training on attentional control, cognitive style, and affect. *Cognitive Therapy and Research, 32*(3), 303–322.

Clarke, P., MacLeod, C., & Shirazee, N. (2008). Prepared for the worst: Readiness to acquire threat bias and susceptibility to elevate trait anxiety. *Emotion, 8*, 47–57.

Coelho, H. F., Canter, P. F., & Ernst, E. (2007). Mindfulness-based cognitive therapy: Evaluating current evidence and informing future research. *Journal of Consulting and Clinical Psychology, 75*, 1000–1005.

Corbetta, M., & Shulman, G. L. (2002). Control of goal-directed and stimulus-driven attention in the brain. *Nature Reviews Neuroscience, 3*, 201–215.

Dandeneau, S. D., Baldwin, M. W., Baccus, J. R., Sakellaropoulo, M., & Pruessner, J. C. (2007). Cutting stress off at the pass: Reducing vigilance and responsiveness to social threat by manipulating attention. *Journal of Personality and Social Psychology, 93*, 651–666.

Derryberry, D., & Reed, M. A. (2002). Anxiety-related attentional biases and their regulation by attentional control. *Journal of Abnormal Psychology, 111,* 225–236.

Ehrenreich, J. T., Fairholme, C. P., Buzzella, B. A., Ellard, K. K., & Barlow, D. H. (2007). The role of emotion in psychological therapy. *Clinical Psychology: Science and Practice, 14,* 422–428.

Eysenck, M., Derakshan, N., Santos, R., & Calvo, M. (2007). Anxiety and cognitive performance: Attentional control theory. *Emotion, 7,* 336–353.

Fan, J., McCandliss, B. D., Sommer, T., Raz, A., & Posner, M. I. (2002). Testing the efficiency and independence of attentional networks. *Journal of Cognitive Neuroscience, 14,* 340–347.

Foa, E. B., Huppert, J. D., & Cahill, S. P. (2006). Emotional processing theory: An update. In B. O. Rothbaum (Ed.), *Pathological anxiety: Emotional processing in etiology and treatment* (pp. 3–24). New York: Guilford Press.

Foa, E. B., & Kozak, M. J. (1986). Emotional processing of fear: Exposure to corrective information. *Psychological Bulletin, 99,* 20–35.

Fredrickson, B. L. (2001). The role of positive emotions in positive psychology: The broaden-and-build theory of positive emotions. *American Psychologist, 56,* 218–226.

Gable, S. L., Reis, H. T., & Elliot, A. J. (2000). Behavioral activation and inhibition in everyday life. *Journal of Personality and Social Psychology, 78,* 1135–1149.

Gronwall, D. M. (1977). Paced auditory serial-addition task: A measure of recovery from concussion. *Perceptual and Motor Skills, 44,* 367–373.

Gross, J. J. (1998). Antecedent- and response-focused emotion regulation: Divergent consequences for experience, expression, and physiology. *Journal of Personality and Social Psychology, 74,* 224–237.

Gross, J. J. (2001). Emotion regulation in adulthood: Timing is everything. *Current Directions in Psychological Science, 10,* 214–219.

Hariri, A. R., & Holmes, A. (2006). Genetics of emotional regulation: The role of the serotonin transporter in neural function. *Trends in Cognitive Sciences, 10*(4), 182–191.

Harvey, A., Watkins, E., Mansell, W., & Shafran, R. (2004). *Cognitive behavioural processes across psychological disorders: A transdiagnostic approach to research and treatment.* Oxford, UK: Oxford University Press.

Hofmann, S. G., & Asmundson, G. J. G. (2008). Acceptance and mindfulness-based therapy: New wave or old hat? *Clinical Psychology Review, 28,* 1–16.

Isaacowitz, D. M. (2005). The gaze of the optimist. *Personality and Social Psychology Bulletin, 31,* 407–415.

Jha, A. P., Krompinger, J., & Baime, M. J. (2007). Mindfulness training modifies subsystems of attention. *Cognitive, Affective and Behavioral Neuroscience, 7,* 109–119.

Joormann, J., & Gotlib, I. H. (2007). Selective attention to emotional faces following recovery from depression. *Journal of Abnormal Psychology, 116,* 80–85.

Joormann, J., Talbot, L., & Gotlib, I. H. (2007). Biased processing of emotional information in girls at risk for depression. *Journal of Abnormal Psychology, 116,* 135–143.

Kabat-Zinn, J. (2003). Mindfulness-based interventions in context: Past, present, and future. *Clinical Psychology: Science and Practice, 10,* 144–156.

Kabat-Zinn, J., Massion, A. O., Kristeller, J., Peterson, L. G., Fletcher, K. E., Pbert,

L., et al. (1992). Effectiveness of a meditation-based stress reduction program in the treatment of anxiety disorders. *American Journal of Psychiatry, 149*, 936–944.

Kendler, K. S., Neale, M. C., Kessler, R. C., & Heath, A. C. (1993). Major depression and phobias: The genetic and environmental sources of comorbidity. *Psychological Medicine, 23*, 361–371.

Li, S., Tan, J., Qian, M., & Liu, X. (2008). Continual training of attentional bias in social anxiety. *Behaviour Research and Therapy, 46*, 905–912.

Linehan, M. M. (1993). *Cognitive-behavioral treatment of borderline personality disorder.* New York: Guilford Press.

Lydiard, R. B., & Monnier, J. (2004). Pharmacological treatment. In R. G. Heimberg, C. L. Turk, & D. S. Mennin (Eds.), *Generalized anxiety disorder: Advances in research and practice* (pp. 351–379). New York: Guilford Press.

Ma, S. H., & Teasdale, J. D. (2004). Mindfulness-based cognitive therapy for depression: Replication and exploration of differential relapse prevention effects. *Journal of Consulting and Clinical Psychology, 72*, 31–40.

MacLeod, C., & Hagan, R. (1992). Individual differences in the selective processing of threatening information, and emotional responses to a stressful life event. *Behaviour Research and Therapy, 30*, 151–161.

MacLeod, C., Mathews, A., & Tata, P. (1986). Attentional bias in emotional disorders. *Journal of Abnormal Psychology, 95*, 15–20.

MacLeod, C., Rutherford, E., Campbell, L., Ebsworthy, G., & Holker, L. (2002). Selective attention and emotional vulnerability: Assessing the causal basis of their association through the experimental manipulation of attentional bias. *Journal of Abnormal Psychology, 111*, 107–123.

Mathews, A., & MacLeod, C. (1994). Cognitive approaches to emotion and emotional disorders. *Annual Review of Psychology, 45*, 25–50.

Mathews, A., & MacLeod, C. (2005). Cognitive vulnerability to emotional disorders. *Annual Review of Clinical Psychology, 1*, 197–225.

McEvoy, P. M., & Perini, S. J. (2009). Cognitive behavioral group therapy for social phobia with or without attention training: A controlled trial. *Journal of Anxiety Disorders, 23*, 519–528.

McNally, R. J. (1995). Automaticity and the anxiety disorders. *Behaviour Research and Therapy, 33*, 747–754.

Mulkens, S., Bögels, S. M., de Jong, P. J., & Louwers, J. (2001). Fear of blushing: Effects of task concentration training versus exposure *in vivo* on fear and psychology. *Journal of Anxiety Disorders, 15*, 413–432.

Ochsner, K. N., & Gross, J. J. (2007). The neural architecture of emotion regulation. In J. J. Gross (Ed.), *Handbook of emotion regulation* (pp. 87–109). New York: Guilford Press.

Ochsner, K. N., & Gross, J. J. (2008). Cognitive emotion regulation: Insights from social cognitive and affective neuroscience. *Current Directions in Psychological Science, 17*, 153–158.

Papageorgiou, C., & Wells, A. (1998). Effects of attention training on hypochondriasis: A brief case series. *Psychological Medicine, 28*, 193–200.

Papageorgiou, C., & Wells, A. (2000). Treatment of recurrent major depression with attention training. *Cognitive and Behavioral Practice, 7*, 407–413.

Pashler, H. (1998). *The psychology of attention.* Cambridge, MA: MIT Press.

Pessoa, L. (2008). On the relationship between emotion and cognition. *Nature Reviews Neuroscience, 9,* 148–158.

Pessoa, L., McKenna, M., Gutierrez, E., & Ungerleider, L. (2002). Neural processing of emotional faces requires attention. *Proceeding of the National Academy of Sciences USA, 99,* 11458–11463.

Posner, M. I. (1988). Structures and function of selective attention. In T. Boll & B. K. Bryant (Eds.), *Clinical neuropsychology and brain function: Research, measurement, and practice* (pp. 173–202). Washington, DC: American Psychological Association.

Posner, M. I., Rothbart, M. K., & Sheese, B. E. (2007). Attention genes. *Developmental Science, 10,* 24–29.

Roemer, L., & Orsillo, S. M. (2007). An open trial of an acceptance-based behavior therapy for generalized anxiety disorder. *Behavior Therapy, 38,* 72–85.

Rottenberg, J., Kasch, K. L., Gross, J. J., & Gotlib, I. H. (2002). Sadness and amusement reactivity differentially predict concurrent and prospective functioning in major depressive disorder. *Emotion, 2,* 135–146.

Segal, Z. V., Williams, J. M. G., & Teasdale, J. D. (2002). *Mindfulness-based cognitive therapy for depression: A new approach to preventing relapse.* New York: Guilford Press.

Schmidt, N. B., Richey, J. A., Buckner, J. D., & Timpano, K. R. (2009). Attention training for generalized social anxiety disorder. *Journal of Abnormal Psychology, 118*(1), 5–14.

Shiffrin, R. M., & Schneider, W. (1977). Controlled and automatic human information processing: II. Perceptual learning, automatic attending and a general theory. *Psychological Review, 84,* 127–190.

Siegle, G. J., Ghinassi, F., & Thase, M. E. (2007). Neurobehavioral therapies in the 21st century: Summary of an emerging field and an extended example of cognitive control training for depression. *Cognitive Therapy and Research, 31,* 235–262.

Suslow, T., Schonauer, K., & Arolt, V. (2001). Attention training in the cognitive rehabilitation of schizophrenic patients: A review of efficacy studies. *Acta Psychiatrica Scandinavica, 103,* 15–23.

Teasdale, J. D. (1999). Emotional processing, three modes of mind, and the prevention of relapse in depression. *Behaviour Research and Therapy, 37,* S53–S77.

Teasdale, J. D., Segal, Z. V., Williams, J. M. G., Ridgeway, V. A., Soulsby, J. M., & Lau, M. A. (2000). Prevention of relapse/recurrence in major depression by mindfulness-based cognitive therapy. *Journal of Consulting and Clinical Psychology, 68,* 615–623.

Tugade, M. M., & Fredrickson, B. L. (2004). Resilient individuals use positive emotions to bounce back from negative emotional experiences. *Journal of Personality and Social Psychology, 86,* 320–333.

Valmaggia, L., Bouman, T. K., & Schuurman, L. (2007). Attention training with auditory hallucinations: A case study. *Cognitive and Behavioral Practice, 14,* 127–133.

Wadlinger, H. A., & Isaacowitz, D. M. (2008). Looking happy: The experimental manipulation of a positive visual attention bias. *Emotion, 8,* 121–126.

Weierich, M. R., Treat, T. A., & Hollingworth, A. (2008). Theories and measurement of visual attentional processing in anxiety. *Cognition and Emotion, 22,* 985–1018.

Wells, A. (2000). *Emotional disorders and metacognition: Innovative cognitive therapy.* Chichester, UK: Wiley.

Wells, A., & Mathews, G. (1994). *Attention and emotion: A clinical perspective.* Hove, UK: Erlbaum.

Wells, A., & Matthews, G. (1996). Modeling cognition in emotional disorder: The S-REF model. *Behaviour Research and Therapy, 32,* 867–870.

Wells, A., & Papageorgiou, C. (1998). Social phobia: Effects of external attention on anxiety, negative beliefs, and perspective taking. *Behavior Therapy, 29,* 357–370.

Wells, A., White, J., & Carter, K. E. P. (1997). Attention training: Effects on anxiety and beliefs in panic and social phobia. *Clinical Psychology and Psychotherapy, 4,* 226–232.

Williams, J. M. G., Russell, I., & Russell, D. (2008). Mindfulness-based cognitive therapy: Further issues in current evidence and future research. *Journal of Consulting and Clinical Psychology, 76,* 524–529.

Williams, J. M. G., Watts, F. N., MacLeod, C., & Mathews, A. (1997). *Cognitive psychology and emotional disorders* (2nd ed.). New York: Wiley.

Witkiewitz, K., Marlatt, A. G., & Walker, D. (2005). Mindfulness-based relapse prevention for alcohol and substance use disorders. *Journal of Cognitive Psychotherapy, 19,* 211–228.

Woody, S. R. (1996). Effects of focus of attention on anxiety levels and social performance of individuals with social phobia. *Journal of Abnormal Psychology, 105,* 61–69.

Yantis, S. (1998). Objects, attention and perceptual experience. In R. Wright (Ed.), *Visual attention* (pp. 187–214). New York: Oxford University Press.

CHAPTER 17

• — • — • — •

Working with Emotion and Emotion Regulation in Behavioral Activation Treatment for Depressed Mood

Matthew R. Syzdek, Michael E. Addis, and Christopher R. Martell

In this chapter, we consider the core conceptual and technical aspects of behavioral activation through the lens of emotion regulation. We begin with an overview of the empirical support for behavioral activation and then describe its origins in behavioral analysis and cognitive-behavioral therapy. Next, we discuss the role of emotion in behavioral activation. In particular, we focus on how assessment strategies in behavioral activation facilitate clients' increased awareness of emotion–behavior relationships. Finally, we apply the core treatment components of behavioral activation to problems in emotion regulation using the framework set out by Gross and colleagues (Gross, 1998b, 1999; Gross & Thompson, 2007).

It should be noted that although behavioral activation has been developed primarily as treatment for major depressive disorder (MDD), the treatment techniques and their relationship to emotion regulation processes can be linked conceptually to other disorders. Depressed mood is a common feature of social anxiety disorder, posttraumatic stress disorder (PTSD), generalized anxiety disorder, and dysthymia, as indicated by high comorbidity rates, high correlations among symptoms measures, and loadings on a shared, higher order factor (Brown, Campbell, Lehman, Grisham, & Mancill, 2001; Cox, Clara, & Enns, 2002; Krueger, 1999; Sellbom, Ben-Porath, & Bagby, 2008; Watson, 2005). Behavioral activation, although not a treatment for all aspects of these disorders, may be an important complement to standard treatments by providing a set of skills for managing depressed mood. For example, the skills learned during behavioral activation (e.g., countering avoidance) may reinforce the skills necessary to target avoidance and emotional suppression present in other anxiety and mood disorders. Accordingly, behavioral activation has been applied as a stand-alone treatment for comorbid anxiety and depression, PTSD, eating disorders, smoking cessation, substance abuse, comorbid depression and obesity, and the prevention of mental health disorders in college students (Anderson & Simmons, 2008; Bercaw, 2008; Daughters et al., 2008; Hopko, Lejuez, & Hopko, 2004; Jakupcak et al., 2006; Pagoto et al., 2009; Schneider et al., 2008). In the following section, we describe behavioral activation's roots as a treatment for depression, and later we discuss how behavioral activation can treat depressed mood occurring across different disorders.

The Development of Behavioral Activation

In the late 1960s and early 1970s, the predominant understanding of depression was based on psychodynamic theory, which viewed depression as a type of anger turned inward against the self. Dollard and Miller (1950) had explained many of the psychodynamic notions in behavioral terms, and Wolpe (1958) had developed his psychotherapy by reciprocal inhibition, but these works did not concern depression directly. Wolpe had specified avoidance behavior as characteristic of many neurotic disorders. C. B. Ferster (1973) wrote a behavioral analysis of depression, and around the same time Peter Lewinsohn and colleagues were explaining depression as the result of low levels of response-contingent positive reinforcement or from response-contingent punishment (Lewinsohn, Biglan, & Zeiss, 1976; Lewinsohn & Libet, 1972).

Rather than considering depression to be characterized by internal conflicts as the psychodynamic theorists did, these behavioral researchers considered the impact of person–environment interactions. According to both Ferster and Lewinsohn, behaviors that are antidepressant in nature are not positively reinforced, and this contributes to the development and maintenance of depression. Lewinsohn and colleagues paid particular attention to the limited number of pleasant events in the lives of depressed clients (Lewinsohn & Libet, 1972). Likewise, Ferster (1973) noted that it was actually the absence of behavior, or the inertia, frequently seen in depressed clients that needed to be the target of treatment. These two clinical researchers were the first to suggest that activating depressed clients, increasing engagement in pleasant activities, and combating avoidance behaviors were necessary and sufficient components of treatment.

During this same period, Beck, Rush, Shaw, and Emery (1979) proposed a comprehensive cognitive theory of depression. Rather than seeing negative cognition as merely symptomatic of depression, Beck considered the negative thinking of people with depression as the cause. As Beck's cognitive therapy for depression developed, it included both behavioral activation scheduling as well as methods for restructuring clients' negative beliefs and attitudes (Beck et al., 1979). Beck and colleagues also recognized that it was important to activate people with severe depression, and that this was often the first intervention in a comprehensive cognitive therapy. The behavioral and the cognitive treatments continued to be practiced throughout the next two decades, but cognitive therapy became the more popular approach.

In the early 1990s, Neil Jacobson and colleagues (1996) proposed that it was activation that accounted for positive outcomes in cognitive therapy for depression. They conducted a component analysis of cognitive therapy and found that behavioral activation alone was as efficacious as the full cognitive therapy protocol. The study was limited by the lack of a no-treatment control group, and subsequently a large-scale, randomized controlled trial was conducted comparing behavioral activation, cognitive therapy, paroxetine, and a pill placebo control group (Dimidjian et al., 2006). During the course of this project, behavioral activation was conducted as a stand-alone treatment (Addis & Martell, 2004; Martell, Addis, & Jacobson, 2001), and the results of this trial suggested that behavioral activation was superior to cognitive therapy and as efficacious as antidepressant medication in the acute treatment of MDD (Dimidjian et al., 2006).

A Behavioral Conceptualization of Depression

Consistent with the earlier formulations of Ferster and Lewinsohn, current approaches to behavioral activation consider person–environment interactions to be paramount in the development and maintenance of depression (Martell et al., 2001). In many cases, negative life events trigger depression. In other cases, lifelong stress, coupled with biological–hereditary vulnerabilities, can lead to the development of depression. As Lewinsohn noted, this leads to a decrease in response-contingent positive reinforcement (Lewinsohn, 2001). For vulnerable individuals, a natural reaction to decreases in response-contingent positive reinforcement is to develop the affective symptoms of depression. It, therefore, makes sense that someone feeling blue, lethargic, and anhedonic and losing interest in activities would begin to decrease his or her activities. However, responding to negative affect through inactivity and withdrawal only serves to worsen the client's mood and keep him or her from opportunities for pleasurable experiences that may actually increase response-contingent positive reinforcement. The client's inertia and avoidance behaviors thus become secondary problems in themselves. These are the targets of behavioral activation.

Behavioral activation targets inertia and avoidance in order to help clients engage in life to increase chances that active, antidepressant behavior will be positively reinforced and increased. Behavioral repertoires characterized by escape and avoidance are often maintained via negative reinforcement. A person with depression often feels relief from emotional distress by withdrawing from the world, even though this increases apathy. As the behavioral repertoire of the client narrows, there is less and less that the client feels motivated to do. Without environmental reinforcement for activating and engaging, the client's motivation continues to decline, and there is a vicious cycle of depression leading to inactivity and then to more depression.

In the following sections, we present the interventions comprising behavioral activation that have been used primarily to target decreases in response-contingent positive reinforcement and increases in avoidance. These behavioral processes not only affect the onset and maintenance of depression but also depressed mood more generally. In our discussion of the treatment components, we attend to how behavioral activation can also be conceptualized as a treatment for problems in emotion regulation that contribute to and exacerbate depressed mood. For conceptual clarity, we organize the interventions into six core components: assessment, activation, countering avoidance, attention to experience, and acceptance. We begin by examining how behavioral activation approaches emotions theoretically and in treatment. We also draw connections between current theories of emotion that are consistent with the metaphor of "emotions as data" underlying assessment strategies in behavioral activation. Finally, we conceptualize how the remaining treatment components can remediate deficits in emotion regulation identified by Gross and colleagues (Gross, 1998a, 1999; Gross & Thompson, 2007).

The Word *Emotion* in Behavioral Activation

Historically, behaviorists tried to avoid conceptualizing emotion as an internal state independent of behavior. One might, therefore, expect that a treatment focused on changing behavior would not have much use for the concept of emotion. However, more recent behavioral and philosophical approaches to language emphasize how the meaning of a word is a function of the context in which it is used (Gifford & Hayes, 1999; Rorty, 1982). In behavioral activation, it is possible to use the concept of emotion clinically in the service of the interventions without committing to a particular ontological view of emotion at a scientific or theoretical level.

There are three ways in which the concept of emotion is most commonly used in behavioral activation. First, emotion is not seen as an internal state but as a repertoire of activity; "emotion" becomes "emoting." For example, sadness can be conceptualized as a set of behaviors (e.g., crying, ruminating about unresolved conflicts, withdrawing from social situations) that one engages in while verbally reporting sadness. This conceptualization of emotion avoids mentalistic explanations that locate emotions "inside" the person as an entity of some sort. From this perspective, emotions and the ways one regulates them are one and the same. This is helpful when considering the function of emoting. By conceptualizing the setting, behavior, and consequences of emoting as acts-in-context, therapists can often ascertain the function of clients' emoting.

Another approach to emotion is viewing "emotions as data." This use of the word highlights how emotions are data or information about person–environment relationships. Emotions can tell people whether positive reinforcement or aversive conditioning is maintaining their actions. This use of the word is consistent with the frequent focus on assessment of behavior–environment–mood relationships in behavioral activation.

Emotions can also be thought of as discriminative stimuli. In this way, the experience of negative and positive emotion can cue different behavioral responses. Sadness may be a cue for seeking social support or for social withdrawal depending on a person's learning history. This conceptualization is consistent with models of emotion regulation that view emotions as stimuli themselves that occasion different types of responses. Each of these three metaphorical conceptualizations of emotion has potential clinical utility depending on the particular interventions therapists use with different clients.

We distinguish emotions from moods, where moods are a more general affective experience extending across contexts and time, perhaps several hours, days, weeks, or months (Gross, 1998b). As a goal of treatment, behavioral activation targets depressed mood and not isolated emotional episodes. At the same time, identifying specific emotional episodes can be helpful for clients in learning the association between what they do and how they feel.

Emotions as Data in Assessment

The concept of core affect is conceptually related to the metaphor of emotions as data used in the assessment component of behavioral activation (Russell & Barrett, 1999). Barrett (2006) theorized that core affect underlies all emotional experience. Core affect is defined as "the constant stream of transient alterations in an organism's neurophysiological state that represent its immediate relationship to the flow of changing events" (Barrett, 2006, p. 21). Core affect consists of two components: valence (positive or negative) and arousal (activation/deactivation). It can be thought of as a "neurophysiological barometer" capturing person–environment relationships that measures how positive or aversive the current context is (p. 21). Barrett further theorizes that core affect is a primarily biological process that is present since infancy.

In behavioral activation, assessment strategies direct the clients' attention to their emotional barometer. Clients are taught that their emotions are data that suggest how the current context is affecting them. In particular, the therapist and the client examine how the clients' activities influence their emotional barometer, raising and lowering positive and negative affect. Data gathered from assessment are then used to guide adaptive behavior.

The Process of Assessment

In treatment, assessment is carried out using self-monitoring, symptom inventories, and functional analyses. All of the therapeutic work in behavioral activation is informed by assessment data, and the other treatment components cannot be used effectively without continuous, accurate assessment information. Except for assessing mood, surveys are less frequently used in the assessment process than in some other treatment approaches because it can be difficult to discern the function of a behavior from a survey. Instead, more ideographic methods like self-monitoring and functional analyses are used.

Martell and colleagues (2001) delineate several specific functions for activity monitoring. Early in treatment, activities and mood are tracked so the client can observe how activity and emotion are usually synchronized. Therapists rely on these data when teaching clients how to analyze the function of their own behaviors. It is important for the clinician to assist the client in seeing how emotion fluctuates over a normal day and to identify which activities enhance mood. Mood and activity data are also important information for assessing how restricted the client's behavioral repertoires and mood are.

After the first few sessions, self-monitoring can be used to evaluate how new activities influence mood. In addition, data from self-monitoring can measure progress toward life goals and reveal whether new activities are positively reinforced. Later in treatment, clients are introduced to activity monitoring as a first step during relapse. In this case, self-monitoring can be helpful in diagnosing problematic behavioral patterns that may be exacerbating mood and contributing to relapse. For example, a client previously treated with behavioral activation was experiencing increased stress at work and problems at home. When these events occurred, she tended to stop listening to enjoyable music, started watching more television, and withdrew from friends. Self-monitoring in this situation helped her notice how these activities were negatively affecting her mood, and she adjusted her activities to prevent a relapse.

Symptom inventories such as the Beck Depression Inventory–II (BDI-II) and Beck Anxiety Inventory (BAI) are important metrics for measuring anxiety and depressed mood over a 1- to 2-week period (Beck, Epstein, Brown, & Steer, 1988; Beck, Steer, & Garbin, 1996). Data from these measures indicate how current activities are influencing mood over time. In some cases, data from symptom inventories can reveal interesting discrepancies. For example, some clients will be very active yet find their BDI-II or BAI continuing to increase. These findings may indicate that their active lifestyle is functioning to avoid other aversive feelings and situations rather than to contact potential positive reinforcers. Other clients may be active in activities that, from a topographical perspective, should be mood enhancing but are not functioning this way. This is informative for a different reason, because it may be that current activities are not consistent with life goals. Data from symptom inventories can be a big-picture barometer of person–environment relationships.

The final component of assessment is conducting a functional analysis. Functional analysis is a hallmark of behavioral activation that teaches clients how to identify factors maintaining their mood disturbance. This requires no new data collection but instead involves a careful analysis and interpretation of existing data. Many clients are unaware of the antecedents and consequences of their behaviors. For example, they may sit in front of the television for most of the evening without ever realizing that this has deleterious effects on their mood. By enhancing awareness of the function of different mood-regulating behaviors, clients can then be more deliberate in how they want to approach activities affecting their mood.

The therapist directs clients in using self-monitoring data to assess how specific behaviors influence mood. A functional analysis approaches this task by investigating the antecedents and consequences of a behavior. A clinician may ask several questions, including "What happened before you did this?", "What was going on and how were you feeling?", "What happened after you took that action?", "How were you feeling during and after?" By answering these types of questions and sifting through their assessment data, the client and therapist can discover how different activities are maintaining depressed mood.

Emotion Regulation in Behavioral Activation

Different uses of the word "emotion" in behavioral activation lead to different conceptualizations of the relationship between emotion and emotion regulation. Following from the perspective of emotions as behavior, emotion regulation and emotion are not conceptually distinct. Emoting behavior is a response to environmental stimuli and entails what is traditionally called *emotion* and *emotion regulation*. For instance, thinking about an anxiety-provoking situation and even reappraising the potential threat of the situation can both be parts of "emoting anxiety" rather than a consequence or antecedent of some internal state called *anxiety*. This definition is consistent with assumptions of behavioral theory that locate causal elements in the environment and not in internal entities or states. Consequently, interventions targeting emoting behavior are directed at modifying the environment and not at modifying internal states.

For pragmatic reasons, it can also be helpful to parse emotion and emotion regulation. By viewing emotions as a psychophysiological barometer and simultaneously as a discriminative stimulus, emotion and emotion regulation become separate processes. One advantage of this approach is its ability to account for the role of private events like psychophysiological arousal and activation in behavior. This approach also allows emotion regulation to be broken down further into the antecedent-focused and response-focused strategies, consistent with those proposed by Gross (1998b).

Gross and Thompson (2007) define emotion regulation as a process comprising different strategies used by individuals to alter the incidence and intensity of an emotion. In this model, emotions emerge along a continuum, including situation, attention, appraisal, and response (Gross, 1998b; Gross & Thompson, 2007). Emotion regulation strategies are on a parallel continuum and are classified according to their location on the emotion generation continuum (Gross, 1998b). Emotion regulation strategies consist of situation selection, situation modification, attentional deployment, cognitive change, and response modulation. Along the emotion regulation continuum are several points of potential intervention for behavioral activation. In the following sections, we describe each of the emotion regulation strategies, identify overlapping concepts shared by emotion regulation and behavioral theory, and detail the associated core treatment components.

Situation Selection

Gross (1998b) contends that altering situations can be a potent form of emotion regulation. Situations are assumed to set the stage for emotions, and some situations are associated with more desirable emotions while other situations bring about less desirable emotions. Because of this, people approach and avoid situations based on their history of experiences with situations and emotions. Gross argues that the cost and benefits of situation selection may differ over time. In some cases, selecting a situation can bring about a desirable change in emotions in the short term yet be maladaptive over time.

This form of maladaptive situation selection identified by Gross can be thought of as a negative reinforcement contingency. Behavioral theory explains that through the process of negative reinforcement, avoidant behavior tends to relieve negative affect momentarily. Such behavior then becomes more likely in the future. A person with depressed mood may thus begin to stay at home to avoid a pile of work in the office and feelings of guilt and incompetence. In the short term, the feelings of guilt and incompetence will likely subside. Over time, though, avoidance can lead to a narrowed repertoire, reduced contact with positive experiences, and increased negative consequences, as in the case of avoiding work, which may lead to job loss, social isolation, and more depressed mood. Social withdrawal can also be conceptualized as another form of maladaptive situation selection that functions to regulate sadness and to avoid interpersonal rejection in the short term (Campbell-Sills & Barlow, 2007). As these examples suggest, it can be more adaptive in the long term to approach some aversive situations and feelings rather than to avoid them.

Behavioral activation connects participants to situations that produce more adaptive behaviors that will eventually be positively reinforced by the environment. Skinner (1971) noted that behavior maintained by positive reinforcers rather than negative reinforcers is associated with people feeling free and in control. The opposite is true for negative reinforcement and punishment, which are associated with feeling controlled and helpless. Thus, it is more desirable for situation selection to occur by a history of receiving reward, feeling pleasure, and reaching meaningful goals than by a vicious cycle of avoiding punishment and negative affect.

Clinically, this theory suggests that the clinician should direct effort toward altering the client's context to give rise to adaptive situation selection by means of positive reinforcement. This can be accomplished by placing the client in contact with positive reinforcing contexts or by the therapist verbally reinforcing the client until the client habituates to the situation or until natural reinforcers begin to maintain the behavior (e.g., accomplishing work in the office, feeling mastery, and receiving praise from supervisors).

Therapists can foster adaptive situation selection by implementing three interventions in behavioral activation. First, the assessment process for clients elucidates how situation and emotion are inextricably linked. General trends in emotion can be observed as well as times of the day and problematic situations associated with negative affect. On the basis of this information, therapists and clients will isolate problem areas for closer examination. It is possible that assessment alone may even be beneficial for clients, because the ability to differentiate emotions is associated with better negative emotion regulation (Barrett, Gross, Christensen & Benvenuto, 2001).

Second, behavioral activation teaches clients how to analyze the function of their situation selection and identify avoidant behavior. TRAP is a useful acronym that therapists use to summarize the three steps leading to avoidance. Triggers are internal or external events of emotional significance such as losing a job, a colleague's interpersonal slight, or thinking of past failures. Responses are emotional experiences following a triggering event. The specific emotional response (e.g., feeling anxious, sad, lonely) depends on the type of trigger. Avoidance Patterns are functionally related sets of behaviors that alleviate an aversive emotional experience in the short term while often maintaining the aversive emotional experience in the long term. Using the TRAP acronym, therapist assist clients in identifying avoidance patterns and in recognizing the short-term and long-term consequences of the situation selection.

Therapists pay particular attention to how a client's activities influence different types of consequences. It is important to note that emotional consequences and goal-oriented consequences of a behavior (e.g., mending a broken relationship, finding employment) may not always agree. For example, when a client avoids a difficult situation, he or she may feel some positive affect while, at the same time, it further displaces the client from his or her goals. In contrast, engaging in an uncomfortable situation may do the inverse, increasing short-term negative affect while facilitating long-term goal achievement. In cases similar to the latter situation, the therapist may need to revisit the treatment rationale with the client in order to motivate him or her to select situations previously avoided. The treatment rationale can accomplish this by laying out how contingencies maintain the client's behavior, by providing an alternate pathway for overcoming the immediate punishment of the aversive situation, and by setting up more distal rewards.

The third strategy for enhancing adaptive situation selection is activity scheduling. Using the findings from assessment, clients will begin scheduling activities into their week and monitoring the emotional and goal consequences of their situation selections. The clients will then begin to adjust their routine to include activities that function to bring them closer to their goals and, in the long term, to reduce negative affect and increase positive affect.

Situation Modification and Attentional Deployment

The second point on the continuum of emotion regulation is situation modification. Although situations may set the stage for emotions, situations themselves are mutable and thus are the associated emotions. Gross (1998b) posits that people can adaptively or maladaptively modify their environment with diverging effects on their emotions.

For instance, Campbell-Sills and Barlow (2007) construe safety signals in anxiety-provoking situations, such as the use of items like medication, cell phones, and food, as maladaptive situation modification when such safety signals function to dampen anxiety (see also Corcoran, Farb, Anderson, & Segal, Chapter 14, this volume). Safety signals are argued to be maladaptive in the long term because they interfere with habituation and maintain fear of the situation. In cases more indicative of depression, a person may be in an antidepressive context and yet not actually be engaging in the situation and reaping the benefits of the potentially mood-enhancing situation.

Gross (1998b) differentiates situation modification from attentional deployment, referring to the latter as attempts at modifying internal experiences and to the former as direct attempts to modify the external environment. This discrepancy arises from the assumption that mechanisms causing behavior are internal processes such as attention and cognition. From a behavioral perspective, there is little difference between attentional deployment and situation modification. Both attentional deployment and situation modification characterize how actions in a situation influence the generation of emotion.

An implicit consensus has emerged across theories of emotion and psychopathology concluding that rumination consists of multiple maladaptive processes leading to considerable deleterious mood and anxiety sequelae. From a behavioral perspective, rumination is self-focused attention that takes the form of recalling past failures and memories or of worry related to anticipated problems and events. The lack of effectiveness and progress toward goals differentiates rumination from problem solving (Lyubomirsky & Nolen-Hoeksema, 1995; Watkins & Baracaia, 2002). Nolen-Hoeskama and colleagues built a program of psychopathology research investigating rumination (Nolen-Hoeksema, Wisco, & Lyubomirsky, 2008). Thus far, a large body of correlational and experimental work links rumination to increased risk for negative affect, depressed mood, depression onset, relapse following positive treatment outcomes, and poor treatment response (Lyubomirsky, Caldwell, & Nolen-Hoeksema, 1998; Moberly & Watkins, 2008; Nolen-Hoeksema & Morrow, 1993). As with avoidance, rumination can be relatively insidious and intractable. Rumination can also negate the positively reinforcing function of activities. In interpersonal interactions, rumination interrupts active social exchanges, and in other activities, it spawns negative feelings that may overshadow a positively reinforcing context. These examples illustrate how rumination occurs in context, not only in a person's mind.

As a consequence of viewing behaviors in context, the interventions for maladaptive situation modification and attentional deployment differ very little. Alternative adaptive behavioral responses are fostered to replace prior behaviors that intensified negative affect and reduced positive affect. Assessment data are used to identify problematic situations. In session, the therapist and the client can analyze the function of the client's behaviors and generate more adaptive responses to situations. These new responses can be included in the activity schedule if the situation occurs periodically or can be role-played if the situation is intermittent in nature.

Behavioral activation also draws on more basic behavioral interventions that modify situations to produce the greatest likelihood of success. When an adaptive action is initially too complex and difficult for a client, the therapist can disassemble the activity into manageable tasks. Graded task assignments are therapeutic techniques that teach clients how to achieve complex and formidable goals one step at a time. Similar to exposure hierarchies used in anxiety treatments, long-term goals are operationalized into concrete activities that help achieve the larger the goal. These activities are then rated for difficulty and organized hierarchically. As treatment progresses, activities are selected with increasing difficulty. Recurring activities can be included each week as an activity goal until the client has achieved the goal several weeks in a row and appears to have successfully integrated the behavior into his or her repertoire. More difficult or intimidating tasks may require verbal rehearsals or role-playing. A therapist may ask a client to imagine the activity, including the steps involved and potential barriers to completing the task. More challenging tasks, or ones that involve interpersonal interactions, may necessitate role-playing the situation. Here the therapist can reinforce effective interpersonal behavior, give feedback to a client about less effective behavior, and offer opportunities for the client to try different approaches.

Attention to Experience

Attention to experience is the second core treatment component in behavioral activation. This set of interventions interrupts maladaptive attentional deployment and facilitates adaptive situation modification. Often ruminative thinking patterns serve an escape or avoidance function that can exacerbate situations and mood. Attention to experience exercises counter passive rumination by teaching clients how to fully engage in activities. Such exercises are akin to mindfulness techniques used in a number of contemporary behavioral therapies. Mindfulness originated in Eastern traditions and was more recently incorporated into several different psychotherapy approaches (see Hayes, Follette, & Linehan, 2004). Attention to experience provides a strategy for clients to engage in lived experience rather than go through the motions while ruminating about distress (Martell et al., 2001).

Before attention to experience work can begin, a functional analysis is usually carried out to identify contexts where rumination occurs and what its consequences are. Once clients and their therapist have come to a consensus about the occurrence and consequences of rumination, a simple rule is introduced to aid in identifying rumination when it is occurring. The rule states "If you find yourself thinking about a particular topic over and over, continue do what you are doing and see if you have made progress in 2 minutes" (Addis & Martell, 2004). If clients do this and answer "No," they are encouraged to tell themselves, "You're ruminating." For some situations, identification alone is sufficient to redirect attention to the present moment. For other situations, the cycle of ruminative thoughts can be dislodged by engaging in the current context. There are several different ways to do this. For interpersonal contexts, engagement can involve attending to what the other person is saying, wearing, and doing. In other contexts, clients are taught to attend to the physical environment, including sights, sounds, smells, tastes and so on. It is usually necessary to assign a specific activity as homework and discuss different behaviors for the clients to do to engage in the present moment.

Cognitive Change

The fourth point on the continuum of emotion regulation is cognitive change. Considerable empirical and theoretical work has investigated the role of appraisal in emotion regulation (Gross & Thompson, 2007; John & Gross, 2004). The assumption underlying this research is that situations do not directly influence emotion; instead, cognitive processes mediate the pathway between situation and emotion (Gross, 1998b). Researchers cite empirical work indicating that positively reappraising negative situations is associated with lower levels of negative affect (Gross, 1998a). However, it could also be the case that positive reappraisal is an outcome of emotion regulation. In other words, cognitive appraisals may be a parallel process to behavioral and emotional responses to a situation but not the cause of the behavior or emotional response.

Consistent with this explanation, treatment outcome research has questioned the necessity of targeting cognitive processes in treatments for depression and anxiety (Dimidjian et al., 2006; Jacobson et al., 1996). As discussed earlier, Jacobson and colleagues (1996) dismantled cognitive-behavior therapy into cognitive and behavioral components. The treatments including cognitive components were found to be no more effective than behavioral activation, which proscribed interventions targeting the content of people's cognitions. Of particular interest to this discussion was the finding that attributional style and explanatory flexibility, both hypothesized cognitive mediators, were affected by behavioral activation (Fresco, Schumm, & Dobson, 2007; Jacobson et al., 1996). Specifically, posttreatment scores indicated that participants viewed the causes to their problems less pessimistically and as more context specific.

Consequently, behavioral activation does not intervene at the point of cognitive appraisal to alter the content of thinking. Rather, a therapist may decide to focus on the process and function of a client's thinking (e.g., focusing on rumination as discussed previously). Thinking behavior like worry and rumination can serve people very poorly if it prevents them from engaging in situations and progressing toward their goals. Behavioral activation simply modifies maladaptive thinking behavior rather than maladaptive appraisals of situations. In general, the question as to the efficacy of these behavioral interventions in promoting adaptive emotion regulation, particularly in comparison to cognitive interventions, can best be answered empirically.

Response Modulation

Until now, we have discussed regulatory processes occurring prior to emotion generation. In contrast, response modulation refers to processes that regulate behavioral, physiological, and experiential components of emotion after an emotion is generated (Gross & Thompson, 2007). Research indicates that how a person responds to an emotion produces different emotional consequences. For instance, it has widely been demonstrated that expressing an emotion is associated with a small increase in the self-reported experience of an emotion (Izard, 1990; Matsumoto, 1987).

Researchers have also investigated the effects of suppressing emotions. Deliberate attempts to mask emotional experience have been shown to reduce positive affect, to have mixed effects on negative affect, and to increase sympathetic activation (Campbell-Sills, Barlow, Brown, & Hofmann, 2006b; Gross, 1998a; Gross & Levenson, 1997). Additionally, both mood and anxiety disorders are associated with increased use of emotional suppression (Campbell-Sills, Barlow, Brown, & Hofmann, 2006a). Kring and Werner (2004) posit that deficits in response modulation maintain negative affect and may function as a diathesis for depression.

A response to an emotion not only modulates the current emotional experience but also shapes future emotional experiences (Gross & Thompson, 2007). Behavioral conceptualizations of response modulation focus on the interrelatedness and cyclical nature of response modulation and emotional experience. For example, avoiding an emotional experience not only reinforces the avoidant behavior in the future but also increases the likelihood that the emotion will occur again in the presence of the stimulus. With regard to depression and anxiety, it is plausible that pathological levels of avoidant behavior and emotional suppression are essentially the same process at different levels of analysis.

The behavioral approaches to emotion discussed earlier can be applied to explain the interconnectedness of response modulation and emotion. An aversive situation, or an aversive stimulus more globally, can set in motion a constellation of experiential, physiological, and behavioral responses that function to mitigate the aversive stimulus. This process is labeled "suppression" when emotions are monitored and "avoidance" when behaviors are monitored. Consequently, adaptive changes made in emotional responses will not only benefit current emotional experiences but also the next cycle of emotion and emotion regulation.

Three core components of behavioral activation target the maladaptive use of response modulation. First, behavioral activation coaches clients to increase engagement in their lives through activation strategies. Second, interventions aimed at countering avoidance are included to reduce negative affect and consist of generating alternative forms of coping with negative emotions. Third, behavioral activation fosters acceptance of emotions to facilitate goal-directed action.

Activation

It has been suggested that activation alone is the active ingredient of behavioral activation (Lejuez, Hopko, LePage, Hopko, & McNeil, 2001). Low energy, low levels of positive affect, and diminished response to positive experiences are primary symptoms and perpetuators of depression (Kring & Werner, 2004; Sloan, Strauss, & Wisner, 2001). Behavioral activation teaches clients how to respond differently to depressed mood and how to make progress in their life in spite of feeling lethargic and helpless. From an emotion regulation perspective, activation strategies function to generate alternative, active responses to depressed mood to replace maladaptive, sedentary responses that exacerbate mood. These active responses interrupt depressed mood by introducing experiences that increase positive affect.

Obviously, activation is a tall task to ask of a person who is feeling down and low in energy. The role of a therapist in behavioral activation is to coach a client through the process of reengaging in their life. Good coaching involves anticipating obstacles, enhancing motivation, and providing helpful feedback and advice. Activation is not an end in itself, nor are pleasurable activities. Instead, activation is a means to living a more fulfilling life, guided by one's goals and not by deprivation. Activation, in its ideal form, is also not motivated by prizes and rewards or avoidance of other more aversive situations. Therapists assist clients in selecting activities that potentially could be positively reinforced by the environment. Self-monitoring data are good indicators of what activities have a history of being mood enhancing and the potential to be positively reinforced.

Behavioral activation uses several therapeutic techniques to motivate the client and increase the likelihood of sustained activation. During each session, the therapist and client collaborate in selecting and scheduling activities for the client to complete between sessions. The therapist usually frames these activity goals as a means both to reengage in life and to empirically establish which activities enhance mood. Akin to acceptance and commitment therapy (Hayes, Strosahl, & Wilson, 1999), the client makes a commitment to complete the activity. Depending on the level of difficulty and prior successes, the client can commit by simply listing a day and time to complete the activity on the activity-monitoring sheet or by making a verbal commitment to the therapist, friends, or family members. To increase motivation, it is essential that the therapist present scheduled activities as commitments. In a meta-analysis, activity scheduling alone evidenced a large effect on depression symptoms and did not differ significantly from cognitive therapy (Cuijpers, van Straten, & Warmerdam, 2007).

When sending a client off with activity experiments, several skills can be useful in combating obstacles like feeling overwhelmed, low energy, depressed mood, and "good intentions but poor follow-through." Graded task assignments discussed earlier can be helpful not only in modifying responses to situations but also in increasing active responses to depressed mood. A hierarchy can be created with activities differing in the amount of activation required to complete them, and each week the client is assigned a new, more difficult task. In some cases, feeling down and lethargic can preclude a client from even starting the first task on the hierarchy. "Doing the next best thing" is a rule taught in behavioral activation, stating "When you feel like you cannot do a task, just commit to doing the very first part of it." Consider an example of a client who struggled to activate and complete school homework. To counter the feelings of lethargy, she would set up her work space as the next best thing to completing her homework. This slight shift in mood following minimal activation may provide sufficient motivation to take further steps toward completing the larger task.

The acronym ACTION used in behavioral activation integrates findings from functional analyses and activation strategies: Assessing whether the behavior is approach or avoidance, Choosing to either activate or avoid, Trying the new behavior, Integrating the behavior into a routine, Observing the consequences of the behavior, and Never giving up. The "I" and the "N" steps are the most difficult for many clients. By tracking several occurrences of a behavior, though, the therapist and client can more accurately infer the function of the behavior and determine whether it is currently adaptive in their present context.

Countering Avoidance

Behavioral activation teaches clients how to counter avoidant responses to emotions and situations and regain control of their lives. Countering avoidance is a particularly difficult task that involves breaking entrenched patterns of behavior, depriving oneself of immediate relief from aversive stimuli, and exposing oneself to uncomfortable thoughts, feelings, and experiences. Strategies are used to connect clients with more distal, positively reinforcing contingencies and to disconnect them from more proximal, negative reinforcing contingencies. These contingencies are usually first identified while reviewing self-monitoring and completing functional analyses. Careful functional analyses are critical to treatment outcomes because they may reveal behaviors associated with pleasure that still function, in an insidious way, to avoid more aversive feeling and situations.

TRAC is the second acronym used for avoidance work following the identification of avoidance patterns using the acronym TRAP, discussed earlier. When in the presence of a **T**riggering event and the corresponding emotional **R**esponse, clients are taught to break the avoidance cycle with **A**lternative **C**oping. In short, therapist use the phrase "Get out of the TRAP, and get back on TRAC(K)" (Martell et al., 2001, p. 102). Alternative coping is "activation" applied to avoidance patterns. Naturally, the therapist can draw upon activation strategies such as activity scheduling, graded task assignments, role-plays, and so on, as tools for building active coping repertoires. The therapist and client apply the TRAC acronym to current situations to teach alternative forms of modulating emotions. The transition from TRAP to TRAC is a shift from coping to avoid negative emotions (e.g., not going to the gym because of fear of what others will think) to pursuing the experience of pleasure, mastery, and meaning in one's life.

Acceptance

Acceptance interventions are directed at maladaptive forms of response modulation. Acceptance is a fundamental shift in response modulation away from many people's natural inclination to directly dampen their experience of aversive emotions and toward the lived experiencing of their emotions. It can also been seen as a shift away from investing energy into fighting one's own psychophysiological barometer, which is a battle against one's own body, toward investing energy in goal-directed action. This can happen once emotions are no longer cues for emotional suppression and avoidance. Instead, when individuals are more accepting of their aversive emotions, they can take steps in goal-driven activity that are independent of their emotions.

A stance of acceptance may seem counterintuitive when, as a psychological treatment for depressed mood, feeling better is a desirable outcome. Behavioral activation views bad feelings as part and parcel of life and not as causes of depressed behavior or things to be directly altered. Instead, the therapist speaks of feelings as signs of depressed behavior. In fact, feelings are considered helpful cues that something in the context is either positively reinforcing or aversive. At first glance, a positive treatment outcome of feeling better appears to contradict the notion of acceptance. However, this confuses long term goals and mechanisms of change. In the long term, therapists want clients to feel better. This is measured by active pursuit of goals and fewer depression and anxiety symptoms. However, this is accomplished by acceptance of emotion. Acceptance is conceptualized as engagement in goal-driven behavior despite one's emotional state. As treatment progresses, clients shift from mood dependency to mood independence, where, at the end of treatment, negative emotions and moods are no longer cues for depressed and anxious behavior.

Acting from the "outside in" is an easy-to-understand way to describe acceptance (Martell et al., 2001). Clients are taught that moods on the "inside" are best affected by engaging in meaningful activity on the "outside." "If only I had more motivation or felt better, I would do . . . " is a phrase endemic to depressed mood that captures mood dependency. When clients attribute their inactivity to lack of motivation or depressed mood, the therapist can draw on data from a functional analysis that contradicts this statement or can invite the clients to experiment with mood-independent behavior as homework. Using verbal rehearsals, the clients walk through alternative responses to feelings of depression or anxiety that are consistent with their goals. This may entail engaging in behaviors that are not mood enhancing (e.g., cleaning the house) but are consistent with goals (e.g., selling a house). If acceptance behaviors are successively reinforced by the environment, clients will learn how to change behavior without changing mood.

Future Directions

Behavioral activation evolved from programs of research applying principles of radical behaviorism to the treatment of depression. Consequently, many of the conceptual links between behavioral activation and emotion regulation described in this chapter are best viewed as hypotheses in need of empirical evaluation. Foremost is our application of behavioral activation to depressed mood present in different disorders. Although there is a nascent body of literature investigating the effects of behavioral activation on different disorders, this area of research is in its infancy (Anderson & Simmons, 2008; Bercaw, 2008; Daughters et al., 2008; Hopko et al., 2004; Jakupcak et al., 2006; Pagoto et al., 2009; Schneider et al., 2008). More research is needed to build on the present body of pilot studies examining behavioral activation as a treatment for individual and comorbid disorders. This research can use a truly transdiagnostic approach that examines the effectiveness of behavioral activation in treating depressed mood occurring across disorders.

Future research grounded in an emotion regulation framework may shed light on processes occurring in behavioral activation. There are several possible mechanisms of change in behavioral activation (e.g., increased response-contingent behavior, reduced social withdrawal); however, researchers have not explicitly examined emotion regulation processes as potential mechanisms of change. In addition, using concepts from emotion regulation research provides a common language for clinical researchers to compare and contrast mechanisms of change across treatments. Different treatments may affect different emotion regulation strategies, or different treatments could affect the same emotion regulation strategies using distinct interventions.

At the same time, emotion regulation research can benefit from the contextual perspective underlying behavioral activation. By investigating emotions and emotion regulation in context, researchers can better understand the complexity of emotional phenomena without parsing the emotion generation and regulation process into mechanisms. A more functional approach to emotion will focus the field on aspects of emotion that can be controlled in the environment and that are amenable to intervention.

Summary

In this chapter, we conceptualized behavioral activation as a treatment for problems in emotion regulation. We conceptualized emotions as data about person–environment interactions and as discriminative stimuli that cue particular behavior–environment relationships. We then illustrated how each of the treatment components of behavioral activation can shape more adaptive emotion regulation. Finally, we highlighted future avenues of investigation that can synthesize theory, methodology, and technology from behavioral activation and basic emotion research to answer critical questions confronting the field. Because theory on both emotion regulation and behavioral activation rests on foundations of strong empirical finding, an integration of these fields can be a catalyst for innovation in understanding and treating psychopathology.

References

Addis, M. E., & Martell, C. R. (2004). *Overcoming depression one step at a time: The new behavioral activation approach to getting your life back.* Oakland, CA: New Harbinger.

Anderson, D. A., & Simmons, A. M. (2008). A pilot study of a functional contextual treatment for bulimia nervosa. *Cognitive and Behavioral Practice, 15,* 172–178.

Barrett, L. F. (2006). Are emotions natural kinds? *Perspectives on Psychological Science, 1*(1), 28–58.

Barrett, L. F., Gross, J., Christensen, T. C., & Benvenuto, M. (2001). Knowing what you're feeling and knowing what to do about it: Mapping the relation between emotion differentiation and emotion regulation. *Cognition and Emotion, 15*(6), 713–724.

Beck, A. T., Epstein, N., Brown, G., & Steer, R. A. (1988). An inventory for measuring clinical anxiety: Psychometric properties. *Journal of Consulting and Clinical Psychology, 56*(6), 893–897.

Beck, A. T., Rush, A. J., Shaw, B. F., & Emery, G. (1979). *Cognitive therapy of depression.* New York: Guilford Press.

Beck, A. T., Steer, R. A., & Garbin, M. G. (1996). *Manual for the Beck Depression Inventory–II.* San Antonio, TX: Psychological Corporation.

Bercaw, E. L. (2008). A behavioral activation approach to smoking cessation for depressed mothers at veterans' affairs medical centers. *Dissertation Abstracts International, 68*(8-B), 55–57.

Brown, T. A., Campbell, L. A., Lehman, C. L., Grisham, J. R., & Mancill, R. B. (2001). Current and lifetime comorbidity of the DSM-IV anxiety and mood disorders in a large clinical sample. *Journal of Abnormal Psychology, 110*(4), 585–599.

Campbell-Sills, L., & Barlow, D. H. (2007). Incorporating emotion regulation into conceptualizations and treatments of anxiety and mood disorders. In J. J. Gross (Ed.), *Handbook of emotion regulation* (pp. 542–559). New York: Guilford Press.

Campbell-Sills, L., Barlow, D. H., Brown, T. A., & Hofmann, S. G. (2006a). Acceptability and suppression of negative emotion in anxiety and mood disorders. *Emotion, 6*(4), 587–595.

Campbell-Sills, L., Barlow, D. H., Brown, T. A., & Hofmann, S. G. (2006b). Effects of suppression and acceptance on emotional responses of individuals with anxiety and mood disorders. *Behaviour Research and Therapy, 44*(9), 1251–1263.

Cox, B. J., Clara, I. P., & Enns, M. W. (2002). Posttraumatic stress disorder and the structure of common mental disorders. *Depression and Anxiety, 15*(4), 168–171.

Cuijpers, P., van Straten, A., & Warmerdam, L. (2007). Behavioral activation treatments of depression: A meta-analysis. *Clinical Psychology Review, 27*(3), 318–326.

Daughters, S. B., Braun, A. R., Sargeant, M. N., Reynolds, E. R., Hopko, D., Blanco, C., et al. (2008). Effectiveness of a brief behavioral treatment for inner-city illicit drug users with elevated depressive symptoms: The life enhancement treatment for substance use (LETS Act!). *Journal of Clinical Psychiatry, 69*(1), 122–129.

Dimidjian, S., Hollon, S. D., Dobson, K. S., Schmaling, K. B., Kohlenberg, R. J., Addis, M. E., et al. (2006). Randomized trial of behavioral activation, cognitive therapy, and antidepressant medication in the acute treatment of adults with major depression. *Journal of Consulting and Clinical Psychology, 74*(4), 658–670.

Dollard, J., & Miller, N. (1950). *Personality and psychotherapy.* New York: McGraw-Hill.

Ferster, C. B. (1973). A functional analysis of depression. *American Psychologist, 28*, 857–870.

Fresco, D. M., Schumm, J. A., & Dobson, K. S. (2007). *Explanatory flexibility and explanatory style: Modality-specific mechanisms of change when comparing behavioral activation with and without cognitive interventions.* Manuscript under review.

Gifford, E. V., & Hayes, S. C. (1999). Functional contextualism: A pragmatic philosophy for behavioral science. In W. O'Donohue & R. Kitchener (Eds.), *Handbook of behaviorism* (pp. 285–327). San Diego, CA: Academic Press.

Gross, J. J. (1998a). Antecedent- and response-focused emotion regulation: Divergent consequences for experience, expression, and physiology. *Journal of Personality and Social Psychology, 74*(1), 224–237.

Gross, J. J. (1998b). The emerging field of emotion regulation: An integrative review. *Review of General Psychology, 2*(3), 271–299.

Gross, J. J. (1999). Emotion regulation: Past, present, future. *Cognition and Emotion, 13*(5), 551–573.

Gross, J.J., & Levenson, R. (1997). Hiding feelings: The acute effects of inhibiting negative and positive emotions. *Journal of Abnormal Psychology, 106*(1), 95–103.

Gross, J. J., & Thompson, R. A. (2007). Emotion regulation: Conceptual foundations. In J. J. Gross (Ed.), *Handbook of emotion regulation* (pp. 3–24). New York: Guilford Press.

Hayes, S. C., Follette, V. M., & Linehan, M. M. (2004). *Mindfulness and acceptance: Expanding the cognitive-behavioral tradition.* New York: Guilford Press.

Hayes, S. C., Strosahl, K. D., & Wilson, K. G. (1999). *Acceptance and commitment therapy: An experiential approach to behavior change.* New York: Guilford Press.

Hopko, D. R., Lejuez, C. W., & Hopko, S. D. (2004). Behavioral activation as an intervention for coexistent depressive and anxiety symptoms. *Clinical Case Studies, 3*(1), 37–48.

Izard, C. E. (1990). Facial expressions and the regulation of emotions. *Journal of Personality and Social Psychology, 58,* 487–498.

Jacobson, N. S., Dobson, K. S., Truax, P. A., Addis, M. E., Koerner, K., Gollan, J. K., et al. (1996). A component analysis of cognitive-behavioral treatment for depression. *Journal of Consulting and Clinical Psychology, 64*(2), 295–304.

Jakupcak, M., Roberts, L. J., Martell, C., Mulick, P., Michael, S., Reed, R., et al. (2006). A pilot study of behavioral activation for veterans with posttraumatic stress disorder. *Journal of Traumatic Stress, 19*(3), 387–391.

John, O. P., & Gross, J. (2004). Healthy and unhealthy emotion regulation: Personality processes, individual differences, and life span development *Journal of Personality, 72*(6), 1301–1334.

Kring, A. M., & Werner, K. H. (2004). Emotion regulation and psychopathology. In P. Philippot & R. S. Feldman (Eds.), *The regulation of emotion* (pp. 359–385). Mahwah, NJ: Erlbaum.

Krueger, R. F. (1999). The structure of common mental disorders. *Archives of General Psychiatry, 56*(10), 921–926.

Lejuez, C. W., Hopko, D. R., LePage, J. P., Hopko, S. D., & McNeil, D. W. (2001). A brief behavioral activation treatment for depression. *Cognitive and Behavioral Practice, 8*(2), 164–175.

Lewinsohn, P. M. (2001). Lewinsohn's model of depression. In W. E. Craighead & C. B. Nemeroff (Eds.), *The Corsini encyclopedia of psychology and behavioral science* (3rd ed., pp. 442–444). New York: Wiley.

Lewinsohn, P. M., Biglan, A., & Zeiss, A. S. (1976). Behavioral treatment of depression. In P. O. Davidson (Ed.), *The behavioral management of anxiety, depression, and pain* (pp. 91–146). New York: Brunner/Mazel.

Lewinsohn, P. M., & Libet, J. (1972). Pleasant events, activity schedules, and depressions. *Journal of Abnormal Psychology, 79*(3), 291–295.

Lyubomirsky, S., Caldwell, N. D., & Nolen-Hoeksema, S. (1998). Effects of ruminative and distracting responses to depressed mood on retrieval of autobiographical memories. *Journal of Personality and Social Psychology, 75*(1), 166–177.

Lyubomirsky, S., & Nolen-Hoeksema, S. (1995). Effects of self-focused rumination on negative thinking and interpersonal problem solving. *Journal of Personality and Social Psychology, 69*(1), 176–190.

Martell, C. R., Addis, M. E., & Jacobson, N. S. (2001). *Depression in context: Strategies for guided action.* New York: Norton.

Matsumoto, D. (1987). The role of facial response in experience of emotion: More methodological problems and a meta-analysis. *Journal of Personality and Social Psychology, 52,* 769–774.

Moberly, N. J., & Watkins, E. R. (2008). Ruminative self-focus and negative affect: An experience sampling study. *Journal of Abnormal Psychology, 117*(2), 314–323.

Nolen-Hoeksema, S., & Morrow, J. (1993). Effects of rumination and distraction on naturally occurring depressed mood. *Cognition and Emotion, 7*(6), 561–570.

Nolen-Hoeksema, S., Wisco, B. E., & Lyubomirsky, S. (2008). Rethinking rumination. *Perspectives on Psychological Science, 3*(5), 402–426.

Pagoto, S. L., Bodenlos, J., Schneider, K., Olendzki, B., Spates, C. R., & Ma, Y. (2009). Initial investigation of behavioral activation treatment for co-morbid major depressive disorder and obesity. *Psychotherapy: Theory, Research, Practice, Training, 45*(3), 410–415.

Rorty, R. (1982). *Consequences of pragmatism.* Minneapolis: University of Minnesota Press.

Russell, J. A., & Barrett, L. F. (1999). Core affect, prototypical emotional episodes, and other things called emotion: Dissecting the elephant. *Journal of Personality and Social Psychology, 76*(5), 805–819.

Schneider, K. L., Bodenlos, J. S., Ma, Y., Olendzki, B., Oleski, J., Merriam, P., et al. (2008). Design and methods for a randomized clinical trial treating co-morbid obesity and major depressive disorder. *BMC Psychiatry, 8,* 77.

Sellbom, M., Ben-Porath, Y. S., & Bagby, R. M. (2008). On the hierarchical structure of mood and anxiety disorders: Confirmatory evidence and elaboration of a model of temperament markers. *Journal of Abnormal Psychology, 117*(3), 576–590.

Skinner, B. F. (1971). *Beyond freedom and dignity.* New York: Knopf.

Sloan, D. M., Strauss, M. E., & Wisner, K. L. (2001). Diminished response to pleasant stimuli by depressed women. *Journal of Abnormal Psychology, 110*(3), 488–493.

Watkins, E., & Baracaia, S. (2002). Rumination and social problem-solving in depression. *Behaviour Research and Therapy, 40*(10), 1179–1189.

Watson, D. (2005). Rethinking the mood and anxiety disorders: A quantitative hierarchical model for DSM-V. *Journal of Abnormal Psychology, 114*(4), 522–536.

Wolpe, J. (1958). *Psychotherapy by reciprocal inhibition.* Stanford, CA: Stanford University Press.

CHAPTER 18

• ——— • ——— • ——— •

Toward an Affective Science
of Insomnia Treatments

**Allison G. Harvey, Eleanor McGlinchey,
and June Gruber**

In Chapter 11 in this volume van der Helm and Walker present compelling evidence that a critical function of sleep in humans is the regulation of emotion and that sleep loss has serious costs for next-day emotional functioning. This evidence raises the intriguing possibility that by simply improving sleep the world would be a more emotionally regulated place!

The goal of this chapter is to consider how to apply advances in affective science to the treatment of insomnia. Given that there is considerable room for improvement in current treatment approaches for insomnia, we suggest that the application of methods and theory relating to affect will be an important propeller for the development of the next wave of theories of, and novel treatments for, insomnia.

Definitions

In this chapter we use the term *emotion* to refer to a *brief* response to specific encounters with salient environmental events that includes coordinated changes in subjective experience, behavior, and physiology (Rottenberg, 2005). An emotion can be distinguished from a mood. A *mood* is defined as a *diffuse, slow-moving, typically long-lasting state* (Gross, 1998). A mood lacks an intentional object; in other words, it is not associated with an eliciting stimulus. We use the term *emotion regulation* to refer to a process by which individuals influence which emotions they have, when they have those emotions, and how they express and experience them (Gross, 1998). Importantly, we use the term *affect* as an umbrella term that covers emotion, mood, and emotion regulation (Gross, 1998). This umbrella term is particularly useful in a discussion of insomnia given that the process of distinguishing between the different affective states, including the role of emotion regulation, has not yet begun.

What Is Insomnia?

Insomnia is a chronic difficulty that involves problems getting to sleep, maintaining sleep, or waking in the morning not feeling restored. It is one of the most prevalent psychological health problems, reported by 10% of the population (Roth & Ancoli-Israel, 1999). The consequences for the sufferer are severe and include functional impairment, work absenteeism, impaired concentration and memory, and increased use of medical services (Roth & Ancoli-Israel, 1999). Furthermore, there is evidence that insomnia significantly heightens the risk of having an automobile accident (Ohayon, Caulet, Philip, Guilleminault, & Priest, 1997) and the risk of subsequently developing another psychiatric disorder, particularly an anxiety disorder, depression, or substance-related disorder (Harvey, 2001). It is, therefore, regarded as a serious public health problem.

Insomnia Is a Transdiagnostic Process

The rates of comorbidity between chronic insomnia and other psychiatric disorders are high. The *Diagnostic and Statistical Manual of Mental Disorders* lists insomnia as a symptom in 14 Axis I disorders and in four disorders included for further study (American Psychiatric Association, 2000). In addition, insomnia is an associated feature across a range of other psychiatric disorders, including social phobia, panic disorder, autism, chronic pain, and eating disorders. Average rates of comorbidity between insomnia and other psychiatric disorders are 53% among those presenting to a health facility and 41.7% among community samples (Harvey, 2001).

In other words, insomnia can be the sole presenting problem or a condition that is comorbid with another psychiatric or a medical disorder. There is accruing evidence that when insomnia is comorbid, it is not an epiphenomenon of the other disorder. Instead, it appears to be an important transdiagnostic mechanism in the onset, relapse, and maintenance of the comorbid psychiatric disorder (Harvey, 2008). Accordingly, we suggest that the application of affective science to insomnia treatment may have implications for a broad range of patients with other psychiatric disorders.

Emotion in Theories of Insomnia

Insomnia has typically been conceptualized as a nighttime disorder. As will become evident in the following discussion of current treatment approaches, most theoretical analyses of the causes of insomnia include the constructs of arousal, anxiety, and worry. These constructs likely overlap with affective processes. However, they are loosely defined and not clearly operationalized. Hence, we suggest that a priority for future empirical and theoretical work will be to clarify the relationship between the existing nighttime constructs (i.e., arousal, anxiety, worry) and tightly defined and operationalized concepts from affective science (i.e., emotion response, emotional regulation, mood). We now outline literature suggesting that daytime, in addition to nighttime, emotional states play an important role in insomnia.

Daytime Emotion as a Contributor to Insomnia

There are competing hypotheses as to the impact of daytime emotion on nighttime sleep. One hypothesis is that insomnia patients are emotionally suppressed during the day. This is based on evidence that people with insomnia appear to inhibit or internalize their emotions (Wegner, Schneider, Carter, & White, 1987). It has been suggested that inhibition and suppression may be strategies adopted to cope with worry and escalating anxiety throughout the day (Rachman, 1980). The combined picture from the thought control literature (Harvey, 2003), along with theorizing relating to emotional processing (Rachman, 1980), is that inhibition and suppression of emotional material during the day will prevent emotional processing. Consequently, the unfinished business will later intrude during the presleep period, fueling worry and anxiety (Harvey, 2003). Bootzin and Rider (1997) observed that bedtime may be "the first quiet time during the day available to think about the day's events and to worry and plan for the next day" (p. 318).

The competing hypothesis is that insomnia patients are *more* emotional during the day. The Multiple Sleep Latency Test (MSLT) indexes daytime sleepiness by measuring the speed of falling asleep on each of five naps throughout one day. Most studies using the MSLT have been unable to detect evidence of heightened sleepiness in people with insomnia relative to good sleepers (e.g., Reidel & Lichstein, 2000; Stepanski, Lamphere, Badia, Zorick, & Roth, 1984). In fact, some of the MSLT studies have reported that insomnia patients are *less* sleepy relative to controls (Edinger, Means, Carney, & Krystal, 2008). This has led to the hypothesis that insomnia patients are hyperaroused in the day. As mentioned earlier, the concept of hyperarousal is not well defined or operationalized but may capture an emotional state. To the best of our knowledge, no published studies have used more compelling measures of emotion.

Regardless of which hypothesis is ultimately supported, it seems likely that a theoretical framework of the role of emotion in insomnia will include a bidirectional vicious cycle (Figure 18.1). Specifically, there may be two paths by which daytime emotion may contribute to nighttime insomnia. First, given the well-established paradoxical effects of thought suppression (Harvey, 2003), if insomnia patients suppress their emotions during the daytime, we would expect a rebound in emotion during the night, which, in turn, fuels insomnia. Second, if insomnia patients are hyperaroused during the daytime, they may be experiencing high-amplitude emotional responses in the day and do not have the skills to emotionally deactivate in order to fall asleep. The following section outlines the flip side of the vicious cycle: how nighttime sleep disturbance contributes to daytime emotion.

Daytime Emotion That Is a Consequence of Insomnia

In Chapter 11, van der Helm and Walker present the evidence base for the critical function of sleep in the effective regulation of emotion and for sleep loss having serious costs for next-day emotional functioning. Hence, it seems reasonable to hypothesize that the effects of chronic insomnia will include difficulties relating to emotion the subsequent day. Of the few studies focusing on the daytime emotional consequences of insomnia, heightened anxiety and depression have been reported as characteristic of

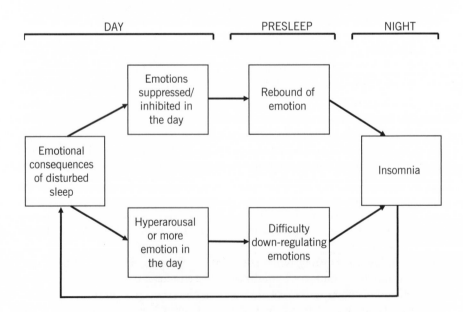

FIGURE 18.1. Bidirectional vicious cycle of emotion and insomnia.

insomnia (Zammit, 1988). Given our earlier definition of emotion versus mood, these measures are best categorized as measures of mood. Hence, an open question for future research is to identify the emotional consequences of insomnia. Later in this chapter we offer several methods for filling this gap.

Empirically Supported Treatments for Insomnia

Over the past few decades, several treatments have been tested for insomnia. In this section we focus on the approach that has been most empirically evaluated: cognitive-behavioral therapy for insomnia (CBT-I). As will become evident, the theoretical perspectives just offered implicating emotion difficulties during the day as contributors to insomnia are minimally explicitly targeted within this treatment approach. They focus entirely on the night. CBT-I is a multicomponent cognitive-behavioral treatment for insomnia. The components that are included under the umbrella of CBT-I are briefly described next.

Stimulus control refers to an intervention in which the patient is instructed to go to bed only when tired, limiting activities in bed to sleep and sex, getting out of bed at the same time every morning. When sleep onset does not occur within 15 to 20 minutes, patients are instructed to get up out of bed and go to another room. The rationale underlying this treatment component is that insomnia is the result of maladaptive conditioning between the environment (bed/bedroom) and sleep-incompatible behaviors (e.g., anxiety, arousal, frustration at not being able to sleep). The stimulus control intervention aims to reverse this association by limiting the sleep-incompatible behaviors engaged within the bedroom environment.

The *sleep restriction* component aims to maximize sleep efficiency and the association between the bed and sleep. The treatment begins by restricting the time spent in bed to the person's estimated average amount of nighttime sleep. The aim is to bring the total amount of time in bed as close as possible to the total sleep time. As such, subsequent instructions may involve the time spent in bed being either increased (as the sleep becomes consolidated) or decreased (to further maximize sleep efficiency).

Sleep hygiene training involves providing education about behaviors known to interfere with sleep such as intake of caffeine, alcohol and nicotine, daytime napping, variable sleep scheduling, exercise within 4 hours of bedtime, and reading while in bed. After the initial education session, monitoring these sleep-unfriendly behaviors on a daily basis is conducted to ensure patients improve the compatibility of their lifestyle with sleep.

Relaxation training can include progressive muscle relaxation, diaphragmatic breathing, autogenic training, biofeedback, meditation, yoga, and hypnosis. These interventions are designed to reduce nighttime psychophysiological arousal.

Paradoxical intention involves explicitly instructing the patient to try to stay awake when they get into bed. The rationale is that the paradoxical instruction reduces the anxiety associated with trying to fall asleep, causing the patient to relax and fall asleep faster.

Cognitive restructuring aims to alter irrational beliefs about sleep and typically involves education about sleep.

Empirical Evidence

In a review of the evidence for each component, the Standards of Practice Committee of the American Academy of Sleep Medicine has concluded that there was sufficient evidence to justify the use of stimulus control, progressive muscle relaxation, paradoxical intention, and sleep restriction. There is a moderate amount of evidence associated with this multicomponent therapy package (Morin et al., 2006). A limited number of the studies reviewed included measures of mood symptoms or measures of daytime functioning. In those that have, self-reported depression was improved after CBT-I in seven studies (four studies reported no significant change). Anxiety improved in three studies (five studies reported no significant change) (Morin et al., 2006).

Does This Treatment Approach Target Emotion?

Paradoxical intention is the only component that explicitly seeks to reduce an affective state, namely anxiety. Although behavioral theory underpins the stimulus control and relaxation components of the treatment, minimal research has tested the mechanisms predicted by these theories to be the cause of insomnia. Hence, it remains possible that these components operate via a change in affective functioning. In stimulus control, perhaps getting out of bed and going to another room provides a distraction from escalating negative emotion. In fact, Manber, Hydes, and Kuo (2004) found that patients who learned to accept their current sleep state and let go of the need to stay in bed while following stimulus control instructions benefited the most from CBT-I. Similarly, perhaps the relaxation component functions by decreasing arousal.

Newer Approaches to Treating Insomnia

Although there is no doubt that CBT-I is effective (Morin et al., 2006), there is substantial room for improvement. For example, there is a subset of patients who do not improve (19–26%). The average overall improvement is 50 to 60% (Morin, Culbert, & Schwartz, 1994), which suggests that a minority of patients become good sleepers. As such, several directions are being pursued in an attempt to improve outcome.

Cognitive Therapy for Insomnia

Cognitive therapy for insomnia (CT-I) was derived from a cognitive model of insomnia (Harvey, 2002), an approach that applies and adapts the cognitive theory of Aaron T. Beck to insomnia (e.g., Barlow, 1998; Beck, 1976; Clark, 1997; Ehlers & Clark, 2000). This approach suggests that insomnia is maintained by a cascade of cognitive processes that operate at night *and* during the day. The five cognitive processes that comprise the cascade are worry (accompanied by arousal and distress), selective attention and monitoring, misperception of sleep and daytime deficits, unhelpful beliefs, and counterproductive safety behaviors that maintain unhelpful beliefs. Predictions from the model have begun to accrue empirical support (see Harvey, 2005, for further examples). The treatment approach aims to reverse the cognitive processes that comprise the model. It is delivered in three phases. In Phase 1, case formulation involves deriving an individualized version of the cognitive model (Salkovskis, 1991): one for a typical recent night of insomnia and one for a typical recent day of insomnia. In Phase 2, the maintaining processes that feature in the model are reversed. In Phase 3, the goal is to consolidate treatment gains, set goals to ensure continued progress, and make plans for preventing relapse. Several of the procedures used during Phase 2 that tap into affective processes are now described.

Intervention to Reduce Worry and Rumination

First, patients are taught to identify and evaluate their sleep-related worrisome thoughts (following Beck, 1995). Second, the strategies often used by patients to manage worry (e.g., thought suppression) are assessed and, if unhelpful strategies are identified, altered. Third, if patients hold positive beliefs about worry (e.g., "Worrying while trying to get to sleep helps me get things sorted out in my mind"), guided discovery and individualized experiments are used to examine and test their validity. From an affective science perspective, these interventions may aim to reduce the use of unhelpful emotion regulation strategies.

Intervention to Reduce Attentional Bias and Monitoring for Sleep-Related Threat

Types of monitoring engaged in by the patient (e.g., monitoring the clock, monitoring for signs of fatigue) and homework assignments to direct attention to the broadest range of stimuli and away from sleep-related threat are then implemented (for further details, see Ree & Harvey, 2004; Tang & Harvey, 2006).

Intervention to Reduce Unhelpful Beliefs about Sleep

Morin (1993) has proposed the importance of unhelpful beliefs about sleep. During the course of therapy, individualized experiments are devised to test the validity and utility of unhelpful beliefs and to collect data on new beliefs (see Ree & Harvey, 2004, for examples).

Intervention to Reduce Use of Safety Behaviors

A safety behavior is an overt or covert action that is adopted to avoid feared outcomes. The problem is that these behaviors (1) prevent people from experiencing disconfirmation of their unrealistic beliefs and (2) may make the feared outcome more likely to occur (Salkovskis, 1991). Guided discovery is used to identify the advantages and disadvantages of using the safety behavior, and individualized experiments are then planned to observe the consequences of dropping or reversing the safety behavior (see Ree & Harvey, 2004, for examples).

Empirical Support

There is preliminary support for CT-I from an open trial of 19 patients with chronic insomnia (Harvey, Sharpley, Ree, Stinson, & Clark, 2007). Assessments were completed pretreatment, posttreatment, and at 3-, 6-, and 12-month follow-ups. The significant improvement in both nighttime and daytime impairment was retained up to the 12-month follow-up. However, this approach awaits replication in a randomized controlled trial that includes appropriate control for attention from a therapist, patient expectation, and passage of time.

Does This Treatment Approach Target Emotion?

The essence of Beck's cognitive model is that negative thoughts (and other cognitive processes) serve to fuel negative emotion. This idea is core to the CT-I treatment approach just described. Hence, we predict that specific measures of emotional responding and regulation may be sensitive to outcome in CT-I. Unfortunately, the open trial did not include measures of emotion, although measures of mood (depression and anxiety) did improve at posttreatment, and these improvements were retained at 12-month follow-up.

Mindfulness

Several variants have been discussed in the literature, including mindfulness-based stress reduction to target sleep disturbance (Britton, Shapiro, Penn, & Bootzin, 2003; Carlson & Garland, 2005), mindfulness-based cognitive therapy for insomnia (Heidenreich, Tuin, Pflug, Michal, & Michalak, 2006), acceptance and commitment therapy for insomnia (Åkerlund, Bolanowski, & Lundh, 2005), and mindfulness meditation with CBT-I (Bootzin & Stephens, 2005; Ong, Shapiro, & Manber, 2008).

These approaches have in common that they conceptualize insomnia as an inability to cognitively, emotionally, and physiologically deactivate or disengage (Lundh, 2005). Acceptance of the thoughts, rather than control and suppression of the thoughts, has been argued to facilitate deactivation and, in turn, promote sleep. In some ways, this is similar to CT-I. However, whereas cognitive therapy teaches patients to change dysfunctional thoughts that may be promoting wakefulness at night, mindfulness and acceptance techniques teach patients to accept their thoughts and feelings in a nonjudgmental and nonstriving way, which may promote a shift in perspective away from trying too hard to combat thoughts and instead lead to an increase in cognitive and emotional flexibility (Ong et al., 2008).

To date, there is no consensus on how mindfulness- and acceptance-based treatments for insomnia should be delivered. Ong and colleagues combined mindfulness meditation with several behavioral techniques (sleep restriction, stimulus control, sleep education, sleep hygiene) (Ong et al., 2008). The treatment was delivered as a 6-week group intervention with seven to eight participants per group. Participants received guided formal meditation training involving breathing meditation, body scan, walking meditation, and eating meditation. Additionally, instructions for stimulus control and sleep restriction were delivered.

Empirical Evidence

Ong and colleagues (2008) reviewed data from 27 patients. A significant reduction in total wake time, sleep-onset latency, and wake after sleep onset was observed. Furthermore, there were significant reductions in presleep arousal as measured by a weekly self-report scale that assesses cognitive and somatic arousal right before bed. Both areas of arousal were significantly reduced across the 6-week intervention. Furthermore, there was a trend toward less trait arousal. Another pilot study (*n* = 14) using mindfulness meditation along with cognitive therapy for insomnia (Heidenreich et al., 2006) reported a significant increase in total sleep time and a reduction in sleep-onset latency.

Åkerlund and colleagues (2005) carried out a small pilot study (*n* = 10) of a five-session acceptance- and mindfulness-based treatment of insomnia. A significant decrease from to pre- to posttreatment for insomnia severity was observed along with a large and significant decrease on cognitive presleep arousal. On sleep diary measures, however, there were no significant differences from pre- to posttreatment. In other words, although the intervention did not improve sleep parameters such as total sleep time or sleep-onset latency, it did reduce cognitive arousal and the self-reported severity of the insomnia symptoms.

Lundin and Tsur (personal communication, 2008) carried out a randomized controlled trial in which they compared three groups: standard CBT (three group sessions, which included stimulus control, sleep restriction, cognitive restructuring, and psychoeducation), the same form of standard CBT with the addition of mindfulness training (in total, seven group sessions), and a wait-list control group. Both CBT groups showed significant improvements on insomnia severity, sleep latency and restorative sleep and on the Insomnia Severity Index. There was no evidence, however, that the mindfulness training had any additional effect beyond that of standard CBT.

Do These Treatment Approaches Target Emotion?

These approaches are thought to help patients accept their thoughts, emotions, and arousal. It is assumed that acceptance will lead to deactivation of emotional states, which, in turn, will promote sleep. Preliminary data are consistent with this possibility. Bootzin and Stevens (2005) observed a reduction in worry following treatments that include mindfulness. Furthermore, Ong and colleagues (2008) reported that significant reductions in self-reported presleep cognitive and somatic arousal and reductions in trait arousal were significantly correlated with a greater number of meditations. Thus, the addition of mindfulness techniques to treatments for insomnia may specifically act to reduce arousal.

Summary and Future Directions

To summarize, we have highlighted the potential value of applying advances in knowledge and methods from affective science to the conceptualization and treatment of insomnia. Throughout this chapter, several gaps in the literature have been noted and theories that implicate affect have been described. The latter provide testable predictions and a framework for guiding future research. In the hope of cultivating research in this domain, we offer a range of other avenues that we see as particularly fruitful.

Incorporate Measures of Emotional Functioning

To date, the measures of emotion used in the insomnia treatment literature have been limited to measures of self-reported mood. Hence, there is a need to develop and validate measures of all facets of affective functioning and to adapt these measures to the study of insomnia during the daytime as well as during awakenings in the night and during sleep. Such measures will be able to answer critical questions: Which aspects of affective functioning need to be targeted in treatments for insomnia? Do current treatments alter affective functioning? Do the mechanisms by which existing and future treatments bring about change include alterations in affective functioning? In the section that follows, we briefly review a range of measures in the hope that future work will seek to validate and use these measures in patients with insomnia.

Daytime Emotional Functioning

Self-report scales, such as the Positive and Negative Affect Schedule (PANAS—Watson, Clark, & Tellegen, 1998; Zohar, Tzischinsky, Epstein, & Lavie, 2005), are one method for assessing emotional experience. The PANAS is a widely used well-validated scale containing 20 items designed to assess positive affect and negative affect. Participants are instructed to indicate "To what extent do you feel this way now?" on a 5-point Likert scale (1 = *very slightly or not at all*, 5 = *extremely*). By modifying the initial instructions, it is possible to derive state ("To what extent do you feel this way now?") and trait ("To what extent do you feel this way in general?") versions. The short form of the PANAS is a 10-item measure that lists several adjectives (Mackinnon et al., 1999) rated on the same 5-point scale. Of all of the measures we discuss here, this is most amenable to use in a clinical setting because it is easy to administer, inexpensive, and quick to complete. However, it provides a limited view that relies on the assumption that individuals can accurately introspect about and report on their emotional state.

More sophisticated methods to elicit emotion response include the use of standardized or normative stimuli presented via an external medium such as films or slides containing emotion-eliciting content. Film clips have been widely used and are regarded as reliable elicitors of neutral, positive, and negative emotional states (Rottenberg, Ray, & Gross, 2007). Static photo images from the International Affective Picture System (Lang, Bradley, & Cuthbert, 1998) as well as standardized images of prototypical facial displays of emotion (Ekman & Friesen, 1978) are also considered reliable elicitors of emotion. Emotional responses to such stimuli can be measured at multiple, intersecting levels, including experiential (e.g., self-report), behavioral (e.g., coding facial displays of emotion), and physiological (both peripheral and central nervous system) responses.

For more naturalistic and ecologically valid indicators of emotional functioning, idiographic stimuli that contain person-specific emotional themes have been developed, of which three examples are presented. First, autobiographical memory recall procedures involve the person being asked to recall emotionally salient life events. Several adaptations of this procedure include asking the person to describe the details of the event (Rottenberg, Gross, & Gotlib, 2005), imagining the event until a maximally positive or negative mood state is achieved (Eich, Macaulay, & Ryan, 1994), or manipulating the vantage perspective from which the emotional event is recalled (Kross, Ayduk, & Mischel, 2005). Second, social interaction paradigms enable the examination of spontaneous emotion under a controlled condition without compromising ecological validity (Roberts, Tsai, & Coan, 2007). Third, experience-sampling methodologies (ESM) aim to capture emotional functioning in the everyday lives of participants outside the laboratory. ESM involves asking people to complete a diary at quasi-random intervals throughout the course of the day. Such procedures have already begun to be used in the study of the relationship between emotions and sleep in healthy populations (Zohar et al., 2005) as well as daytime emotional functioning in insomnia (Scott & Judge, 2006). The latter study observed an association between insomnia and increased daytime hostility and decreased feelings of joy and attentiveness.

In the context of insomnia, stimuli need to be used to assess the range of facets of emotional responding, including the amplitude of the emotional response (i.e., emotional reactivity), the degree to which participants can regulate their emotional responses while viewing evocative stimuli (Wilson, Watson, & Currie, 1998), as well as the temporal course of emotional responding, including the time to reach peak intensity and time to recover from an emotional response (Davidson, 1998). In these paradigms, it is important to use a multimethod approach to carefully assess emotional functioning at intersecting subjective (e.g., PANAS), behavioral (e.g., coding of facial displays of emotion), and physiological (e.g., autonomic physiology, functional magnetic resonance imaging, electroencephalogram [EEG]) levels of assessment.

Emotional Functioning during Wakings in the Night

It may be possible to extend the paradigms just described to examine emotional functioning immediately before sleep and during awakenings in the night. For example, physiological measures of emotional responding can be added to polysomnography (the current gold standard measure of sleep). Then portable devices such as laptops could be used to present emotional material while in bed. Alternatively, patients with insomnia could be asked to imagine emotional memories while trying to get to sleep. Examining presleep emotional functioning will enable researchers to directly examine the impact of emotion on sleep dysregulation.

Mood Measures

As discussed earlier, an emotion is a brief response to specific encounters with salient environmental events, and a mood is defined as a diffuse, slow-moving, typically long-lasting state. We also highlighted that the reality of most psychiatric disorders will be a unique and complex interaction between moods and emotions. As such, the development and inclusion of measures of mood will be important in future research.

Emotional Functioning during Sleep

Autonomic measures of skin temperature and heart rate have been associated with specific emotion states (Levenson, 1992) and could be measured during sleep. There is also potential value in assessing REM sleep in patients with insomnia. REM variables have long been hypothesized to have an important role in emotion regulation (Perlis & Nielsen, 1993) in both healthy (Cartwright, Luten, Young, Mercer, & Bears, 1998) and mood-disordered (Benca, Obermeyer, Thisted, & Gillin, 1992) populations. The extent to which abnormalities exist in REM in insomnia patients remains an open question. Finally, an intriguing finding in the insomnia literature is the presence of heightened beta-EEG evident during sleep in insomnia patients (Perlis, Mercia, Smith, & Giles, 2001). It is possible that this heightened beta-EEG may be a neural correlate of excessive emotion during sleep.

Transdiagnostic Treatment for Sleep Disturbance

At the beginning of this chapter, we presented evidence for high rates of comorbidity between insomnia and other psychiatric disorders. Much of the treatment research has been conducted on "pure" insomnia samples (i.e., the presence of psychiatric comorbidity has been exclusionary). Relatively little is known about the relationship between comorbidity and response to treatments for insomnia, although there is some evidence in other disorders that the presence of comorbid insomnia predicts poorer outcome (Verbeek, Schreuder, & Declerck, 1999).

One approach to treating comorbid cases has been to apply evidence-based therapies sequentially (Kraemer, Wilson, Fairburn, & Agras, 2002). For example, if a patient presents with depression and insomnia, the sequential approach would involve treating the depression first and then moving on to treat the insomnia, or vice versa. This approach perhaps makes the most sense if the co-occurring disorders are independent and additive. However, if the disorders mutually maintain each other, the sequential approach may not be maximally efficient (Westen, Novotny, & Thompson-Brenner, 2004). Given increasingly compelling evidence for mutual maintenance between insomnia and its commonly comorbid disorders (Bateson, 2004), it may be more efficient to treat the comorbid disorders simultaneously. Manber and colleagues (2008) showed impressive results with a combined approach. This study compared treating the depression only versus treating *both* the depression (with escitalopram, an antidepressant) *and* the insomnia (with cognitive behavior therapy for insomnia). The combined approach was superior for *both* depression and insomnia outcomes. Another way this might be achieved is by treating maintaining mechanisms that are shared by the insomnia and the comorbid disorder (i.e., transdiagnostic mechanisms). For example, the targets of

CT-I are worry, dysfunctional beliefs, attentional bias, and misperception. Because these are also mechanisms known to maintain the disorders most commonly comorbid with insomnia, namely selected anxiety disorders and depression (for a review, see Harvey, Watkins, Mansell, & Shafran, 2004), it is possible that CT-I will be effective in reducing the insomnia *and* the symptoms and emotional distress associated with these comorbid disorders. If the hypothesis that problems relating to emotion are important transdiagnostic processes is confirmed, there will be potential for developing other comorbid treatment approaches for comorbid cases.

Future research is also needed to explore the potentially wide-reaching public health implications of developing a truly transdiagnostic intervention for insomnia. Depending on the emergence of evidence relating to the role of emotion and emotion regulation in insomnia, it is possible that this intervention may need to target transdiagnostic affective processes. A series of interesting research questions need to be answered here. First, is it possible to develop one treatment protocol—a transdiagnostic treatment—that effectively treats insomnia in all psychiatric disorders, or will disorder-specific adaptations be required? If the former, this would have the great advantage of easy dissemination. This is important, because developing and disseminating transdiagnostic treatment protocols (as opposed to disorder-specific treatment protocols) would reduce the heavy burden on clinicians, who must already learn multiple treatment protocols that often share common theoretical underpinnings and interventions. Second, given the association between poor sleep and impaired quality of life, does improving sleep improve the functioning of individuals with a range of psychiatric disorders? Finally, if insomnia and the symptoms/processes of psychiatric disorders are mutually maintaining, does a transdiagnostic treatment also reduce symptoms and processes associated with the comorbid psychiatric disorder? Future research will be needed to determine the extent to which such exciting possibilities are realistic and to establish which affective processes will need to be targeted and how (see Harvey, in press, for further discussion).

Mechanisms of Treatment Change

Although there is evidence supporting the efficacy of various approaches to the treatment of insomnia, there is little information about the active therapeutic mechanisms responsible for sleep improvements. In a follow-up study of patients who had completed CBT for insomnia, Harvey, Inglis, and Espie (2002) identified self-reported use of stimulus control and sleep restriction to be the best predictor of improvement in sleep, followed by cognitive restructuring. Two other studies have reported reduction in dysfunctional beliefs to be associated with the maintenance of improvement in sleep (Edinger, Wohlgemuth, Radtke, Marsh, & Quillian, 2001; Morin, Blaise, & Savard, 2002). Moreover, Verbeek and colleagues (1999) found that there were more treatment responders among those who received the cognitive therapy component (83%) than among those who did not receive it (56%). To date, however, no study has conducted a formal analysis of treatment mediators and moderators of treatments for insomnia using recent statistical advances. If we can identify mediators of treatment outcome, these aspects of the treatment can be intensified and refined while inactive or redundant elements can be discarded, thereby improving outcome and efficiency. The question that arises from this chapter is the extent to which current treatments operate via a mechanism involving one or more domains of affective functioning.

Medication Treatments

It would be interesting and informative to consider medication treatments for insomnia, most of which target the gamma-aminobutyric acid-A—GABA(A)—receptors, the major inhibitory neurotransmitters in the brain. Space limitations preclude us from doing so, but we wish to briefly note that several medications targeting the GABA(A) receptors are efficacious treatments for insomnia. The impact of these medications specifically on the affective functioning of insomnia patients should be explored using the methods discussed earlier. Consideration should also be given to the possibility that some of the side effects of these treatments may be in the domain of affective functioning. For example, feeling sedated the next day may have the effect of reducing the experience of positive emotion.

Implications for Other Kinds of Sleep Disturbance

In this chapter we have focused on insomnia, the most common sleep disturbance. However, we emphasize that the manifestations of sleep disturbance in psychiatric disorders are numerous and include hypersomnia, delayed sleep phase, circadian dysregulation, nightmares, and nocturnal panic attacks. It seems highly likely that each of these impact the affective functioning of sufferers.

Positive Emotion Interventions

We noted earlier the empirical finding of decreased feelings of joy and attentiveness among patients with insomnia. Hence, there is budding interest within the insomnia literature in integrating interventions to enhance positive emotions. Brewin (2006) noted that CBT assumes that vulnerability to psychiatric disorders is based in negative memory representations that are activated by triggering events and that maintain negative mood. Traditional CBT theories assume that CBT intervenes by directly modifying the negative information in memory. Drawing from evidence in the animal literature, conditioned fear reactions can easily be reinstated or renewed by reexposing the animal to the unconditioned stimulus and placing it in a new context and then re-presenting the conditioned stimulus. On this basis, Brewin suggests that CBT does not directly modify negative information in memory. Instead, he argues that there are multiple memories involving the self that compete to be retrieved at any one point in time. CBT produces a change in the relative activation of the positive versus negative representations such that the positive ones are assisted to win the retrieval competition. Importantly, he suggests that more explicitly training the positive representations may result in a generation of even more effective treatments. Perhaps by incorporating interventions we may be able to increase the strength of the positive representation so that it is more likely to win in the retrieval competition. Positive interventions have already been included in a new treatment for adolescents with sleeping difficulties, and the most recent version of CT-I includes a savoring intervention (based on McMakin, 2007; McMakin, Siegle, & Silk, 2009). Before we describe this approach, we note that the utility of this addition to the multicomponent treatment awaits empirical testing.

The savoring intervention trains patients to focus on the positives in their life. This is a strategy that has begun to be used across disorders in recognition of the potential value of building rapid associative connections with the positive. Savoring consists of attending to, appreciating, and enhancing positive experiences that patients have had during the day. They can savor an everyday event like looking out the window and noticing the lovely trees and flowers, reminiscing over a favorite vacation, or anticipating a family reunion or a date with one's spouse/partner. Patients train in focusing on the positive experience, and when negative thoughts arise, they gently disengage from those thoughts and return to savoring the positive experience. We have extended this to include honoring patients' personal resources and strengths in everyday actions (e.g., cooking a great evening meal) to larger concepts (e.g., being a great parent or a resourceful human). The rationale is to train an association between bedtime and positive affect.

Conclusion

The lack of empirical evidence—and the great potential—is palpable. We believe the application of advances in affective science to the treatment of insomnia has potential to contribute to the development of novel and more effective interventions for this high-prevalence, crippling public health problem. In the true spirit of the transdiagnostic approach, one source of research hypotheses as we move forward to fill in the many gaps will be the promising findings reported in this volume in the context of other psychiatric disorders.

References

Åkerlund, R., Bolanowski, I., & Lundh, L. G. (2005). *A pilot study of an act-inspired approach to the treatment of insomnia.* Unpublished data.

American Psychiatric Association. (2000). *Diagnostic and statistical manual of mental disorders* (4th ed., text rev.). Washington, DC: Author.

Barlow, D. H. (1988). *Anxiety and its disorders: The nature and treatment of anxiety and panic.* New York: Guilford Press.

Bateson, A. N. (2004). The benzodiazepine site of the GABAA receptor: An old target with new potential? *Sleep Medicine, 5*(Suppl. 1), S9–S15.

Beck, A. T. (1976). *Cognitive therapy and the emotional disorders.* New York: International Universities Press.

Beck, J. S. (1995). *Cognitive therapy: Basics and beyond.* New York: Guilford Press.

Benca, R. M., Obermeyer, W. H., Thisted, R. A., & Gillin, J. C. (1992). Sleep and psychiatric disorders: A meta-analysis. *Archives of General Psychiatry, 49,* 651–668.

Bootzin, R. R., & Rider, S. P. (1997). Behavioral techniques and biofeedback for insomnia. In M. R. Pressman & W. C. Orr (Eds.), *Understanding sleep: The evaluation and treatment of sleep disorders.* Washington, DC: American Psychological Association.

Bootzin, R. R., & Stevens, S. J. (2005). Adolescents, substance abuse, and the treatment of insomnia and daytime sleepiness. *Clinical Psychology Review, 25,* 629–644.

Brewin, C. R. (2006). Understanding cognitive behaviour therapy: A retrieval competition account. *Behaviour Research and Therapy, 44*(6), 765–784.

Britton, W. B., Shapiro, S. L., Penn, P. E., & Bootzin, R. R. (2003). Treating insomnia with mindfulness-based stress reduction. *Sleep, 26,* A309.

Carlson, L. E., & Garland, S. N. (2005). Impact of mindfulness-based stress reduction (MBSR) on sleep, mood, stress and fatigue symptoms in cancer outpatients. *International Journal of Behavioral Medicine, 12,* 278–285.

Cartwright, R., Luten, A., Young, M., Mercer, P., & Bears, M. (1998). Role of REM sleep and dream affect in overnight mood regulation: A study of normal volunteers. *Psychiatry Research, 81,* 1–8.

Clark, D. M. (1997). Panic disorder and social phobia. In D. M. Clark & C. G. Fairburn (Eds.), *Science and practice of cognitive behaviour therapy* (pp. 121–153). Oxford, UK: Oxford University Press.

Davidson, J. R. T. (1998). The long-term treatment of panic disorder. *Journal of Clinical Psychiatry, 59,* 17–21.

Edinger, J. D., Means, M. K., Carney, C. E., & Krystal, A. D. (2008). Psychomotor performance deficits and their relation to prior nights' sleep among individuals with primary insomnia. *Sleep, 31,* 599–607.

Edinger, J. D., Wohlgemuth, W. K., Radtke, R. A., Marsh, G. R., & Quillian, R. E. (2001). Does cognitive-behavioral insomnia therapy alter dysfunctional beliefs about sleep? *Sleep, 24,* 591–599.

Eich, E., Macaulay, D., & Ryan, L. (1994). Mood dependent memory for events of the personal past. *Journal of Experimental Psychology: General, 123,* 201–215.

Ehlers, A., & Clark, D. M. (2000). A cognitive model of posttraumatic stress disorder. *Behaviour Research and Therapy, 38,* 319–345.

Ekman, P., & Friesen, W. V. (1978). *Facial action coding system: A technique for the measurement of facial movement.* Palo Alto, CA: Consulting Psychologists Press.

Gross, J. J. (1998). The emerging field of emotion regulation: An integrative review. *Review of General Psychology, 2*, 271–299.

Harvey, A. G. (2001). Insomnia: Symptom or diagnosis? *Clinical Psychology Review, 21*, 1037–1059.

Harvey, A. G. (2002). A cognitive model of insomnia. *Behaviour Research and Therapy, 40*(8), 869–893.

Harvey, A. G. (2003). The attempted suppression of pre-sleep cognitive activity in insomnia. *Cognitive Therapy and Research, 27*, 593–602.

Harvey, A. G. (2008). Insomnia, psychiatric disorders, and the transdiagnostic perspective. *Current Directions in Psychological Science, 17*, 299–303.

Harvey, A. G. (in press). A transdiagnostic approach to treating sleep disturbance in psychiatric disorders. *Cognitive Behavior Therapy.*

Harvey, A. G., Sharpley, A., Ree, M. J., Stinson, K., & Clark, D. M. (2007). An open trial of cognitive therapy for chronic insomnia. *Behavior Research and Therapy, 45*, 2491–2501.

Harvey, A. G., Watkins, E., Mansell, W., & Shafran, R. (2004). *Cognitive behavioural processes across psychological disorders: A transdiagnostic approach to research and treatment.* Oxford, UK: Oxford University Press.

Harvey, L., Inglis, S., & Espie, C. A. (2002). Insomniacs' reported use of CBT components and relationship to long-term clinical outcome. *Behavior Research and Therapy, 40*, 75–83.

Heidenreich, T., Tuin, I., Pflug, B., Michal, M., & Michalak, J. (2006). Mindfulness-based cognitive therapy for persistent insomnia: A pilot study. *Psychotherapy and Psychosomatics, 75*(3), 188–189.

Kraemer, H. C., Wilson, G. T., Fairburn, C. G., & Agras, W. S. (2002). Mediators and moderators of treatment effects in randomized clinical trials. *Archives of General Psychiatry, 59*, 877–883.

Kross, E., Ayduk, O., & Mischel, W. (2005). When asking "why" doesn't hurt: Distinguishing rumination from reflective processing of negative emotions. *Psychological Science, 16*, 709–715.

Lang, P., Bradley, M., & Cuthbert, B. (1998). Emotion, motivation and anxiety: Brain mechanisms and psychophysiology. *Biological Psychiatry, 44*, 1248–1263.

Levenson, R. W. (1992). Autonomic nervous system differences among emotions. *Psychological Science, 3*, 23–27.

Lundh, L. G. (2005). The role of acceptance and mindfulness in the treatment of insomnia. *Journal of Cognitive Psychotherapy, 19*, 29–39.

Mackinnon, A., Jorm, A. F., Christensen, H., Korten, A. E., Jacomb, P. A., & Rodgers, B. (1999). A short form of the Positive and Negative Affect Schedule: Evaluation of factorial validity and invariance across demographic variables in a community sample. *Personality and Individual Differences, 27*, 405–416.

Manber, R., Edinger, J. D., Gress, J. L., San Pedro-Salcedo, M. G., Kuo, T. F., & Kalista, T. (2008). Cognitive behavioral therapy for insomnia enhances depression outcome in patients with comorbid major depressive disorder and insomnia. *Sleep, 31*(4), 489–495.

Manber, R., Hydes, N., & Kuo, T. (2004). What aspects of cognitive-behavioral therapy for insomnia do patients find helpful? *Sleep, 27*, A282.

McMakin, D. L. (2007). *Positive emotion regulation coaching for depression.* Unpublished doctoral dissertation, University of Denver.

McMakin, D. L., Siegle, G. J., & Silk, S. R. (2009). *Positive emotion regulation coaching for depression.* Manuscript submitted for publication.

Morin, C. M. (1993). *Insomnia: Psychological assessment and management.* New York: Guilford Press.

Morin, C. M., Blais, F., & Savard, J. (2002). Are changes in beliefs and attitudes about sleep related to sleep improvements in the treatment of insomnia? *Behaviour Research and Therapy, 40*(7), 741–752.

Morin, C. M., Bootzin, R. R., Buysse, D. J., Edinger, J. D., Espie, C. A., & Lichstein, K. L. (2006). Psychological and behavioral treatment of insomnia: An update of recent evidence (1998–2004). *Sleep, 29,* 1396–1406.

Morin, C. M., Culbert, J. P., & Schwartz, S. M. (1994). Nonpharmacological interventions for insomnia: A meta-analysis of treatment efficacy. *American Journal of Psychiatry, 151,* 1172–1180.

Ohayon, M. M., Caulet, M., Philip, P., Guilleminault, C., & Priest, R. G. (1997). How sleep and mental disorders are related to complaints of daytime sleepiness. *Archives of Internal Medicine, 157,* 2645–2652.

Ong, J. C., Shapiro, S. L., & Manber, R. (2008). Combining mindfulness meditation with cognitive-behavior therapy for insomnia: A treatment-development study. *Behavior Therapy, 39,* 171–182.

Perlis, M. L., Merica, H., Smith, M. T., & Giles, D. E. (2001). Beta EEG in insomnia. *Journal of Sleep Medicine Reviews, 5,* 365–376.

Perlis, M. L., & Nielsen, T. A. (1993). Mood regulation, dreaming and nightmares: Evaluation of a desensitization function for REM sleep. *Dreaming, 3,* 243–257.

Rachman, S. (1980). Emotional processing. *Behaviour Research and Therapy, 18,* 51–60.

Ree, M., & Harvey, A. G. (2004). Insomnia. In J. Bennett-Levy, G. Butler, M. Fennell, A. Hackman, M. Mueller, & D. Westbrook (Eds.), *Oxford guide to behavioural experiments in cognitive therapy* (pp. 287–305). Oxford, UK: Oxford University Press.

Riedel, B. W., & Lichstein, K. L. (2000). Insomnia and daytime functioning. *Sleep Medicine Reviews, 4,* 277–298.

Roberts, N. A., Tsai, J. L., & Coan, J. A. (2007). Emotion elicitation using dyadic interaction tasks. In J. A. Coan & J. J. B. Allen (Eds.), *Handbook of emotion elicitation and assessment* (pp. 106–123). Oxford, UK: Oxford University Press.

Roth, T., & Ancoli-Israel, S. (1999). Daytime consequences and correlates of insomnia in the United States: Results of the 1991 National Sleep Foundation Survey. II. *Sleep, 22,* S354–S358.

Rottenberg, J. (2005). Mood and emotion in major depression. *Current Directions in Psychological Science, 14,* 167–170.

Rottenberg, J., Gross, J. J., & Gotlib, I. H. (2005). Emotion context insensitivity in major depressive disorder. *Journal of Abnormal Psychology, 114,* 627–639.

Rottenberg, J., Ray, R. D., & Gross, J. J. (2007). Emotion elicitation using films. In J. A. Coan & J. J. B. Allen (Eds.), *The handbook of emotion elicitation and assessment* (pp. 9–28). London: Oxford University Press.

Salkovskis, P. M. (1991). The importance of behaviour in the maintenance of anxiety and panic: A cognitive account. *Behavioural Psychotherapy, 19,* 6–19.

Scott, B. A., & Judge, T. A. (2006). Insomnia, emotions, and job satisfaction: A multilevel study. *Journal of Management, 32,* 622–645.

Stepanski, E., Lamphere, J., Badia, P., Zorick, F., & Roth, T. (1984). Sleep fragmentation and daytime sleepiness. *Sleep, 7*(1), 18–26.

Tang, N. K. Y., & Harvey, A. G. (2006). Altering misperception of sleep in insomnia: Behavioral experiment versus verbal explanation. *Journal of Consulting and Clinical Psychology, 74*, 767–776.

Verbeek, I., Schreuder, K., & Declerck, G. (1999). Evaluation of short-term nonpharmacological treatment of insomnia in a clinical setting. *Journal of Psychosomatic Research, 47*, 369–383.

Watson, D., Clark, L. A., & Tellegen, A. (1998). Development and validation of brief measures of positive and negative affect: The PANAS scales. *Journal of Personality and Social Psychology, 54*, 1063–1070.

Wegner, D. M., Schneider, D. J., Carter, S. R., III, & White, T. L. (1987). Paradoxical effects of thought suppression. *Journal of Personality and Social Psychology, 53*(1), 5–13.

Westen, D., Novotny, C. M., & Thompson-Brenner, H. (2004). The empirical status of empirically supported psychotherapies: Assumptions, findings, and reporting in controlled clinical trials. *Psychological Bulletin, 130*, 631–663.

Wilson, K. G., Watson, S. T., & Currie, S. R. (1998). Daily diary and ambulatory activity monitoring of sleep in patients with insomnia associated with chronic musculoskeletal pain. *Pain, 75*, 75–84.

Zammit, G. K. (1988). Subjective ratings of the characteristics and sequelae of good and poor sleep in normals. *Journal of Clinical Psychology, 44*, 123–130.

Zohar, D., Tzischinsky, O., Epstein, R., & Lavie, P. (2005). The effects of sleep loss on medical residents' emotional reactions to work events: A cognitive-energy model. *Sleep, 28*, 47–54.

Index

Page numbers followed by *f* indicate figure, *t* indicate table

447